Restraint and Handling of Wild and Domestic Animals

Restraint
of Wild AND

THIRD EDITION

AND Handling Domestic ANIMALS

MURRAY E. FOWLER

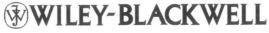

WILEY-BLACKWELL

A John Wiley & Sons, Inc., Publication

Murray E. Fowler, DVM, is Professor Emeritus of Zoological Medicine at the School of Veterinary Medicine, University of California at Davis, Davis, CA. Most recently, he has been a consultant of Ringling Brothers, Barnum and Bailey's Circus. His previous publications include *Zoo and Wild Animal Medicine, Fifth Edition* (2003); *Restraint and Handling of Wild and Domestic Animals* (Blackwell Publishing, 1995); *Medicine and Surgery of South American Camelids* (Blackwell Publishing, 1998); and *Biology, Medicine and Surgery of South American Wild Animals* (Blackwell Publishing, 2001).

Edition first published 2008
© 2008 Murray E. Fowler

Blackwell Publishing was acquired by John Wiley & Sons in February 2007. Blackwell's publishing program has been merged with Wiley's global Scientific, Technical, and Medical business to form Wiley-Blackwell.

Editorial Office
2121 State Avenue, Ames, Iowa 50014-8300, USA

For details of our global editorial offices, for customer services, and for information about how to apply for permission to reuse the copyright material in this book, please see our website at www.wiley.com/wiley-blackwell.

Library of Congress Cataloguing-in-Publication Data

Fowler, Murray E.
    Restraint and handling of wild and domestic animals / Murray E. Fowler. – 3rd ed.
        p. cm.
    Includes bibliographical references and index.
    ISBN-13: 978-0-8138-1432-2 (alk. paper)
    ISBN-10: 0-8138-1432-4 (alk. paper)
  1. Animal immobilization. I. Title.
    QL62.5.F68 2008
    636.08'3–dc22

                                                    2008012654

A catalogue record for this book is available from the U.S. Library of Congress.

Set in 10 on 12 Times by SNP Best-set Typesetter Ltd., Hong Kong

1 2008

C O N T E N T S

P R E F A C E to the First Edition

The original intent in this book was to deal only with wild animal restraint. However, upon deliberation, it was realized that fundamental principles of restraint apply to both domestic and wild animals, so it was decided to include both groups to present a more comprehensive picture of the subject.

The objectives of this book are to collect under one cover discussions and illustrations of the principles of animal restraint and handling and to describe some restraint practices for diverse species of vertebrate wild and domestic animals. Heretofore no single source has offered information for handling such diverse animals as a 2.5-g hummingbird and an elephant weighing 5,000–6,000 kg. It is hoped that this book will satisfy that need for all who handle animals—particularly veterinarians; animal caretakers; wildlife biologists; wildlife rehabilitators; personnel of zoos, research, and humane society facilities; and any others who deal with animals.

Government regulatory agencies require humane treatment and proper care and handling of all animals in captivity. It is legally necessary for those maintaining wildlife to provide adequate restraint facilities and personnel trained in satisfactory handling techniques to prevent or minimize injuries.

Restraint and handling techniques for domestic animals have long been well documented and described. Although the most recent text[1] was written in 1954, the principles outlined in that excellent publication are still valid.

Wild animal restraint and handling techniques are not as well known nor as widely publicized except in those notorious instances when inhumane and torturous methods used in capture and transport attract the attention of the news media. Some people feel that all wildlife should be returned to the native habitat and left to live and die undisturbed by human beings. This attitude is naive in this day and time. Wild animals have become an integral part of society and will continually be handled. It behooves us to know and use techniques safe for both animal and handler.

The need for understanding restraint principles, particularly for wild animals, is exemplified by the statement of an experienced zoo veterinarian in a recent publication: "It is all very well to plan an operation on a tiger, but the problem that arises is how to catch the beast, and once having caught it, how safely to secure it. Nor is this difficulty restricted to the tiger, it applies in a lesser or greater degree to every type of wild animal in captivity. Not one of them will cooperate in your well-meaning efforts to help them, and no such thing as gratitude exists in their primitive makeup."[2]

This book is not, nor is it meant to be, an exhaustive encyclopedia on animal restraint. The author is well aware that certain individual researchers or biologists may favor one or more techniques or special tools not mentioned here. It is impossible for any individual to acquire a personal knowledge of all possible combinations of restraint and handling procedures for every species or even for groups of species. However, the techniques presented have proved successful in the hands of experienced individuals and should serve as guides for anyone faced with similar problems.

It is only through an enlightened understanding of restraint principles that humane handling with the least amount of stress will be possible for any animal. It is hoped that by bringing all this information together in one source, more people will be able to share in saving wild animals for posterity.

1. Leahy, J.R., and Barrow, P. 1954. Animal Restraint. Ithaca, N.Y.: Comstock.
2. Graham-Jones, O. 1973. First Catch Your Tiger. New York: Taplinger.

P R E F A C E   to the Second Edition

The concluding paragraph of the preface to the first edition states, "It is only through an enlightened understanding of restraint principles that humane handling with the least amount of stress will be possible for any animal. It is hoped that by bringing all this information together in one source, more people will be able to share in the saving of wild animals for posterity."

I have been gratified at the reception of the first edition of *Restraint and Handling of Wild and Domestic Animals*, by animal health technicians, zookeepers, animal owners, wildlife rehabilitators, animal husbandry students, and veterinarians. In the nearly 20 years that have elapsed since the first edition was written, some described procedures and techniques have changed but slightly. Many aspects of physical restraint remain valid. In some other aspects, there have been material changes.

One of the more significant changes in general restraint has been the greater attention paid to avoiding and minimizing stress during restraint. I would like to believe that the first edition contributed to a greater understanding of the absolute need to minimize stress. The design of livestock handling yards, chutes, and loading ramps has become a sophisticated art. Public sentiments demand, even more vociferously than two decades ago, humane care in all aspects of maintaining animals in captivity.

Chemical restraint had been coming to the fore in the decade prior to publication of the first edition, but the two intervening decades have seen the development and marketing of many new drugs. Investigations into the pharmacodynamics of drugs now allow more logical combination of certain drugs, which are used more frequently to capitalize on the desirable effects of each while counteracting undesirable effects. Extensive clinical usage has demonstrated the desirability, and in many cases the necessity, of using drug combinations. There is still no single drug that is the drug of choice for immobilizing all species of animals. Furthermore, no individual has the time or opportunity to deal with more than a few drugs and species of animals, hence the need for sharing.

Now, more than ever, persons contemplating chemical restraint of unfamiliar animals must take the time to communicate with experienced restrainers. Even a review of the literature may fail to provide the most current techniques being used, particularly for sensitive species like giraffe or hippopotamuses. Currently available restraint drugs are discussed at length in this edition. Furthermore, promising drugs that are currently unavailable in the United States but are being used effectively in other countries have been included, with the expectation that they may soon become available here.

South African veterinarians and biologists are leaders in advancing the art of chemical restraint, particularly in free-ranging African mammals, and the literature from South Africa has been freely used to augment the experiences from North America and other countries of the world.

Effective drugs used and methods for chemical restraint of animal groups have been included in this volume. No pretense is made that all suitable procedures have been described. The techniques included have been used by me or by respected colleagues. The literature citations bring chemical restraint up to the present.

Some sections of this volume remain virtually unchanged because the methods described previously are still valid. Other sections have been modified extensively in keeping with new developments in the field, particularly in regard to the increased importance played by private owners and how they handle their animals (camelids, ratites).

No one begins a restraint procedure with the expressed purpose of failing, but failure is the result for many who fail to apply basic principles that determine success. In all facets of my life, I have utilized a formula (5 Ps) for success that has a direct application to restraint. Perhaps it may help others focus on important issues.

Success = Plan + Prepare + Practice + Produce + Persist

You may try to eliminate some aspects of the formula or shortcut the process, but I feel that this formula provides the most efficient and effective pathway for success. There must be a plan. Too often there is no plan, rather the idea seems to be "Let's just go do it." The questions remain, who is to do what and when? Preparation is essential. In preparation, the questions to be answered are: Are all the tools and equipment ready? Has transportation been arranged? Have emergency procedures been planned and necessary equipment provided? What of alternate plans if the situation suddenly changes? If the animal is to be darted, when was the last time target practice was held? Every possible complication or problem should be anticipated. Then the restrainer must carry out the procedure as planned (produce). When the procedure has been completed, the whole process should be evaluated. Setbacks and failures must be offset by persistence in applying fundamental principles.

P R E F A C E to the Third Edition

The third edition is illustrated in color. Modern technology allows printing in color without materially adding to the cost. New chapters added to the third edition include animal behavior, animal welfare, training for restraint procedures, camelidae, and megavertebrates. Several sections have been given chapter status or moved to be consistent with reorganization of sections. For instance, camelidae has been given chapter status and moved to the domestic animal section, and chemical restraint has been moved to the nondomestic animal section. The methods of delivery of chemical restraint agents have been given chapter status.

The chemical restraint chapter has been expanded and new chemical restraint agents added. Each chapter in the wild animal section has a discussion of chemical immobilization for that group of animals, including tables and current references.

Animal welfare must be a constant concern of those who restrain animals. The well-being of an animal should be given the highest priority. Although modern chemical restraint agents have made it possible to accomplish many procedures more efficiently and safely, take time to contemplate all of the effects that may impinge on the animal. Will the animal's condition be improved with the intended procedure? Are there alternative methods to accomplish the same goal? Are all of the needed equipment and supplies to work safely and efficiently ready? Are restraint personnel adequately trained and experienced to deal with any contingency?

Government regulations require that animals receive humane care at all times. It is too bad that regulations must direct us to do what should be our moral obligation and desire to accomplish.

Animals may become overstimulated with an epinephrine rush during restraint procedures. They may be inclined to, and capable of, feats of athleticism beyond imagination. I have seen a giant eland *Taurotragus oryx* jump, from a standing start, an 8-foot fence that had easily contained the animal for years. Furthermore, an American bison *Bison bison* cow climbed a 6-foot fence to avoid capture. A Grevy zebra *Equus grevyi* mare jumped out of a moated enclosure to avoid contact with a newly introduced stallion to the enclosure. Consider all aspects of the environment in which the restraint procedure is to be performed. Maintenance of facilities and equipment must be routine.

ACKNOWLEDGMENTS

I acknowledge the many individuals (colleagues, animal owners, keepers, zoo administrators) and institutions that have contributed to my experiences with procedures and methods for handling animals. I have utilized all of the procedures discussed and illustrated in this volume over a professional lifespan of 5 decades. There may be other methods that accomplish the same purposes, but these work in my hands and I can recommend them.

Once again I am indebted to my wife Audrey for her unfailing support and encouragement. Her copy reading skills were vital to the success of this project. I lovingly dedicate this edition to her.

Restraint and Handling of Wild and Domestic Animals

PART 1

General Concepts

CHAPTER 1

Introduction

Restraint varies from confinement in an unnatural enclosure to complete restriction of muscular activity or immobilization (hypokinesia).[4] Both physical and chemical restraint are now practiced. Anciently only physical restraint was utilized. Just when man learned of chemical immobilization (poison arrows) is not known, but it antedates recorded history.

The physiological effects of restricted movement have been studied. For centuries, extended bed rest for ill or postsurgical human patients was practiced—to the detriment of the patient. Now it is known that many deleterious effects result from this type of immobility. Solitary confinement is known to be extremely devastating for a human being. Similar confinement of social animals produces severe psychological stress.[4]

Restraint practices evolved with the domestication of animals for food, fiber, labor, sport, and companionship.[2,4,6,7,13] Domestication necessitated special husbandry practices. As people began to minister to animals' needs, they found it necessary to restrict activity by placing them in enclosures. If animals resisted when wounds were treated or medication administered, it was necessary to further restrain them. Trial and error combined with the shared experiences of fellow human beings ultimately produced satisfactory practices.[2,3]

A person who undertakes to restrict an animal's activity or restrain the animal is assuming a responsibility that should not be considered lightly.[4,10] Each restraint incident has some effect on the behavior, life, or other activities of an animal. From a humane and moral standpoint, the minimum amount of restraint consistent with accomplishing the task should be used. This should become a maxim for persons who must restrain animals.

Each time it is proposed to restrain an animal, the following questions should first be asked: Why must this animal be restrained? What procedure will produce the greatest gain with the least hazard? When will it be most desirable to restrain the animal? Who is the most qualified to accomplish the task in the least amount of time and with the least stress to the animal? What location would be best for the planned restraint procedure?

WHY RESTRAINT

Everyone must agree that domestic animals require transporting, medicating, and handling. Some contend that all wild animals should be free ranging, without human interference. This philosophy seems naive in the present time.

Wild animals kept in captivity require special husbandry practices. They must be transported, housed, and fed. If they become ill, they must be examined and treated.

Free-ranging animals may have to be translocated, as was necessary when the Kariba dam was built in Southern Rhodesia. The translocation of free-ranging wild animals has become a common method of wild animal management for reducing overpopulation or building a population in a new location. The reintroduction of captive-bred wild animals to a former native habitat or a revitalized habitat is now routine. All of these animals must undergo significant screening, which in turn requires restraint, transport, and eventual release. Diseases in wildlife populations must be monitored, since some have far-reaching consequences for the health of domestic livestock and human beings. Many wild populations are managed. As far as wild animals are concerned, any captive situation involves some form of restraint.[4]

GENERAL CONCEPTS

Four basic factors should be considered when selecting a restraint technique: (1) Will it be safe for the person who must handle the animal? (2) Does it provide maximum safety for the animal? (3) Will it be possible to accomplish the intended procedure by utilizing the suggested restraint method? (4) Can constant observation and attention be given the animal following restraint until it has fully recovered from the physical or chemical effects? Once these four factors are evaluated, a suitable technique can be selected.[4]

Many wild animals can inflict serious, if not fatal, injury. The first concern when dealing with wild animals should be the safety of human beings. To think otherwise is foolhardy, and those who grandstand or show off by manipulating dangerous animals without benefit of proper restraint may injure themselves or bystanders. Those who own or have administrative responsibility for wild animals must recognize that the animal, no matter how valuable, cannot be handled in such a way as to jeopardize the safety of those who must work around it. Techniques are known that when properly used can safeguard both animal and operator.

It is desirable to build proper facilities into areas where wild animals must be kept so that these handling procedures can be safely carried out. It is foolish to pay thousands of dollars for a zoo specimen if facilities are not available in which to handle or restrain the animal for prophylactic measures or treatment of disease or injury.

Certain wildlife populations have become so depleted they are near extinction. We should not practice on these species. It is not economically feasible, nor is there sufficient animal life for each person to gain through personal experience the intimate knowledge of various behavioral patterns and characteristics to enable them to develop expertise in the successful use of restraint procedures. Therefore we must learn from the experiences of others who have dealt extensively with one species or family of animals and utilize their knowledge of the more successful techniques.

To be successful in working with animals, one must understand their behavioral characteristics and the aspects of their psychological makeup that will allow for provision of their best interests. Successful restraint operators must understand and have a working acquaintance with the tools of restraint. They must understand the use of voice, manual restraint, and chemical restraint. Special restraint devices and their application should be thoroughly understood. These are explained in the text, with a major emphasis on physical restraint methods. It has been my experience that an operator who really understands what can be done with physical restraint can build upon this information to carry out more successful chemical immobilization—if it is indicated.

The general principles of chemical restraint will be outlined and specific tables presented to give current usage of chemical restraint agents in various classes of animals. There is a marked swing toward the use of chemical restraint when working with wild animals. Pharmaceutical companies are carrying out research on newer and better restraint agents. This has led to the marketing of new products on a continuing basis. This ongoing activity may lead to the false assumption that applying physical restraint techniques is no longer necessary. Nothing could be further from the truth.

Just as the indiscriminate use of antibiotics may cloud test results and cause the inefficient clinician to make an inaccurate diagnosis, indiscriminate chemical restraint can likewise produce clinical aberrations and is often hazardous to the animal.

Chemical restraint is an extremely important adjunct to physical restraint practices, particularly in regard to wildlife. However, it is far from universally ideal and cannot replace special squeeze cages and other specially arranged facilities for wild animals, which allow them to be approached without imposing undue stress or hazard. Those who work extensively with wild animals know that no single chemical or group of chemical restraint agents fulfills all of the safety and efficacy requirements to qualify for universal application.

The decision whether to use chemical or physical restraint is based on the skill of the handlers, facilities available, and the psychological and physical needs of the species to be restrained. No formula can be given. If in doubt, someone who has had experience should be consulted.

WHEN TO RESTRAIN

One does not always have a choice of times when restraint should be carried out. Emergencies must be dealt with immediately. In the majority of instances, however, planning can be done.

Environmental Considerations

Thermoregulation is a critical factor in many restraint procedures. Hyperthermia and, more rarely, hypothermia are common sequelae. Heat is always generated with muscle activity. During hotter months of the year, select a time of day when ambient temperatures are moderate. Special cooling mechanisms such as fans may be required. Place restrained animals in the shade to avoid radiant heat gain. Conversely, use the sun's heat if the weather is cool. Avoid handling when the humidity is 70–90%. Cooling is difficult under such circumstances.

Take advantage of light and dark. Diurnal animals may best be handled at night when they are less able to visually accommodate. Nocturnal species may be more easily handled under bright lights.

Behavioral Aspects

An animal's response to restraint varies with the stage of life.[4,5,6] A tiger cub grasped by the loose skin at the back of the neck will curl up just as a domestic kitten does. Such a reaction is not forthcoming with adults.

A female in estrus or with offspring at her side reacts differently than at other times. Males near conspecific estrus females may be aggressive.

Male cervids (deer, elk, caribou) go into rut in the fall of the year. By this time the antlers are stripped of velvet and are no longer sensitive. Now the antlers are weapons. Although a handler may safely enter an enclosure of cervids during the spring or summer, it may be hazardous to do so during the rutting season.

Hierarchical Status

Most social animals establish a pecking order. A person trying to catch one animal in an enclosure may be attacked by other members of the group. Dominant male primates are especially prone to guard their band. I have seen similar responses in domestic swine and Malayan otters.

Animals removed from a hierarchical group for too long a time may not be accepted back into the group. At the very least they will have lost a favored position and must win a place in the order.

Infants removed from the dam and kept separated for more than a few hours may be rejected when reunited. Species vary greatly in this behavioral response. An infant Philippine macaque was accepted back by the mother after a 3-month separation. Some species may reject the infant if it has human scent on it. A further hazard of hours-long separation occurs if the dam has engorged mammary glands. The hungry infant may overeat and suffer from indigestion.

Health Status

Recently transported animals are poor restraint risks. Transporting in crates, trucks, and planes is a stressful event. The longer the journey, the more stress. The method of handling and type of accommodations used in transport are also important. If possible, allow the animal time to acclimate to a new environment before carrying out additional restraint.

Sick domestic animals are routinely handled for examination and treatment. It may be more difficult to evaluate the health status of wild animals. Standard techniques of measuring body temperature or evaluating heart and respiratory rate may yield meaningless results because of excitement. Even though a captive wild animal may exhibit some signs of a disease, it may be prudent not to handle it. The following incidents illustrate two such cases.

A nine-year-old child wrote a letter to the president of the United States following a visit to a small zoo. She told him the yak had long hair and long toenails and asked why the zoo didn't give it a haircut and trim its toenails. The letter was answered in an admirable way by a zoo director who explained that the long hair was normal and that it might be more dangerous to catch the yak than to let it be slightly uncomfortable with the long toenails.

In another situation a bison had dermatitis. A decision was made to catch it to check the lesion. The animal died of overexertion during the process.

Deciding when to intervene is difficult. Clinical experience may be the governing factor.

Territoriality

Domestic animals differ in response to handling depending on where they are. A veterinarian attempting to handle a dog in the owner's home will find a more defiant individual than if the same dog is placed in the strange environment of a hospital examining room. Cattle, horses, swine, and sheep likewise respond differently in their own corral or pen than if in a strange place. An animal can sometimes establish its territory rather quickly. A dog placed in a hospital cage may defend it as "home" within a few hours. After removal from the cage the dog may become more docile.

Many wild animals are highly territorial. In order to work on such animals they must be moved to a new enclosure.

HUMANE CONSIDERATIONS

It is incumbent upon a person who takes the responsibility of manipulating an animal's life to be concerned for its feelings, the infliction of pain, and the psychological upsets that may occur from such manipulation.[1,2,3,10,11] One must, however, be able to be objective about such manipulations and realize that the manipulation is for the best interests of the animal. Some feel that to restrict an animal's activity in any way is immoral and inhumane. At the opposite extreme is the person who has a total disregard for the life of animals.

Pain is a natural phenomenon that assists an animal to remove itself from danger in response to noxious influences. No animal is exempt from experiencing pain.[1] Pain is relative; individual persons and animals experience pain in varying degrees in response to the same stimulus. Pain can become so intense, however, that an animal may die from shock induced by pain. We should not minimize the effect of pain, nor should we overemphasize it. Some persons cannot cope with pain in themselves, their children, or their pets.

Working as a medical technologist while a student in veterinary school, I frequently saw mothers bring children into the laboratory for a blood count and tell them, "This isn't going to hurt." Nonsense, it does hurt. Why not face the fact and learn to cope with it? We all experience numerous painful stimuli every day. We live through it and so do animals.

Sensitive people do not like to inflict pain. Veterinarians and others who manipulate animals are morally and ethically obligated to minimize pain in the animals they handle. The animal under restraint is incapable of escaping from pain. The handler must perceive the feelings of the animal and take appropriate steps to alleviate pain.[1,4]

Some of the tools used in restraint practices involve the infliction of mild pain to divert the animal's attention from other manipulative procedures. The equine twitch is an example. The chain is placed over the nose of the horse and twisted down, causing a certain degree of pain. If the horse is preoccupied with the mild pain of the nose, nonpainful manipulative procedures can be carried out elsewhere on the body.

Every restraint procedure should be preceded by an evaluation as to whether or not the procedure will result in the greatest good for that animal. Animals have feelings. People should not look upon animals as machines to be manipulated at will.

It is interesting to peruse a 1912 book on the restraint of domestic animals.[12] One can not read the book without feeling that some of the procedures recommended would cause considerable unpleasantness to the animal and in some cases be inhumane. However, some of the techniques used 96 years ago for physical restraint are similar to those used currently, although modern considerations for behavior and training have diminished the necessity of "brute force."

Albert Schweitzer was one of the foremost proponents of the concept of reverence for life.[10] Human beings may have supreme power over other forms of life on this earth, but unless they recognize a dependence upon other life forms and have an appreciation for their position in the scheme of things, they will fail to develop an attitude that will result in humane care for animals under their charge.[11] Persons who seek to work in animal restraint would do well to read some of the literature of the humane movement so they might become more empathetic in their approach to procedures that involve the infliction of pain and understand the emotional trauma associated with restraint.[1–7]

Plan each restraint episode in detail. Anticipate potential problems. Provide equipment and facilities commensurate with the procedure. Time is crucial—get the job done fast. Follow through with observation and care until the animal is back to normal. If you lack experience in handling a given species, ask for help from someone who does have the experience.

Remember: (1) Safety to the handler. (2) Safety to the animal. (3) Will it do the job? (4) Get the animal back to normal.

DOMESTICATION

Approximately 35 of the nearly 50,000 species of vertebrates have adapted to humans' needs for food, fiber, work, sport, and beauty, and are considered to be domesticated (Tables 1.1, 1.2). All but three or four species were living in harmony with humans before the time of recorded history.[3,6,13]

Domestication is an evolutionary process that involves a gradual (thousands of years) change in the gene pool of a species to allow adaptation to an artificial environment. Domestic animals must cope with buildings, fences, crowding, confinement, lack of privacy, changed photoperiodicity, altered climatic conditions, and different food.

Genetic alteration during the evolutionary process took place by selection for specific characteristics that were economically or esthetically pleasing to humans. Docile animals were selected over aggressive individuals. This may require only a single gene mutation. Other economically important characteristics include higher fertility, rapid growth, efficient food conversion, higher milk production, and disease resistance. Farmers have often selected polled cattle over horned breeds to minimize injury.

There was definite selection to reduce or eliminate undesirable wild characteristics such as territoriality, intra-specific dominance, elaborate food identification and gathering mechanisms, intricate courtship behavior, and fear of humans. This constant selection yielded animals that are much easier to handle. They tolerate the presence of humans without a flight response. If physically restrained they rarely fight to the death, as do some wild species.

Mankind has been able to change the morphology and behavior of some domestic animals to the degree that it is difficult to determine what their wild counterpart might be like. Many breeds of livestock and companion animals have been produced. An overview, with excellent illustrations of breeds of livestock, is found in Sambraus.[8] He lists 55 breeds of cattle, 41 of sheep, 17 of goats, 62 of horses, 4 of donkeys and 15 of swine. There are more than 100 breeds of dogs and cats.

Asian elephants *Elephas maximus* were considered to be a domestic animal in years past. Surely the elephant has been in the service of humans for millennia, but it nevertheless lacks some of the criteria for domestication. Currently the elephant is classified as being in domesticity.

Two insect species are considered domestic animals, those being the European honeybee *Apis melifera* and the silkworm *Bombyx mori*.

TABLE 1.1. Domestic mammals

Common Name	Scientific Name	Family	Order
Mouse	*Mus musculus*	Muridae	Rodentia
Rat	*Rattus norvegicus*		
Guinea pig	*Cavia porcellus*	Cavidae	
Golden hamster	*Mesocricetus auratus*	Cricetidae	
Rabbit	*Oryctolagus cuniculus*	Leporidae	Lagomorpha
Dog	*Canis familiaris*	Canidae	Carnivora
Fox	*Vulpes fulva*		
Cat	*Felis catus*	Felidae	
Mink	*Mustela vdon*	Mustelidae	
Ferret	*Mustela furo*		
Horse	*Equus caballus*	Equidae	Perissodactyla
Ass (donkey)	*Equus asinus*		
Swine	*Sus scrofa*	Suidae	Artiodactyla
Bactrian camel	*Camelus bactrianus*	Camelidae	
Dromedary camel	*Camelus dromedarius*		
Llama	*Llama glama*		
Alpaca	*Llama pacos*		
Reindeer	*Rangifer tarandus*	Cervidae	
Cattle, European	*Bos taurus*	Bovidae	
Cattle, zebu	*Bos taurus*		
Yak	*Bos grunniens*		
Banteng	*Bibos banteng*		
Gayal	*Bibos frontalis*		
Water buffalo	*Bubalus bubalis*		
Musk-ox	*Ovibos moschatus*		
Sheep	*Ovis aries*		
Goat	*Capra hircus*		

TABLE 1.2. Domestic birds

Common Name	Scientific Name	Family	Order
Pekin duck	*Anas platyrhyncos*	Anatidae	Anseriformes
Muscovy duck	*Cairina moschata*		
Goose	*Anser anser*		
Canada goose	*Branta canadensis*		
Mute swan	*Cygnus olor*		
Chicken	*Gallus gallus*	Phasianidae	Galliformes
Ring-necked pheasant	*Phasianus colchicus*		
Coturnix quail	*Coturnix coturni*		
Peafowl	*Pavo cristatus*		
Guinea fowl	*Numida meleagris*	Numidae	
Turkey	*Meleagris gallopavo*	Meleagrididae	
Pigeon	*Columba liva*	Columbidae	Columbiformes
Budgerigar	*Melopsitticus undulatus*	Psittacidae	Psittaciformes
Canary	*Serinus canarius*	Fringillidae	Passeriformes

REFERENCES

1. Caras, R. 1970. Death As a Way of Life. Boston: Little, Brown.
2. Carson, G. 1972. Men, Beasts and Gods. New York: Charles Scribner's Sons.
3. Dembeck, H. 1965. Animals and Men. Garden City, NY: Natural History Press. (Trans. from German)
4. Fowler, M.E. 1995. Restraint and Handling of Wild and Domestic Animals. Second Ed. Ames, Iowa State University Press.
5. Fox, M.W., ed. 1968. The influence of domestication upon behavior of animals. In: Abnormal Behavior in Animals, pp. 64–75. Philadelphia: W.B. Saunders.
6. Hafez, E.S.F. 1968. Adaptation of Domestic Animals, pp. 38–45. Philadelphia: Lea & Febiger.
7. Hume, C.W. 1957. The Status of Animals in the Christian Religion. London: United Federation for Animal Welfare.
8. Sambraus, H.H. 1992. An Atlas of Livestock Breeds. London, Wolfe.
9. Scheffer, V.B. 1974. A Voice for Wildlife. New York: Charles Scribner's Sons.
10. Schweitzer, A. 1965. The Teaching of Reverence for Life. New York: Holt, Rinehart and Winston.
11. Thoreau, H.D. 1965. Walden. New York: Harper & Row.
12. White, G.R. 1912. Restraint of Domestic Animals, Second Ed. Nashville, TN, Williams Printing.
13. Zeuner, F.E. 1963. The History of Domestic Animals. London: Hutchins.

CHAPTER 2
Tools of Restraint

Although some instances of tool use have been described in nonhuman vertebrates, only humans have developed a high degree of skill in the use of tools. Every vocation, profession, or activity in which man engages requires the use of tools. The animal restrainer must become acquainted with a wide variety of tools used to handle animals safely, humanely, and effectively.

Tools may make a job easier or more efficient. The degree of skill attained by the restrainer is directly proportional to the degree of proficiency achieved in the use of tools of the trade. Tools must be kept in good repair; the art and practice of their use must be kept toned up.

Restraint levels may vary from the level achieved by arousing the subordinate feelings of an animal by voice and/or force of personality to the level of complete physical or chemical immobilization (hypokinesia). The tools used in effecting a given degree of restraint vary greatly. Some tools may be desirable for dealing with one species and be contraindicated when working with another. Success in the art of restraint requires both experience and study to know when it is appropriate to use a specific type of restraint. Inappropriate use of certain techniques may be not only unwise but dangerous to animal or human being.

When skilled animal restrainers are asked to share their secrets of success in working with animals, they can seldom give a detailed description of techniques. They have learned and habituated various means of restraint and sometimes do not even recognize the use of a system of techniques and tools. Undoubtedly the use of the tools of restraint has become second nature or instinctive to them.

For ease of discussion, the tools have been placed into seven categories: (1) psychological restraint—understanding a certain biological characteristic enables more satisfactory manipulation of a given animal; (2) diminishing sense perceptions of animals; (3) confinement; (4) lending added strength to or extension of the arms; (5) physical barriers used to protect us or allow closer scrutiny of animals; (6) physical force—used to subdue animals; and (7) chemical restraint—used to sedate, immobilize, or anesthetize animals.

PSYCHOLOGICAL RESTRAINT

The successful restrainer must know a given species' particular behavioral patterns. For instance, to handle swine with a snout rope, one must know that it is the nature of the pig to pull back when the upper jaw is grasped. An elephant will also tend to pull backward from a rope secured around the trunk. This may be useful in directing an elephant to sit down rather than fall to its side during narcotic immobilization. The same technique would be dangerously unsuitable for handling a carnivore, because a carnivore would attack instead of pulling back on the rope.

Each species exhibits its own behavioral pattern, its own degree of nervousness, and other unique traits. (See Chapter 5 for more details.) Knowledge of these patterns enables restrainers to counteract or incorporate them into restraint practices.

Voice is an important tool, frequently overlooked by animal handlers because of its simplicity. Emotional states are reflected in the voice.

Both domestic and wild animals readily perceive fear or lack of confidence. Some scientists believe that a frightened person may actually exude odorous substances, which can be smelled by animals. Others believe that persons betray fear to animals through voice or other behavior, and that animals will not perceive fear hidden by self-confident behavior and voice control.

Students sometimes struggle for many minutes to halter a horse that whirls away each time the head is approached. Another person walks confidently into the box stall, speaks to the horse in a firm tone, then walks up to the animal and places the halter. This is extremely frustrating to students who can see essentially no difference between their mode of approach to the horse and that of the skilled person. They failed because the horse perceived their uncertainty.

Perhaps an excellent teaching tool could be developed by making an audiovisual presentation revealing the differences between the sound of the students' voices and their attitudes in approaching the animal and the voice and attitude of the skilled restrainer.

Voice differences were graphically demonstrated to me in a slightly different situation. I was anesthetizing an African puff adder while making a television teaching tape to demonstrate the restraint technique. Both video and audio recordings were made during the actual procedure. After the procedure was completed I listened to the playback. At the point in the procedure when I grasped the animal by hand at the back of the head, after pinning it, my voice jumped almost half an octave higher in pitch. This was a graphic illustration of an altered emotional pattern being reflected in the voice. Obviously I was somewhat concerned as I grasped this poisonous snake. I did not recognize the change of voice at the time, but it was clearly heard on the playback.

Such subtle changes affect animal behavior in a given situation and signify confidence or lack of it. Perhaps the best advice that can be given is that a handler who lacks confidence in either self or procedure should remain silent.

Other mannerisms of the restrainer also reflect emotional state. Timidity when approaching the animal, the way the hands are held, quickness or slowness in using the hands, and general stance indicate confidence or lack of confidence to the animal.

Be sure animals are aware of your approach. As a boy I came alongside an old cultivating horse and threw a burlap sack over its back, intending to jump on and ride. The startled horse kicked out and flattened me. This was not so much a matter of restraint as failure to make contact with the animal. Contact may be by voice or through sight, but an unstartled animal is easier to manipulate. If the principle of surprise must be utilized to catch the animal, be prepared to cope with the results of fright.

Both domestic and wild animals can be trained to permit the carrying of certain manipulative procedures. Approaching a 5-year-old stallion that has run free on pasture or range since birth is much more difficult than approaching a 5-year-old stallion accustomed to people and trained for riding.

Likewise, wild animals can be trained to perform various acts or allow certain procedures to be carried out. Usually they cannot be trained to allow any procedure inflicting even minimal degrees of pain. Sometimes even this inhibition can be overridden under certain circumstances, at least to the extent of injecting medications or sedative agents to properly trained animals. A killer whale can be trained to lay its flukes on the bank at the side of a pool and lie quietly while a blood sample is withdrawn from a vein.

With wild animals, it is important to recognize that the training may involve establishing dominance over the animal by the trainer. This is a complex behavioral phenomenon, and it is unlikely that a casual person who comes in to manipulate that animal can acquire such dominance in a short time. Thus it is usually necessary for the trainer to perform the manipulative procedure for the clinician or veterinarian who must carry out an examination or make injections.

Hypnosis has been practiced on human beings for many years. Even surgery has been performed on individuals under hypnosis. The same technique has been effectively applied to animals. Many species of animals can be hypnotized. For instance, a chicken blindfolded and placed on its back will lie quietly in that position for a long period. Crocodilians can be manipulated in the same way, relaxing and entering a hypnotic state if placed on the back and stroked on the belly for a moment or two. Animals that "play dead," such as the opossum, enter a state essentially hypnotic. There is reason to believe that a horse may likewise become semihypnotized when the twitch is placed on its nose.

Many tales indicate that various animals hypnotize their prey when capturing food. It is unlikely that these states are bonafide representations of true hypnosis. It may be that entering this torpid state is a phenomenon that permits prey species to become free of the final pain of death when captured by a predator. It is not uncommon for a yet unharmed animal, chased by a predator, to give up and seemingly accept death without struggle. A zebra chased and grabbed by a lion will usually give up without a fight although in many instances the zebra may be fully capable of striking and killing the lion. Instead of doing so, the zebra becomes semicomatose, accepting the inevitable.

This response is utilized by those capturing such wild animals as zebras, giraffe, and some antelope species. For a few minutes immediately following capture by roping, they appear to be in a hypnotic state and can be approached and placed in crates without their kicking or striking. Those same animals, released from the crate into a holding pen, cannot be approached without dire consequences to the unwise person who makes that attempt.

Self-confidence is perhaps the single most important attribute that can be developed by the restrainer. This confidence can be acquired by experience, though some individuals seem to possess such ability almost innately. Some handlers develop the ability to manipulate or handle only one species or group of animals. Others handle many species with ease.

I am acquainted with one individual who possesses a phenomenal ability to work with the large wild felids. He had not worked with these animals extensively prior to a few years ago when, as an adult, he began to acquire an interest in some of the cats. I have seen him enter an enclosure containing mixed species of large, adult, untrained wild cats, including tigers and lions. These cats would wait in line to place their forepaws upon his shoulders and lick his face. He has such a degree of rapport, I am told, that he has entered an enclosure containing a half-dozen adult male African lions to successfully quell a fight.

This man has absolute confidence in his ability to work with these cats. There is no evidence of fear-mastery or dominance over the cats. He has studied their behavior sufficiently to know how to respond to the animals and how to get along with them, although many of the cats were adult when he acquired them. He has also taken lions known to be vicious toward other persons, studied them for a time, and safely entered an enclosure with them, feeling perfectly at ease.

To some this may appear a foolhardy and hazardous undertaking. Certainly it would be foolhardy for a person lacking the great confidence and behavioral skills of this individual to enter such an enclosure. Nonetheless it vividly illustrates what can be accomplished by someone with confidence and skill.

The successful restrainer must acquire detailed knowledge of the anatomy and physiology of the species to be manipulated, including the distance the limbs can reach to kick or strike. It is important to know the degree of agility and speed of the species in question. Techniques such as the use of a half-hitch chest rope to cast bovine species make use of a physiological response. The importance of gaining as much knowledge as possible of the biology and physiology of any species to be restrained cannot be overstated.

The significance of the physiological and behavioral phenomena of social and flight distances must be understood. All animals, including human beings, live with certain social interactions. These interactions involve both intimate and casual relationships. Social distances are inherent in the evolutionary development of a species. Social distances are precise for a given species and cannot be encroached upon without adverse effects. The general relationship of social distance is illustrated in Figure 2.1.

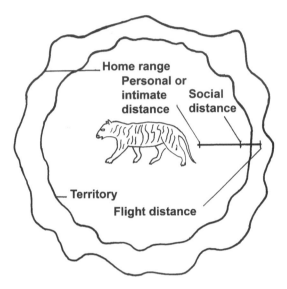

FIG. 2.1. Social distances of animals.

Domestic animals are less intensely affected by the lack of sufficient social distance than are wild species. The process of domestication necessitated that animals allow closer social contact with other individuals of the same species and with many other species.

Wild animals are habituated to social interactions and respond to violations of social distance in a prescribed manner. The usual response of the animal is to fight or flee. For example, a gazelle approached by a cheetah, though obviously aware of the cheetah's presence, stands quietly. But as soon as the cheetah approaches within a narrowly defined distance, the gazelle explodes into flight. This narrowly defined distance is "flight distance."

Flight distance varies among species according to agility, speed, and other behavioral traits and possibly the speed and agility of the enemy. A skilled keeper at a zoo gave me a vivid illustration of how an understanding of flight distance may be applied in restraint. He entered a cage to net some monkeys. As he approached the animals, he showed me that he could come within a certain distance without disturbing them. He then described and illustrated that if he moved one foot another few inches closer, the monkeys were startled and ran from him. This certain distance was the flight distance for that particular species in that situation.

He showed me that by using a long-handled net, he could reach out and catch one of the monkeys without startling it because the animal did not recognize the net as violating the flight distance. Thus by understanding this basic phenomenon, he was able to capture the animal without undue stress for the animal or himself.

Understanding flight and social requirements of various species is an important management tool for zoos and other institutions maintaining captive wild animals. Individuals of the antelope species in particular can be placed under continual severe stress if unable to maintain required social distances from other members of the group, from human beings, or from predator species. Sight barriers may meet these requirements as well as actual distance barriers. Flight distance can be modified by training. Furthermore, flight distance for animals raised in captivity differs from that of animals captured and brought into captivity as adults.

The response of an animal to a violation of flight distance is usually explosive; the animal either flees or attacks at full capacity. A wild animal may fling itself against a wall or into other barriers without regard for the consequences, once the flight response is initiated. An animal with no means of escape may attack without regard for its own safety.

Weapons Used against Humans

All animals have both defensive and offensive mechanisms enabling them to cope with encounters with enemies. In most restraint situations, the restrainer is the enemy, and the response of the animal to the manipulative procedure involves one or another of the mechanisms used by that animal to cope with danger. Thus the restrainer, in addition to understanding behavior, should know the defense and offense mechanisms operating in that species in order to modify or counter the effects of such responses.

Defense mechanisms may involve a display or demonstration of one sort or another, which warns the responsive handler that the animal intends to protect itself. Anatomical structures for defense and offense include claws, talons, feet and legs, teeth, bills or beaks of birds, special glands that exude scent, and the body itself.

Any animal with teeth and/or the ability to open the mouth widely enough to grasp some part of the restrainer's body is capable of biting. Not all who are capable will readily bite. All the carnivores, however, are prone to use the teeth, particularly the large canine teeth, to protect themselves and/or obtain food. The bite of many carnivores is serious and may be fatal. Birds, although not possessing teeth, are capable of biting or pecking. Some of the larger birds, such as the macaw, are able to crush bones with their heavy beaks, and large raptorial species (hawks, eagles) can severely tear tissue. Smaller birds can also inflict serious wounds. Birds with straight bills, such as fish-eating cranes and storks, may peck the eyes of the handler unless handled carefully.

Some animals, particularly invertebrate species, have special stingers with which to defend themselves, which may also be used in gathering food. Bees, wasps, some coelenterates, some marine cones, mollusks, fish, and other species have developed stinging structures that inflict pain and can cause illness or even fatalities in handlers.

Animals possessing horns or antlers can seriously injure by goring. Horns and antlers are used for display in combat with one another and in defense against enemies. Therefore it may be necessary to protect the horns from injury, as well as to prevent injury to animal and handler.

Some animals without sharp horns or antlers are capable of using the head as a battering ram to severely bruise or crush a handler against the wall. The giraffe is particularly prone to butt in defense or offense. Wild sheep also use their heavy horns and heads as battering rams, as do domestic goats and large domestic sheep. In fact, all horned animals, even if dehorned, are capable of crushing a person. Serious injury may result from failure to understand this characteristic.

Large animals such as the hippopotamus, elephant, and rhinoceros can cause serious damage by crushing a handler against walls or posts. Large constrictor snakes do not crush the bones of victims, but kill by suffocation. By throwing their coils around the body, snakes may cause serious injury or death. Even a small constrictor is dangerous if the coils become wrapped around the neck of a handler.

The teeth of most herbivores are not adapted to biting, nor is this a usual fighting technique for these species. Nonetheless these animals may become prone to bite when placed in a captive situation. Deer may reach out and grab a handler if frustrated or frightened. The hippopotamus, which is a grazer, bites in both offense and defense. The teeth of the hippo are formidable, and many persons have succumbed to a hippopotamus bite. Wallaroos often bite.

A few herbivorous species have large canines used for fighting. Male llamas and camels possess canine teeth that are used both in intra-species fighting and offensively against human restrainers. Likewise the small muntjac deer has enlarged canine teeth, used primarily in intra-species fighting but which can be used in defense against handlers.

Hoofed animals are capable of kicking, the only defense mechanism of some species. The response may be reflexive and is often elicited simply by touching the animal anywhere on the body. Knowledge of the length of the leg and the direction of the kick are important in such cases. The horse usually kicks straight backward. However, a few individuals kick forward and outward in a manner similar to the kick of the domestic bovine, referred to as "cow-kicking" by horsemen. As indicated, the cow does kick forward and out, so the most dangerous position for a handler may be just in front of the hind leg.

Novices may believe they can jump away when an animal initiates a kick, but experience will teach that this is not possible. The strength of some animals is phenomenal, and one must keep this in mind at all times. A camel can kick a 10 cm × 10 cm (4 in. × 4 in.) support for a building and break it in two.

Front limbs primarily strike or paw in defense. Many species, including South American camelids (llamas, alpacas), camels, giraffes, and equines, are prone to strike or paw.

Some species, such as the shark, have very rough skin surfaces used to rub against an enemy, inflicting serious abrasions. The handler who does not recognize that the surface is rough may be injured when manipulating sharks, certain lizards, and pangolins.

Poisonous snakes and lizards and some poisonous mammals are capable of envenomating enemies or prey with potent toxins.[1] Handling such species requires the use of highly specialized techniques and should be restricted to those who are fully qualified to do so by experience and inclination.

Some animals utilize the technique of spraying the enemy with urine or other substances. The octopus emits an inky fluid in which to hide itself as it escapes. Some primates, and other species such as the chinchilla, may urinate on the person who is trying to capture them. Such urination may also occur as an anger phenomenon or be used to delineate territory. Defecation may fit into the same category.

Numerous species have scent glands which produce materials objectionable to people. The skunk is the most noteworthy in this regard, but many other species, including carnivores and reptiles, have such glands. The musk gland is usually associated with the anus, and the material is often discharged under excitement. The scent glands sometimes serve purposes other than defense.

Spitting is a means of defense for some species. The expectorant may be composed of saliva, regurgitated stomach contents, or a specialized venom. Some cobra species are notorious for accurately projecting venom for distances up to 3 m (10 ft). Camelids and some apes are spitters. In one unique instance a shark in an aquarium surfaced and spit water on the author.

Regurgitation may occur in response to fright, but it is often a direct response to handling. Camels and llamas may deliberately spew foul-smelling material from the stomach on the handler. Cranes, storks, vultures, and pelicans may emit crop contents. Wolves and other carnivores may regurgitate as a stress response.

Although an elephant may use the tusks to gore or the trunk to grasp and fling an offender, it primarily tramples the enemy. Any large heavy mammal is capable of placing someone under its feet and trampling him. Fatalities from elephants, camels, rhinoceros, hippopotamuses, and other large animals have occurred.

Carnivores and other species may defend by clawing. Claws, whether sharp or dull, can inflict serious injury. Perhaps the worst injury I have received while manipulating animals was caused when a giant anteater drove its two blunted claws into the bone of my wrist. Clawing may result in infected scratches, or severe slashes transecting muscles, skin, blood vessels, and nerves, possibly incapacitating the handler permanently. In addition, the claws may grasp and pull a person into close contact within reach of teeth and strong forelimbs to bite and/or squeeze.

In short, the whole spectrum of the animal kingdom possesses abilities for self-protection. The restrainer must acquire knowledge of these mechanisms and be able to counter them in the restraint procedure. There are safe places to stand next to domestic animals. There are proper distances to recognize in working with animals and many ways to counter offensive and defensive mechanisms. Some specific mechanisms possessed by various animal groups will be described in the appropriate sections.

DIMINISHING SENSE PERCEPTIONS

Reducing or eliminating an animal's visual communication with its environment is an important restraint technique. A parakeet experiences less stress when placed in a darkened room before it is grasped for examination and/or medication. Blindfolding the domestic horse may make it possible to introduce it into a new environment, such as a trailer or a new stall, without engendering fright. Obviously it is impossible to blindfold most wild animals until the animal is already in hand. However, one can frequently place animals in a darkened environment.

If a herd of flighty and nervous black buck antelope are placed in a darkened room, the keeper can usually enter and grasp one animal without causing the pandemonium that develops if such an attempt is made from a herd in a lighted enclosure. It is important to recognize that manipulation of animals in such a restricted environment is somewhat hazardous if the herd includes males with horns.

This technique is contraindicated for species that possess excellent nighttime vision; in a darkened enclosure nocturnal species may well have better eyesight than the handler. It is therefore obvious that a detailed knowledge of the behavior and biology of a species is necessary before attempting any manipulation.

It may be necessary to blindfold an ostrich before it can be approached. Special devices can be constructed to place a blindfold over the head of such an individual. (See Chapter 29.) Most wild animals cannot be blindfolded until after capture. However, subsequent to capture, much stress can be relieved if the animal is blindfolded. A blindfolded animal may lie quietly for a long period while nonpainful manipulations are carried out. Sedation and anesthesia are required for painful procedures. Sedated animals handled in sunlight should be blindfolded to prevent damage to the retina by direct rays of the sun on an eye that cannot accommodate properly.

Sound is important in restraint. The importance of tone and quality of the voice as a restraint technique has already been described. Conversely, excessive sounds of people talking, motors, noisy vehicles, and other strange noises may seriously upset a wild animal. Restraint is easier to achieve if sounds can be dampened and harsh tones of voice eliminated or diminished in proximity to the animal. Cotton plugs in the animal's ears may suffice; however, it is extremely important that they be removed before the animal is released.

The skilled handler of domestic animals can accomplish much by proper use of the hands on the animal. Soothing, by stroking in the proper direction in the proper areas of the body, can be very valuable. Placing a hand firmly on the neck or shoulder of a horse and stroking it elicits desirable responses, while a lighter touch in the flank area may induce kicking. Most trained lions and tigers will frequently rub up against an individual; if one recognizes this as a friendly gesture, much can be accomplished. However, the handler who perceives it as a threat or is frightened will be unable to take advantage of this behavior in restraint.

Most untrained wild animals respond negatively to the touch of a person and institute defense mechanisms in response. Once such an animal is in hand, stress on the animal will be diminished if touching is kept at a minimum.

Cooling diminishes an animal's ability to respond to stimuli, particularly with poikilothermic species. My first experience in handling a large snake involved treating a large python for tail rot. I experienced much trepidation until I arrived at the ranch and found that the animal had been placed in a walk-in refrigerator some 2 hours previously. The animal was torpid and easily manipulated. Hypothermia has been used in the past to render nonvenomous species of snakes and lizards immobile for purposes of surgery, but this technique cannot be recommended. The potential hazard of the development of respiratory infections following prolonged cooling must be recognized. Sedative techniques are available to replace cooling as a technique.

CONFINEMENT

Confinement is a tool of restraint, but the acceptable degree of confinement may vary considerably, depending on the species and the situation. To the free-ranging wild animal, being placed in a large fenced-in area represents confinement, resulting in a certain degree of stress on the adult wild animal. Confinement can be progressively intensified by smaller enclosures. In a zoo situation this may be in an alleyway; for a domestic animal it may be confinement in a stall or shed. Close confinement makes it easier to evaluate clinical signs. The closest and most stressing confinement is that requiring an animal to be placed into a special cage, such as a transfer cage (Fig. 2.2) in a zoo, a special night box or bedroom, a shipping crate, or one of the many different types of squeeze cages (Figs. 2.3 to 2.7).

Squeeze cages are an extremely valuable restraint tool for wild animals. It is important to recognize that no squeeze cage can be adapted for universal use. Animals vary in both anatomical conformation and physiological requirements; the design of the squeeze cage must accommodate these to be safe and useful for carrying out various procedures. Squeeze cages designed for use in particular wild species will be described under those groups. Commercial squeeze chutes are available for domestic sheep, cattle, and swine.

Confinement may likewise be carried out by the use of special bags. The cat bag is useful for handling domestic species and can be adapted for use with many different species of small wild mammals. Similar bags can be constructed for

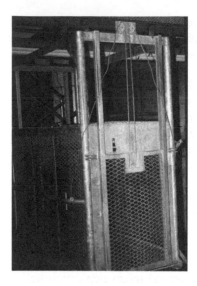

FIG. 2.2. Transfer cage, mounted on an overhead track, designed to fit between two rows of cages. Used to move animals from one cage to another.

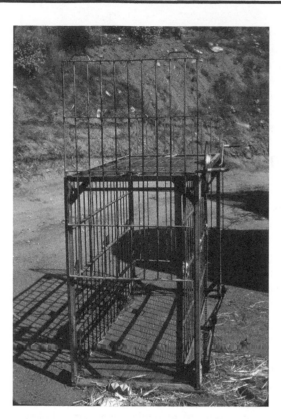

FIG. 2.4. Light squeeze cage for felids.

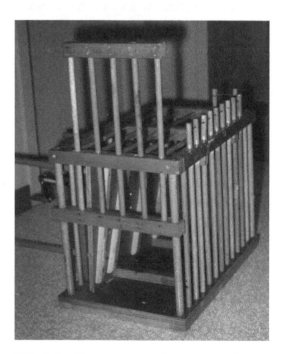

FIG. 2.3. Home-constructed squeeze cage for small mammals.

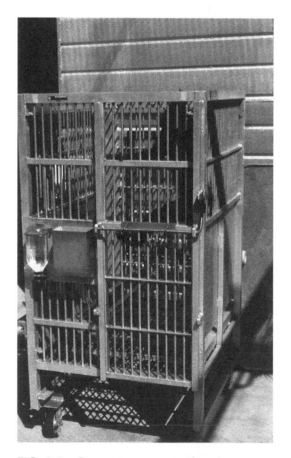

FIG. 2.5. Stronger squeeze cage for primates.

handling almost any kind of animal. If such bags are not available, burlap or jute sacks can be used to protect many species of birds and animals, as well as the handler. A limb or a wing can be extended through a hole in the side or from the partially opened top.

Towels or other flat cloths can be used to wrap animals for short manipulative procedures. This technique is frequently used with parrots, domestic cats, and the young of many carnivorous species. Birds may also be placed in a stockinette or woman's nylon hose.

Reptiles may be restrained for radiographic studies, anesthesia, or other mild manipulative procedures by inserting them into plastic tubes, as shown in Figure 2.8.

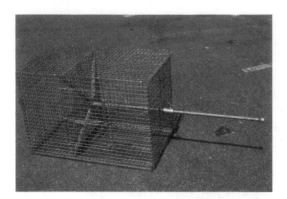

FIG. 2.6.   Portable squeeze cage for small animals.

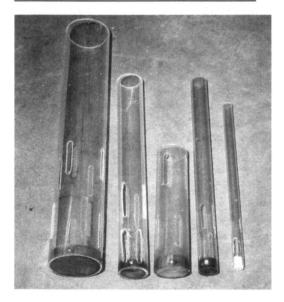

FIG. 2.7.   Squeeze cage for pinnipeds. Squeeze from top.

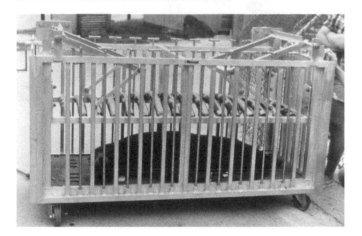

FIG. 2.8.   Plastic tubes used for snake restraint.

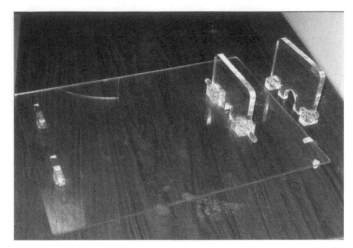

FIG. 2.9.   Plastic restraint board for radiography of birds.

fastened with adhesive or masking tape, or the board can be equipped with Velcro straps to hold the animal (Fig. 2.9). The techniques are similar to those used in a hospital to restrain an infant needing specialized intravenous medication or restriction of movement.

Well-trained domestic cattle and horses may be placed into stocks for examination and manipulative procedures. This is the common method used to restrict movement, medicate, carry out dentistry, or examine a horse.

Confinement can also be accomplished with the use of ropes, cables, or wire panels. Gregarious species such as domestic sheep or cattle may be herded into a restricted chute area and the handler may walk among the animals to urge them into the chute to examine, medicate, drench, or carry out other desired procedures.

EXTENSION OF ARMS

Ropes are an excellent means of extending the arm. Details of rope use are found in Chapter 3.

Snares, hooks, and loops are used to capture and restrain animals in a variety of situations (Fig. 2.10). A snare is an important tool, but used carelessly, it can cause unnecessary pain or suffocate an animal. Commercial snares are usually designed with swivels for more humane and effective manipulation. An excellent snare is produced by the Ketch-all Company of San Diego (Fig. 2.11). It is a quick-release snare that permits the animal to twist without being suffocated. Homemade snares can be constructed from either metal or plastic pipe, using rope or cable. Snares used in obstetrics for extraction of the fetus can be adapted for use in animal handling. Special snares are made for handling swine.

A special combination of a snare and a rope can be made by placing the rope loop at the end of a long bamboo pole, lending rigidity to the rope for placement of the loop.

As soon as the neck is surrounded, the pole is loosed, and one has the animal by the rope. This technique was used

Complete restraint of an animal, usually under sedation, may be carried out with a restraint board (Fig. 2.9). This is routinely used with birds, snakes, and small primates. Such a board may consist of a Plexiglas sheet to which the animal is

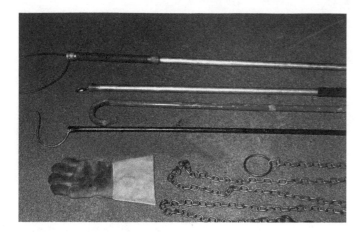

FIG. 2.10.   Some tools of restraint.

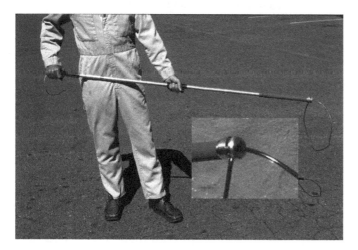

FIG. 2.11.   Commercial cable snare "Ketch-all" pole.

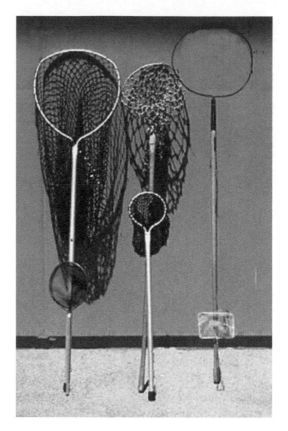

FIG. 2.12.   Nets.

in capturing free-ranging wild ungulates in the past. The animal was pursued in a 4-wheel-drive vehicle and captured, the pole was removed, and the animal was brought to a stop by snubbing it to some part of the vehicle.

Snares are hazardous in the hand of an untrained person. The animal may be suffocated by careless use. When grasped, some animals immediately begin to twist. This is natural behavior for carnivores such as wild felids and for crocodilians. If the handler does not compensate by counter-manipulating the snare, the cable twists up, causing the animal to strangle.

It is desirable to include one front leg through the snare, but it is not always possible to catch the animal in the best position. Catching the animal around the abdomen allows too much mobility of the head, making it possible for the animal to injure the handler. Animals having great dexterity of the forelimbs are not suitable candidates for use of the snare. They push the snare away, preventing application. This is true of some carnivores, such as the raccoon, and most primates. As soon as it is possible to grasp the animal, remove the snare and apply other methods of restraint to minimize the possibility of strangulation.

Nets are important tools for animal restraint. They come in all sizes and shapes (Figs. 2.12, 2.13), from those used to capture tiny insects to the very large cargo net used to restrain a musk-ox. Keep them readily available and in good repair. Obtain a variety of sizes to provide the right net for manipulating a wide range of species. By placing a net on the animal, many manipulative procedures such as injection with sedatives, medication, examination, or obtaining samples for laboratory work can be carried out.

Hoop nets with long handles may be directed at an animal. It is important for the handler to recognize that the hoop edge may injure the animal. It is better to allow the animal to enter the net rather than swing the net at the animal and possibly bang or crush it with the hoop. The net should be of sufficient depth to allow the hoop to be twisted, incarcerating the animal in the bottom of the net. Too shallow a net may permit the captured animal to climb back out of the net. If a net is shallow, immediately placing the hoop against the ground will further restrict the animal and prevent escape. An animal in a net may retain too much mobility. Pressing the animal with a broom, shovel, or stick can further restrict movement.

As shown in Figure 2.14, a net must be deep enough to allow closure with the animal in the bottom of the net. Figure 2.14 shows a net open and closed.

Birds with talons or animals with claws are difficult to handle in large mesh nets. They may poke their limbs through

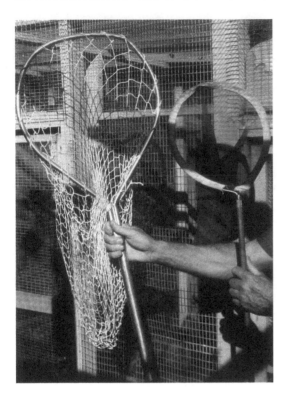

FIG. 2.13. Bird nets.

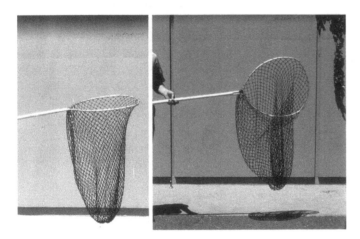

FIG. 2.14. A net must be deep enough to allow closure with the animal in the bottom of the net.

the netting or cling to it, making it extremely difficult to extract them from the net. It is better to utilize a smooth net for some birds, perhaps one made from the plastic sacking now being used for livestock and other animal feeds. If the mesh of a net is too large, the animal may force its head through the mesh and strangle before it can be released. The size of the mesh should correspond to the size of the animal to be netted.

Rectangular nets may be placed in the path of various types of animals. As the animal runs toward it, the net is extended. Since a net is not usually recognized as a barrier, the animal will run into it. The net may then be dropped over it, and the animal will entangle itself. Handlers can then grasp

the animal and proceed with further restraint. This technique has been successfully used on animals of various sizes, up to the size of the musk-ox. The size of the mesh and strength of the rope must be commensurate with the species being manipulated.

Nets may be used to lift animals from precarious spots, such as out of moats into which they have fallen, or transport them for short distances via helicopters or airplanes.

It is important to know the characteristics of the materials with which a net is constructed. Nylon, cotton, and manila are all used, and each will withstand different degrees of stretch and wear. Carnivorous species are apt to chew at netting and may effect escape by chewing holes. The net should be inspected before each use for flaws that may allow the animal to escape at an inopportune time and place or to grasp and injure the handler.

Very fine nets called mist nets are used to capture small birds and bats. Cannon nets are sometimes used to capture animals. The animal is baited to a selected area and a folded net is shot over the top of it to entrap it.

Another technique is to suspend a net over an area such as a salt lick or feeding area. Animals are enticed beneath the net, which is then dropped to entangle them. See Chapter 28.

Special tongs have been developed for working with various species of animals, including swine and certain of the canids, such as the fox. A vise tong is used to grasp the animal at the neck, much as is done with a snare. The tong does not completely encircle the neck but clamps behind the back of the head. Tongs are usually used only to obtain initial hold of the animal; other means are then used to apply further restraint.

Nose tongs are widely used for handling domestic bovine species. See Chapter 11. One may grip the nose with the fingers as improvised nose tongs.

Bulls, particularly dairy bulls, usually have a ring placed through the nose to allow for safer manipulation or handling A special bull lead, which is a pipe with a hook on the end of it, can be used to grasp the ring to guide the animal, allowing the handler to stay away from the animal. See Chapter 11 for details.

The snake hook, in its various forms, is utilized in handling all species of reptiles. Descriptions are found in Chapter 25.

Trained wild animals, particularly the large cats or bears, may be restrained to some extent with the use of chains. The chains either snap into heavy collars on the neck or encircle the neck and snap into a link. For short manipulative procedures, particularly if it is necessary to sedate the individual, the chain may be placed around the neck by the trainer and wrapped around a post or other solid object. The animal can be grasped by the tail and the injection quickly given.

PHYSICAL BARRIERS

Physical barriers may be used to protect handler and animal or to allow the handler closer proximity without alarming the animal.

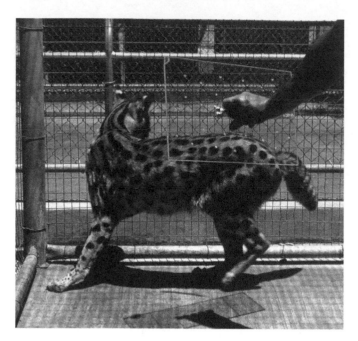

FIG. 2.15.   Plastic shield used to ward off attack by a small mammal or bird while maintaining visual contact.

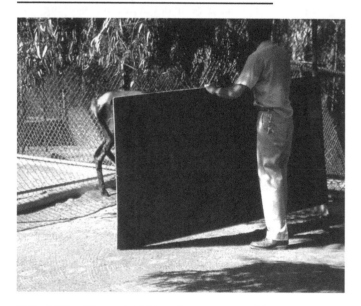

FIG. 2.16.   Plywood shield used to move a wapiti.

Shields are important tools of restraint (Figs. 2.15, 2.16). They may consist of plywood sheets or be constructed with handles on the back to be held by the manipulator. Shields may allow close approach to the animal or may be used between two transfer cages having swinging doors instead of guillotine doors. Plastic shields allow the handler vision without exposing the head. They are useful in handling large nonvenomous reptiles, some of the smaller mammals, and some birds.

A head screen offers protection from extremely agile animals that may become aggressive. The head screen must be made of small enough mesh that birds cannot peck through it or animals cannot reach through to scratch the face. These are especially useful in handling hornbills, cranes, storks, and certain species of primates.

A blanket may be used to shield the animal from the handler. It will also protect the handler from legs, horns, or antlers. A small antelope may frequently be captured by allowing it to jump into a blanket, completely enclosing it, and holding it in the blanket. Small mattresses may be similarly used. A mattress is more solid than a blanket and may be used to press the animal against a wall to inject it with a sedative or to carefully grasp it for additional restraint. A mattress is also valuable to cushion the body and protect the eyes of a restrained animal from trauma caused by thrashing on the ground.

Bales of hay or straw may be used as physical barriers for working on or around animals. Rectal examinations or perineal surgery of mares or stallions may be performed using these devices to prevent injury to the manipulator from kicking. Also, they are soft and do not traumatize the legs of an animal that kicks. Such barriers should be high enough that the animal cannot kick over the top of them.

Wire panels or solid gates may be used to squeeze animals against the walls of buildings or fences. It is important to prevent the animal from sticking a leg through the mesh or slats of such panels. Fractures of the limb are common from slatted panels.

Opaque plastic sheeting is excellent for use as a physical barrier to direct animals to proceed in a desired direction. (See Chapter 28.) Animals recognize an opaque plastic sheet as a barrier, while they may not recognize a wire or wooden fence as such. Thus animals may be directed into loading crates or into chutes with opaque plastic sheeting in a manner heretofore impossible. Plastic sheeting has its greatest application when moving hoofed animals.

Giraffe-like species do not respond well to the barrier type of manipulative procedure. They look over the top or reach the head underneath to look, instead of moving away from the barrier.

PHYSICAL FORCE

The hands are used in most manipulative procedures; the wise restrainer takes every precaution to protect them. The hands may be used alone to grasp an animal. The restrainer must know where and how to grasp the animal to be protected and to accomplish the restraint required.

The pressure required varies with the species. Handling a 50-g parakeet is indeed different than holding onto a 12-kg macaque. The amount of force applied must be appropriate to the species. Suffocation may result from the application of too great a pressure. Limbs or ribs may be fractured by applying too much force.

The greatest protection for the hands is detailed knowledge of the animal. Many people use gloves, which are an important tool of restraint. Gloves vary from thin cotton gloves used to handle small rodents to heavy, double-layered, coarse leather gloves used to handle large primates (Fig. 2.17). Leather welder's gloves are excellent for general use.

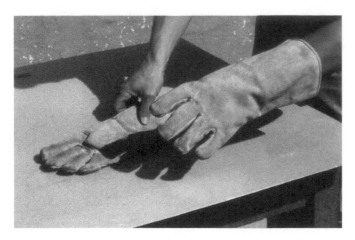

FIG. 2.17. Gauntleted leather welder's gloves.

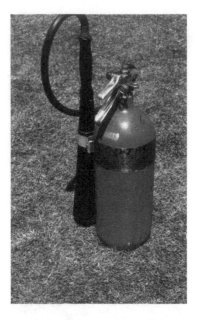

FIG. 2.18. Carbon dioxide fire extinguisher may be used to frighten an animal to move into another enclosure.

The thicker and heavier the glove, the less the ability of the handler to determine how tightly he/she is grasping an animal or to feel the response of the animal. Because of this, many handlers refuse to use gloves.

Carnivorous species can likely bite through the thickest gloves available, so a glove is not an absolute guarantee of protection from biting. Preferably, leather gloves should be loose on the hand so that if an animal bites, the digit can slip sideways and be missed as the canine teeth penetrate the leather.

Gloves do not protect from crushing by powerful jaws. A tiger can crush the bones of the hand, or a large macaw can fracture finger bones without breaking the skin of a gloved hand.

Chain-mail gloves used either alone or within a leather glove offer more protection against the tearing effects of large canine teeth, particularly in regard to primates. Such gloves are useful as restraint aides, but they do decrease tactile discrimination and do not entirely eliminate the crushing effects of the bites of animals with strong jaws.

An animal may be encouraged to move in a given direction by using a rolled up newspaper, a scoop shovel, or a house broom. Using a broom to persuade a horse to enter a trailer is a time-tested technique. All of these devices inflict minimal pain, but the noise of the slap encourages the desired response. These techniques are useful in handling both domestic and wild animals.

Other tools for applying physical force include poles or bars to additionally restrict animals in cages or to press on a netted animal to hold the head down for a short time while injections are being made.

Carbon dioxide-charged fire extinguishers have been utilized to encourage or frighten animals to move out of a den or into another enclosure (Fig. 2.18). Apparently the sound and/or the fog resulting from discharge of the fire extinguishers frighten them into moving away from the source of annoyance. This technique is not infallible but has been successful. It may also be used as a defensive weapon for manipulating such animals should they escape. Burning highway flares will also frighten some animals (e.g., nonhuman primates).

CHEMICAL RESTRAINT

Chemical restraint has been the single most important contribution to the art of animal handling that has occurred in recent years. It enables one to manipulate some species of animals that heretofore simply could not be handled. Many different agents are used for chemical restraint. None of them are satisfactory in all cases. Each has its indications and limitations and each must be used with judicious understanding of what it can and cannot do. Perhaps the greatest evil of the chemical restraint era is for the novice to assume that all that is required to solve all restraint problems is a drug, a syringe, and some method to inject it into the animal. Such is emphatically not the case.

Chemical restraint is such an important tool for restraint that a special chapter is devoted to it.

SPECIAL TECHNIQUES

Slings are not necessarily restraint tools, but are adjuncts to the proper care and management of animals unable to maintain the upright position because of injury or illness. Slinging may also be necessary to extract an animal from a precarious position, such as from a moat or, in the case of free-ranging animals, a bog.

The rope sling described in Chapter 3 is adaptable to most species of quadrupeds. The size of the rope should vary with the size of the animal. Other slings may be purchased commercially, or they may be constructed if one understands the basic anatomy and physiology of the animal. Slings are commonly used for horses and cattle with injuries that necessitate resting one or more limbs. Birds may also be slung, as depicted in Figure 29.37. Bird slings usually must be improvised.

A speculum is used to hold the mouth open for oral examination, dental surgery, or gastric intubation. Specula may be elaborate commercial metal devices (Fig. 2.19) or they may be

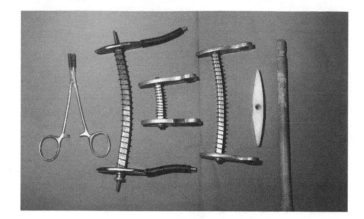

FIG. 2.19.   Dental specula for small mammals.

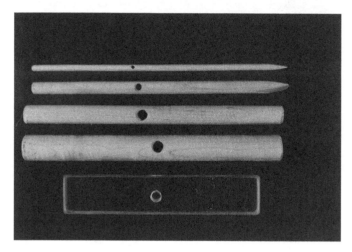

FIG. 2.20.   Hardwood dowels and plastic used for specula.

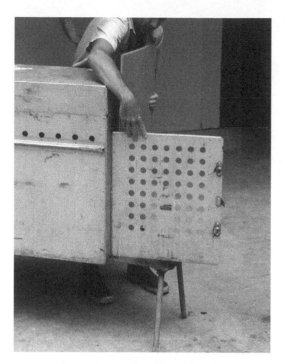

FIG. 2.21.   A plywood shield is used to block the opening of a swinging-door cage until the cage can be pushed up against the door of another cage.

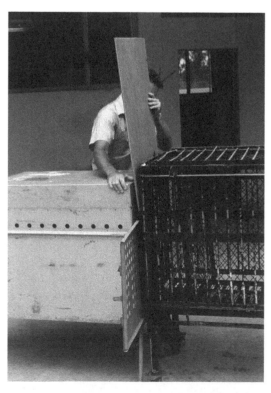

FIG. 2.22.   Removal of the shield to allow passage of animal to a new cage.

constructed from doweling (Fig. 2.20). A set of hardwood dowels 25-cm (10-in.) long of the following dimensions will accommodate birds, reptiles, and mammals up to 10 kg (22 lb): 25 mm (1 in.) with a 13-mm (0.5-in.) diameter hole; 19 mm (0.75 in.) with a 13-mm (0.5-in.) diameter hole; 13 mm (0.5 in.) with a 6-mm (0.25-in.) diameter hole; 6 mm (0.25 in.) with a 3-mm (0.12-in.) diameter hole. Old broom handles serve the need for larger specula. The beveled end of the dowel is gently inserted between the lips and teeth to open the mouth.

Clear plastic may be used to allow a better view of oral structures, but plastic is harder and may be more traumatic to the teeth than wood. The size of the plastic speculum illustrated is 35 mm (1.5 in.) × 15 mm (0.65 in.) × 20 cm (8 in.) with a 13-mm (0.5 in.) hole.

To transfer an animal from a swinging-door cage to another cage, procure a shield to cover the swinging door. Slowly open the door of the cage containing the animal just wide enough to allow insertion of the solid shield behind it. When the shield is in place, open the door (Fig. 2.21). Place the new cage with the opening closely against the shield. Remove the shield, allowing the animal to enter the new cage (Fig. 2.22).

Obviously this technique is highly effective only for small to medium-sized primates, carnivores, rodents, and other small mammals not strong enough to push away the shield.

REFERENCE

1. Fowler, M.E. 1993. Veterinary Zootoxicology. Boca Raton, Florida: CRC Press.

CHAPTER 3
Rope Work

Rope was one of the earliest tools used by humans. Prehistoric humans first used vines but soon began to fashion rope from the fibers of bark, cotton, hides, hair, coconuts, and silk. Braided rope of animal hair was known in southwest Asia prior to 4000 B.C. Every culture has used rope in one form or another to hoist, haul, tie, secure, hunt, fish, build, explore, bridge, sail, and catch.[7]

The Egyptians used rope made from papyrus and camel hair to build pyramids and to hunt hippopotamuses in the Nile. The Incas built rope bridges across the gorges of the Andes. Mayans used rope to haul stones for building temples. North American Indians fashioned ropes from bark and horsehair. Tribes near the ocean hunted whale with ropes of cedar. By the fourteenth century a rope-making guild was formed in England.[7] The western and southwestern areas of the United States were settled by a sturdy lot of cowboys proficient in the use of ropes.

Rope is a basic tool required for many manipulative procedures on wild and domestic animals. Even though drugs and other devices are often used in restraint practice, fundamental knots, hitches, and rope techniques have wide application.

CONSTRUCTION OF A ROPE[6–8]

The fundamental unit of all cordage is the yarn or thread. Plant or synthetic fibers are straightened by combing, then drawn into a small tube and twisted. Individual fibers are overlapped and interlocked during the twisting process to bind and give strength. The hardness of the twist is determined by the number of twists per foot, which varies from 8 to 22. Two or more yarns twisted together in opposite directions to that forming the yarn produces a strand. The final rope is made by twisting three or more strands together.

The twist of the individual strand is opposite to the twist given the strands as they are laid together. The twists are directed so they turn in toward each other to securely bind and prevent untwisting in the final rope. Three or more ropes can be twisted together to form a rope cable. Instead of twisting, strands of soft fibers such as cotton can be machine-braided into a rope. Such ropes are easier to handle than ordinary rope, and annoying twisting is less likely to occur.

Select the proper type and size of rope for the job (Tables 3.1–3.4; Figs. 3.1–3.3). Care for rope as for a precision instrument and it will provide long, useful service. Keep rope clean. Dragging it through dirt and feces or over rough gritty surfaces allows abrasive particles to work into the rope and damage fibers. If the rope becomes soiled, wash it in plain water and dry thoroughly before storing to prevent fungal decay. Avoid using soaps and detergents.[8]

Protect ropes from acids, alkalies, oils, paints, and other agents not chemically neutral. Rinse rope that has been soaked with urine.

Prevent kinks, which cause permanent damage and weakening of the rope. Do not tie knots in hard-twist ropes. Minimize sudden strains or jerking as they may break a rope otherwise strong enough to handle the load. A short glossary of terms is provided at the end of the chapter to acquaint the reader with the terminology used when handling rope.

BASIC ROPE WORK

Figure 3.4A illustrates specific terms used to refer to the parts of a rope. The standing part "w" is the segment not being used; the length "u" is a bight or bend that will be used in procedures or to construct knots; and "v" is the end of the rope used to thread through knots, etc. Figure 3.4B illustrates a loop or half hitch, a fundamental step in building some knots. Figure 3.4C shows an overhand knot.

To prevent unraveling, use one of the methods illustrated in Figures 3.5–3.8. Burn nylon rope at the tip, melting the strands together. This prevents unraveling but does not form a bulge at the end of the rope. The bulge may actually be desirable.

SPLICING ROPE[2,4,6]

Splicing may occasionally be necessary to join or repair ropes. Various types of splices are available (Fig. 3.9). In general, short splices add bulk but little rope is wasted in the splice. A long splice is less bulky but requires a longer segment of rope. A long splice may be necessary if the rope must pass through a block and tackle. The eye splice and back splice have special uses in the construction of rope halters.

A short splice is made by unraveling a sufficient length of the ends of both segments to be joined so that at least three over and unders may be carried out. For a 1/2-in. rope, this should amount to approximately 6 in. (15 cm). The unraveled ends are placed together as illustrated in Figure 3.10A. The strands of one segment are anchored to the other rope with a piece of string or masking tape. Interlace one loose strand over the adjacent strand and under the following strand. Each

TABLE 3.1. Soft fibers used for ropes

Soft Fibers	Common Name of Plant	Scientific Name of Plant	Geographical Source of Fibert	Part of Plant Used for Rope	Advantages	Disadvantages
Cotton	Cotton	*Gossypium* spp.	Worldwide	Fibers attached to seed	Soft, flexible, least likely to cause rope burns, inexpensive, excellent for hobbles	Weak, subject to abrasion, water damage and fungal deterioration
Linen	Flax	*Linum usitatissimum*	Northern Europe	Leaves	Strong	Expensive
Hemp	Marijuana, hemp	*Cannabis sativa*	Middle East, China, Italy, South America	Stems, leaves	Very soft and pliable, twine, excellent for hobbles	Weak
jute	jute	*Corchorus* sp.	Malaysia, India	Stems	Used primarily for burlap and twine	Weak, makes poor rope

TABLE 3.2. Hard fibers used for ropes

Common Name of Fiber	Common Name of Plant	Scientific Name of Plant	Geographical Source of Plant	Part of Plant Used	Advantages	Disadvantages
Manila	Abaca	*Musa textilis*	Philippines, Central America	Sheathing of leafstalks	One of strongest natural known fibers	Fibers are hydroscopic; unless treated, rope becomes unmanageable when wet
Sisal	Agave, sisal	*Agave sisalana*	Mexico, Central America, Africa, Hawaii, Indonesia	Fibers stripped from long, pulpy leaves	Inexpensive, used for twines and ropes where strength not important	80% as strong as manila
Maguey	Maguey sisal	*Agave cantala*	India, Java	Same as sisal	Used for special trick and fancy ropes	Similar to sisal
Mexican maguey henequen	Maguey	*Agave* spp.	Mexico	Same as sisal	Used for twine and cheap rope	Similar to sisal
New Zealand hemp	New Zealand flax	*Phormium tenas*	New Zealand	Leaves	Softer, more flexible than manila	Lacks strength
Coir or sennit	Coconut	*Cocos nucfera*		Tropical Pacifictusk of fruit	Highly water resistant	Availability

TABLE 3.3. Other fibers used for ropes

Name of Fiber	Source of Fiber	Where Used	Advantage	Disadvantage
Nylon	Synthetic, from chemicals derived chiefly from petroleum and natural gas products	Worldwide	Strongest rope available, resists moisture and fungus, only safe rope for handling large bovids and equids	Highly elastic, difficult to take up slack in slings and casting ropes, inflammable, causes rope burns easily
Dacron	Synthetic polyester fiber	Worldwide	Similar to nylon, slightly weaker	Similar to nylon
Polypropylene	Synthetic fiber, produced by polymerization of pro-pylene, a by-product of crude oil refining	Worldwide	Water resistant, will float, resistant to acids and alkalies	Will melt with heat, should not be used where friction is expected
Leather or rawhide	Cured leather or rawhide of many different animals	Mexico. Many cultures have used leather for rope throughout history	Rope is nicely balanced for throwing	Extreme variability in quality and strength, used only with dally system
Horsehair and other animal hair	Tail and mane hairs of horses, etc.	Southwestern United States, other areas of world	Can be fashioned into ornamental ropes, has little use in restraint	Harsh on the hands, causes rope burns easily

TABLE 3.4. Strength comparison of rope

		Breaking Strength[a] (approximate)													
		Manila		Sisal		Cotton		Nylon		Dacron		Polypropylene		Wire Cable[b]	
Diameter (in.)	Diameter (mm)	(lb)	(kg)	(lb)	(kg)	(lb)	(kg)	(lb)	(kg)	(lb)	(kg)	(lb)	(kg)	(lb)	(kg)
3/16	4.8	450	204	360	164	250	114	1,110	504	1,050	477	800	363	2,120	962
1/4	6.4	600	272	480	218	420	191	1,850	840	1,750	795	1,350	613	4,100	1,861
3/8	9.4	1,350	613	1,080	490	890	404	4,000	1,820	3,600	1,634	2,650	1,203		
1/2	12.7	2,650	1,200	2,120	960	1,450	658	7,100	3,220	6,100	2,770	4,200	1,907	17,820	8,090
5/8	15.7	4,400	2,000	3,520	1,600	2,150	976	10,500	4,770	9,000	4,086	5,700	2,588		
3/4	19.1	5,400	2,450	4,320	1,960	3,100	1,408	14,200	6,470	12,500	5,675	8,200	3,723	35,480	16,108
1	25.4	9,000	4,100	7,200	3,270	5,100	2,315	24,600	11,170	20,000	9,800	14,000	6,356	62,400	28,330
1 1/2	38.1	18,500	8,400	14,800	6,720			55,000	25,000	36,000	16,344	29,700	14,484		
2	50.8	31,000	14,100	24,800	11,260			91,000	41,315	61,500	27,921	53,000	24,062		

[a] A safe working load is double the breaking strength.
[b] Ordinary flexible steel cable (6 strands, 19 wires, 1 fiber core).

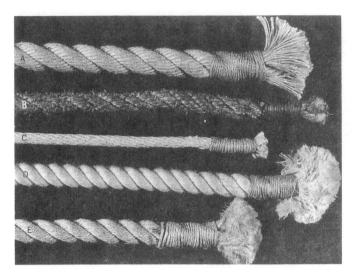

FIG. 3.1. Soft fiber ropes: **A.** Linen (flax).
B. New Zealand flax. **C.** Braided cotton (sash cord).
D. Twisted cotton (7/16 in.) **E.** Hemp.

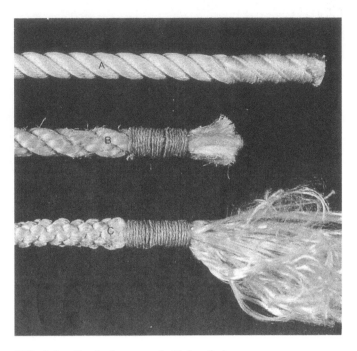

FIG. 3.3. Synthetic ropes: **A.** Nylon (in.).
B. Polypropylene (A6 in.). **C.** Terylene (% in.).

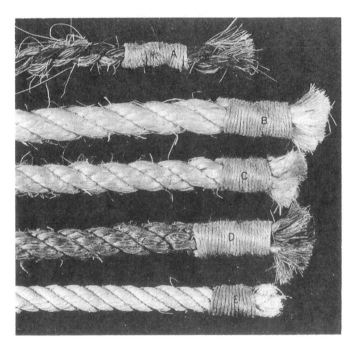

FIG. 3.2. Hard fiber ropes: **A.** Horsehair. **B.** Sisal
(7/16 in.). **C.** Manila (7/16 in.). **D.** Tarred Manila
(7/16 in.) **E.** Maguey.

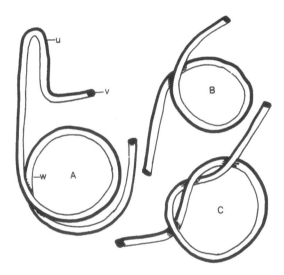

FIG. 3.4. **A.** Parts of a rope: (u) bend or bight;
(v) end or running part; (w) standing part. **B.** Loop
or half hitch. **C.** Overhand knot.

strand, in turn, is handled in this manner until all of the strands
are interlaced over and under three complete times. When one
side is completed, the string or tape is removed and the same
procedure followed on the opposite side. A completed splice
is illustrated in Figure 3.11. Remember that a splice is about
80% as strong as unspliced rope.

A long splice is begun in the same manner as a short
splice except that longer strands must be unraveled. To splice
a 1/2-in. rope, at least 1 ft (0.3 m) should be used. Place the
two ropes together, intermeshing the strands as illustrated in
Figure 3.10A. The splice is continued by unwrapping one
strand while intertwining a corresponding strand from the

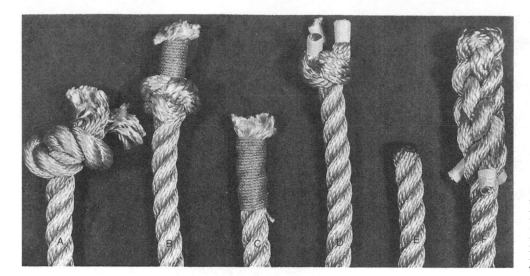

FIG. 3.5. Methods of preventing unraveling: **A.** Overhand knot. **B.** Double crown knot. **C.** Whipping. **D.** Simple crown. **E.** Burned end of nylon rope. **F.** Back splice.

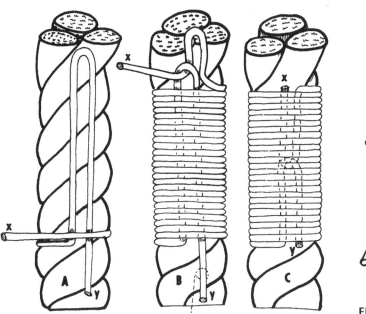

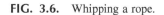

FIG. 3.6. Whipping a rope.

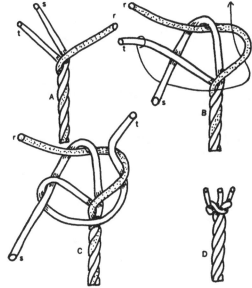

FIG. 3.7. Wall knot.

opposite rope in the place of that strand, as illustrated in Figure 3.10C. This unraveling and relaying of the strands is continued until the relaid strand is used up. Tie an overhand knot in these two strands as shown in Figure 3.10D. At the center of the splice, unravel a strand in the opposite direction, laying the opposite strand in the open track. These two strands are finished like the first two. The third set of strands, left in the center of the splice, are tied in place with an overhand

knot. Cut the ends of the strands, leaving tiny projections to prevent knots from loosening. The completed splice is illustrated in Figure 3.9B.

A back splice is used as a stopper knot and is begun by unraveling the rope and interweaving the strands as illustrated in Figure 3.8A,B. The interweavings are tightened and the basic splicing method of carrying one strand over and under adjacent strands is followed. Again, this procedure is repeated

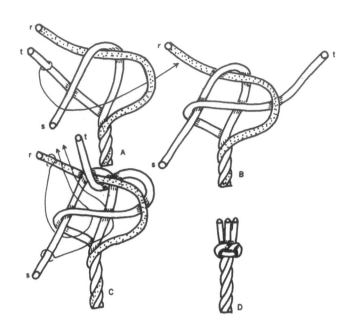

FIG. 3.8.   Matthew Walker knot.

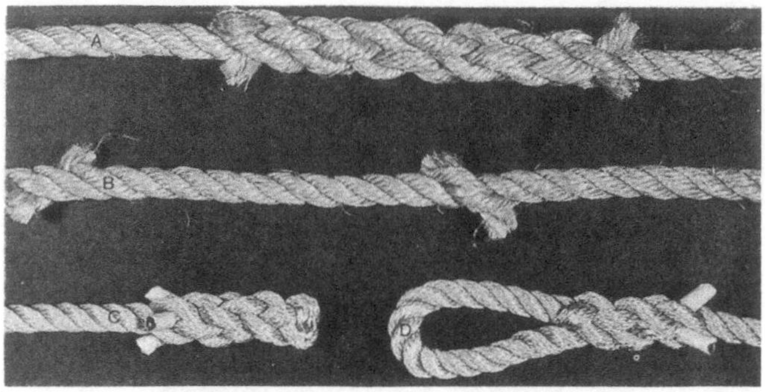

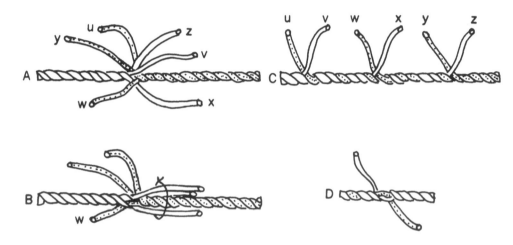

FIG. 3.9.   Splices: **A.** Short splice. **B.** Long splice.
C. Back splice. **D.** Eye splice.

FIG. 3.10.   Construction of short and long splices.

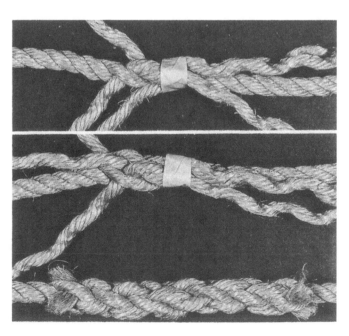

FIG. 3.11.   Making a short splice.

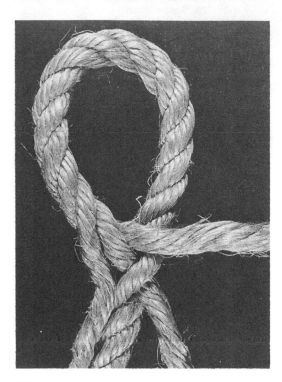

FIG. 3.12. Starting the eye splice. Continue by inserting each free strand alternately under and over subsequent strands in the standing segment.

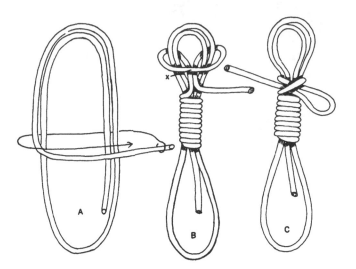

FIG. 3.13. Hanking a rope: **A.** Basic coil. **B.** Securing the end. **C.** Alternate method of securing end.

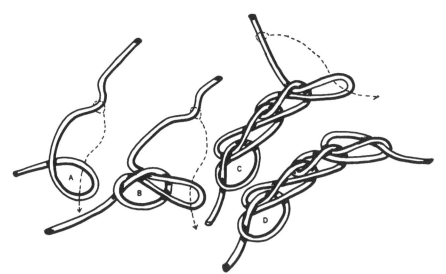

FIG. 3.14. Crocheting loop for storing large rope, block and tackle, and electrical cord.

in triplicate. The completed knot is illustrated in Figure 3.9C.

The eye splice is begun by unraveling the strands and laying the strands across the rope as illustrated in Figure 3.12. The knot is completed by inserting each strand in turn under and over the subsequent strand. When all three strands have been laced through a corresponding strand on the standing part, all strands are pulled tight. The basic splicing over-under

procedure is repeated until the splice is completed (Fig. 3.9D).

HANKING A ROPE

A rope must be kept coiled or secured in some manner to prevent tangling. One method is to hank the rope (Fig. 3.13). First coil the rope. The size of the coil depends on the length and diameter of the rope. To complete the hanking, wrap one end around the coils as shown in Figure 3.13A. Secure the ends as illustrated in Figure 3.13B or C. In B, a loop is grasped at x, put through the coils, and brought back over the top. The standing part (the end) is then pulled tight. A variation is to bring the loop beneath a previous wrap.

Long, heavy ropes, block and tackles, and electrical cord may be stored in a crocheted loop (Fig. 3.14). Lariats and other hard-twist ropes should be coiled only.

KNOTS[2,3,4]

Variations of the square knot are used in many aspects of rope work. It is the basic knot of surgery and has wide application in restraint, especially for securing crates and cages. The basic knot is tied as illustrated in Figure 3.15A–C. In the completed knot, both strands of each loop are parallel and project through the opposite loop on the same side.

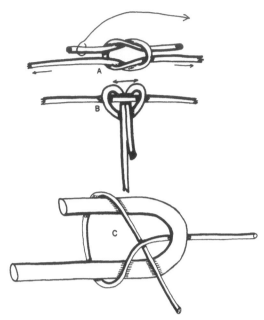

FIG. 3.16. **A, B.** Square knot converted to a slipknot by linear tension. **C.** Sheet bend.

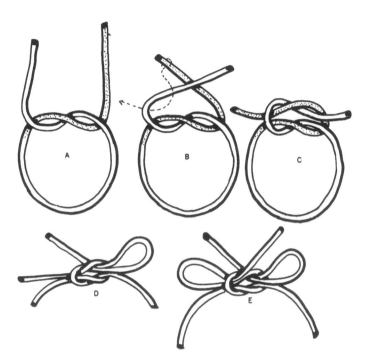

FIG. 3.15. **A, B, C.** Basic square knot. **D.** Single bowknot. **E.** Double bowknot.

A single or double bowknot (used to tie shoelaces) is a variation of the square knot. Bowknots are often used in restraint because they can be quickly untied.

The square knot must not be used where linear tension is applied to the knot. When tension is improperly applied (Fig. 3.16), it becomes a slipknot and is dangerous to use on a loop around the neck or leg of an animal. If the knot becomes a slipknot, the animal may strangle, or if on the leg, gangrene may develop.

A sheet bend is used to join two ropes of unequal size. This knot is tied by forming a bight in the end of the larger rope and interlacing the smaller rope (Fig. 3.16C). A variation of this knot is used as the tail tie. (See Figure 3.33.)

The bowline is the universal knot of animal restraint. It is the basis for many specialized knots and hitches. Temporary rope halters, casting ropes, slings, breeding hobbles, and sidelines all require the bowline. The advantage of the bowline is that it is secure, yet can be easily untied despite excessive tightening.

There are ten or more variations of the bowline, each claimed by its adherents to be easier to tie or better for a particular purpose than the basic knot. However, shortcut methods are usually not adaptable to all situations. Time and effort spent learning the shortcut would be better spent in really understanding and becoming proficient in tying the basic knot.

The knot is begun by forming a loop in the standing part of the rope, leaving an end long enough to encircle the object being secured (Fig. 3.17A). The end is then inserted through the loop (Fig. 3.17B,C). The final knot should be tightened carefully. If a mistake is made in the direction of threading the end through the loop, the knot can still be tied by encircling the other segment of the standing rope. In this instance the direction of pull will be across the knot, but this is usually of little consequence (Fig. 3.17D,E). The same configuration is basic to the tail tie and the sheet bend.

The clove hitch (Fig. 3.18) is frequently used to begin other procedures. This knot can be tied around a leg or post (Fig. 3.19). This hitch is used around the hock to form a temporary breeding hobble. Encircle the object, bringing the end above the standing part to a half hitch (Fig. 3.19A).

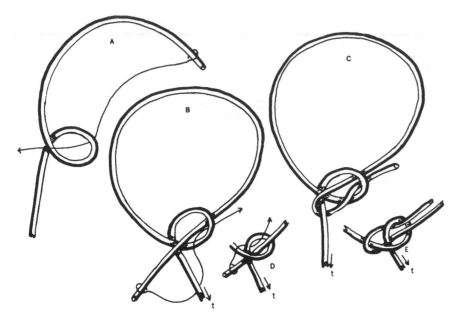

FIG. 3.17. Basic bowline.

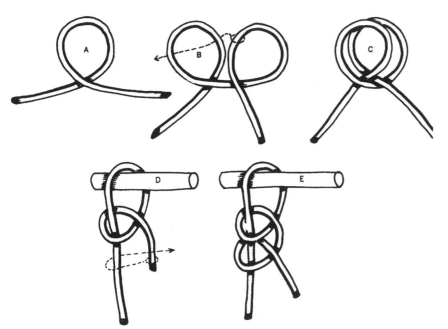

FIG. 3.18. A, B, C. Basic clove hitch.
D, E. Clove hitch around same rope, also called
a double half hitch.

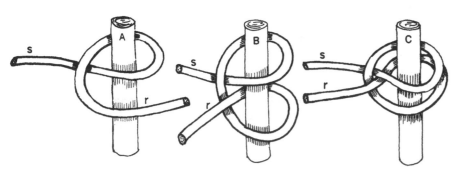

FIG. 3.19. Clove hitch tied around an
object.

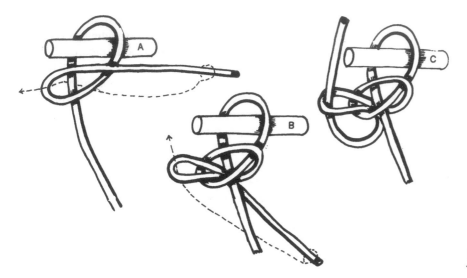

FIG. 3.20. Halter tie.

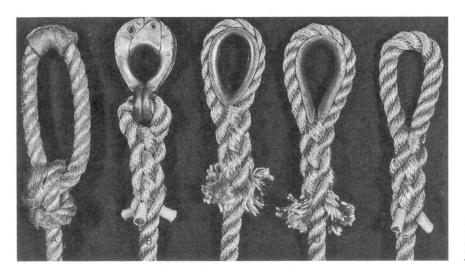

FIG. 3.21. **A.** Honda knot. **B.** Quick release honda. **C.** Brass honda in an eye splice. **D.** Galvanized metal honda. **E.** Eye splice.

Continue around the object in the same direction and thread the end above the second loop (Fig. 3.19B). The clove hitch is not a secure knot. Tension applied on the standing end of the rope, either intermittently or continuously, may slacken the loops and free the animal.

The halter tie has numerous applications in animal restraint, only one of which is to secure an animal to a post, fence, or ring. Tying this knot should become second nature to anyone wishing to become proficient in animal handling. The knot is tied by wrapping the end of the rope around a post or ring, then forming a loop, and laying it over the standing part of the rope as in Figure 3.20A. The end of the rope is then grasped and brought beneath the formed loop and the standing part of the rope, continuing through the loop (Fig. 3.20B).

This is the basic knot. Carry the standing end of the rope through the loop as illustrated in Figure 3.20C to make it less likely that accidentally pulling on the standing end of the rope will release the halter. This knot must be tied close to the object to which the animal is anchored. A major advantage of using the halter tie is that the series of loops allow easy release of the knot. Even if an animal pulls back on the rope, a quick tug on the standing part, after the end has been removed from the loop, releases the knot. This knot is used for forming breeding hobbles, casting ropes, slings, and sidelines.

A honda (Fig. 3.21) forms a small loop through which the standing part of the rope may be passed to form a larger loop for securing or catching an animal. There are many ways of fashioning a honda. To tie the honda knot, a wall or over-hand knot is tied in the end of the rope. Then an overhand knot is tied (Fig. 3.22A). The distance from x to y will be approximately two and a half times the length of the final loop. The knot is finished by gently pulling on the standing

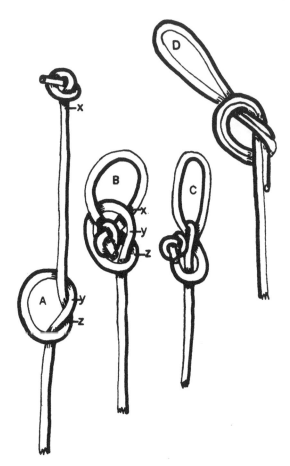

FIG. 3.22. Honda knots: **A, B, C.** Basic knot. **D.** Quick honda knot.

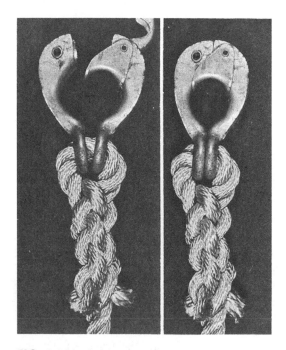

FIG. 3.23. Quick-release honda.

end of the rope until the loop is tightened and the knot is secured. If tied and secured properly, the standing part emerges from the middle of the loop, as depicted in Figure 3.22C.

A very simple honda can be fashioned by doubling the end of the rope and tying an overhand knot in the doubled rope (Fig. 3.22D). A disadvantage of this easily formed knot is that the honda comes off at approximately a 45-degree angle from the rope, producing an imbalance on the rope end.

The weight of a metal honda causes some loss of balance from the rope and is a potential hazard if the honda strikes an eye or the body of an animal. Nevertheless, a quick-release honda is valuable when working with wild animals since the honda can be released by pulling the latch (Fig. 3.23).

THROWING OR TOSSING A ROPE[1,5]

Any type of rope may be thrown at an animal, but it takes little experience to recognize that hard-twist ropes such as manila or nylon are much more efficient for throwing than softer ropes. Hard-twist ropes have better balance and the loop stays open better.

A novice may become frustrated by the amount of practice necessary to acquire proficiency in roping, but persistence yields dividends. Although it is possible to catch most domestic and wild animals without being able to toss a rope, most handlers will find that it is desirable to have mastered this art.

Roping an animal to establish a first contact is an art that was highly developed by old-time cowboys of the southwest and western United States.[1] Their feats are legendary. Roping styles varied from region to region. Vestiges of the glory of the past are now found primarily in the sport of rodeo.

Roping has its greatest application when handling cattle. Nonetheless, horses, sheep, and even swine may be caught under proper circumstances. Wild species are so much faster at dodging the loop than domestics, greater proficiency is required to capture them.

Roping is not without hazard to the animal and the operator. If the rope is used injudiciously and a tightened loop is left around the neck too long, the animal strangles. Bruises or lacerations of the skin or the cornea of the eye may occur when struck by metal hondas. Rope burns are also potential injuries. Animals frightened by roping may injure themselves by jumping against or over fences or walls.

I once roped a weanling foal in a wooded pasture. The loop had settled low on the neck, and as the slack was jerked, the head and neck were drawn to the side, pulling the foal off balance. At that moment the foal ran into a low branch of a tree and fractured its spine.

A properly coiled rope lies smooth and is flexible. As the coil is formed the rope may require twisting or untwisting to conform to the natural twist or lay of the rope. If a coil kinks and fails to lie open and smooth against other coils, it is an indication that the rope must be twisted one way or the other.

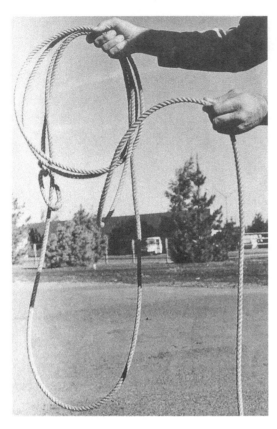

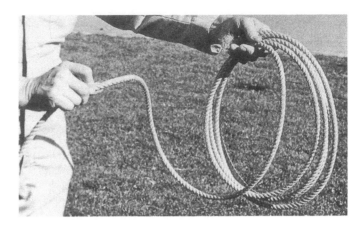

FIG. 3.25. Right-handed roper coiling a rope to his left hand.

FIG. 3.24. Right-handed roper coiling a rope to his right hand. Appropriate twist is made with left thumb and forefinger to make the coil lie properly.

A right-handed roper can coil the rope in either hand. When coiling in the right hand, first build a loop (Fig. 3.24). Then grasp the standing part of the rope with the left thumb and forefinger and form a coil of the desired diameter. As the coil is brought to the right hand, remove twists or kinks by rolling the rope one way or the other between left thumb and forefinger until the coil is smooth. Continue the same motion until the entire rope is coiled.

To coil into the left hand, grasp the end of the rope in the left hand and grasp the standing part with the right thumb and forefinger. Bring the coil over, untwisting as necessary, and place it in the left hand (Fig. 3.25). Notice the direction of the coiling. This is important. Continue coiling until the honda is reached.

As the rope is coiled, a specific twist is built into each coil. If one simply grasps the honda and pulls out a loop without untwisting the rope, kinks will form in the loop that cannot be shaken out (Fig. 3.26). The loop may be untwisted after forming or the kink may be prevented by feeding the honda backward around each coil until the loop is the desired size. Because of the built-in twist, a left-handed roper cannot use a rope coiled by a right-handed roper, or vice versa.

Two methods of throwing a rope are pertinent to animal restraint: the drag toss and the swing toss. The drag toss is

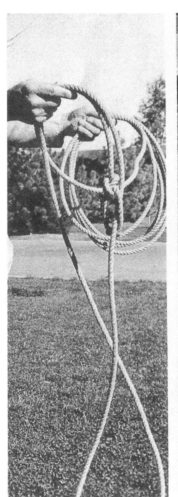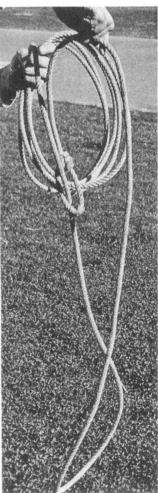

FIG. 3.26. Twisted loop. Twist cannot be shaken out. Remove twist by rotating the honda end in the appropriate direction.

less likely to frighten the animal than the swing, but less speed is generated for the throw and the animal may more easily dodge the loop. The techniques described and illustrated are for a right-handed roper. The loop is grasped so that the honda hangs approximately halfway down the loop (Fig. 3.27) and is carried behind the body at the side (Fig. 3.28). The coil is held loosely in the opposite hand with the end of the rope held firmly between thumb and forefinger. At the appropriate moment, the loop is brought forward as the arm is thrown toward the head of the animal. The loop is opened by a quick forward thrust of the wrist (Fig. 3.29). As it settles around the animal the loop is tightened by drawing the unused coils back sharply. This is called "jerking the slack."

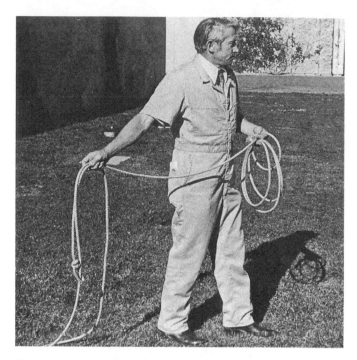

FIG. 3.28.   Initial position for drag-toss method of roping. Wrist is bent back and to the right.

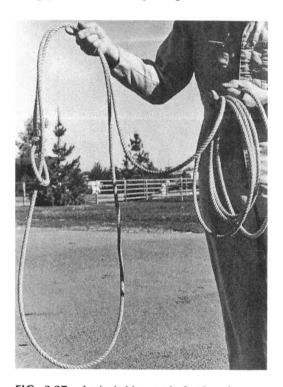

FIG. 3.27.   Lariat held properly for throwing.

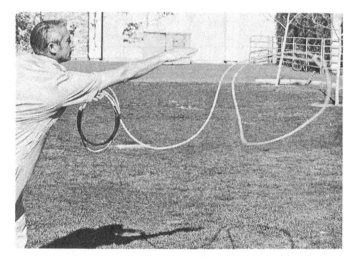

FIG. 3.29.   Drag-toss throw. Arm is brought forward and directed at the object to be roped. Hand is brought forward and to the left to flip the loop open.

The swing toss is used when the rope must be thrown a greater distance or a fast-moving animal must be caught. Hold the rope as for the drag toss. The loop is kept open by twisting with the proper wrist action. The hand must rotate in a circle at the wrist. To practice opening a loop, hold your arm in front of your body. Keep the arm steady and rotate your hand. For the right-handed person, this is performed by bending the hand to the right as the wrist is flexed back. Then the hand is bent toward the left while a quick snap of the wrist upward completes the rotation. Practice this motion with a small loop held waist high. Keep the arm stationary. You should learn to swing an open loop indefinitely, using wrist action only. The quick snap of the wrist upward is the key to maintaining an open loop. When the wrist action is mastered, arm movement can be added to develop more momentum. The wider the arc the more momentum acquired. The rapidity of the swing also affects momentum.

Timing of the throw and release is critical. Practice throwing at a stationary object. Swing the rope over the head (Fig. 3.30). As the loop is rotated forward, direct the arm toward the object. When the arm is at maximum stretch, open the hand and let the loop fly (Fig. 3.31). Throwing a rope is much like throwing a baseball. The rope will go in the direction the arm is pointed. Follow-through with the arm is of prime importance.

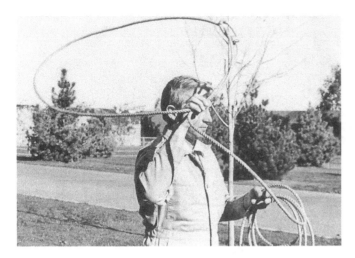

FIG. 3.30. Initial position of swing-throw method of roping.

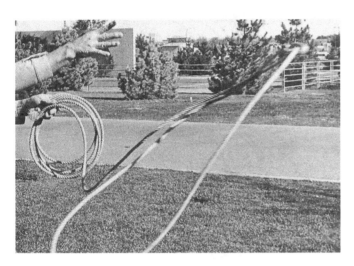

FIG. 3.31. Swing-throw release. Right hand follows through to the object being roped. Coils play off the fingers of the left hand.

The coils in the opposite hand are allowed to play out freely from a partially opened hand. As the loop drops over the object, the slack is jerked. This should be done each time the rope is thrown, to establish a habit. Key factors for the swing and toss follow:

1. No twists in the loop
2. Wrist action to keep the loop open
3. Directing the arm at the target
4. Follow through
5. Jerking the slack immediately

A third method of roping used by professional animal capturers is by means of a loop hung from the end of a long bamboo pole. The loop is attached to the pole by a light string

that will break easily. The animal is usually pursued in a vehicle. The roper stands in the back. When the vehicle comes alongside the animal, the roper places the loop over the head, the pole breaks away, and the vehicle slows down to stop the animal.

Catching the animal is only half the problem. The animal must be stopped and subdued before it strangles itself or injures the roper. Obviously this should be planned for before roping begins.

A large animal must be dallied to a post or ring. The rope must be long enough to reach the anchor. To stop a smaller animal, the roper presses the rope across the body or legs while standing in a braced position (Fig. 3.32). Be prepared to be jerked off balance. A light pair of gloves will protect against rope burns.

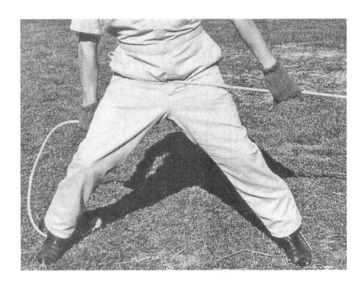

FIG. 3.32. Bracing for stopping a roped animal.

Domestic animals are easily subdued from this position since they habitually pull back and stand until grabbed. Wild animals are unpredictable. They are as likely to jump forward or to the side as to pull back. If a dally can be taken and the animal snubbed up before contact is made, injuries are likely to be fewer.

If two ropers of sufficient skill are available, the animal can be stretched by simultaneously roping the neck and the hind legs and pulling in opposite directions. This method may be the only way to subdue larger bovids in order to trim feet or collect laboratory samples.

The tail tie is frequently used to prevent the tail from swishing and striking the operator, but it may also be used in certain instances to restrain an animal or to lift it. When the tail tie is used to lift an animal, be sure the particular species can be lifted by the tail. In equine species the tail can be used to support the hindquarters. In bovine species the tail will break.

The knot is tied by bending the switch of the tail back on itself, forming a bight. The rope used to complete the knot

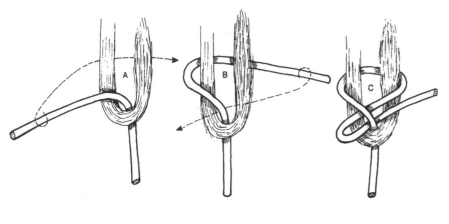

FIG. 3.33. Tail tie.

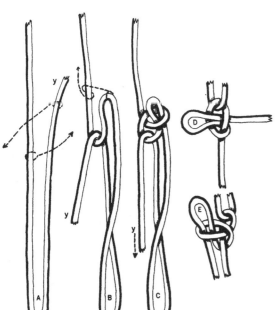

FIG. 3.34. Trucker's hitch.

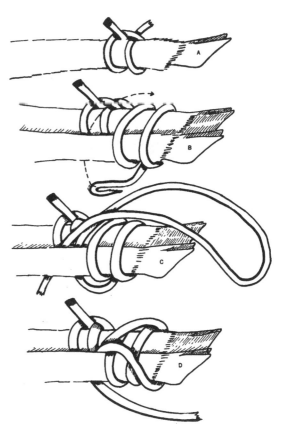

FIG. 3.35. Foot hitch: Start with clove hitch around one leg. **A.** Wrap both legs two times. **B.** Form loop in the standing part and anchor as in **C.** and **D.**

is brought through the bight, circled behind both segments and brought forward across the bight, and looped underneath the previously placed strand (Fig. 3.33). The basic configuration of this knot is similar to that of the bowline. Thus the knot is secure and is also easily untied, no matter what degree of tension is placed on it. Its disadvantage is that if tension is not constantly maintained, the knot may loosen and fall off. The bight or bend in the tail can only be made when there is sufficient hair to form the loop. Do not bend and tie the coccygeal vertebra.

A trucker's hitch can be tied either at the end of a rope or at any point along a rope to remove slack. It can also be used to stretch the legs of a cast animal. Since the end is never threaded through a loop, this hitch is easily untied, and tension on the hitch is adjustable. If the animal moves, slack can be taken up or released. Tension must be constantly applied to the hitch to keep it tied. This hitch is tied by passing the rope around a post or hook and bending the rope back on itself.

Form another bend in the standing segment and loop the running end over it (Fig. 3.34A, B). Form a half hitch in the standing segment and place it over the bend. If there is to be excessive tension over a prolonged period, a double half hitch may be used. Pulling on the free end places tension on the whole hitch (Fig. 3.34C).

When an animal must be stretched, a foot hitch is desired that will sufficiently secure the feet, yet be easily untied (Fig. 3.35). First a clove hitch or a honda knot is placed on one of

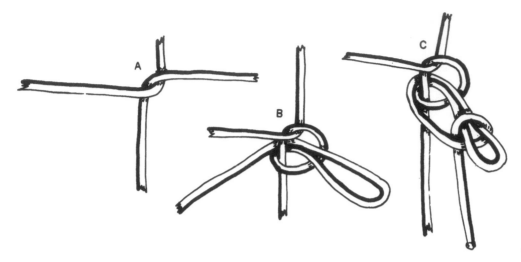

FIG. 3.36. Anchor hitch.

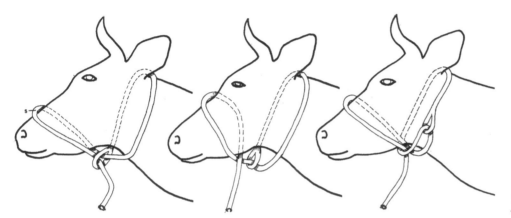

FIG. 3.37. Temporary rope halters.

the legs. Next both legs are encircled with the rope. Then a loop of the standing part of the rope is brought between the legs and placed over both feet. The standing part is then anchored to a post or ring. A trucker's hitch can be used to hold the tension satisfactorily. As the animal struggles, the knot is tightened, but when the animal relaxes, the knot will loosen. The release of the knot is accomplished by simply taking the loop back over the feet, pulling on the loop, and unwrapping. No secure knot is used in this procedure.

The anchor hitch is used to secure a part of a complex roping procedure, allowing the standing part to continue on or change direction. Suppose a rope is used to lash an animal to a board or table. If you wish to anchor the rope to take up slack or change direction, apply the anchor hitch (Fig. 3.36). To tie an anchor hitch, bring the standing part of the rope around either another segment of rope or around any handy object such as a post. The slack is taken up and an overhand knot tied, using a loop instead of the end of the rope (Fig. 3.36B). In order to continue using the standing part of the rope, a half hitch must be placed over the loop. Then the standing part can proceed in any direction and produce tension

in a different manner. The loop can also be used as a pulley or a fulcrum on which to tie other knots. This knot is easily undone by releasing the half hitch and pulling on the standing part of the rope.

ROPE HALTER

Rope halters are used to lead animals, tie them up, secure the head to operating tables during surgery, or steady the head when manipulating under chemical restraint. Excellent rope halters are available commercially for most domestic animals. Temporary rope halters (Fig. 3.37) can be adapted to any species. The size of the rope should be varied to suit the strength of the animal.

No animal should be left tied with any of these halters without supervision, as the nose loop may slacken and fall from the nose, freeing the animal or, worse, strangling it.

A more permanent rope halter is easily constructed (Figs. 3.38, 3.39). The rope size and length of the nose piece can be varied to make a halter suitable for either a small domestic calf or a bull elk.

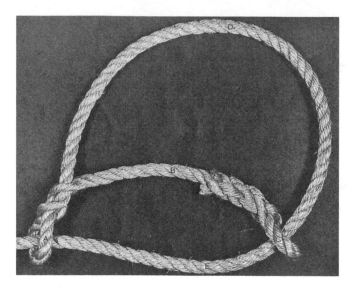

FIG. 3.38.   Rope halter: **B** goes over the nose, **D** behind the ears, **E** under the chin. Distance **A-B-C** must vary with the size of the animal. Loop at **A** is formed first, then an eye splice is made at **C.**

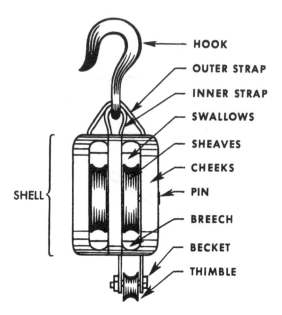

FIG. 3.40.   Terminology used for a block. (Courtesy, Tubbs Cordage Company.)

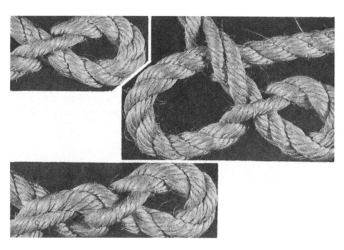

FIG. 3.39.   Rope halter cheek loop: First establish location of this loop on the rope. Allow enough distance to construct the eye splice. Form the loop by running long segment of the rope under one strand of the short segment (**A**). Complete the loop by inserting short segment through long segment and pulling it tight (**B,C**).

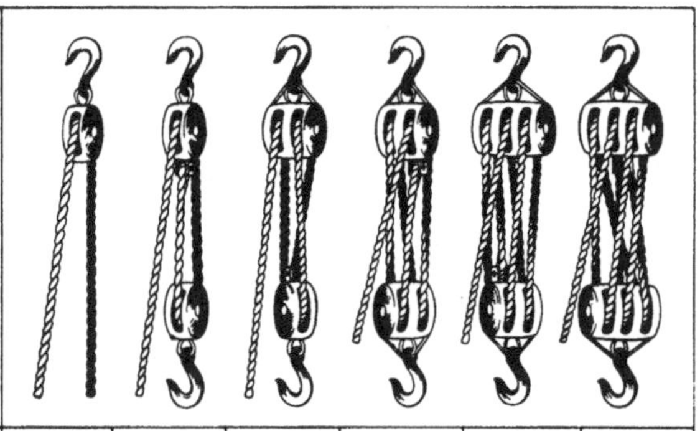

BLOCK AND TACKLE USAGE

A block and tackle (Fig. 3.40) provides a mechanical advantage for slinging animals, lifting crates, or casting an animal such as an elephant. Various types of block and tackle are represented in Figures 3.41 and 3.42. One sheave does not provide any mechanical advantage but changes the direction of the pull. Multiple sheaves provide a significant mechanical advantage. Multiple-sheaved blocks may easily become tangled if not stored properly. The crocheting loop illustrated

ROPE SIZE (DIAMETER)	ONE SHEAVE one single block	TWO SHEAVES two single blocks	THREE SHEAVES double and single or two and one	FOUR SHEAVES double and double or two and two	FIVE SHEAVES triple and double or three and two	SIX SHEAVES triple and triple or three and three
½″	475	850	1,200	1,400	DO NOT USE ½″	
¾″	970	1,800	2,400	3,000	3,500	
1″	1,620	3,000	4,050	5,000	6,000	6,700
1¼″	2,430	4,500	6,075	7,500	9,000	10,000
1½″	3,330	6,100	8,500	10,500	12,000	13,500

FIG. 3.41.   Safe loads when used with a given rope size and type of block and tackle. (Courtesy, Tubbs Cordage Company.)

in Figures 3.14, 3.43, and 3.44 is excellent for this purpose. Extend the block and tackle to the maximum and proceed as illustrated.

Crates are usually moved manually or with a forklift. Large crates for rhinoceroses or hippopotamuses must be

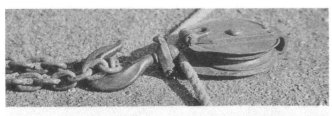
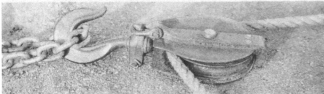

FIG. 3.42. Snatch block. Used to change direction of pull in a rope without threading rope through the block.

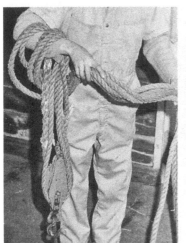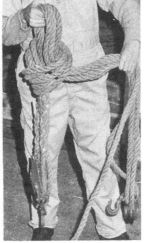

FIG. 3.43. Storage of block and tackle: Beginning of crocheting loop, left. Continuation of crocheting loop, right.

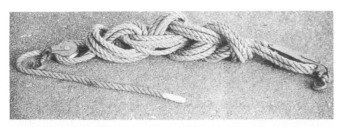

FIG. 3.44. Block and tackle ready for storage.

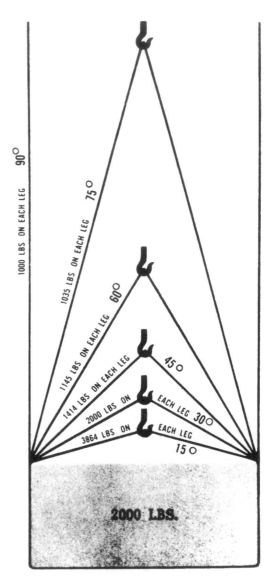

FIG. 3.45. Weights borne by supporting ropes when lifting crates. All weights indicate the load borne by each leg of sling at the various angles of lift. (Courtesy, Tubbs Cordage Company.)

moved with a crane. Be certain the cables used are of sufficient size to accommodate the load. The angle of attachment of the guy wire to the load is important in distributing the load (Fig. 3.45). Work with a large safety margin.

An excellent sling can be built with rope. The diameter and length of the rope used are dependent on the size of the animal. A 50-ft, 1/22-in. nylon rope is suitable to lift a 100-lb horse. The sling is illustrated as applied to a standing horse. In practice it can be put on a recumbent animal as well.

First form a neck loop in the doubled rope and a bowline at the base of the chest. Bring the running segment between the front legs and back through the corresponding side of the neck loop (Fig. 3.46). Cross the ropes over the back, then bring the ropes between the hind legs. Be certain not to cross ropes underneath the animal. The ropes should pass on either

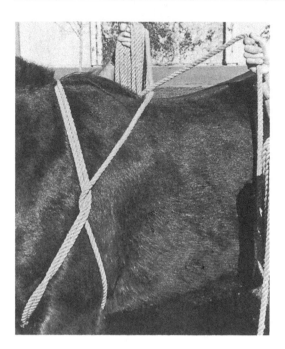

FIG. 3.46. Beginning a rope sling.

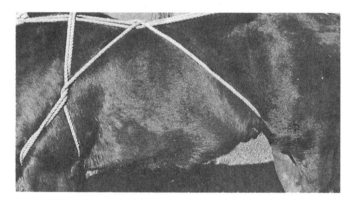

FIG. 3.47. Continuation of rope sling.

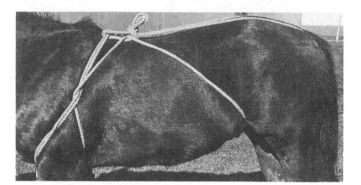

FIG. 3.48. Completed rope sling.

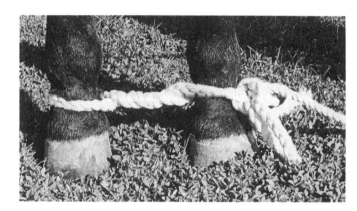

FIG. 3.49. Temporary rope hobble constructed of braided cotton rope.

side of the tail and underneath all the ropes on the back (Fig. 3.47). Take all slack out of the ropes and complete the sling by doubling the running ends back and tying with a halter tie (Fig. 3.48). An attempt should be made to place the lifting site over the approximate center of gravity of the animal. Even if this is not done the animal can still be lifted, since each leg is in its own sling loop. The animal cannot slip out of the sling.

Rope may be used to hobble an animal to prevent it from kicking, striking, or wandering away (Fig. 3.49). I have seen this technique used to prevent a camel cow from kicking at a newborn calf. Soft cotton rope is the most suitable for hobbles, but other fibers may be used.

A trained animal may be hobbled with a short rope. A longer rope is necessary with dangerous species. Make the tie

with a bow knot so it can be released quickly if the animal fights too hard or falls down. Do not leave the ends long enough to step on lest the knot be released.

ROPE AND CORDAGE TERMS

Bight: The part of a rope that is curved, looped, or bent—the working part of the line.

Binder twine: Single oiled or treated yarn, usually sisal, used for binding sheaves in harvesting; generally in 5- or 8-lb balls.

Block: The framework into which sheaves or pulleys are fitted, over which rope may be led to reduce power necessary for lifting. Blocks are designated as single, double, etc.

Cord: Two or more yarns twisted together much the same as a strand, used to tie bundles and whip ropes.

Dally: Placing tension on a rope by wrapping it around an object without securing the rope. The friction produced provides the anchoring necessary but also allows for some slackening if the tension is likely to be greater than the strength of the rope.

Heaving line: A small rope weighted at one end that is thrown across the water to assist in moving a larger rope.

Hitch: Type of knot used for making a rope fast to an object, usually for a temporary purpose.

Lariat: In general usage, this is any rope used to form a loop and throw at an animal to catch it. Specifically, it is a rope constructed with an extremely tight or hard twist. The fiber is either manila or nylon. The hard twist provides more "body" to the rope and helps keep the loop open. The lariat is used only for catching and holding an animal. Knots are difficult to tie in a lariat because of the stiffness of the rope. In fact, tying knots in such a rope will put kinks in it and minimize its usefulness as a lariat.

Lay: A term used to designate the amount of turn or twist put in a rope, such as soft, medium, or hard lay.

Laying rope: The operation of twisting together three or more strands into rope.

Line: The term used by sailors for rope.

Sheet bend: A form of knot to fasten two ropes together.

Snatch block: A special block with one side of the shell capable of being opened to allow a cable or rope to be placed in the block without having to thread it. Useful in restraint to change the direction of pull in inconvenient situations (Fig. 3.42).

Splicing: To unite ends of ropes by interweaving the strands.

Standing part: The principal part of the rope as compared with the working part.

Tackle: A combination of rope and blocks for the purpose of decreasing the power necessary in lifting or moving loads.

Whipping: Binding the strands at the ends of the rope to prevent unraveling.

Twine: A simple yarn, usually made from sisal and not tightly twisted.

REFERENCES

1. French, W.M. 1940. Ropes and roping. Cattleman 26(May): 17–30. (excellent presentation of techniques of roping animals).
2. Gibson, C.E. 1953. Handbook of Knots and Splices. New York: Emerson Books.
3. Graumont, R., and Hensel, J. 1952. Encyclopedia of Knots and Fancy Rope Work, 4th ed. Cambridge, MD: Cornell Maritime Press.
4. Leahy, J.R., and Barrow, P. 1953. Restraint of Animals, 2nd ed., pp. 6–37. Ithaca, NY: Cornell Campus Store.
5. Mason, B.S. 1940. Roping. New York: A.S. Barnes. (trick and fancy).
6. McCalmont, J.R. 1943. Care and use of rope on the farm. USDA, Farmer's Bull. 1931.
7. Some Brief Facts of Life about Rope. Its Origins, Development, Uses and Characteristics. (ND.) Auburn, NY: Columbian Rope.
8. Tubbs Technical Reference on Rope. (ND.) San Francisco: Tubbs Cordage.

CHAPTER 4
Thermoregulation

Life is dependent on energy. Animals obtain energy through the chemical action of ingested nutrients plus radiant energy from the sun. Products of energy use within the body are further chemical action, heat, and work. The animal body is an energy transformer, utilizing energy to produce work, locomotion, growth, maintenance, reproduction, and useful products such as wool and milk. Excess heat must be dissipated from the body by radiation, conduction, convection, or evaporation.[6]

For practical purposes, the body temperature of a given animal is understood to be the temperature recorded on a thermometer inserted into the rectum deeply enough to reflect the core or deep temperature of the animal. Other temperatures may be of concern to the animal restrainer (Fig. 4.1). The temperature at the skin surface may be either higher or lower than core temperature. Heat may be lost or gained, depending on the temperatures of the skin and the surface upon which the animal is placed. The coat temperature of well-insulated species will likely be close to ambient air temperature. The effect of insulating layers, both external and internal, on body temperatures is of critical importance during restraint.

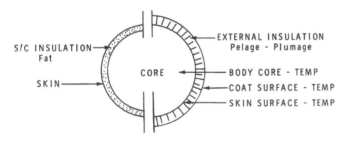

FIG. 4.1. Schematic of insulation methods and their relationship to temperatures.

Homeotherms (endotherms), including most birds and mammals, are capable of physiological responses that initiate heat production or conservation.[5,8,10,12,15,17,19] Body temperatures usually remain within narrow limits. The body temperatures of poikilotherms such as reptiles, amphibians, fishes, and invertebrates fluctuate with the ambient temperature. The primary source of heat for these animals must be external. The primary method available to poikilotherms for cooling, if the ambient temperature rises to a point incompatible with life, is to move into a cooler environment. Thus heat regulation in this class of animals is behavioral.

During restraint, thermoregulatory problems of wild animals are likely to be more difficult to prevent than those of domestic species. Domestic animals, bred for docility and accustomed to people, usually accept restraint practices. Wild animals, on the other hand, usually struggle against restraint until completely exhausted. Violent muscular activity generates significant quantities of heat. Unless the animal is physiologically and physically in a position permitting heat dissipation, hyperthermia will result. Unalleviated hyperthermia can cause death in a matter of minutes.

The degree of temperature elevation is directly related to the duration and intensity of muscular activity modulated by inherent heat regulatory mechanisms. Small species overheat more quickly than large species, as a result of a higher metabolic rate.

Restraint of animals during periods of high ambient air temperatures and/or high relative humidity is fraught with danger. Under such conditions muscular activity will generate heat more rapidly than it can be dissipated.

PHYSIOLOGY

Many physiological and behavioral mechanisms are involved with heat regulation in animals (Fig. 4.2). Details can be obtained from the references.

Hot and cold receptors in the skin act as detectors, alerting the body to environmental conditions that may be destructive. When the appropriate receptor is stimulated, the impulse is relayed to special cells in both the anterior and posterior hypothalamus. The temperature of blood flowing through the hypothalamus may directly affect thermosensitive cells.

Information is integrated with specific motor responses to either increase heat production and/or conserve heat, or increase heat loss (Fig. 4.2). The whole system functions as a thermostat.

Heat Production

Heat is gained by increased production or by absorption from the environment. The body produces heat through basal metabolic activities, muscle tone, shivering, exercise, fever (disease), and by utilization of special energy stores such as brown fat. Heat from the environment is absorbed by radiation, conduction, and convection (Figs. 4.3, 4.4).

Heat and Moisture Conservation

Heat conservation mechanisms are not as important to the animal restrainer as are mechanisms of heat production,

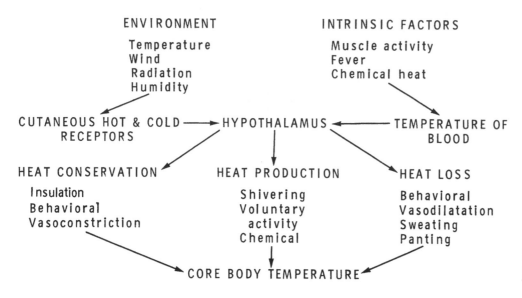

ENVIRONMENT

Temperature
Wind
Radiation
Humidity

INTRINSIC FACTORS

Muscle activity
Fever
Chemical heat

CUTANEOUS HOT & COLD → HYPOTHALAMUS ← TEMPERATURE OF
RECEPTORS   BLOOD

HEAT CONSERVATION   HEAT PRODUCTION   HEAT LOSS

Insulation   Shivering   Behavioral
Behavioral   Voluntary   Vasodilatation
Vasoconstriction   activity   Sweating
                                    Chemical   Panting

CORE BODY TEMPERATURE

FIG. 4.2. Thermoregulatory physiologic mechanisms.

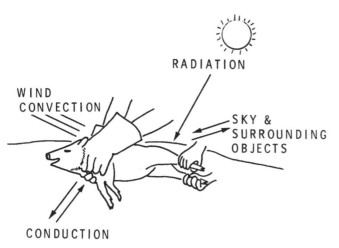

RADIATION

WIND
CONVECTION

SKY &
SURROUNDING
OBJECTS

CONDUCTION

FIG. 4.3. Thermal influences on a restrained animal.

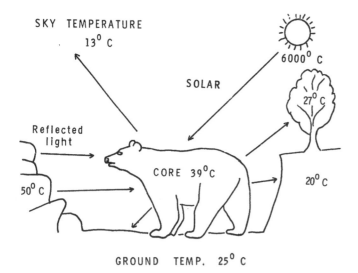

SKY TEMPERATURE
13° C

SOLAR

6000° C

27° C

Reflected
light

50° C

CORE 39°C

20° C

GROUND TEMP. 25° C

FIG. 4.4. Radiant heat flow to and from an animal.

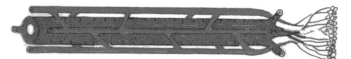

FIG. 4.5. Diagram of countercurrent heat exchange system. Peripheral arteries and veins are adjacent to one another. Warm arterial blood coming from the core gives up heat to cooler venous blood coming from the capillary bed. Central body temperature is not jeopardized.

except in a negative way. An animal that is an efficient heat conserver may require special attention to provide cooling if it overheats during restraint. Heat is conserved through vascular responses such as peripheral vasoconstriction and by countercurrent heat exchange systems (Fig. 4.5).

Peripheral vasoconstriction is important for heat conservation; it allows the skin temperature to drop without jeopardizing the core temperatures. Arteriolar constriction decreases blood flow to the skin. Venous constriction increases the velocity of blood flow, which decreases the exposure time of the blood to cold. All species are capable of peripheral vasoconstriction to some degree, but arctic species, highly adapted to cold, exhibit a marked ability to respond in this manner.

Countercurrent heat exchange systems are also highly developed in animals living in extremely cold environments.[6] The animal restrainer must not interfere with these systems but should take advantage of them when handling such species. Captivity in unnatural habitats may adversely alter an animal's ability to acclimate to extremely cold situations. For instance, in winter, gulls can walk on ice at −30°C (−22°F) without harm. If gulls are acclimated to warm laboratory conditions and then allowed to walk on ice, their feet freeze.[6] Animals in zoos often live in unnatural environments. Such animals should not be expected to respond in the same manner as free-ranging wild animals.

Piloerection is also a mechanism that conserves heat by increasing the thickness of the pelage or plumage insulation layer.

Desert species use one or more of the following mechanisms to conserve moisture: voiding of highly concentrated urine, production of dry feces, allowing body temperature to elevate during the heat of the day (heat storage), peripheral vasoconstriction, and insulation or piloerection to prevent evaporation.

Mechanisms for Cooling

Heat is dissipated through conduction, convection, radiation, evaporation, and excretions such as urine and feces. The conversion of moisture to water vapor (evaporation) requires 0.58 kcal of heat for each gram of water converted.[14] Evaporation takes place from the skin surfaces of all species to a limited degree (insensible heat loss), as long as the relative humidity is not so high that the air is already saturated with moisture.[13]

Species with numerous cutaneous sweat glands, such as the horse and humans, maintain effective cooling mechanisms as long as the volume of water intake is sufficient. Surface evaporation can be augmented by smearing the skin with saliva (marsupials) or sponging it with water (elephants).

Evaporation also takes place from the lungs of all breathing animals. Some species such as the dog pant, increasing evaporative cooling from the respiratory tract. Panting is more than rapid breathing. Otherwise the dog would hyperventilate and become alkalotic. The open-mouth breathing of an ungulate may assist in dissipating heat, but other metabolic changes harmful to the animal may also take place.

Morphological Adaptations for Cooling

The large ears of the African elephant increase the surface area for cooling by evaporation, simple conduction, convection, and radiation. The ears are kept moving to assist in heat dissipation. Desert species such as the fennec or bat-eared fox also have large ears to aid in thermoregulation.

It has been demonstrated that the horns of bovid species function in thermoregulation.[18] Do not cover horns for prolonged periods during restraint procedures, since this may inhibit cooling and cause the brain temperature to rise to a dangerous level.

Behavioral changes often allow animals to exist in microclimates within an environment that is generally assumed to be incompatible with the animal's ability to control body temperature. Nocturnal species are active when it is cool. Rodents burrow during the day when the above-ground ambient temperature is too high for comfort. The hippopotamus forages at night when it is cool and submerges in water during the hotter part of the day. Desert bovines seek any available shade during the heat of the day to lessen heat gain from the hot desert environment.[15] Many other species rest quietly during the hotter part of the day and forage or move about in the cooler morning and evening.

The crocodile reverses the process. During daylight hours the crocodile basks on the shore, absorbing heat to maintain body temperature during the night when it feeds in the water.

THERMOREGULATORY MEDICAL PROBLEMS

Hyperthermia (heat exhaustion, heat cramps, sunstroke, overheating)

DEFINITION.   Hyperthermia is excessive elevation of the body temperature.

ETIOLOGY.   Predisposing factors to the development of hyperthermia include prolonged high ambient temperatures, high humidity, dehydration, mycotoxins and drugs that inhibit thermoregulation, and excessive muscular exertion or metabolic activity. Muscular exertion is a particularly important source of heat production during restraint and is more dangerous in fat or heavily insulated animals.

Placing animals in poorly ventilated shipping crates exposed to high ambient temperatures is sure to cause hyperthermia. A brachycephalic dog is less able to cool by panting because it cannot move sufficient air through its narrowed upper airway. Temperatures in enclosed automobiles parked in the sun quickly reach 49–54°C (120–154°F). Pets left in cars may die from hyperthermia.

Dehydration, lack of salt, adrenal insufficiency, and the use of vasodilatory drugs (such as alcohol) contribute to overheating. Additional contributing factors include reduced cardiac efficiency or cardiac failure. Reduced cardiac efficiency may be the result of malnutrition, lack of exercise, infection, or intoxication.

Trauma (extensive contusions, fractures, or lacerations) causes the release of pyrogens as products of tissue destruction. This reaction also takes place following surgery, so a slight elevation in body temperature may be expected. Although usually not dangerous, this slight elevation may tip the balance if body temperature is already at a precariously high level because of heat produced during restraint for the surgery.

The temperature elevation seen in animals suffering from infectious diseases results from increased metabolic activity and enhances phagocytosis and immune body production; it also decreases the viability of disease organisms. Prolonged elevation of temperature for days causes the development of certain physiological conditions that affect restraint practices. Stores of liver glycogen are depleted, with resultant decreased energy stores and potential hypoglycemia. The animal may be forced to call upon body protein for energy, resulting in weight loss, weakness, and increased nonprotein nitrogen in the blood. Elevated body temperature increases the need for fluid intake. If the need is not met, the animal dehydrates.

Restraint techniques may inhibit heat-dissipating mechanisms. Canids use panting for evaporative cooling. As the body temperature elevates, the normal resting respiratory rate of approximately 30 changes to 300–400, increasing the rate of evaporative cooling from the respiratory mucous membranes. It is a common practice to muzzle dogs and other canids to prevent biting. With the muzzle in place, the animal cannot pant. With high ambient temperatures and a struggling animal, hyperthermia is inevitable.

Another example is the use of stockinettes to restrain the wings of hawks. Hawks dissipate heat by extending their wings, exposing lightly feathered areas beneath the wings to the air for convection cooling. By clasping the wings close to the body and adding a layer of insulation in the form of the stockinette or nylon hose, heat dissipation is effectively prevented.

Pathophysiology of Hyperthermia[4,9,11,20,22]

Hyperthermia increases metabolic activity and cellular oxygen consumption (10% for each degree C rise in humans).[8] In mammals at body temperatures above 41°C (105.8°F), oxygen utilization exceeds the oxygen supplied by normal respiration, initiating hypoxic cellular damage. The brain, liver, and kidneys are most likely to manifest such damage. Protein begins denaturing at approximately 45–47°C (113–116.8°F) in all species.[7,14] Normal body temperatures of birds are 40–42°C (104°–107.6°F); thus a struggling bird has a narrow temperature safety margin.

The effects of hyperthermia on organ systems may be profound, and if heat stress has been severe or prolonged, residual effects may alter organ function and even kill the animal long after the core body temperature has returned to normal. The central nervous system (CNS) is the most sensitive to hyperthermia. Effects on the CNS may be initiated by direct heat, causing necrosis of neurons, or by secondary factors, such as hypotension, causing cerebral hypoxia or effects on the cardiovascular and hemic systems (hemorrhage, disseminated intravascular clotting [DIC]), causing lesions within the CNS.

Hyperthermia in the pregnant female may cause fetal CNS damage, resulting in various congenital anomalies or even death of the fetus.[11] These anomalies are the result of excessive heat acting on the embryonic cells of the CNS at a crucial time, early in gestation. In humans the critical period is between 40 and 44 days following fertilization. The crucial period in other species is unknown, but it is likely to be comparative.

Other effects on the female include diminished intensity of receptivity and anestrus. During pregnancy, the more profound effects are seen as fetal damage, including inhibition of embryonic cleavage and implantation, initiation of teratogenesis, and abortion.[11] Fetal effects have been noted in animals when the core body temperature of the dam rises above 40.1°C (104.2°F) for prolonged periods.

Excessive heat is spermicidal, at the primary spermatocyte stage. Although not yet studied in most species, at least 35 days and up to 60 days are required for spermatogenesis to produce mature viable sperm once the heat stress is decreased.

Elevation of the core body temperature initiates a shift in the blood supply from the viscera to the skin. Decreased blood flow to the stomach and intestine results in diminished digestive function. Gastrointestinal motility is decreased, as is rumination. In addition to the shift of blood from the viscera, heart rate is increased and central venous pressure is decreased, along with a relative decrease in blood volume (potential for hypotension and hypovolemic shock). Hypovolemia may result in decreased glomerular filtration and loss of kidney function (prerenal uremia), followed eventually by renal shutdown, which may be complicated by DIC. Generalized hemolysis overloads the kidney with hemoglobin, which exacerbates any kidney malfunction or may directly cause kidney malfunction.

Hyperthermia results in hemoconcentration, electrolyte imbalances, increased fragility of erythrocytes, leukocytosis, and metabolic acidosis. Platelet counts are decreased. Effects on the coagulation cascade may be profound and lethal. Prothrombin time is increased, and there is an increased consumption of coagulation factors and fibrin split factors, resulting in hemorrhage and, potentially, DIC.

Sequence of Events during Hyperthermia

Following is the probable sequence of events during a severe hyperthermic episode in an animal.

1. Elevation of the core body temperature.
2. Accelerated heart rate.
3. Increased respiratory rate.
4. Redness of skin surface.
5. Sweating.
6. Hemoconcentration.
7. Body fluid shift from viscera and muscle to skin.
8. Decreased glomerular filtration.
9. Dehydration.
10. Decreased central venous pressure.
11. Effects on the CNS, including cerebral hypoxia and coagulative necrosis.
12. Effects on the embryo and fetus.
13. Coagulation defects (DIC).
14. Other organ system damage.

CLINICAL SIGNS. Clinical signs of hyperthermia include increased heart and respiratory rates, accompanied by open-mouth breathing (Fig. 4.6). Species capable of sweating, sweat and salivate profusely in the early stages. Llama and alpaca males with hyperthermia may have a pronounced scrotal edema (Fig. 4.7). As the temperature continues to elevate, the animal dehydrates, and both sweating and salivation decline and may cease. As hyperthermia accelerates, the pulse becomes weak and the animal shows signs of restlessness, dullness, and incoordination. Convulsions (cerebral anoxia) and collapse, rapidly followed by death, result if temperatures rise and remain for long above 42–43°C (107.6–109.4–F).

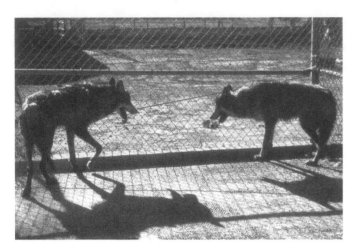

FIG. 4.6. Wolves showing open-mouth breathing associated with hyperthermia.

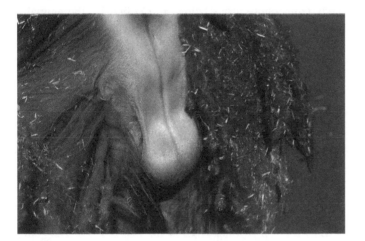

FIG. 4.7. Scrotal edema in a hyperthermic llama.

Other metabolic and pathological changes associated with hyperthermia include hypoxemia, metabolic acidosis, hypercalcemia, myoglobinuria, hemoglobinuria, disseminated intravascular coagulation, hemolytic anemia, and renal shutdown.

Hyperthermia produces signs similar to those of septicemia, high fevers, and other convulsive syndromes. These should be considered in differential diagnosis.

THERAPY. Cool the animal as quickly as possible. Techniques for cooling include spraying the body surface with cold water or immersing small animals in cold water. In those species having a dense coat, ruffle the hair to allow the water to penetrate to the skin. Cold water enemas and alcohol baths may be beneficial. The animal can be packed in crushed ice. Provide adequate ventilation—circulating air with a fan if necessary—to assist in convection heat removal.

Hypovolemic shock should be treated with rapid administration of cold lactated Ringers and corticosteriods. Sodium bicarbonate should be given to counteract metabolic acidosis. Supplemental oxygen is required to combat hypoxemia. Hyperthermia may devitalize tissues, resulting in delayed illness such as pneumonia or nephritis. Monitor or observe the animal for several days following a known hyperthermic episode.

Hypothermia (cold stress, freezing, exposure)

DEFINITION. Hypothermia is a decreased body temperature caused when heat loss exceeds heat gain. Hypothermia is normally less damaging to animals than hyperthermia, but if the body temperature of homeotherms falls below 34°C (93.2°F), thermoregulation is impaired, requiring artificial rewarming. Below 30°C (86°F) thermoregulation is completely eliminated.[14,P.1068]

ETIOLOGY. Predisposing factors include exposure to wind (convection cooling) (Tables 4.1 and 4.2), a soiled or moistened coat, restraint on a cold surface, and restricted exercise. Another important cause is impairment of central thermoregulatory controls by anesthetics or chemical restraint drugs.

Two roloway monkeys were chemically restrained with ketamine hydrochloride for routine tuberculin testing. Upon completion of the test, each monkey was returned to a large outdoor enclosure and laid on a cold concrete slab. The environmental temperature was 15–18°C (60–65°F). Normally,

TABLE 4.1. Wind chill chart, United States. Temperature degrees Fahrenheit, wind speed miles per hour

		Temperature (Degrees Fahrenheit)															
Wind	5	36	31	25	19	13	7	1	−5	−11	−16	−22	−28	−34	−40	−46	−52
Speed	10	34	27	21	15	9	3	−4	−10	−16	−22	−28	−35	−41	−47	−53	−59
Miles	15	32	25	19	13	6	0	−7	−13	−19	−26	−32	−39	−45	−51	−58	−64
Per	20	30	24	17	11	4	−2	−9	−15	−22	−29	−35	−42	−48	−55	−61	−68
Hour	25	29	23	16	9	3	−4	−11	−17	−24	−31	−37	−44	−51	−58	−64	−71
	30	28	22	15	8	1	−5	−12	−19	−26	−33	−39	−46	−53	−60	−67	−73
	35	28	21	14	7	0	−7	−14	−21	−27	−34	−41	−48	−55	−62	−69	−76
	40	27	20	13	6	−1	−8	−15	−22	−29	−36	−43	−50	−57	−64	−71	−78
	45	26	19	12	5	−2	−9	−16	−23	−30	−37	−44	−51	−58	−65	−72	−79
	40	26	19	12	4	−3	−10	−17	−24	−31	−38	−45	−52	−60	−67	−74	−81
	55	25	18	11	4	−3	−10	−18	−25	−32	−39	−46	−54	−61	−68	−75	−82
	60	25	17	10	3	−4	−11	−19	−26	−33	−40	−48	−55	−62	−69	−76	−84

Source: U.S. NOAA's Weather Service, 2007.

TABLE 4.2. Wind chill chart, United States. Temperature degrees, Celsius, wind speed kilometers per hour

Wind Chill Chart (Metric)												
Temperature (Degrees Celsius)												
Wind Speed Km Per Hour	5	0	−5	−10	−15	−20	−25	−30	−35	−40	−45	−50
Calm	5	0	−5	−10	−15	−20	−25	−30	−35	−40	−45	−50
5	4	−2	−7	−13	−19	−24	−30	−36	−41	−47	−53	−58
10	3	−3	−9	−15	−21	−27	−33	−39	−45	−51	−57	−63
15	2	−4	−11	−17	−23	−29	−35	−41	−48	−54	−60	−66
20	1	−5	−12	−18	−24	−30	−37	−43	−49	−56	−62	−68
25	1	−6	−12	−19	−25	−32	−38	−44	−51	−57	−64	−70
30	0	−6	−13	−20	−26	−33	−39	−46	−52	−59	−65	−72
35	0	−7	−14	−20	−27	−33	−40	−47	−53	−60	−66	−73
40	−1	−7	−14	−21	−27	−34	−41	−48	−54	−61	−68	−74
45	−1	−8	−15	−21	−28	−35	−42	−48	−55	−62	−69	−75
50	−1	−8	−15	−22	−29	−35	−42	−49	−56	−63	−69	−76
55	−2	−8	−15	−22	−29	−36	−43	−50	−57	−63	−70	−77
60	−2	−9	−16	−23	−30	−36	−43	−50	−57	−64	−71	−78
65	−2	−9	−16	−23	−30	−37	−44	−51	−58	−65	−72	−79

Source: Meteorological Service of Canada, The Green Lane, 2007.

after ketamine immobilization, an animal revives in 20–40 minutes and is then capable of increased muscle activity to assist internal heat production. One and a half hours later, the attendant found both animals still comatose. The rectal temperature of each animal had dropped below 32°C (90°F). One animal died, the other recovered following intensive treatment.

A chemically restrained animal may be incapable of shivering to generate heat in a cold environment. Hypothermia may quickly ensue.

Newborns are particularly susceptible to hypothermia because of undeveloped thermoregulatory systems. In a cold wet environment, the unattended or neglected newborn may quickly become hypothermic and may die. Adults of small species become hypothermic more rapidly than those of large species because of the relatively larger surface area exposed by a small animal.

Animals subjected to surgery in addition to restraint may become hypothermic because of heat loss from cold tables, exposure of large surgically prepared areas, large open incisions, and the use of vasodilatory drugs (acepromazine) and general anesthesia (halothane).

Excessive application of cleansing solutions and alcoholic skin disinfectants is detrimental to the patient's thermal status, particularly in small species.

Animals in shock become hypothermic quickly. Any hypoxic condition predisposes to hypothermia.[21,vol.2]

Just as excessive muscular activity associated with physical restraint may produce hyperthermia, so prolonged immobility may induce hypothermia, particularly in poorly insulated species.[1,2,3,16]

CLINICAL SIGNS. Shivering is a standard sign in animals not sedated or anesthetized. Sometimes it is difficult to differentiate between the shivering that occurs with fright or anger and that of hypothermia. Hypothermic animals are usually dull in reaction and slow to respond to stimuli. The primary sign of hypothermia is an excessive drop in body temperature. Temperatures may decrease below the limits of an ordinary clinical thermometer. Critical evaluation of body

temperature with a broader calibrated thermometer may reveal that the temperature is as low as 29.5°C (85°F). When the body temperature drops below 32°C (89.6°F), the animal is likely to become comatose and unable to respond to any stimulation. Accidental hypothermia may decrease the amount of anesthetic agent required and lead to the assumption that a patient is anesthetized when in reality it is simply hypothermic.

A decrease in body temperature is accompanied by a decrease in cardiac output, heart rate, blood pressure, and glomerular filtration rate. Blood viscosity and hematocrit levels increase. Signs noted with temperatures below 30°C (86°F) may include slow and shallow breathing, metabolic acidosis, "sludging" in the microcirculation, ventricular fibrillation, and coagulation disorders.

THERAPY. Rapid warming of the whole body is essential to maintain life. Local heat applications to the limbs are insufficient for warming the whole body. The most effective way is to immerse the animal in a warm water bath (Fig. 4.8). Water temperature should be maintained between 40.5°C (105°F) and 45.5°C (114°F). Hold the animal's head out of

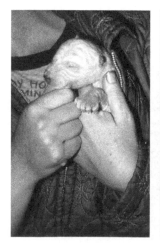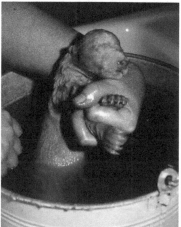

FIG. 4.8. Warming an infant polar bear.

the water and ruffle the hair coat to make sure that heat exchange is taking place at the skin surface. Large animals that cannot be immersed in water baths can be sprayed with warm water or wrapped in warm blankets and the body surface massaged. Warm water enemas are helpful. Warm broth or other liquids given via stomach tube are indicated. Intravenous infusions of warm saline are effective in raising the body temperature. Surgical exposure of a suitable vein may be necessary to effect intravenous administrations because of the decreased blood pressure.

Small animals can be rubbed dry and warmed by being placed next to the skin of the attendant until more effective warming techniques can be applied.

If a surgical patient becomes hypothermic, the incision site can be flushed with warm (not over 42°C or 82°F) saline. Circulating water-type heating pads are effective in preventing hypothermia in surgical patients and in treating accidental hypothermia. Electric heating pads or blankets are not recommended because they can easily become too hot. Hypothermic and shock patients normally suffer from skin vasoconstriction and are thus incapable of carrying intense heat away from the skin. Electric heating pads have caused skin burns and sloughs. Be cautious when applying heat directly to the skin.

Hot water bottles can be used to raise the ambient air temperature in a small enclosed area (heat tent). A hot water bottle should be wrapped in a towel if it is to be used near the skin. Plastic milk cartons or plastic bags can be used in lieu of a standard hot water bottle.

The air surrounding the patient can be warmed with infrared heat lamps, forced-air driers, electric floor heaters, surgical lamps, or commercial radiant heat infant warmers.

When an animal has been warmed with water, be sure the coat is thoroughly dried with a hand-held hair dryer as soon as the temperature equilibrates. Damp hair chills the skin. Monitor the temperature frequently during warming to prevent overheating. Observe the animal for a sufficient time following equilibration to be certain it is thermoregulating on its own.

DEFINITION OF TERMS

Basal metabolism (BMR): The metabolic rate necessary to produce the energy required by an animal (in a thermo-neutral and postabsorptive state) to carry out basic maintenance functions while at rest. These include blood circulation, respiration, kidney function, and specific dynamic action. BMR is related to body size and surface area. Animals with high BMRs represent a greater risk for hyperthermia during restraint.

Conduction: Direct transfer of heat between an animal and contiguous objects. The rate of transmission of heat is proportional to the temperature gradient. The direction of flow is from higher to lower temperature. An animal lying on hot soil absorbs heat. Contrarily, an animal lying on a cold concrete surface loses heat.

Convection: The transmission of heat by movement of a medium surrounding or within an object. An animal may either absorb or dissipate heat because of air or water movement over the surface of the body. Blood carries heat to and from organs by convection.

Countercurrent heat exchange system: An anatomical arrangement of adjacent veins and arteries that warms the blood at the periphery, which assists in stabilization of core body temperature (Fig. 4.5).

Critical temperature: Those ambient temperature levels above and below which life is threatened. High and low critical temperatures vary with the species of animal; one cannot extrapolate critical levels for other species from information concerning humans.

Dehydration: A decrease of tissue and cellular body fluids.

Evaporation: The conversion of liquid to vapor. Water absorbs 0.58 kcal for every gram of water evaporated. This is an extremely important cooling mechanism for many animals.

Frostbite: A condition resulting when living tissue is frozen. Gangrene usually develops in the affected tissue. Frostbite commonly affects the extremities of the limbs, the tail, and the tips of the ears.

Heat cramps: Spasms of muscles following reduction of sodium chloride levels in the plasma. Spasms may be part of the syndrome of heat exhaustion or may occur independently.

Heat exhaustion: A state of collapse brought on by insufficient blood supply to the cerebral cortex as a result of dilatation of the blood vessels in response to heat. The disease is not as acute nor so rapidly fatal as heat stroke.

Heat stroke or sun stroke: Inability of the heat regulatory mechanisms to maintain body temperature. It is characterized by acute onset and extremely high body temperatures up to 42–45°C (108–113°F).

Homeostasis: (1) That group of mechanisms functioning to produce stability of the internal environment of an organism. (2) The maintenance of body functions within ranges compatible with life, reached by actions or reactions initiated in response to environmental change.

Homeotherm or endotherm: An animal capable of thermoregulation by intrinsic mechanisms. The term "warm-blooded" is sometimes used but is neither descriptive nor accurate.

Hyperthermia: Any disorder resulting in an elevated body temperature. Hyperthermia is not necessarily a fever. A fever is hyperthermia plus toxemia, in many cases associated with an infectious process.

Hypothermia: A state characterized by subnormal body temperatures.

Poikilotherm: An animal that must rely primarily on external sources for heat or coolness to maintain a suitable body temperature. Behavioral adaptations provide primary thermoregulatory mechanisms. These animals are popularly referred to as "cold-blooded," an inaccurate term.

Radiation: All rays within the electromagnetic wave spectrum transfer energy through space without heating the intervening air. The sun is the most important source of radiant heat. However, all warm objects, including animals, emit radiant energy. The direction of flow depends on the temperature gradient.

Thermoneutral zone: The ambient temperature range within which an animal can carry out normal body functions while at rest without resorting to special heating or cooling mechanisms.

REFERENCES

1. Bartlett, R.O., and Miller, M.A. 1956. The adrenal cortex in restraint hypothermia. Endocrinology 14:181–87.
2. Bartlett, R.G., and Quimby, F.H. 1958. Heat balance in restraint (emotionally) induced hypothermia. Am J Physiol 193:557–59.
3. Bartlett, R.G., Bohr, V.C., and Helmendoch, R.H. 1956. Comparative effect of restraint (emotional) hypothermia on common laboratory animals. Physiol Zool 29:256–59.
4. Blood, D.C., and Radostits, O.M. 1989. Hyperthermia (Heat stroke). In: Veterinary Medicine, 7th ed. London: Bailliere Tindal.
5. Calder, W.A., and King, J.R. 1974. Thermal and caloric relations of birds. In: D.S. Farner and J.R. King, Eds. Avian Biology, vol. 4. New York: Academic Press.
6. Dill, D.B., ed. 1964. Adaptation to the environment. Handbook of Physiology, sec. 4. Washington, D.C.: American Physiological Society. (This is an extremely valuable general reference.)
7. Gordon, M.S. 1968. Animal Function: Principles and Adaptations. New York: Macmillan.
8. Guyton, A.C. 1971. Body temperature, temperature regulation, and fever. In: Textbook of Medical Physiology, 4th ed., p. 842. Philadelphia: W.B. Saunders.
9. Hales, J.R.S., and Richards, D.A.B., eds. 1987. Heat Stress, Physical Exertion and the Environment. Amsterdam: Excerpta Medica.
10. King, J.R., and Farner, D.S. 161. Energy metabolism, thermoregulation, and body temperature. In: A.J. Marshall, ed. Biology and Comparative Physiology of Birds, vol. 2. New York: Academic Press.
11. Moberg, G.P. 1985. Influences of stress on reproduction: Measure of well-being. In: G.P. Moberg, ed. Animal Stress. Bethesda, MD: American Physiological Association.
12. Prosser, G.L., ed. 1973. Temperature. In: Comparative Animal Physiology, 3rd ed. Philadelphia: W.B. Saunders.
13. Richards, S.A. 1973. Temperature Regulation. London: Wykenham Publications.
14. Ruck, T.C., and Patton, H.D. 1965. Physiology and Biophysics, 19th ed. Philadelphia: W.B. Saunders.
15. Schmidt-Nielsen, K. 1964. Desert Animals. London: Oxford Univ. Press.
16. Squires, R.D., Jacobson, F.H., and Bergey, G.E. 1971. Hypothermia in cats during physical restraint. Naval Air Development Center, Crew Systems Dep. NADC-CS-7 117.
17. Swan, H. 1974. Thermoregulation and Bioenergetics. New York: American Elsevier.
18. Taylor, C.R. 1963. The thermoregulatory function of the horns of the family bovidae. Ph.D. diss., Harvard University.
19. Taylor, C.R., and Rountree, V.J. 1973. Temperature regulation and heat balance in running cheetahs: A strategy for sprinters? Am J Physiol 224:848–51.
20. White, S.L. 1990. Alterations in body temperature. In: B.P. Smith, ed. Large Animal Internal Medicine. St. Louis: CV Mosby.
21. Whittlow, G.C., ed. 1970, 1971, 1973. Comparative Physiology of Thermoregulation. Vol. 1, Invertebrates, Fish, Amphibians, Reptiles, Birds; Vol. 2, Mammals; Vol. 3, Special Aspects of Thermoregulation. New York: Academic Press.
22. Yousef, M.K. 1985. Stress Physiology in Livestock. Vol. 1, Basic Principles. Boca Raton, FL: CRC.

CHAPTER 5

Understanding Behavior for Restraint Purposes

An understanding of animal behavior is crucial to the successful application of restraint procedures with minimal stress.[3,15] Each species or animal group has a repertoire of actions that astute observers are capable of evaluating and classifying. For purposes of this book, behavior is defined as all aspects of an animal's total activity, especially that which may be externally observed.[11,12,14–16] Behavior may be controlled by genetics[1], in which case the action is innate, but may also be learned or modified by individual experiences.

Animal handlers of livestock and companion animals must learn to understand the behavior of their charges.[11,12] Zoo and wildlife veterinarians may deal with hundreds of species of animals, each with their own behavioral characteristics.[8–10,13,20] How can animal handlers, keepers, and clinical veterinarians know all of the subtleties of behavior that would allow them to apply optimal restraint? In short, they can't, but there are basic behavioral patterns that are shared by most mammals. Birds have their own patterns, as do reptiles and amphibians.

Veterinary students become well-versed in physical examination and laboratory detection of illness, but many receive little training or experience in simply observing normal behavior in a natural setting for domestic animals, let alone wild species. So how does one acquire the skills that will enable a person to detect behaviors that affect restraint, or the early stages of illness? One may read about behavior, but it takes time just looking at the species in a collection to learn enough to determine even minor variations from "normal" behavior. Another method is to listen to experienced owners, trainers, or keepers, but observation is the key.

WHY BE CONCERNED ABOUT ACQUIRING OBSERVATIONAL SKILLS?

- To be able to select appropriate restraint procedures
- To be able to detect incipient illness[3]
- To detect stress in the lives of animals[3,4,16]
- To assist in the welfare and well-being of animals[2]

NORMAL BEHAVIOR

Restrainers must first understand normal to detect abnormal.[5,18,19,21] Behaviors to be emphasized for restraint purposes are methods of offense and defense, communication (vocalization, body language, facial expression), hierarchical status, locomotion, recumbency, and getting up and down.

As examples, some behaviors of South American camelids (SAC) and elephants will be discussed.

Offense and Defense

SOUTH AMERICAN CAMELIDS. A person restraining any species of animal should know how that animal defends itself or how it may respond to a perceived threat. Offense and defense weapons used by camelids include kicking, charging, chest-butting, biting, and spewing stomach contents (spitting) on other camelids or people.[4,5,7]

Veterinarians and animal handlers must be aware of abnormal behavior that may develop in hand-raised camelid neonates (cria is the Spanish term for baby animal). Camelid neonates that are bottle-fed and kept without social interaction with other camelids may become imprinted on people and while young are submissive (Fig. 5.1). As they mature, the resulting abnormal behavioral characteristics are more critical in male camelids, but may also occur in females. When the hand-raised male reaches sexual maturity, he may begin to treat humans as he would another male camelid. He will

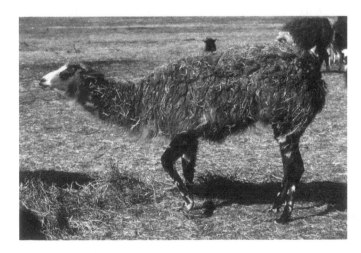

FIG. 5.1. Submissive posture in a llama.

charge and chest-butt a person who will likely be knocked down and then bitten. When male camelids fight other male camelids, they attempt to bite each other on the legs, neck, or more seriously the scrotum, castrating the victim.[4]

"Spitting" behavior is one of the few things that the general public knows about SACs. They are capable of projecting the foul-smelling stomach contents a distance of 1–2 meters. Llamas and alpacas are generally placid around people and spitting at people is rare. However, spitting is the ultimate response in social interaction between SACs, if more mild threat displays are disregarded.

The behavioral sequence of spitting begins with the ears laid back against the neck; accompanied by a gulping or gurgling sound from the throat region. A bolus of food is then regurgitated from compartment one of the stomach.

It has been the author's experience that alpacas are more prone to spitting than are llamas, but individual llamas may develop a dislike for a particular person. Veterinarians often bear the brunt of such disfavor.[4,5]

SAC usually "cow kick" reaching forward and outward. Alpacas tend to be more prone to kicking than llamas.

Male camelids have formidable canine teeth and are capable of inflicting serious or fatal injury.

ELEPHANT. No one except a trained, qualified elephant handler should approach, come in contact with, or command an elephant. Elephants will generally not listen to or follow the commands of a stranger. Elephants use several methods for offense and defense, including biting, slapping with the trunk, grasping with the trunk, and pulling, pushing, or throwing.[19] As an offensive or defensive weapon, the trunk is without equal in the animal world. Handlers must appreciate the reach of the trunk and know the danger from the trunk of an angry elephant.

Elephants may purposely step on a person's foot. They are adept at kicking and can easily balance on one front and one hind leg. Extreme aggression may be exhibited by the elephant kneeling and head-pressing upon what they perceive as a threat, inconvenience, or a toy. Even an elephant in an elephant restraint device or on tethers may injure a person unfamiliar with an elephant's reach or its signals of aggressive intent.[19]

Although the swinging tail is usually not considered an offensive weapon, it must be considered when administering medication in the rear quarters or when tethering a hind leg. Being soundly struck is painful, and a blow to the face or head may be injurious.

COMMUNICATION

An effective means of communication is vital for the survival of any population of wild or domestic animals, just as it is in human society. South American camelids communicate with each other, humans, and other animals by vocalization and body language.[5,8–10]

Vocalization

Although SACs are not highly vocal, they do have a repertoire of sounds. Alpacas are generally more vocal than llamas. The most common sound has been described as humming (bleating). The pitch and tone of the humming is significant in SAC communication. Franklin[6] describes the **contact hum** as an auditory contact between herd members and especially between a mother and her cria. **Status humming** is a deeper tone that communicates contentedness, tension, discomfort, pain, or relief. The **interrogative hum** is higher pitched and has an inflection at the end. Other variations in intonation are described as a **separation hum** or a **distress hum**.[5]

Llamas emit a snort characterized by a short burst of air through the mouth with loose lips. The snort indicates mild aggression. A clicking sound can be made with the tongue, which also indicates mild aggression. A grumbling threat is emitted when a feeding animal is approached too closely by another, or when an aggressor is about to regurgitate onto an offender.

Screaming indicates extreme fright. Some llamas and alpacas scream continuously when restrained for diagnostic or therapeutic procedures. Screeching is a loud squealing sound, usually made by males chasing one another during a territorial dispute or a fight.

The SAC alarm call is emitted when a male or female perceives danger to be near. The approach of strange dogs or other predators may trigger an alarm call. The alarm call is a high-pitched series of sounds and has been variously described as whistling or neighing, and by some as similar to the braying of a hoarse donkey. When the alarm call is sounded, other SACs within hearing become alerted and turn toward the source of the sound.

ELEPHANTS. Vocalizations to be aware of during elephant restraint procedures include the following:[17]

Bellow. A loud fear- or pain-related call.

Blow. An audible air blast from the trunk, or a visual blast containing dust or food particles.

Scream. Produced when an elephant is extremely excited or angry.

Trumpet. Loud, high frequency, pulsating sound.

Trunk tapping. Elephants may amuse themselves or exhibit slight irritation by tapping on a smooth, flat surface with the tip of the trunk, producing a hollow thumping sound.

Musth rumble. This is a deep-throated, guttural, or bubbly vocalization that is loud and low. Musth is a normal periodic behavior in mature male elephants. For safety, handlers must recognize the primary signs of musth, including aggressive behavior, drainage from the temporal glands, dribbling urine from the prepuce, and unusual vocalization (musth rumble). Other signs that are not unique to musth but commonly occur during musth, are anorexia, dehydration, and somnolence. A bull elephant in musth is dangerous and should be handled only from behind a protective barrier.

Body language

SACs.   Body language, including ear and tail position, is a sure indicator of the mental state of a SAC and many other species of mammals. Various degrees of aggression are communicated between herd-mates by ear, head, and tail positions, usually displayed in concert (Figs. 5.2, 5.3). The ears of a contented, un-aroused SAC are in a vertical position and turned forward.[4] In the alert animal, the ears are cocked forward. Relaxed SACs may allow the ears to lie horizontal to the rear. This is a normal position and should not be considered to indicate aggression when other signs of aggression are absent. In some individuals the ears may appear to spread sideways from the top of the head. This ear position may be used when listening to something going on behind them or just for relaxation. Asymmetrical ear positions may also be seen. Ear and tail position may be in a continual sate of flux, especially when animals are fed, if feeding stations lack adequate space for all herd members.

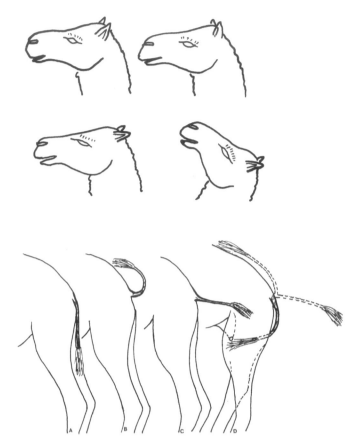

FIG. 5.3.   Ear and tail positions of a camel.

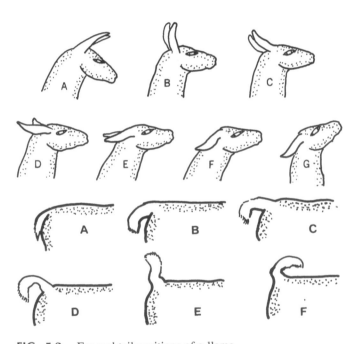

FIG. 5.2.   Ear and tail positions of a llama.

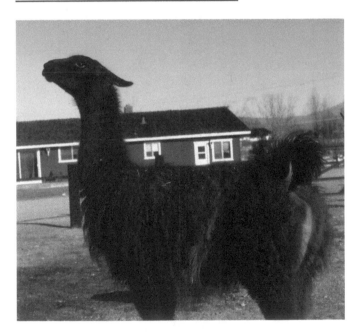

FIG. 5.4.   Intense aggression in a llama.

Mild to moderate aggression is signaled by the head being held horizontal with the ears positioned above the horizontal. As aggression increases the ears move below the horizontal and may be flattened against the neck. Intense aggression is exhibited by the nose being pointed in the air and the ears flattened against the neck (Fig. 5.4).[4,5]

Tail position also communicates social information. In the un-aroused SAC, the tail lies flat against the body. Mild aggression or alertness is indicated by the tail being slightly elevated, but below the horizontal. As the degree of agitation escalates, the tail may be carried horizontal, curled above the horizontal, or vertical. Basically the higher the tail, the higher the level of aggression. The tail may also be seen to wave from side to side, especially in males that are slightly agitated.

These aggressive behaviors are employed by social animals to minimize outright fighting.

Submissiveness in the llama, guanaco, and alpaca is indicated by curving the tail forward over the back, with the head and neck held low, the ears in a normal to above horizontal position, and the front limbs slightly bent. This behavior is frequently seen in SACs that become imprinted on humans. The submissive crouch of a vicuña is with the tail curved forward but with the head curved back over the body.

Llamas generally move at normal gaits with the head held vertically or slightly forward. The alpaca's normal neck position is approximately 70 degrees above horizontal. When either of these species rush or charge at dogs, coyotes, other SACs, or humans, they do so with the neck held almost horizontal. This position may be used for balance as it is also the head and neck position used when running downhill.

ELEPHANTS. All personnel working with elephants should understand basic elephant body language behaviors.[19] Particular attention should be paid to the ears and trunk to assess the mood of an elephant. The elephant is unique by possessing a highly mobile trunk that has many important functions including eating, drinking, breathing, lifting, vocalizing, social discipline, and manipulating tools. Furthermore, the trunk is used to deliver volatile and nonvolatile odorants to olfactory center receptors in a specialized nasal cavity and cribriform plate. Finally, the trunk may be used aggressively (Fig. 5.5).

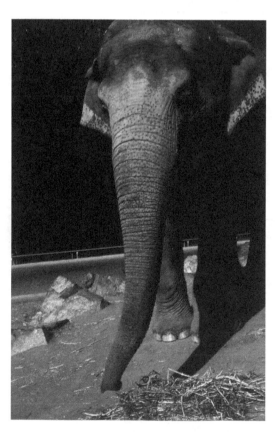

FIG. 5.5. Elephant trunk.

Following are elephant behaviors that may be exhibited associated with restraint procedures:[11]

Alert. The elephant stands facing a person with the head raised, ears spread, tail raised, trunk raised or turned in a "sniff" position.

Wariness. The elephant is in heightened alertness, and with eyes wide open, glances at other elephants.

Sniff. The trunk is extended down and forward in a "J" shape, with the tip out horizontally to sniff another elephant, or person (Fig. 5.6).

Mock charge. The elephant runs toward another elephant or a person with ears extended, head and tusks held high, tail may or may not be elevated, and the trunk extended (Fig. 5.7). The charging elephant stops before reaching the target and usually trumpets.

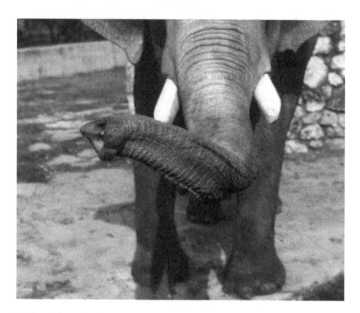

FIG. 5.6. Elephant trunk in the sniff position.

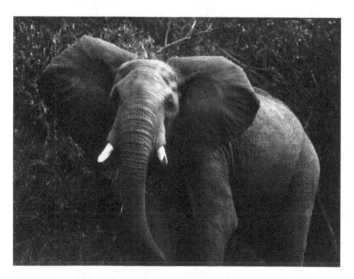

FIG. 5.7. Elephant in a threat or mock charge posture.

Real charge. The trunk is tucked under the head, the head is up and attempts to contact the target. The ears are usually close to the head and usually there is no trumpeting.

Slap. An elephant strikes another elephant with the trunk.

Kick. An elephant may strike forward with a forelimb or toward the side or rearward with a hind limb.

HIERARCHICAL STATUS

A group of SACs, be they all males, all females, or of mixed sexes, quickly establishes a hierarchy (pecking order). Hierarchical status may be determined by seniority in the herd, age, or sex and relatedness. Once established, the rules are obeyed or action is taken by the dominant over a subordinate individual. The action may be a threat only or carried to a conclusion by spewing stomach contents at the offender. Adult males may engage in vigorous combat.[4,5]

Miscellaneous Camelid Behaviors

Alpacas like to play in water.[4] If water is provided in tubs, buckets, or tanks, they will joyously splash. Both llamas and alpacas seek out water during hot weather. If a pond or large water tank is available, they may stand in the water up to their abdomen. Both species are capable of swimming, but do so only when forced. However, they will stand or lie down in shallow ponds or streams to cool themselves. Heavy fiber normally covers the legs of alpacas down to the fetlocks. In hot weather they may stand in water so long that the leg fiber becomes macerated and sheds, leaving a blocked haircut appearance on the upper leg.

Recumbency

SACs.   Sternal recumbency is the most common position for rest and relaxation for llamas and alpacas. In fact, that position is considered the default position for them when faced with an unpleasant situation such as toenail trimming or blood collection. When lying sternally, the front legs are usually folded beneath the chest, but SACs have the unique capability to lie with the forelimbs extended forward.[4]

South American camelids have a pronounced callosity over the sternum, and they may remain recumbent sternally for hours to days without compromising the circulation of the limbs. Lateral recumbency is also a normal camelid position, with the animal apparently sleeping or sunning itself via the thermal window.

ELEPHANTS.   Elephants do not rest comfortably in sternal recumbency. Pressure on the abdomen exerts visceral pressure forward and prevents the diaphragm from effectively participating in respiration. This knowledge must be understood when carrying out restraint procedures. However, most elephants will sleep in lateral recumbency for a few hours each night and even at rest during the day.

When lying down, the elephant sits down on one hind leg, with the front legs extended forward (stretch position). Then it lowers the body to the floor and rolls over on its side. When arising, the first action is to rock the upper fore and hind leg forward and backward to give momentum for lifting the body to the stretch position. Then the front limbs are straightened followed by each hind limb. The space between the fore and hind limb is dangerous when standing near a recumbent elephant. A keeper at a zoo had several ribs fractured when he was rocked between the limbs of an elephant trying to arise.

Eye

SACs.   The large expressive eyes of SACs immediately attract everyone's attention. A good deal may be learned by attentive evaluation of the eye (eyeball, eyelids). It has been said that the eye is the window to the emotional state of an animal. Observant people are quick to perceive a person's emotional state or illness on the basis of eye clarity, pupillary dilatation or constriction, and eyelid position. Often a mother has only to look into the eyes of a child to sense excitement, apathy, depression, or guilt of a misdeed. The eyes of healthy or ill animals are also revealing. It is difficult to describe an apathetic look or a pained expression, but these are present in animals as well as humans.

The eyes of a healthy SAC should be clear and bright. The pupils should respond quickly to extra light. Poking a finger toward the eye should produce a blink reflex. The appearance of the eyes provides the basis for abnormal countenance (facial expression).

ELEPHANTS.   Elephants have small eyes, and facial expressions are overshadowed by ear and trunk movements. Nonetheless, the degree of alertness is indicated by the openness of the eyelids. Eyes should be clear and bright. Elephants don't have tear ducts, so excess lacrimal secretion flows from the conjunctival sac and down the cheek. It is important to differentiate this clear fluid from the opaque and discolored drainage associated with conjunctivitis or keratitis.

BEHAVIORAL CHANGES ASSOCIATED WITH RESTRAINT

Knowing normal behavior allows evaluation of the emotional and physical status of an animal before, during, and after restraint procedures. Many of the behavioral changes are an exaggeration of normal behavior. Remember that the objective of any restraint procedure is to return an animal to its normal daily activity as quickly as possible.

Devious Behavior

Immobilization of an adult male polar bear had to be conducted in an outside enclosure. A Palmer-dart was loaded with a dose of phencyclidine and projected to the bear using a Palmer short-range rifle. The placement of the dart was good. The bear immediately walked to a corner and lay down and exhibited signs of immobilization.

The induction was much too rapid and caused the clinician to question that immobilization had occurred. The bear was prodded by a long piece of electrical conduit from the top of the night quarters. There was no response from repeated prodding. The clinician still questioned the immobilization and prepared another dart with the same initial dose. This was also delivered by remote injection. After an appropriate time for induction to have taken place, the clinician entered the enclosure and approached the bear again with prodding.

Finally the darts were removed. It was then determined that the first dart had not expelled any of the agent into the bear. Had a person gone in with the polar bear after an appropriate time, one can only surmise what action the bear may have taken.

Animals sense when activities are being carried out at an unusual time, and may refuse to enter the night house. As an example, an adult polar bear required frequent immobilization for treatment of audicoptic mange. Keepers attempted to entice him into the night enclosure, but he wouldn't move entirely in. He would stand with a rear leg extended through a doorway, preventing closure of a sliding metal door. Ultimately it was decided to keep the bear in the night house after normal feeding in the morning until clinicians could immobilize the bear.

REFERENCES

1. Alcock, J. 2005. Animal Behavior an Evolutionary Approach, 8th Ed. Sunderland, Massachusetts, Sinauer Associates.
2. Anonymous. 2005. Animal Welfare Act and Animal Welfare Regulations. United States Department of Agriculture, Animal and Plant Health Inspection Service.
3. Fowler, M.E. 1995a. Stress. In: Fowler, M.E. 1995. Restraint and Handling of Wild and Domestic Animals. 2nd Ed. Ames, Iowa State University Press. pp. 57–66.
4. Fowler, M.E. 1999. Llama and alpaca behavior—A clue to illness detection. Journal Camel Practice and Research 6(2):135–152.
5. Fowler, M.E. 2008. Behavioral clues for detection of illness in wild animals: Models in camelids and elephants. In: Fowler, M.E., and Miller, R.E. 2008. Zoo and Wild Animal Medicine, Current Therapy, 6th Ed. St. Louis, Saunders/Elsevier, pp. 33–59.
6. Franklin, W.L. 1982. Biology, ecology, and relationships to man of South American camelid. Limesville, Pennsylvania, Pymatuning Laboratory of Ecology, University Pittsburgh, Special Publication 6, pp. 457–489.
7. Grandin, T. 2000. Habituating antelope and bison to cooperate with veterinary procedures. J Applied Animal Welfare Science 3(3):253–261.
8. Grier, J.W. and Burk, T. 1992. Biology of Animals Behavior. St. Louis, Missouri, Mosby.
9. Hediger, H. 1955. The Psychology and Behaviour of Animals in Zoos and Circuses. New York, Dover Publications.
10. Hediger, H. 1964. Wild Animals in Captivity. New York, Dover Publications.
11. Hediger, H. 1969. Man and Animal in the Zoo. New York, Seymour Lawrence/Delacorte Press.
12. Houpt, K.A. 2005. Domestic Animal Behavior for Veterinarians and Animal Scientists, 4th Ed. Ames, Iowa, Blackwell Publishers.
13. Jensen, P. Editor. 2002. The Ethology of Domestic Animals: An Introductory Text. Wallingford, Oxon, United Kingdom, CABI Publishing.
14. Markowitz, H. 1982. Behavioral Enrichment in the Zoo. New York, Van Nostrand Reinhold.
15. Mazur, J.E. 2002. Learning and Behavior, Prentice-Hall.
16. Moberg, G.P. 1985. Biological response to stress: Key to assessment of animal well-being. In: G.P. Moberg, ed., Animal Stress, Bethesda, MD, American Physiological Society.
17. Moberg, G.P. 2000. Biological response to stress: Implications for animal welfare. In: Moberg, G.P. and Mench, J.A. 2000. The Biology of Animal Stress, Basic Principles and Implications for Animal Welfare. New York, CABI Publishing, pp. 1–22.
18. Olson, D. Ed. 2004. Behavioral management. In: Olson, D., Ed.. 2004. Elephant Husbandry Resource Guide. Silver Springs, Maryland. Published jointly by the American Zoo and Aquarium Association Elephant Taxon Group, The Elephant Manager's Association and the International Elephant Foundation, pp. 93–122.
19. Price, E.O. 2002. Animal Domestication and Behavior. Wallingford Oxon, CABI Publishers.
20. Reichard, T.A. 2008. Behavioral training for medical procedures. In: Fowler, M.E., and Miller, R.E. 2008. Zoo and Wild Animal Medicine, Current Therapy, 6th Ed. St. Louis, Saunders/Elsevier, pp. 66–67.
21. Schulte, B. 2006. Behavior. In: Fowler, M.E., and Mikota, S.K., Eds. Biology, Medicine and Surgery of Elephants. Ames, Iowa, Blackwell Publishing, pp. 35–43.
22. Tresz, H. 2006. Behavioral management at the Phoenix Zoo: New strategies and perspectives. J Applied An Welfare Science 90(1):65–70.
23. Wilson, E.O. 1980. Sociobiology—The Abridged Edition. Cambridge, Massachusetts, Harvard University Press.

CHAPTER 6

Training for Restraint Procedures

Modern animal management practices require that the stress (distress) of any procedure be minimized to optimize animal welfare. Training is the pathway by which the animal becomes accustomed to a procedure in a methodical manner. Domestic animals require training for their well-being and optimal interrelationship with people. There is a marked difference in handling range cattle compared to dealing with a herd of dairy cows that are being milked twice daily. The difference is a matter of accustoming the cattle to a closer association with people. Farmers or ranchers may not realize it, but they are indeed training their animals to enter a chute or be placed in a stanchion. However, that training is required for their proper husbandry.

Training is basically teaching an animal certain procedures or actions. Parents train their children to look both ways before crossing a street, how to tie their shoes, and how to act in society. Dog owners send their pets to obedience school to prepare them to become more desirable pets. Horses are taught to allow a person to ride on their backs or be harnessed to pull a cart. Oxen may be paired as calves and trained to obey verbal and touch commands. Animals gather information from many sources and respond positively or negatively, which is called learning. If a person initiates and coordinates the process, it is called training.

Modern animal management programs emphasize training based on positive reinforcement that makes the animal a willing participant in the handling procedures.[14] Free-ranging wild antelope may be trained to be herded into another enclosure by methodically and quietly moving them back and forth from one place to another without any procedures being performed. They become less inclined to charge the fence or attempt to jump a chute wall.

Before discussing training further, consider the reasons we may wish to train an animal. Training provides physical exercise and mental stimulation. Training, when done properly, produces an animal with a more cooperative behavior, which is important in training for medical or restraint procedures. Training also provides a more fulfilling life and a less stressful environment for the animal and their handlers. Secondary reasons for training include educating or entertaining the public and to allow certain research procedures to be performed. Since the dawn of civilization animals have worked for people, which usually requires special training (for example, guide dogs for helping the blind, search and rescue dogs, draft animals, capuchin monkeys *Cebus appella* used to assist quadraplegic individuals). Animals are also trained for sporting events (dog and horse racing). Training is the cornerstone of a good animal care program.[14]

This chapter is not meant to be a definitive treatise on training of animals, and its presentation here is not meant to attempt to turn veterinarians or animal handlers into trainers. However, understanding the need for and process for training will assist in the well-being of their charges. For more details see the books by Adams; Bennett and Tellington-Jones; Clyde, Bell, Kahn, Rafert, and Wallace; and Ramirez.[1-3,14] Training may be an integral part of many successful animal handling programs. Most vertebrate animals are capable of learning many procedures if trainers use proper procedures and are consistent.

Training an animal may be challenging, as it completely relies on effective communication between the animal and the trainer, using the language of actions and consequences. It is highly recommended that one handler only be given the responsibility of training a new behavior. Using more than one handler to train may introduce inconsistencies in the training process, which may cause confusion and anxiety on the part of the animal.

OVERVIEW OF ANIMAL TRAINING

First the person doing the training must really want to improve the well-being of the animal. An ego trip or a desire for power over an animal is not conducive to the development of trust between the animal and the trainer, which is essential for success. The trainer must have or acquire an understanding of general animal behavior and basic training principles.

Terms, such as, operant conditioning, positive reinforcement, bridging, targeting, and cuing must be incorporated into one's vocabulary.[14] Attendance at training workshops or better still, working with or observing an experienced animal trainer in action to gain some experience, is highly desirable. It is absolutely necessary for the trainer to know about the normal behavior of the animal to be trained.

Providing a proper environment for training to take place is crucial. Adequate time must be allocated on a consistent basis to make any training feasible. The trainer must likewise be consistent in cuing and giving rewards. Success in any endeavor, but especially in training, is based on preparation, practice, producing, and persistence.

Elephants as an Example of Training

Each species of animal will require a different training protocol, but for this chapter, consider the elephant. Optimal elephant management in captivity requires that the animal be trained.[1,7,11,17] Handling elephants directly (free contact) or through a barrier (protected contact) requires different training regimens, but the end result is to be able to carry out a procedure in a safe and efficient manner for both the elephant and humans. Some institutions use a hybrid of these two management strategies.

Having a well-trained elephant requires that the trainer also be trained and experienced.[11] The person must be dedicated to improving the well-being of his or her charges and be willing to learn from others and attend training seminars and workshops. Elephant caretakers should be permanently assigned to work with elephants so that mutual respect and trust may be fostered.

A trained elephant is likely to be safe to work around with a minimum of physical or chemical restraint required. Training the elephant to position its body, ears, limbs, tail, or head to allow examination, collection of laboratory samples or administration of medication greatly enhances the care that may be provided (Fig. 6.1).

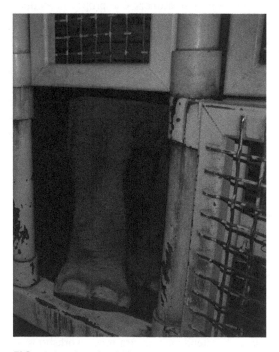

FIG. 6.1. A trained elephant placing a foot through a protective barrier.

The key to an optimal training program is to facilitate opportunities for the elephant to make associations through consequences that enhance understanding of the handler's requests.

Operant conditioning is a learning method in which a particular response is elicited by a stimulus because that response produced desirable consequences (reward). As an example, if a desired behavior is followed by something the elephant seeks (praise, food, treat), it is more likely to repeat that behavior and even to enhance the behavior. This is called positive reinforcement. The presentation of the reinforcement must be given to the elephant at the exact moment the elephant performs the behavior in order to communicate to the elephant that the behavior was the one being requested.

Timing is important. Using the foregoing logic, a trainer may move an elephant into an Elephant Restraint Device (ERD) by slowly but consistently asking the elephant to move forward and reinforcing (rewarding) the behavior. See Table 6.1 for some selected terms used in training.

TABLE 6.1. Selected training terms

Term	Definition
Conditioned response	A type of learned response that occurs through association with a specific stimulus.
Desensitization	The process of accustoming an animal to a new stimulus through gradual exposure to it.
Cue	A stimulus that precedes a behavior, signaling that a specific response will be reinforced if performed correctly. The result is that the stimulus will consistently elicit only that particular response.
Negative reinforcement	A process in which a response increases in frequency due to the avoidance, escape, or removal of an aversive stimulus from the animal's environment.
Operant conditioning	A type of learning in which behavior is determined by its consequences; strengthened if followed by reinforcement (positive or negative) and diminished if followed by punishment. The animal's behavior is instrumental in acquiring the desired response.
Positive reinforcement	The process of following an action or response with something that the animal wants, thereby causing an increase in the frequency of occurrence of that behavior.
Punishment	An act that occurs immediately after a behavior it is meant to affect, and causes a decrease in the frequency of that behavior.
Reinforcer	Anything that occurs immediately following a behavior that tends to increase the likelihood that the behavior will occur again.
Stimulus	Anything that elicits or affects a behavioral response.
Time-out	Cessation of all reinforcement immediately following an inappropriate or undesirable response. A gentle type of punishment of short duration.
Unconditioned stimulus	A stimulus that elicits a particular response without any prior association, that is, it is not a learned association; it is a reflex.

Reinforcers may be positive or negative. Positive reinforcement increases response probability by the presentation of a positive stimulus following a response. Negative reinforcement does the same in reverse, through the removal, reduction, avoidance, or prevention of an aversive stimulus following a response.

Verbal commands may be accompanied by touching a specific area of the body (Table 6.2). Trainers working with an elephant behind a barrier usually use a whistle or a clicker as a bridge for reinforcement. The bridge is used as a signal

TABLE 6.2. Commands used in elephant management[*11]

All right—Release from previous command
Back up—Move backward in a straight line
Come here—Move to the handler
Come in—Move laterally toward the handler
Ear—Present ear forward or through an ear hole in a barrier
Foot—Front leg, foot to elbow parallel to the ground; rear leg foot to stifle parallel to ground; present foot for tethering; move foot into the foot hole in protected contact
Get over—Move laterally away from handler
Give—Hand object to the handler
Lean in—Position body parallel to and in contact with a barrier in protected contact
Leave it—Drop whatever is in the trunk
Lie down—Assume lateral recumbency
Move up—Move forward in a straight line
No (quit)—Stop unwanted behavior
Open—Open the mouth wide for visual inspection
Salute—Raise trunk and foot simultaneously
Steady—Freeze
Stretch—Assume sternal recumbency
Target—Move toward target, touched with target pole
Trunk down—Drop trunk straight down to the ground
Trunk up—Curl trunk up to touch the forehead
Turn—Pivot in a circle, right or left

* These verbal commands may be accompanied by touching an appropriate spot on the head, body, or legs.

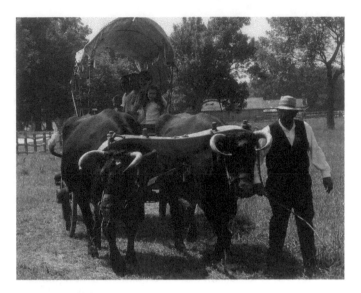

FIG. 6.2. Trained oxen.

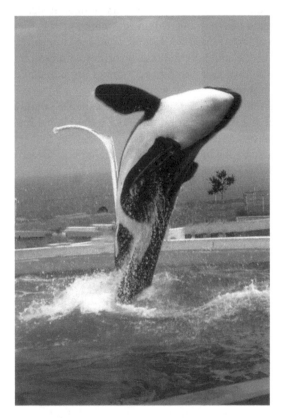

FIG. 6.3. A killer whale jumping out of the water voluntarily.

to the elephant that the requested behavior has been performed and the reward is forthcoming when the reward cannot be presented immediately.

Elephants may also learn by observing other elephants carrying out the desired behavior. It is interesting to watch young circus elephants mimic their elder companions during playtime.

It may be helpful if a veterinarian is familiar with some of the commands used by trainers to induce an elephant to perform various behaviors that have relevance to restraint and/or physical examination.

By knowing commands and the appropriate response of the elephant, a veterinarian may be able to evaluate the competence of the trainer/handler. However, the veterinarian should not make the mistake of trying to issue commands. If the elephant is not responding to the handler's commands, it is unsafe for interaction and the veterinarian should leave the elephant area immediately.

Training Other Animals

The author had an opportunity to work with a team of trained oxen for a summer (Fig. 6.2). These animals had been trained as a team as calves to respond to seven vocal commands: Gee = turn right, Haw = turn left, Come up = start moving, Easy = slow down, Whoa = stop, Back = back up, Step out = move away from the tongue, and Step in = move toward the tongue. Specific touch cues were used to reinforce the verbal command. Various drivers worked this team, and it was apparent that the tone of voice of the driver made a difference in the response of the oxen. Mules and horse may be trained to respond to the same verbal commands.

Zoo and seaquarium animals may be trained by enhancing normal behaviors (Fig. 6.3). Many marine mammals are trained to present themselves for blood collection and urinary catheterization for obtaining urine samples. See Chapter 25.

TRAINING FOR VETERINARY PROCEDURES

Husbandry is defined as the care and management of animals using the best scientific principles and knowledge available.[14] Husbandry includes providing a healthy environment, proper nutrition, proper social structure, sound behavioral management, systematic record keeping, and professional veterinary care. It is in the last category that time should be spent learning the procedures used to train animals to accept restraint and to carry out medical procedures.

By teaching an animal to cooperate in its own health care, life becomes less stressful for the animal, the caretaker, and the veterinarian. Husbandry training facilitates good health care by allowing the veterinarian better access to the animal.[2-6,8,10,12-16,18] Animals may be taught to position themselves properly for an examination, including rectal examination, genital tract evaluation, ultrasound, blood and urine collection, body temperature, respiration, and cardiac function measurements and for moving from one enclosure to another.[14]

Training for restraint and medical procedures involves the process of desensitizing an animal to a new stimulus or group of stimuli. This is done by exposing the animal to the novel stimulus in gradually increased increments.[14] Most medical procedures necessitate touching the animal. In nearly all wild animals and untrained domestic animals, touching initiates a voluntary motor response causing immediate employment of the animal's defense or offensive repertoire. With this tactile response, minimized training for many tasks may be accomplished.

Use caution when training dangerous animals to allow medical procedures to be carried out unless there is the possibility of a protective barrier between the handler and the animal. Procedures lending themselves to being less stressful to the animal and yet avoiding risky anesthesia include visual and physical examination, measurement of baseline physiological parameters, collection of samples for diagnostic purposes, and parenteral administration of vaccines, antibiotics, and other medications. Long-term administration of medications such as insulin has heretofore been difficult or impossible. Minor surgical procedures, wound care, and bandage changes may be accomplished with little restraint and/or under local anesthesia.[17] Foot care is a constant challenge in zoos, but problem animals may be trained to allow lifting the feet, inspecting them, and carrying out nonpainful procedures (hoof and nail trimming).

Training animals to move between exhibit enclosures, night quarters, or squeeze cages aids in introducing an individual animal into a new group, cleaning and sanitizing quarters, observing closely, isolating for immobilization or medication, and separating for breeding and/or birthing. Having animals trained to step onto a platform scale is an extremely valuable procedure for calculating dosages for medication and immobilizing agents or monitoring the condition of animals.

If training for restraint and medical procedures is to be carried out in a zoo, a coordinator should be appointed and each member of the concerned staff be assigned specific responsibilities. The procedures to be trained for and the species to be involved should be prioritized. The staff must be trained to carry out the training. Zoo administrators must be involved in the planning and support the projects. Time must be allocated for the trainers to carry out their task.

TRAINING FOR TRANSPORTING

Transporting an animal to another exhibit in a zoo or between zoos has the potential to be extremely distressful to a wild animal. Both captive and free-ranging wild animals may be trained to load into crates. This may take considerable time, but the rewards of avoiding traumatic injury and stress may mean the difference between life and death of an animal.

The following example illustrates the value of proper training. An adult female elephant under free-contact management lost her enclosure mate and was to be transported to another zoo to become a member of a herd. Without proper training, an elephant truck was backed into the elephant area and the elephant was brought to the ramp to enter the truck. The elephant was tethered by both front legs with ropes leading up the ramp to the front of the truck. By alternating pressure on each limb, the elephant was inched into the truck and tethered to floor anchors.

The journey had proceeded for only 30 kilometers (19 miles) when the driver of a zoo car following behind noticed that the elephant's trunk was protruding through the floor of the truck. After the truck was stopped and inspected, a hole approximately 30 cm (12 in.) in diameter was found in the 5 cm (2 in.) thick oak flooring. The elephant had repeatedly fallen to her knees until she broke the hole in the floor. The elephant was returned to the zoo and off-loaded.

Another opportunity to place the elephant developed, but this time a container unit for shipping cargo was strategically placed in the elephant area and situated so that a truck could eventually back up to it. Using proper training methods, the elephant was fed and watered in the container and ultimately confined and tethered inside for variable periods of time. After weeks of training it was deemed safe to initiate the transport.

The elephant willingly moved into the container and was confined there until the truck could be situated. When all the doors were opened, she walked directly into the truck and was tethered for transport. She was moved nearly 4,000 km (2,484 miles) across the United States and was successfully off-loaded. One of the elephant's keepers rode in a passenger cubicle in visual and audible contact with the elephant.

REFERENCES

1. Adams, J.L. 1981. Elephant training. In: Wild Elephants in Captivity. Arson, California, Center for the Study of Elephants, pp. 168–200.
2. Bennett, M.M., and Tellington-Jones, L. 1992. Lllama Handling and Training: the TEAM approach. Dundee, New York, Zephyr Farms Publishing.
3. Clyde, V.L., Bell, B., Kahn, P., Rafert, J.W., and Wallace, R.S. 2002. Improvement in the health and well-being of a bonobo *Pan paniscus* troop through a dynamic operant conditioning

program. Proc Am Assn Zoo Vet, Milwaukee, Wisconsin, pp. 45–49.

4. Dumonceaux, G.A., Burton, M.S., Ball, R.L., and Demuth, A. 1998. Veterinary procedures facilitated by behavioral conditioning and desensitization in reticulated giraffe *Giraffa camelopardalis* and Nile hippopotamus *Hippopotamus amphibious.* Proc Am Assn Zoo Vet and Am Assn Wildlife Vet, Omaha, Nebraska, pp. 388–92.

5. Grandin, T. 2000. Habituating antelope and bison to cooperate with veterinary procedures. J Applied Animal Welfare Science 3(3):253–61.

6. Heidenreich, B. 2004. Training birds for husbandry and medical behaviors to reduce or eliminate stress. In: American Association of Zoos and Aquariums, Conference Proceedings, Silver Springs, Maryland.

7. Kempe, J.E. 1950. The training of elephants. Country Life 107(Jan. 27):228–9.

8. Laule, G.E., and Desmond, T.J. 1990. Use of positive behavioral techniques in primates for husbandry and handling. Proc Am Assn Zoo Vet, South Padre Island, Texas, pp. 269–73.

9. Laule, G.E., and Whitaker, M.A. 1998. The use of positive reinforcement techniques in the medical management of captive animals. Proc Am Assn Zoo Vet and Am Assn Wildlife Vet, Omaha, Nebraska, pp. 383–7.

10. Miller, M., MacPhee, M.S., and Mellen, J. 2002. Proactive development of an integrated behavioral husbandry program in a large zoological setting. Proc Am Assn Zoo Vet, Milwaukee, Wisconsin pp. 59–62.

11. Olson, D., Ed. 2004. Elephant Husbandry Resource Guide. Published jointly by the American Zoo and Aquarium Association (AZA), Elephant Manager's Association and the International Elephant Foundation.

12. Phillips, M., Grandin, T., Graffam, W., Iribeck, N., and Cambre, R. 1998. Crate conditioning of bongo for veterinary and husbandry procedures at the Denver Zoological Gardens, Zoo Biology 17:25–32.

13. Pryor, K. 1999. Don't Shoot the Dog. The New Art of Teaching and Training. Revised edition. New York, New York, Bantam Books.

14. Ramirez, K. 1999. Animal Training: Successful Animal Management Through Positive Reinforcement. Chicago, Published by the Shedd Aquarium.

15. Reichard, T.A., Shellabarger, W., and Laule, G. 1993. Behavioral training of primates and other zoo animals for veterinary procedures. Proc Am Assn Zoo Vet, St. Louis, Missouri, pp. 65–69.

16. Reichard, T. 2008. Behavioral training for medical procedures. In: Fowler, M.E., and Miller, R.E., Eds. Zoo and Wild Animal Medicine, 6th Ed. St. Louis, Saunders/Elsevier, pp. 66–67.

17. Steele, B. 1992. Training elephants. In: Shoshani, J., Ed. Elephant Majestic Creatures of the Wild. Emmaus, Pennsylvania, Rodale Press, pp. 155–7.

18. Stringfield, C.E., and McNary, J.K. 1998. Operant conditioning of diabetic primates to accept insulin injections. Proc Am Assn Zoo Vet, and Am Assn Wildlife Vet, Omaha, Nebraska, pp. 396–7.

19. Wiebe, S.C. 2002. Phlebotomy through operant conditioning in captive tigers Panthers tigris. Proc Am Assn Zoo Vet, Milwaukee, Wisconsin, pp. 65–67.

CHAPTER 7
Stress

Stress is the cumulative response of an animal to interaction with its environment via receptors[6] or as another author defines it, "stress is the biological response elicited when an animal perceives a threat to its homeostasis" (Fig. 7.1).[12] The threat is a stressor (stress-producing factor), and it is important to recognize that a psychological perception of a threat may be as important as the response to a physical stressor.

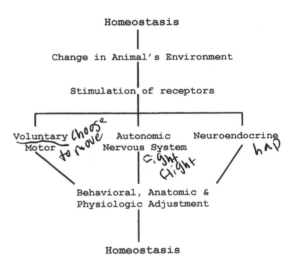

FIG. 7.1. Homeostasis mechanisms.

The biological responses brought about by stress are adaptive, directed at coping with environmental change, and every animal is subject to stress whether free-ranging or in captivity. Intense or prolonged stimulation may induce detrimental responses (distress).[12]

Species vary in their perception of a threat and how they process the information received to evoke a physiologic response. It is not possible to use any single laboratory parameter to determine the stress status of an animal.

Little significant research has been conducted of stress in wild animals, so the following discussion is based on research in some domestic animals and human beings. It is important to understand that animals do become distressed.

A stressor is any stimulus that elicits a biological response when perceived by an animal (Table 7.1).[6,7,8] A listing of some of the potential stressors acting on animals may direct attention to consideration of these important factors when handling animals. Somatic stressors (stimulation of the physical senses) include temperature changes, strange sights, unfamiliar sounds

TABLE 7.1. Receptors responding to stressors

Teleceptors (Stimuli received from a distance)
  Sight (visual)
  Sound (auditory)
  Odor (olfactory)
Exteroceptors (Cutaneous stimuli)
  Heat (thermal)
  Cold (thermal)
  Touch
  Pressure (proprioceptor)
  Pain (nociceptor)
Interceptors (Visceral and internal stimuli)
  Hunger
  Thirst
  Taste (chemoceptor)
  Oxygen and Carbon Dioxide tension (carotid body)
  Deep pressure
  Body position (vestibular)

and touches, or odors, thirst, and hunger (Fig. 7.2). Stimulation of receptors during restraint may occur by actions illustrated in Figure 7.3.

Psychological stressors include anxiety, fright, terror, anger, rage, and frustration. Closely allied are behavioral stressors, including overcrowding, lack of social contact, unfamiliar surroundings, transport, and lack of appropriate foods. Miscellaneous stressors include malnutrition, toxins, parasites, infectious agents, burns, surgery, and drugs.

It is becoming more and more important to recognize that stimulation of visual and auditory senses have a marked bearing on accumulative stress. Modern interpretation makes no distinction between specific and nonspecific responses,

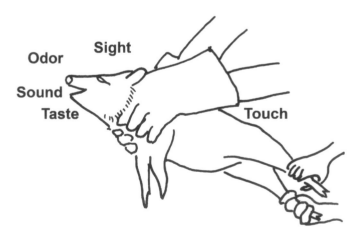

FIG. 7.2. Physical sensory stressors that may be stimulated during restraint.

Restraint responses

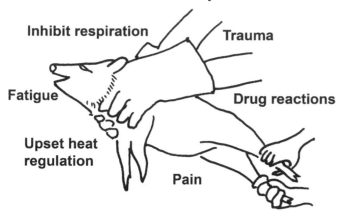

FIG. 7.3.   Actions that may occur during restraint.

Adrenaline response

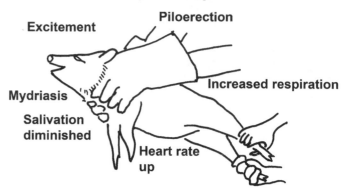

FIG. 7.4.   Epinephrine (Adrenaline) responses.

because there is marked species variation in how organisms process and act upon stimuli.[3,9] There may even be varying responses from an individual, depending upon which stimuli are acting upon it at a given time and the experience, hierarchical status, nutrition status, or history of a previous adaptation to the stimulus.[6,10,13]

BODY RESPONSE TO STRESS STIMULATION

The central nervous system (CNS) receives messages from receptors, processes the information, and initiates a biological response through one or more of the following pathways: behavior, autonomic nervous system, neuroendocrine system, or immune system.[6]

Animals respond in appropriate ways to stimulation of specific receptors. For instance, when cold receptors are stimulated, the body experiences a sensation of coolness. Various somatic and behavioral changes occur that conserve heat and stimulate increased heat production. The animal is adjusting to a new situation (homeostatic accommodation). If heat is the stressor, the animal tries to take steps to cool itself.[6]

The autonomic nervous system deals with short-term stress responses (flight or fight scenario); however, any tissue

innervated by autonomic nerves may be affected (such as, increased peristalsis) (Fig. 7.4, Table 7.2). The autonomic nervous system is of lesser importance in distress because the duration of stimulation is usually short, but if prolonged, it may become a factor.

The neuroendocrine system is a major pathway for the development of distress. Often this pathway is thought to be the hypothalamic-pituitary-adrenocortical (HPA) pathway (Fig. 7.5). However, modern research has conclusively demonstrated that all systems modulated by the hypothalamic-pituitary axis may be affected (growth, reproduction, immunity, metabolism, behavior).

Individual animals and species vary in the primary pathway utilized to cope with change. The pathways used by most wild animals are unknown. However, continuous adrenal cortex stimulation and excessive production of cortisol elicit many adverse metabolic responses. Psychological as well as physical changes may occur. The clinical syndromes of adrenocortical stimulation have been identified in some species (human, dog, horse, laboratory animals). There is much still to learn about the effects of hypercorticism in wild animals. However, the basic biologic effects of cortisol should be understood.[3,6,9,10]

Protein catabolism and lipolysis contribute to the pool for glyconeogenesis. Slight to moderate hyperglycemia has a diuretic effect, producing polyuria and polydipsia. Prolonged

TABLE 7.2.   **Detailed effects of sympathetic stimulation**

Effector Organ	Norepinephrine Response (α receptors)	Epinephrine Response (β receptors)
Eye	Mydriasis	Relaxation of ciliary muscle for far vision
Heart	No response	Increased heart rate Contractility increased
Blood vessels		
Coronary	Vasodilatation	Vasodilatation
Skin	Vasoconstriction	Vasodilatation
Skeletal muscle	Vasodilatation	Vasodilatation
Abdominal viscera	Vasoconstriction	No response
Lung		
Bronchial muscles	No response	Relaxation
Intestines		
Motility and tone	Decrease	Relaxation
Sphincters	Contraction	No response
Skin		
Pilomotor	Contraction	No response
Sweat glands	Slight localized secretions	No response
Salivary glands	Thick, viscous secretion	Amylase secretion

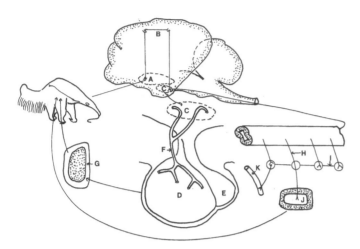

FIG.–7.5. Neuroendocrine pathways (Hypothalamic Adenohypophyseal Pathways [HAP]). **A.** Thalamus. **B.** Neocortex. **C.** Hypothalamus. **D.** Anterior pituitary. **E.** Posterior pituitary. **F.** Hypothalamic adenohypophyseal portal vein. **G.** Adrenal cortex. **H.** Preganglionic fibers of sympathetic nerves. **I.** Sympathetic trunk. **J.** Adrenal medulla. **K.** Intestine.

hyperglycemia stimulates the beta cells of the pancreas to produce more insulin.

Cortisol reduces the heat, pain, and swelling associated with the inflammatory response, an effect useful in the treatment of many diseases. The anti-inflammatory action of cortisol is brought about by reducing capillary endothelial swelling, thus diminishing capillary permeability. Additionally, capillary blood flow is decreased by the action of cortisol. Both of these actions are helpful in shock therapy.

The integrity of lysosomal membranes is enhanced by cortisol. Under such circumstances, bacteria and other particulate matter are engulfed by phagocytes, but hydrolytic enzymes (which would destroy the organisms) are not released from the lysosomes.

Within a few hours of a cortisol stress response, there is a reduction in the number of circulating lymphocytes (50% or greater). Lymphocyte levels return to normal within 24 to 48 hours following cessation of stress. The effect of stress on the total leukocyte count varies with the species, and depends upon the normal relative leukocyte distribution. Species with normally high percentages of lymphocytes, such as mice, rabbits, chickens, and cattle, respond with a lymphopenia and neutrophilia and a decrease in total leukocytes. Dogs, cats, horses, and human beings, having relatively low lymphocyte counts, respond with an increase in leukocytes.[6]

Eosinophil production decreases in response to elevated levels of cortisol. Eosinophil production is directly related to histamine production, such as occurs in the event of tissue injury or allergic reactions. Cortisol neutralizes histamines and inhibits re-granulation of mast cells, thus further reducing histamine production. The elevated production of cortisol

during stress results in eosinopenia. Catecholamines also cause eosinopenia; thus emotional stress may elicit a stress hemogram. In addition, cortisol stimulates increased production of circulating erythrocytes. Serum calcium levels decrease through inhibition of calcium absorption from the gastrointestinal tract.

Stress ulceration of the gastrointestinal system is a well-known syndrome in humans, rats, and marine mammals. Whether or not stress is a factor in wild animal ulcers is unknown, but studies have determined the basic effect of cortisol on the digestive system. Most of the studies have been performed on humans and laboratory animals, and as there may be significant species differences, direct extrapolation is unwise. The pathogenesis of gastric stress ulcers in humans and marine mammals is multifactorial. Hypercortisolism causes hypersecretion of acid and digestive enzymes. A duodenal reflux introduces substances from the duodenum into the stomach (lysolecithin) that reduces the effectiveness of the mucous membrane barrier. A third factor is vasoconstriction of the vasculature of the stomach, which in turn causes local hypoxia and a deficiency of adenosine triphosphate. These also contribute to the reduction of the mucous membrane barrier. Whether these factors operate in wild animals is unknown, but the possibility should be considered.

Catecholamines (epinephrine) contribute to the production of gastric secretions, so stimuli mediated via the sympathetic nervous system (fear, anxiety, frustration, anger) may have a potential effect on ulcerogenesis.

OTHER ENDOCRINE RESPONSES TO STRESS REPRODUCTION

Intense and prolonged stressor stimulation has been found to be detrimental to the normal reproductive cycle.[4,11] Acute response to stress caused by restraint or transportation has been found to inhibit ovulation in livestock.[11,13] Stressor stimulation may prevent ovulation by inhibition of the preovulatory secretion of luteinizing hormone (LH). Another mechanism may be via the HPA axis, which may inhibit corticotropin-releasing hormone, which is essential for the production of gonadotropin-releasing hormone (GnRH), which, in turn, is essential for ovulation to occur.

METABOLISM

Metabolic changes associated with stress may shift resources that are needed for basic functions such as growth, especially during critical growth stages. Suppression of thyroid function occurs as a result of neuroendocrine derangement.

IMMUNITY

Several mechanisms may act on the immune system to inhibit normal immunocompetence.[2,6,9,10] Interference with

DNA synthesis causes atrophy of lymphoid tissue throughout the body. Cell-mediated immune responses are diminished, an effect that may interfere with appropriate response to vaccination and tuberculin-testing programs. Lymphopenia decreases the number of leukocytes available to combat infection.

DIAGNOSIS OF STRESS

Signs vary with the pathway stimulated. Since few studies have been conducted on stress in wild animals, it is unlikely that a diagnosis can be made on the basis of signs. No single laboratory determination is definitive as a diagnostic tool for distress, but plasma cortisol levels are commonly used as an indication of stress.[14] However, just the collection of blood from a wild animal for analysis may cause an increase in plasma cortisol. Steroid levels in feces and urine are used as indicators in some wild animals, and salivary cortisol has been used as a noninvasive method to monitor stress in elephants.

In one captive Asian elephant cow, salivary cortisol predictably rose from a baseline of 6.17 ± 1.43 nmol/L to 31.8 nmol/L following introduction into a new herd.[5] Plasma cortisol is only one measure of stress. Of equal importance to this study was that the stressor stimulation was of short duration (2 days) after which cortisol levels returned to baseline levels. Thus the introduction into a new herd did not produce lasting distress in this elephant.

Stress response protein (SRP) profiling is a novel technique currently under investigation in elephants as a method to detect chronic physiologic stress and disease.[1] It is based on measuring levels of 40 stress response proteins using immunohistochemical staining and image analysis. Stress-related alterations in SRP profiles are similar among the mammalian species studied thus far and appear capable of differentiating healthy animals from those with disease or physiological stress.[1]

PATHOLOGY

The lesions produced by distress (harmful stress) are difficult to document. Pathologists often negate a diagnosis of death caused by stress. Many of the effects of stress are functional, leaving no definitive lesion to mark their presence. Nonetheless, it is known that tissues and organs are weakened by prolonged insult, lowering resistance to disease. Classic lesions are lymphoid tissue atrophy, adrenal cortical hyperplasia, and gastrointestinal ulceration. Though the actual cause of death may be pneumonia, parasitism, or starvation, stress may have paved the way for development of these terminal ailments.[14]

SUMMATION

Stress is ever present in both free-ranging and captive wild animals. It is crucial that stress remains at levels that are beneficial to the animal and do not rise to become distress, which is detrimental to animal well-being. Veterinarians providing health care for any animal should consider stress as a contributory factor in specific diseases. Husbandry practices should be evaluated and correction of those that may be harmful recommended. Some wild animals are social animals. Isolation for therapy or recuperation may be counterproductive. Malnutrition is a stressor, as are repeated and prolonged restraint episodes.

The stress response mechanisms employed by most wild animals are unknown, which should make research on the effects of stress a high priority. More detailed information about stress may be obtained from the references.

REFERENCES

1. Bechert, U.S., and Southern, S. 2002. Monitoring environmental stress in African elephants *Loxodonta africana*, through molecular analysis of stress-activated proteins. Proc Am Assoc Zoo Vet, pp. 249–53.
2. Blecha, F. 2000. Immunity system response to stress. In: Moberg, G.P., and Mench, J.A. 2000. The Biology of Animal Stress, Basic Principles and Implications for Animal Welfare. New York, CABI Publishing, pp. 11–118.
3. Breazile, J.E. 1987. Physiologic basis and consequences of distress in animals. J Am Vet Med Assoc 10:1212.
4. Coubrough, P.I. 1985. Stress and fertility, a review. Onderstepoort J Vet Res 52:153.
5. Dathe, H.H., Kucelkorn, B., and Minnemann, D. 1992. Salivary cortisol assessment for stress detection in the Asian elephant *Elephas maximus*: a pilot study. Zoo Biology 11:285–289.
6. Fowler, M.E. 1995. Stress. In: Fowler, M.E. 1995. Restraint and Handling of Wild and Domestic Animals. 2nd Ed. Ames, Iowa State University Press. pp. 57–66.
7. Fowler, M.E. 1998. Stress. In: Fowler, M.E. Medicine and Surgery of South American Camelids, 2nd Ed. Ames, Iowa State University Press, pp. 232–42.
8. Fowler, M.E. 2006. Multisystem disorders (stress). In: Fowler, M.E., and Mikota, S.K., Eds. Biology, Medicine and Surgery of Elephants. Ames, Iowa, Blackwell Publishing, pp. 243–53.
9. Hattingh, J., and Petty, D. 1992. Comparative physiological responses to stressors in animals. Comparative Biochemistry and Physiology A-Comparative-Physiology 101(1):113–16.
10. Moberg, G.P. 1985. Biological response to stress: Key to assessment of animal well-being. In: Moberg, G.P., Ed., Animal Stress, Bethesda, MD, American Physiological Society.
11. Moberg, G.P. 1985. Influences of stress on reproduction: Measure of well-being. In: Moberg, G.P., Ed., Animal Stress, Bethesda, MD, American Physiological Society, pp. 27–50.
12. Moberg, G.P. 1987. Problems of defining stress and distress in animals. J Am Vet Med Assoc 191:1207–11.
13. Moberg, G.P. 2000. Biological response to stress: Implications for animal welfare. In: Moberg, G.P., and Mench, J.A. 2000. The Biology of Animal Stress, Basic Principles and Implications for Animal Welfare. New York, CABI Publishing, pp. 1–22.
14. Spraker, T.R. 1993. Stress and capture myopathy in artiodactylids. In: Fowler, M.E. 1993. Zoo and Wild Animal Medicine, Current Veterinary Therapy, 3rd Ed. Philadelphia, W.B. Saunders, pp. 481–88.

CHAPTER 8

Animal Welfare Concerns During Restraint

All animals maintained in captivity should be treated humanely and provided with potable water, nutritious food, proper handling, health care, and a proper environment. Furthermore, all animals should be treated with respect. Fear, pain, suffering, and distress should be kept to a minimum. From a humane and moral standpoint, the minimum amount of restraint consistent with accomplishing a necessary task should be used. It is incumbent upon a person who assumes the responsibility for managing domestic and either captive or free-ranging wildlife to be concerned about the animal's well-being. Everyone would agree that animal's well-being is an important issue.[1,3,6–9,12–15,17,21,23,25,26,28]

DEFINITION OF TERMS

Many terms are used by different individuals and organizations to describe human associations with animals.[4,5,19,20,24]

Animal welfare: Providing for the physical and mental well-being of an animal (health, readiness to breed and reproduce, appropriate behavior for the species, and willingness to work). Criteria for judging the health of an animal include appropriate weight, appetite, feeding a proper diet, normal body functions (breathing, defecating, urinating), and normal life span. Ultimate judgment of health requires full knowledge and understanding of an animal's biology, natural behaviors, and life in its native environment.

Animal well-being: Maintaining an animal in optimal health (physical and mental) includes minimizing stress.

Animal rights: A system, advocated by some, that animals should have legal rights equal to those guaranteed people by the United States Constitution.

Animal Rights Advocates: Advocates who make proposals concerning animal rights issues. Some advocates believe that no animal should ever be in captivity; that all zoos and circuses should be eliminated; and that people should not have pets, companion animals, or farm animals. They espouse vegetarianism and are against the use of animal products (leather, silk, wool). They are also against the use of animals in research and are essentially against conservation.

Animal Rights Activists: Persons acting in support of a cause. They usually are vegetarian and have animal-friendly habits. They proselyte for their cause and may be active in organized peaceful disruption of animal activities.

Animal Rights Extremists: Individuals who advocate animal rights and may participate in acts of violence such as liberating captive animals, destroying property, sabotage, harassing people, and even threatening humans with death. Several extremist organizations are listed by the Federal Bureau of Investigation (FBI) as being domestic terrorist groups.

WHAT DOES ANIMAL RIGHTS ACTIVISM HAVE TO DO WITH RESTRAINT?

Restraint is absolutely necessary for many animal husbandry procedures and certainly for many veterinary procedures.[26–28] Some restraint procedures may be considered forms of animal abuse by misinformed individuals. Therefore, it is incumbent upon those who care for animals to use appropriate procedures and with the minimal amount of restraint necessary to accomplish a task. A restraint procedure should be chosen based on what has to be done and should be humane and safe for both animal and handlers.

Zoos have special challenges, because many procedures must be done in view of the public, who may be critical if the procedure seems to inflict pain or unnecessary roughness. It may be necessary for a knowledgeable zoo spokesperson to be present to explain what and why certain procedures are necessary.

The visiting public and animal rights organizations are quick to pick up on what they perceive as behavioral abnormalities, such as stereotypic behavior, weaving, head-bobbing, self mutilation, and aggressiveness, some of which may actually be physiologic. For example, shifting in elephants (shifting weight from one leg to the leg on the opposite side) is thought by some to be only a stereotypic behavior. In reality it may serve a necessary physiologic function. The venous return of blood from the foot back to the heart is facilitated by a periodic compression of the digital cushion, which in turn compresses the veins and helps propel the blood back to the heart.

WHAT ARE ZOOS DOING TO PROMOTE ANIMAL WELL-BEING?

The American Zoos and Aquariums Association (AZA) has a program for accrediting zoos that meet high standards of animal care, including having adequate veterinary services.[12-16] Keepers are being trained (in-house and externally). Enclosures are being upgraded. Many zoos are participating in the conservation of free-ranging wild animals away from the zoo and are cooperating in Species Survival Plans (SSP) with captive populations. Scientific research is promoted by AZA.

The economic resources of a zoo should be allocated first to animal well-being. If appropriate enclosures or other facilities (restraint chutes, protection from adverse environmental influences, water quality) are not available, zoo managers should refrain from exhibiting a species until the criteria have been met.

Poor animal care is indicated by reduced life expectancy, impaired growth, impaired reproduction, injury, disease, immunosuppression, behavioral anomalies, self-narcotization, unresponsiveness, and stereotypes.

Public Relations

Unfortunately, some animals are abused by their owners. Some animal rights activists insist that any animal kept in captivity is abused. It is hard to counteract unwarranted criticism.[18] Zoos have some special challenges with public relations issues. Following are some suggestions to minimize conflicts with the public:

- Establish trust with the public (visitors, media, humane societies) by being friendly, cooperative, and honest.
- Educate by assuming that critics have been misinformed as to the true facts or lack of knowledge.
- Practice the Golden or Silver Rule: Treat others as you would like to be treated.
- Identify a person to speak for the institution.
- Make time for meetings with media personnel.
- Invite media to spend time at the zoo, especially for unique occasions.
- Prepare short news releases on zoo happenings.
- Clear all communications with the P.R. person and make sure the director is appraised.
- Be loyal to the institution you represent.

Misinformation

The author was in charge of the veterinary monitoring team for a 100-mile equine endurance trail ride. A person with a video camera closely observed as horses were being examined at various checkpoints. Later, adverse comments were added to the edited video, which was then sent to third-party "specialists" for their evaluation. Without having seen any of the animals, but accepting the narration and edited video provided, these "specialists" made a scathing report stating that these horses were abused. The editors had included close ups of minor scratches on the leg as an example of horrible wounds inflicted on the trail. White hair spots on the withers were cited as evidence of saddle sores inflicted on the ride. No video was taken of a horse that came into a checkpoint in a near-exhausted state, but which recovered nicely with rest. It was obvious that the cameraperson knew nothing about horses.

Following the ride I received a telephone call from the president of a national humane association who proceeded to tell me how terrible we were to subject those horses to such abuse. He claimed that the horses were forced to go on the ride and were in pain and agony throughout the ride. I asked him if he had ever seen a trail ride. "No, but people told me how bad they are." "Do you own a horse?" "No." "Have you ever ridden a horse?" "No." He was told that the horses were well-trained and enjoyed the activity. He was asked to call back later when he knew a little more about horses and what they could and could not do.

FARM ANIMAL WELFARE

Animals used for food and fiber or work were domesticated before recorded history. People became intimately acquainted with the behavior of their animals and adopted husbandry and restraint procedures that served the needs of both the animals and the people.[22] The animals were generally kept in environments that allowed the animals to express their normal behavior patterns. Procedures were usually applied that provided for good animal welfare.

It wasn't until the advent of intensive animal production, approximately 50 years ago, that the general public and animal rights organization began to question whether or not some intensive practices are consistent with animal welfare. It is not the intent of the author to dwell on the conflict between producers and animal rights activists. The literature on this subject is voluminous, and there is minimal "middle ground." Research, to explore sound alternative management practices, is critical to solving the dilemma.[10,22]

It is necessary for cattle handlers to understand behavior. Many people in the cattle business lack knowledge of flight distance, balance point, and reasons for balking.

Poor restraint and handling of beef cattle is fostered by "cowboying" the cattle. This is a cultural and attitudinal problem[22], because cattle may be trained to enter chutes or they can be poked, prodded, and yelled at. Proper animal welfare should encourage gentleness. Proper design of chute systems fosters cattle compliance without elevated stress levels.

Transporting animals is a significant stressor in livestock operations. Loading and unloading are especially hazardous. Roughness, electrical shocking (hot-shot, cattle-prod), and shouting should be avoided. Fright is a known psychological stressor.[11]

Poor equipment, poor maintenance of equipment, and improper use of restraint facilities contributes to poor animal handling, hence poor animal welfare. This is an area that should be researched to develop more animal-friendly restraint devices.[11]

GOVERNMENTAL REGULATION OF ANIMAL WELFARE

Local, state, and federal legislation exist for animal welfare in many countries of the world, including the United States (Table 8.1). In the United States, privately owned companion animals and farm animals are protected by anti-cruelty laws, which may entail confiscation by Animal Control agencies of animals being abused or mistreated. The Federal Animal Welfare Act (AWA) was first enacted in 1966 and has been revised several times since.[2] This act was meant to protect animals used in research and on exhibit. It includes regulation standards for dogs, cats, guinea pigs, hamsters, rabbits, nonhuman primates, and marine mammals (Code of Federal Regulations 9 Part 3, sub-parts A thru E). Sub-part F covers general standards for other warm-blooded animals not otherwise covered in the other parts. Sub-part F covers animals used in research but also those exhibited in licensed facilities covered by the Animal Care division of the Animal and Plant Health Inspection Service (APHIS) of the United States Department of Agriculture (USDA). Local and state governments may enact more stringent regulations.

TABLE 8.1. Agencies Responsible for Animal Welfare in the United States

Federal
U.S. Department of Agriculture (USDA), Animal and Plant Health Inspection Service (APHIS)
Animal Welfare Act (1970) for exhibit and research animals
U.S. Department of Interior (USDI)
U.S. Department of Fisheries and Wildlife
Endangered Species Act
U.S. Department of Commerce
Marine Mammal Act
State, County, and City regulations

REFERENCES

1. Anetelyes, J. 1986. Animal rights in perspective. J Amer Vet Med Assoc 189:757–59.
2. Anonymous. 2005. Animal Welfare Act and Animal Welfare Regulations, Washington, D.C. United States Department of Agriculture, Animal and Plant Health Inspection Service.
3. Appleby, M. 1999. What should we do about animal welfare? Oxford, Blackwell Sci 1999:36–37.
4. Baggot, S.M. 2006. Veterinarians as advocates for animal rights. J Am Vet Med Assn 229(3):350–52.
5. Blum, D. 1994. The Monkey Wars. New York, Oxford University Press.
6. Broom, D.M. 1991. Animal welfare: concepts and measurements. J Animal Sci 69:4167–75.
7. Drayer, M.E., Ed. 1998. The Animal Dealers. Washington, D.C., Animal Welfare Institute.
8. Duncan, I.J.H. 1981. Animal rights-animal welfare: A scientist's perception. Poultry Sci 60:489–99.
9. Duncan, I.J.H. 1996. Animal welfare defined in terms of feelings. Acta Agric. Scand. Section A, Animal Sci. Supplementum 27:29–35.
10. Grandin, T. 2000. Livestock Handling and Transport, 2nd Ed. Wallingford, Oxon, U.K. CABI Publishing.
11. Grandin, T. 2000. Habituating antelope and bison to cooperate with veterinary procedures. J Applied Animal Welfare Science 3(3):253–61.
12. Hutchins, M., Smith, B., and Allard, R. 2002. In defense of zoos and aquariums: The ethical basis for keeping wild animals in captivity. J Am Vet Med Assoc 223(7):958–65.
13. Kirtland, J. 2000. Animal welfare activist or animal rights extremist: Whose side are you on? J Elephant Managers' Association 11(3)164–69.
14. Koontz, F.W. 1995. Wild animal acquisition ethics for zoo biologists. In: Norton, B.G., Hutchins, M., Stevens, E.F., and Maple, T.L., Eds. Ethics in the Ark, Washington, D.C., Smithsonian Institution Press, pp. 127–45.
15. Laule, G.E. 2002. Positive reinforcement training and environmental enrichment: enhancing animal well-being. J Am Vet Med Assoc 223(7):969–72.
16. Maple, T.L. 2002. Strategic collection planning and individual animal welfare. J Am Vet Med Assoc 223(7):966–68.
17. Norton, B.G., Hutchins, M., Stevens, E.F., and Maple, T.L., Eds. 2002. Ethics on the Ark: Zoos, Animal Welfare and Wildlife Conservation. Washington, D.C. Smithsonian Institution Press.
18. Oliver, D.T. 1999. Animal Rights: The Inhumane Crusade. Bellevue, Washington, Merrill Press.
19. Regan, T. The case for animal rights. Berkeley, University of California Press.
20. Regan, T., and Singer, P., Eds. 1989. Animal Rights and Human Obligations. 2nd ed. Englewood Cliffs, New Jersey, Prentice-Hall.
21. Rollins, B.E. 1992. Animal Rights and Human Morality, Revised ed. Buffalo, New York, Prometheus Books.
22. Rollins, B.E. 1995. Farm Animal Welfare: Social, Bioethical, and Research Issues. Ames, Iowa State University Press.
23. Scigaliano, E. 2002. Love, War, and Circuses: The Age-old Relationship Between Elephants and Humans. Boston, Houghton Mifflin Company.
24. Singer, P., Ed. 1985. In Defense of Animals. Oxford, U.K. Basil Blackwell, Inc.
25. Spedding, C. 2000. Animal Welfare. London, Earthscan Publications.
26. Tannenbaum, J. 1995. Veterinary Ethics, Animal Welfare, Client Relations, Competition and Collegiality, 2nd Ed. St. Louis, Missouri, CV Mosby Co., pp 166–70, 173.
27. Tresz, H. 2006. Behavioral management at the Phoenix Zoo: New strategies and perspectives. J Applied An Welfare Science 90(1):65–70.
28. Wielebnowski, N. 2003. Stress and distress: evaluating their impact for the well-being of zoo animals. J Am Vet Med Assoc 223(7):973–76.

CHAPTER 9

Medical Problems During Restraint

Persons who are responsible for restraint procedures must be continually alert to prevent or deal with medical problems or emergencies arising during restraint. Emergencies may arise even under ideal conditions. The behavior of any animal is unpredictable when it is excited as a result of a restraint procedure. Injuries may occur or metabolic changes, inapparent to the eye, may take place. Either or both may result in incapacitation or death.

It is not my intent to discourage the use of animal restraint techniques by dwelling on the myriad adverse conditions that may arise therefrom; rather, it is to emphasize some severe potential problems in order to encourage restrainers to take precautions to prevent or alleviate them. Prevention must be the byword. To prevent medical problems, it is important to recognize and minimize the animal's exposure to potential etiological hazards. When emergencies arise, the restrainer should be prepared to take immediate remedial action.

The objective of this chapter is to provide for the person untrained in veterinary medicine an overview of medical problems and to review basic medical techniques for the veterinary clinician. Further details may be obtained from standard veterinary medical texts and references.[1,3,5,6,12,15,16,21]

PREPARATION FOR RESTRAINT PROCEDURES

The restrainer should plan carefully and anticipate problems, thinking through in detail each section of the procedure. A written plan may be necessary for the novice. In any case, possible counteractions should be planned for every conceivable contingency. Think safety—first, for people involved in the procedure; second, for the animal. Consider whether or not the designed procedure will permit completion of the necessary task.

All tools should be on hand and in proper repair. It is tragic to snare an animal only to find that the release mechanism is malfunctioning. The animal may strangle before a tight snare can be released.

Severe hemorrhage and respiratory arrest are two conditions requiring immediate attention. Digital pressure and pressure bandaging will usually control hemorrhage until ligation and/or suturing can be done. The restrainer should always be prepared to clear airways, assist respiration, and provide supplemental oxygen.

Peracute Death from Restraint
Ventricular fibrillation
Cholinergic bradycardia
Anoxia—Strangulation
Hemorrhage
Hypoglycemia
Brain concussion or contusion

Animals sometimes die during restraint. The text boxes in this chapter list the most common causes of death, based on rapidity of mortality. Each will be discussed in some detail. These killers should be kept uppermost in mind when preparing for a restraint procedure.

Of only slightly less concern to the animal restrainer are animals that become unconscious during the manipulative period. The conditions likely to result in unconsciousness are provided in the following text box. Note that many of these conditions may end in death if proper therapeutic measures are not quickly instituted.

Hypnosis is not a medical problem but rather a tool that may be used by the restrainer. (See Chapter 2.) However, hypnosis complicates differential diagnosis in an unconscious animal.

Acute Death from Restraint
(Minutes to hours)
Adrenal insufficiency
Gastric dilation—Bloat
Hyperthermia
Acidosis
Hypocalcemia
Hypoglycemia
Fracture of cervical vertebrae

Delayed Death from Restraint (Hours/Days)
Capture myopathy—Cardiac necrosis
Gastric dilation—bloat
Gangrenous pneumonia—regurgitation

Continued

Hypothermia
Shock—trauma
Causes of Unconsciousness in a Restrained Animal
Adrenal insufficiency
Anoxia
Brain concussion
Cholinergic bradycardia
Ventricular fibrillation
Hemorrhage
Hypnosis
Hypoglycemia
Hypothermia
Shock

TRAUMA

Hemorrhage (bleeding)

DEFINITION. Hemorrhage is loss of blood from the vascular system. Hemorrhage may be internal, taking place within tissues (hematoma), organs (as into the intestine), or into body cavities; or external, in which vessels are opened to the surface, allowing blood to escape.

ETIOLOGY. Lacerations are the most common cause of hemorrhage during restraint. Disruption of small vessels and capillaries is of little consequence to larger animals, but transection of large arteries or veins may be life threatening to any animal. Contusions may likewise result in extensive blood loss, because many animals have pliable skin that stretches to accommodate large quantities of subcutaneous fluid. Hemorrhage leading to the development of a hematoma may originate from capillary oozing or rupture of a single large vessel.

Hemorrhage accompanies fractures. If sharp bone ends are not quickly immobilized, they may sever arteries and veins coursing near the free ends of the bone. Fractures of the femur are especially dangerous because of potential laceration of the large femoral artery, which would result in rapid exsanguination.

CLINICAL SIGNS. Surface hemorrhage is obvious, but it is difficult for the inexperienced person to assess the extent of blood loss. Blood dispersed over the floor or walls of an enclosure appears to be more voluminous than it really is. Animal owners often become highly excited at seeing such blood and assume the animal is dying. Except when major arteries and veins are transected, larger animals rarely die because of lacerations. Any blood loss is much more dangerous for tiny animals.

Blood volume in vertebrates, as a percentage of body weight, varies from species to species, from 5 to 16%.[7,18] The average blood volume for humans is reported as 7.7% body weight.[7] The blood volume of birds varies from 5 to 13%, depending on species, age, sex, and functional status.[9] Loss of 15–20% of the blood volume produces no clinical signs in

humans. Loss of 30–35% may be life threatening, and loss of 40–50% is usually fatal. The blood volume of a 4,500-kg (9,900-lb) elephant is approximately 360 L (95 U.S. gal.). A 50-g parakeet circulates 4 ml of blood. A 20% loss amounts to 0.8 ml. As can be seen, a few drops of blood lost from a parakeet is a matter of serious concern, whereas a loss of 80 L is inconsequential to an elephant.

Internal hemorrhage is not visible to the eye, but the consequences are equally as dangerous as those of external hemorrhage. Clinical signs associated with internal hemorrhage are pale mucous membranes and a rapid, shallow pulse. The most serious complication of hemorrhage is shock from vascular hypovolemia. Clinical signs are the same as above. Large hematomas that can be seen or palpated externally may develop from internal hemorrhage. With limb fractures, the swelling may be evident. Hematomas over the stifle or on the head are also apparent and may be easily identified by tapping with a large-bore needle, following customary surgical preparation at the site.

THERAPY. Identify the source of hemorrhage and stop the bleeding. Standard first aid techniques, taught for use in human beings and domestic animals, may be impossible to apply to a wild animal. Pressure bandages, digital pressure, or tourniquets—to constrict the blood vessels—are important techniques for stopping hemorrhage. When major vessels have been severed, it is necessary to isolate the vessel and ligate it. All these techniques require the animal to be in hand and quiet. With wild animals, this is the first problem to solve.

It is especially important that blood vessels be securely ligated and hemorrhage control is complete before releasing wild animals, since a second restraint to control subsequent bleeding magnifies stress. Wild animals also suffer from greater catecholamine response, with its accompanying higher blood pressures. When the animal is released, elevated blood pressure may destroy the clot, reinstituting hemorrhage.

If a developing hematoma is noticed, a pressure wrap or cold therapy may prevent further hemorrhage. When hemorrhage into a hematoma ceases, the serum gradually separates from the formed clot and the lesion becomes a seroma. This process may take 1–2 days. Small seromas may be resorbed. Seromas over 4 cm require incision for drainage. Little drainage can be accomplished with a needle and syringe. Usually it is prudent to wait 3–5 days before incising to allow healing of the ruptured vessel and adequate separation of the serum from the clot. If hemorrhage into the hematoma continues, consider the possibility of a coagulation defect. If the blood coagulates normally, it may be necessary to make a large incision to search for the ruptured vessel and ligate it to stop the bleeding. This is drastic therapy, instituted only as a last resort.

Institute replacement therapy if sufficient blood has been lost to threaten life. Although replacing a loss of blood volume with saline, dextrose, or other electrolyte solutions may help alleviate shock, whole blood is required when massive hemorrhage has occurred. Whole blood may be extremely difficult to obtain in the case of wild animals. Nearby zoos and research facilities have heretofore responded quickly to an urgent call for blood to save the life of a valuable and rare animal.

Cross matching should be carried out whenever possible, though little is known about the blood groups of most wild animals. Even if simple cross matching shows extreme incompatibility, at least one blood transfusion may be indicated in a life-threatening situation. The clinician must make a value judgment in this instance. It is unlikely that one transfusion will induce fatal anaphylactic shock, a common result of mismatched transfusions in humans. It is highly improbable that a wild animal has been exposed to many types of blood proteins. A second blood transfusion may be much more hazardous because the animal may have developed antibodies against such blood.

A hemogram is of little value in determining the extent of acute blood loss. The ratio of blood constituents remains essentially the same even following massive hemorrhage and a pronounced drop in total volume.

Laceration (wound, cut, bite, puncture, goring)

DEFINITION. A laceration is a wound resulting from disruption of the integrity of the skin, exposing underlying muscles, blood vessels, nerves, bones, and other tissue. Lacerations are a common result of restraint procedures.

ETIOLOGY. Many objects tear or incise the skin. Objects protruding into a cage or pen are extremely hazardous to animals, particularly during restraint when the excited animal exercises little caution to avoid them. Pieces of wire used to mend fencing, bolts on doors, and boards with rough edges or exposed ends are all potential sources of lacerations. It is important to recognize that objects need not be sharp to inflict such wounds. Blunt objects can severely lacerate when struck with the terrific force exerted by a frightened animal attempting to escape.

Other types of lacerations include those inflicted by the bites or scratches of cage mates during the excitement of capture.[4] This is a particular problem when dealing with primates in groups.

Hierarchical status may be upset as an animal attempts to elude capture. Free fighting may occur if one animal tries to hide behind another. An animal may even bite itself during these stressful periods. This behavior is known as "displacement activity;" that is, the animal is unable to escape so it resorts to other types of objectionable behavior such as biting itself or cage mates.

Goring wounds may be caused by animals with horns or antlers. Serious or fatal wounds may be inflicted when animals become impaled on objects in or around enclosures. Animals may jump onto the tops of fences and become impaled on posts or other objects attached to the top of the fence. One horse was fatally injured when it jammed the center divider pole of a trailer into the thoracic cavity, rupturing the anterior vena cava.

THERAPY. If only superficial structures have been exposed, standard wound treatment with debridement, suturing, or leaving the wound open may suffice. The wound should be given more intensive treatment if vital structures such as joint capsules, tendons, nerves, or arteries are exposed.

Antibiotics are of questionable value in the treatment of most lacerations. However, certain wounds seem prone to become highly septic, requiring antibiotic treatment. Bites from primates and snakes are particularly septic and should be treated with debridement and by establishing drainage—in addition to treatment with antibiotics. Many wounds resulting from bites and tears do not heal with first intention. Establish satisfactory drainage and leave the wound open to heal by granulation.

The severity of goring or other puncture wounds is difficult to assess. Sometimes, though not always, it is possible to establish the extent of the lesion with a blunt probe. The wound should be cleaned as thoroughly as possible and the animal should be monitored to determine whether vital structures have been penetrated. Punctures into thoracic and abdominal cavities are particularly dangerous and life threatening. Standard techniques of therapy are detailed in surgical textbooks.

Abrasion (scrape)

DEFINITION. An abrasion is a wound caused by erosion.

ETIOLOGY. Abrasions are frequently caused during restraint and may be self-inflicted through escape attempts. Abrasions may occur as an animal bolts against a fence or wall. A common mistake in the construction of animal enclosures is to place the posts on the inside of the fence, providing objects that are potential weapons for producing abrasions, contusions, and lacerations.

Abrasions may be inflicted by the restrainer. Animals immobilized with drugs are frequently grasped and dragged from one spot to another, abrading the undersurface. Large animals that are impossible to lift should be moved on a large, heavy canvas or a piece of plywood used as a stoneboat so that hair and skin are not eroded by dragging.

An animal fleeing capture may slip, fall, and slide along a rough concrete surface, seriously damaging the skin and underlying structures. A horse fell through a trailer floor while being transported and ground off the soles of its feet. Escaping animals frequently run without regard for the pain caused by erosion of their feet. Some panicked animals have worn hoofs or nails off to the bone. It is impossible to repair such injuries. In one instance a group of foals, frightened by handling for medication, escaped through an open gate and ran down a highway. Before the animals could be stopped and rounded up, two foals had worn the hoofs away, exposing the third phalanx. Both animals had to be euthanized.

CLINICAL SIGNS. Abrasions vary from the minimal damage of hair scraped off the surface to the severe trauma of total erosion of the skin, exposing or even eroding such vital structures as nerves, arteries, and bones.

THERAPY. Abrasion should be treated according to its severity. Obviously, in the case of simple hair loss, no therapy is needed. Many abrasions may be treated by simply cleaning the wound and applying soothing ointments. Abrasions involving vital structures must be treated surgically as well as medically.

Contusion (bruise)

DEFINITION. A contusion is injury to a tissue without laceration of the skin.

ETIOLOGY. Contusion results from a blow to the body surface, either self-inflicted (as when an animal collides against an object) or by an object striking the animal. Contusions often result when animals attempt to elude capture. They also may be inflicted by the handler hitting the animal with a stick or the metal hoop of a net. A contusion caused by a light blow may be limited to the skin and subcutaneous tissue. Heavier blows may seriously damage the periosteum of the bone or crush blood vessels and nerves, resulting in permanent disability.

CLINICAL SIGNS. Bruising may not be evident immediately following injury. Sometimes no surface injury is visible, even when deep structures have been severely damaged. Contusion of bone may result in a periostitis that may not be apparent for several days after occurrence of the injury.

Usually within moments following a blow, extravasation of blood or serum into the damaged area causes swelling, pain, and sometimes discoloration, depending on the thickness of the skin and the degree of pigmentation. Heat is another sign of contusion, as the inflammatory response develops quickly.

The color of a contusion varies with the length of time since the injury. Color is usually associated with hemorrhage. As hemoglobin progresses through various degenerative stages and is converted to other metabolites, various shades of red, blue, and green may be seen. Discoloration is not necessarily indicative of tissue necrosis.

PATHOGENSIS OF THE LESION. A contusion traumatizes cells, rupturing capillaries and other blood vessels and destroying cells through simple mechanical damage. Within moments the damaged area fills with extravasations of either plasma or whole blood escaping from the damaged vascular system. Such extravasation will continue until clotting mechanisms function or sufficient pressure develops to inhibit the further escape of fluids. How quickly this occurs depends on the location of the contusion.

In enclosed spaces such as the calvarium, the hoof, or next to the bone, pressure from extravasation may inhibit the actions of vital nerves, interfere with circulation, or interfere with brain function. When clotting takes place, serum in the area incites inflammation.

THERAPY. Immediately apply cold compresses and/or ice packs. Cold inhibits the extravasation of fluids into the area, reducing swelling and pain. It allows time for the normal protective mechanisms of the body to close off damaged vessels and may prevent the massive swelling that causes pressure damage. Ice may be applied directly or in a plastic bag. Do not, under any circumstances, put salt into ice and water, because salt lowers the temperature to the freezing point, damaging tissue. An animal may resent the temporary pain of the initial application of cold, but as the coolness anesthetizes the area, the pain subsides.

Simple contusions, not secondarily involving broken skin, usually do not require antibiotics as adjunct therapy.

Rope Burn

DEFINITION. Rope burn is an abrasive injury caused by the friction and heat generated as a rope moves rapidly over the body.

ETIOLOGY. The etiology of rope burn involves the entangling of an animal in lariats or nets used for restraint. Rope burns are usually inflicted during operations requiring the roping of animals or when hobbles are applied. Improper placement of hobbles or ropes used for casting may cause rope burns if the animal has sufficient freedom to rapidly kick against the rope, sawing it back and forth against the skin.

PATHOGENESIS OF THE LESION. The damage caused by rope burn is a combination of abrasion and the excessive heat generated by friction. The resulting injury is as serious as a burn produced by cautery or open flame. Deeper tissues are injured as well as surface structures.

CLINICAL SIGNS. Abrasion follows the path of the rope over the body or limb. Hair is removed and the skin discolored. In cases of severe rope burn, the skin may be penetrated, exposing subcutaneous structures. Within minutes after the injury is inflicted, fluid exudes from the surface. Swelling and inflammation quickly ensue.

THERAPY. Cold water or ice packs applied immediately to the surface is major first aid. The packs should be maintained for at least an hour. Once the initial effect has been overcome, apply ointment to soften the skin surface and prevent extravasation of fluids. Limbs should be dressed to keep dirt and other debris from contaminating open wounds.

HEAD AND NECK INJURIES
Brain Concussion and Contusion

DEFINITION. Concussion is the transient loss of brain function as the result of a blow to the head. It is a functional condition with no gross structural changes. A contusion is an extension of the concussion, wherein the brain sustains physical damage (hemorrhage, edema).

ETIOLOGY. Any blow to the head may result in concussion. Blows may be self-inflicted when an animal flings itself against a wall or ceiling. Birds frequently injure themselves by flying into glass walls or windows unperceived as barriers.

The use of sight barriers is extremely important when dealing with wild animals. Many wild animals do not perceive a chain link fence to be a barrier and may severely injure themselves if suddenly moved into an enclosure surrounded by this type of fence. Animals in flight may also attempt to escape through openings too small to accommodate them.

CLINICAL SIGNS. Immediate unconsciousness caused by a blow to the head is the primary clinical sign of concussion. Unconsciousness may be transitory or prolonged. If it persists longer than 24 hours, it is likely that organic damage has been done. Other signs are transitory vasomotor and respiratory malfunction, immediate loss of reaction to stimuli, loss of the corneal reflex, dilated pupils, and flaccid muscles. Vomiting occurs in some cases.

The clinical signs of contusion of the brain include either immediate or delayed unconsciousness. If the animal is not rendered unconscious initially, hemorrhage into the cranial cavity may produce delayed unconsciousness. Additional signs of brain contusion are seizures, ophisthotonus, absence of pupillary response, signs of cranial nerve damage, and failure of vital respiratory and cardiac functions.

THERAPY. The animal should be protected from further injury during the recovery period and shaded from sun and light. Such an animal usually has impaired thermoregulatory ability and may become either hyperthermic or hypothermic if not protected from exposure. The animal may be disoriented upon regaining consciousness and needs protection from hazards such as ponds, lakes, low fences, moats, and so on. A darkened, quiet stall or cage will reduce stimulation. Cold compresses applied to the head have initial value but are of little benefit once clinical signs have developed.

Usually little can be done medically to aid recovery of a wild animal suffering from a serious head injury. Although principles of neural surgery used in small animal practice may be applied, the prognosis is grave when dealing with wild species.

Fractures of the Skull

DEFINITION. A fracture is a break in the continuity of bone.

ETIOLOGY. Skull fractures may result from any blow to the head. Blows on the side of the skull (temporal region) or at the back of the head (occipital or nuchal region) are particularly dangerous. Animals that throw themselves over backward may strike the back of the head on surrounding objects or on the ground. Basilar skull fractures are a usual consequence.

CLINICAL SIGNS. Depression on the surface of the skull is the clinical sign of a fracture involving the calvarium. Rarely will crepitation be present. One should not palpate vigorously because of the danger of further depressing the fracture. Radiographs are the basis for a definitive diagnosis of fracture.

The animal with a fractured skull will exhibit varying degrees of central nervous involvement, such as paralysis or, if certain basal functions are disrupted, respiratory or cardiovascular failure. The animal will probably be unconscious. A superficial wound exposing the bone may or may not be seen.

THERAPY. The treatment of skull fractures is exceedingly difficult and must be conducted by a veterinary orthopedic surgeon. General treatment consists of protecting the animal from extremes of environment and preventing further injury from thrashing or convulsions. Vital functions should be monitored and respiratory and cardiovascular systems supported.

Horn and Antler Damage

Appendages of the head are frequently liable to injury as a result of restraint practices. Some of these structures are designed for active combat and will withstand considerable pressure. The bighorn sheep has massive horns capable of withstanding heavy blows. On the other hand, the slender horns of some antelope species are easily fractured or traumatized.

Antlers are bony extensions of the frontal bones developed by members of the family Cervidae. These structures are shed annually. As the antler begins to develop, it is covered with a highly vascularized epithelium known as "velvet." When the antler is mature the velvet is scraped off, leaving a highly polished, hard, branched structure on the head.

The antler is soft and easily broken during the developmental stage. Grasping immature antlers as handles during restraint or banging them against a wall or chute may easily fracture them. When developing antlers are fractured, extensive hemorrhage may result from laceration of the velvet. Less severe injuries during the velvet period may produce disfigured and asymmetrical antler growth.

When the velvet has been scraped off, the antler is hard and may serve as a handhold for the head, but if too much pressure is applied, the mature antler will also fracture. Since mature antlers are avascular, the only damage is deformity until the animal sheds again. Mature antlers of males may be sawed off a few inches from the skull to reduce danger to persons or other animals.

A horn is a specialized cornified epithelium overlying a bony core extension of the frontal bone of members of the family Bovidae.

Two types of horn injuries may occur during restraint. The first is contusion of the horn, resulting in separation of the outer covering from the bony core. The second type of injury is fracture of the bony core, separating it from the frontal bone.

ETIOLOGY. The horns of such species as the American bison are prone to injuries that pull the horn off the cornual process of the frontal bone. When these animals are confined in a chute for tuberculin testing or collecting blood samples, they may tear off the horn by raking the head up and down the side of a chute. Bleeding usually stops without treatment. The outer covering grows from the base of the horn at the corium and regenerates in time.

Antlers and horns may be damaged if an animal strikes its head against fences, walls, cages, or shipping crates. An animal may fracture a horn caught in a fence or in a crack in a door or wall. Delicate horns and antlers may be broken by grasping them as handholds. If horns or antlers must be used as handholds, the base of the horn or antler should be grasped to minimize the danger of injury.

CLINICAL SIGNS. Deformity of the structure is the most prominent sign of a fracture. Increased mobility may be either observed or palpated. Hemorrhage may be present, depending on the stage of development of antlers or whether the outer covering has been torn off the bony core of a horn.

When making a clinical examination of a fractured horn or antler, it is important to determine whether or not the skull has been fractured. Usually only the bony core of the horn fractures, but occasionally the frontal bones also fracture. Frontal bone fractures are serious because the frontal sinus is involved. Furthermore, such a fracture may open into the brain cavity.

THERAPY. It is impractical to attempt to repair fractures of antlers. Amputate the distal segment. Incise and remove the distal segment of an antler in velvet and apply a pressure bandage to the proximal segment to control hemorrhage.

A horn shell torn off the bony core cannot be reattached because the blood supply has been destroyed. If the bony core is intact, apply a soothing ointment such as antimicrobial ointment. In time a new horny shell will develop. If the horny shell is still in place but the bony core is fractured, attempt to stabilize the horn by clamping it to the opposite horn. A good clamping technique is to insert wooden blocks between the two horns and bind them together. Another technique is to wrap plumber's tape or perforated metal tape around the horns. Attach one to the other with a turnbuckle. Splinting the horn and wrapping the head with bandage and cotton may sufficiently stabilize the horn of a young animal.

Fractures of the frontal bone must be carefully reduced, the horn set into its proper place, and fixed with an appropriate splint or fixation device. It is important to recognize that injuries to the horn often result in hemorrhage from the nose because of the respiratory connection via the cornual process of the horn into the frontal sinus, thence to the maxillary sinus, and into the nose.

Facial Paralysis

Definition. Facial paralysis is a clinical syndrome produced by the disruption of facial nerve function. The facial nerve innervates muscles of the eyelid, cheek, and upper lips.

ETIOLOGY. During restraint, a blow to the jaw or to the side of the head may injure the facial nerve, especially if the blow strikes at a point where the nerve courses near a bone. A blow to that nerve may result in either temporary or permanent cessation of function.

CLINICAL SIGNS. Signs noted are dependent on the location of the damage to the nerve. If it occurs at the base of the ear, all the classical signs may be present. These are closure of the upper eyelid, inability to clear food from the cheek pouches, and pulling of the upper lip to the side of the face opposite the injury. Additionally, the facial nerve supplies some ear muscles. If the injury occurs near the ear, the ear may droop or fail to prick in response to auditory stimulation. Swelling over the lateral aspect of the face or jaw may or may not appear.

A second potential cause of facial paralysis is infection or abscess in or near the point at which the facial nerve emerges from the skull, near the base of the ear. An abscess may be noticed before restraint is begun, or it may be discovered as a result of the restraint practice.

A temporary or permanent rope halter left on an animal in prolonged lateral recumbency may produce point pressure on the facial nerve.

THERAPY. Most facial paralyses are transient, self-correcting in a few hours to a few days. In persistent paralysis, hot compresses may mobilize the constituents causing pressure on the nerve. Otherwise little can be done. Some clinicians recommend the use of large doses of steroids to slow the inflammatory process, but others feel such therapy is of little benefit.

Paralysis from Stretching the Neck

DEFINITION. Impaired neural or muscular function as a result of stretching the head and neck into abnormal positions.

ETIOLOGY. It is not unusual for the restrainer to grasp the head or neck when attempting to control an animal. Nerves and muscles of the head may be damaged by excessive stretching or twisting.

CLINICAL SIGNS. The head may be carried in a peculiar position. Onset may be noted immediately or several hours after restraint has been carried out. The animal may be unable to elevate the head, or the head may be deviated to one side as the result of unilateral damage to a nerve or muscle.

The most serious manifestation of neck injury is "wobbler syndrome" (idiopathic ataxia) of foals. Many affected foals have been injured by mishandling during restraint procedures for medication or examination. The cervical vertebrae have been twisted, resulting in a subluxation. Pressure is exerted on the spinal cord, causing disruption of motor function in the hindquarters.

THERAPY. No specific therapy has been found to be effective for conditions produced by damage to the neck. Symptomatic and/or supportive therapy is indicated.

LIMB INJURIES

Fracture (broken bones, a break)

DEFINITION. A fracture is disruption in the continuity of a bone. A complete discussion of various types of fractures, with clinical signs and recommendations for treatment, is not appropriate for this book, but it is important to know that the limbs of many species are easily fractured during restraint procedures. Extreme care must be exercised to minimize the pressures exerted on fragile bones by heavy-handed restrainers.

Fractures occur when limbs are caught in chutes, stanchions, walls, cargo doors, screen mesh, or wires. Bones may also be broken by injudiciously slamming the hoop of a capture net into an animal or by an animal jumping against trees, walls, or cages. Some fractures are a result of the stress inherent in capturing or moving groups of animals, which frequently leads to increased aggression, manifested by kicking or butting.

A startled animal usually initiates flight with a sudden jump. If the footing is poor the animal may fall. A fall as an animal attempts to whirl away on one leg may result in fracture of the femur or tibia in both wild and domestic species, particularly equine species.

Fractures may occur through unusual accidents. In one instance, when removing a Siberian ibex from a crate, a handler reached into the front and grabbed the horns. The animal bolted out of the crate and two or three people immediately jumped on it. In the scuffle the animal's tibia was broken.

In another instance, a horse was being cast for surgery. The animal was pulled into lateral recumbency, but the hind limbs were not flexed and pulled up tightly enough against the body. The animal was able to extend its hind leg and exert sufficient pressure to fracture its femur.

If animals become twisted and pinned into peculiar positions, fractures are likely to occur.

CLINICAL SIGNS. Fractures of the distal extremities are usually easy to recognize because of the extreme abnormal mobility and abnormal positioning of the limb. In many cases crepitation or grating of the bone ends may be discerned. Fractures of the upper limbs, particularly of heavy-bodied animals, are extremely difficult to diagnose. In many instances radiographs of these bones cannot be made; diagnosis is based on the continued inability of the animal to support weight on the limb.

THERAPY. Treatment of fractures is a complicated procedure requiring the special talents of the veterinary surgeon.

Fractures are emergencies, requiring quick treatment to prevent trauma to contiguous vessels and nerves from the jagged bone ends. In the case of domestic animals, immediately apply a splint to immobilize the leg. In wild species, it is usually necessary to sedate or immobilize the animal before applying a splint.

When dealing with wild animals, any suspected fracture should be fully evaluated before the animal is released from restraint. Once it has been released, efforts to recapture it may cause further damage of sufficient magnitude to result in complete disuse of the limb and perhaps the death of the animal.

Sprain

DEFINITION. A sprain is damage of the ligaments and tendons surrounding a joint, caused by twisting and pulling. A sprain may be more serious than a fracture and result in prolonged incapacitation.

ETIOLOGY. Joint injuries are caused in the same manner as bone fractures. A sprain results when a joint is twisted in such a manner as to tear the collateral ligaments, joint capsules, or other tendinous structures supporting the integrity of the joint.

CLINICAL SIGNS. Sprains are usually indicated by disuse of the limb and therefore are seldom observed until after a restrained animal has been released. The joint may swell because of the stretching of collateral ligaments, tendons, joint capsules, and other tissues around the area. Additional clinical signs include heat, pain, and immobility.

DIFFERENTIAL DIAGNOSIS. Most sprains are noticed a few hours to days after a restraint procedure. Other conditions may simulate a sprain. An abscessed joint, arthritis, contusion of a joint, and circulatory conditions resulting in edema of the structures are typical ailments, with symptoms similar to those of sprain.

THERAPY. Therapy is similar to that for fracture.

Laminitis (founder)

DEFINITION. Laminitis is inflammation of the highly vascular laminae attaching the bone of the digit to the horny covering of the hoof.[13,16] Laminitis is associated with severe pain and dysfunction of the limb involved. It is a common disease of the horse, but any species with laminae in the hoof or toenail (elephant, llama) may develop laminitis. Species with toenails rather than an enclosed hoof are less likely to suffer from the more serious chronic effects of laminitis.

ETIOLOGY. Restraint laminitis is caused by contusion of the hoof. Trauma to the hoof may occur through an animal's attempt to escape by banging the hoofs against a solid surface such as a concrete or wooden wall or against the side of a truck. During manipulative procedures in chutes, animals often thrash, striking any object in the way. Contusions of the hoof wall are a possible consequence. Animals chased for some distance on a hard surface may develop laminitis.

PATHOGENESIS OF THE LESION. Contusion of the hoof wall results in congestion as a result of the increased blood supply to the area. The hoof is a finite space, and engorgement exerts pressure on sensitive tissues, causing severe pain. Severe trauma at a single point may result in a hematoma beneath the hoof wall similar to that suffered when a thumbnail is struck with a hammer. Usually, following the initial congestion, the body resorbs the excess blood, and structures are undamaged. If pressure from congestion continues, the tissues of the lamina may atrophy, causing the hoof to separate from the digit of the foot. Chronic laminitis is a common ailment of the horse.

CLINICAL SIGNS. Laminitis is characterized by severe pain, heat over the affected hoof or toenail, and disuse. Unfortunately laminitis caused by restraint is seldom evident until after the animal has been freed. Adequate subsequent observation and/or examination usually defines the injury of a domestic animal, but in wild species a subsequent examination requires re-subjecting the animal to restraint. Furthermore, it is difficult to make a correct diagnosis because there is no evidence of swelling or discoloration of the hoof. Since complete disuse of the limb is the only sign, laminitis must be differentiated from sprains, fractures, and nerve injuries.

THERAPY. The most valuable immediate treatment for per-acute or acute traumatic laminitis is the application of cold water or ice for at least an hour. The difficulty lies in making the original diagnosis quickly. Usually by the time the diagnosis is definite, it is too late for cold water to have much value. In fact, at this stage, alternate hot and cold applications are indicated to relieve the congestion of the hoof.

Traumatic laminitis does not readily respond to medication. Phenylbutazone may be administered (intravenously or orally only) at the following dosage: equine: 4.0–8.0 mg/kg orally or 3.0–6.0 IV twice daily; camelids: 2.0–4.0 mg/kg orally or IV once daily.[13] Phenylbutazone reduces inflammation, and its analgesic action allows the horse to walk, which is important in improving circulation in the foot. Unfortunately, phenylbutazone should be given either intravenously or orally, so that its use in wild animals is minimal.

For equids, elevate the heel to diminish tension on the toe to minimize separation of the hoof wall laminae from the corresponding laminae of the third phalanx. In camelids or elephants, shorten the toenail so that there is no contact of the toenail with the ground.

Additionally, promote digital circulation with acepromazine 0.02–0.04 mg/kg IM. This has a vasodilation effect and also encourages the animal to lie down, thus reducing pain and tension on the laminae.

Detailed discussion of laminitis therapy is found in standard veterinary medicine text books.[16,21]

Nerve Injury (paralysis, radial paralysis, perineal paralysis, brachial paralysis)

DEFINITION. Nerve injury is diminished function of either or both sensory and motor nerves.

ETIOLOGY. Nerve injury may result from the same types of accidents as those that cause fractures, sprains, or contusions. Nerves are injured during the restraint process by excessive stretching of the limbs or head or by a blow to the nerve as it crosses a bony prominence. In attempting to control or place limbs in less-active positions, they may be unduly stretched, disrupting normal nerve function.

Delayed paralysis may result when heavy-bodied animals are immobilized and kept in lateral recumbency for long periods. Two mechanisms may be involved in this phenomenon. The first operates through anoxia, caused by excessive pressure on the arterial blood supply—familiar to us as the foot "going to sleep." This occurs when a heavy-bodied animal lies against a lower leg, causing ischemia. Usually the ischemia is transient and is alleviated as soon as the animal gets up. Temporary paralysis may be apparent, but function of the limb returns within moments.

The second mechanism operating in cases of delayed paralysis is also associated with ischemia. This type often occurs during equine surgery, when the horse is restrained in lateral recumbency. If an animal under general anesthesia or restrained by immobilizing agents is totally relaxed, pressure on blood vessels in the brachial plexus results in ischemia. If ischemia lasts for 1–2 hours, the endothelium of the capillaries may be slightly damaged. As the animal recovers and arises, blood rushes into the ischemic areas. Because of the damaged endothelium, capillary permeability is increased, allowing extravasation of plasma into the area, which exerts pressure on nerves.

Thus an animal may experience paralysis immediately after arising from anesthesia or immobilization. The use of the leg quickly returns, only to become dysfunctional again in an hour or so as a result of swelling in or around the nerve site (brachial plexus).

Radial paralysis may result from a blow to the forearm over the radius and ulna at the point where the radial nerve lies in close approximation to the bone.

Peroneal paralysis is commonly noted in animals trussed up in a casting harness or rope in such a manner that the hind limb is tightly flexed for a long time. The problem may also be caused by excessive stretching or by continued pressure on the nerve.

Paralysis associated with pressure on the brachial nerve seldom occurs in a partially conscious animal. The struggling of such an animal involves sufficient muscular activity to support normal blood circulation in the limb and maintain capillary integrity. The problem develops only in a recumbent animal that is kept entirely relaxed for a long time.

CLINICAL SIGNS. The most prominent signs are those of motor malfunction. Animals with brachial paralysis cannot use the forelimb. They stagger and may fall when they try to walk. Most wild animals are able to support themselves on three legs, but some refuse to do so. Radial paralysis is indicated by the inability of the animal to extend the front leg forward without dragging the hoof along the ground. Peroneal paralysis is characterized by the inability of the animal to support weight on the hind limb. The joint knuckles at the fetlock, and the animal may walk or attempt to walk on the anterior surface of the fetlock. Sensory perception is usually disrupted as well. Sensory disruption may easily be identified if the animal is in hand but is less easily evaluated with a free wild animal.

THERAPY. Most nerve injuries are temporary in nature, but the animal may injure itself further, and, more seriously, before nerve function returns. In the case of peroneal paralysis, it is important to support the leg and protect the anterior aspect of the fetlock to prevent joint trauma. Wild animals are particularly difficult to treat in these cases because they will not tolerate slings or other supports. Generally therapy is aimed at protecting soft tissue structures and bones from trauma until nerve function returns. Unfortunately little can be done to assist the animal afflicted with permanent nerve injury. The process of nerve regeneration is long and drawn out; it is usually not possible to provide a wild animal with adequate nursing care for a sufficient length of time to allow regeneration to take place.

Differential diagnosis of nerve injuries must include fractures, sprains, and capture myopathy (discussed later in this chapter).

Injury to Toenails, Claws, and Hoofs

Toenails, claws, and hoofs may be contused, or torn from the digit.

ETIOLOGY. A hoof may be torn from the foot if the foot is entangled in fences or in cracks or crevices in walls. Claws or toenails are frequently torn as animals scratch or claw while attempting to escape.

CLINICAL SIGNS. Signs of claw injury include hemorrhage and loss of the claw from the surface of the digit or the hoof from the foot. In some instances the nail remains attached by the corium. In other cases it is torn completely away from the foot. Abrasions of the nails occur from prolonged scratching at hard surfaces in attempts to escape. In these cases the shape of the claw is changed and bleeding from the tip of the nail may be noted.

THERAPY. If the nail or claw has been entirely torn away, control the hemorrhage and protect the bed of the nail by applying bandages as long as is necessary for regrowth of the nail. In some instances a damaged coronary band prevents regeneration, and amputation of the digit becomes necessary.

DAMAGE TO FEATHERS AND SCALES

The skin appendages of birds, reptiles, and fish are as liable to damage as is the hair of mammals. All these structures are protective in nature. Abrasions that remove such

structures expose more sensitive tissues and may allow infections to penetrate the body.

Mature feathers are avascular, except at the tip of the follicle. Removal of certain feathers or cutting them at the tip to inhibit flight is a routine clinical procedure. A newly developing feather (pin feather), however, is intensely vascular. Exercise special caution when handling birds known to be developing new feathers. Manipulation of an animal at the time feathers are erupting may tear the feathers and cause serious hemorrhage. If a pin feather is torn, the feather shaft remaining in the follicle must be removed completely to stop hemorrhage. If the shaft extends beyond the skin surface, grasp the shaft with a forceps (preferably a needle forceps) and pull straight out. If the shaft is broken off flush with the skin, the shaft must be separated from the follicle wall with a hemostat to allow grasping with the forceps.

METABOLIC CONDITIONS

Stress and Thermoregulatory Problems

Stress is the ever-present cloud that plagues both animal and restrainer. The concept is difficult to understand, yet of great significance. Chapter 7 is devoted to this topic.

Hyperthermia and hypothermia are both significant medical problems occurring during restraint procedures. The medical importance of these conditions warrants a detailed separate discussion. (See Chapter 4.)

Acidosis

DEFINITION. Homeostasis necessitates maintenance of a delicate acid-base balance in the blood. Normal mammalian blood pH varies between 7.35 and 7.45. Minor changes in either direction trigger serious metabolic consequences: pH less than 7.35 = acidosis; pH greater than 7.45 = alkalosis.[8,11,22,24]

ETIOLOGY. The prime cause of acidosis in restrained animals is excessive muscular activity associated with excitement, chase, and resistance to handling.[8] Acidosis is the result of lactic acid buildup during anaerobic oxidation in the muscle cells. One minute of exhaustive exercise may cause a drop to a pH of 6.8.[10,11,17] Other respiratory and metabolic activities of the body contribute to the acid-base balance. A malnourished animal, for example, is utilizing its own protein reserves for energy and has usually developed ketosis with excessive hydrogen ion production. Metabolic acidosis may also be induced by starvation, chronic interstitial nephritis, acute renal insufficiency, diarrhea, and dehydration.[8] Thus evaluation of the disease state of any animal to be restrained is important to permit the clinician to guard against aggravation of a preexisting acidosis.

Respiratory acidosis may develop whenever there is interference with normal respiratory function. Airways are frequently obstructed during restraint. Pneumonia, emphysema, and anesthesia without forced or assisted respiration may contribute to the development of acidosis.

Acidosis may contribute to other serious metabolic and electrolyte upsets. Acidosis associated with exercise persists for several minutes after running or struggling has ceased, even if animals are trying to accommodate by hyperventilation. Thus animals are commonly manipulated or anesthetized while in an acidotic state. In the acidotic state, serum calcium is elevated, which, combined with hypoxia, sensitizes the cardiac muscle to the effects of catecholamines. Ventricular fibrillation and death may be the sequel to such a double metabolic insult.

CLINICAL SIGNS. Neurological signs are primary indicators of acidosis. The animal is listless and exhibits mental confusion. It may lapse into coma and/or suffer from seizures progressing to convulsions. The skin is frequently characterized by lack of turgor since dehydration is commonly associated with acidosis. The animal breathes rapidly to exhale excessive carbon dioxide.

THERAPY. It is important to establish open airways and assist respiration to eliminate carbon dioxide. Direct therapy for correcting acidosis is intravenous infusion of sodium bicarbonate solution (4–6 mEq/kg), usually in conjunction with other parenteral fluids such as saline or dextrose.

Alkalosis

Alkalosis is of minimal importance as a restraint problem. Respiratory alkalosis may be produced by hyperventilation, but usually this is possible only by forced breathing while an animal is on an anesthetic machine. Metabolic alkalosis is common in certain digestive tract diseases associated with pyloric obstruction, gastritis, gastric foreign bodies, vomiting, and abomasal disease in cattle. Additional disease conditions characterized by alkalosis include salt poisoning, hyperadrenalism (which may be a factor in stress), and certain brain stem diseases.

Hypoxia/Anoxia

DEFINITION. Hypoxia is decreased availability of oxygen in the tissues. Anoxia is total absence of oxygen. Hypoxia may be general, in which all tissues lack sufficient oxygen, or it may occur only in localized organs such as the brain and cardiac muscles, which are particularly susceptible to insufficient oxygen.

ETIOLOGY. Some species can breathe through both mouth and nostrils; others breathe primarily through the nose (horses, elephants, llamas, alpacas). Elephants have no pleural space, hence no negative pressure in the thorax. Respiration is accomplished by movement of the diaphragm and chest wall. If an elephant is immobilized in sternal recumbency, the abdominal viscera push cranially to inhibit the movement of the diaphragm. Airways may be obstructed by tight ropes or snares around the neck, too tight a grip by a handler, or by twisting the neck. Strangulation can occur easily if an animal sticks its head through a net or a webbing containing spaces

too large for that species. Do not obstruct the nostrils of any animal during restraint. Gloves diminish tactile discrimination and may mask excessive pressure applied to the thoracic cavity while gripping the animal (Fig. 9.1).

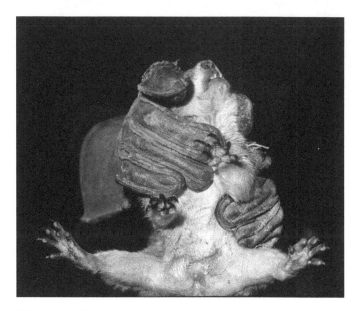

FIG. 9.1. Gloves decrease tactile sense and may result in an animal being squeezed to the point of suffocation.

Birds breathe with a bellows type of respiration that necessitates movement of the keel or sternum forward and down for inspiration and backward and up for expiration. (See Fig. 24.1.) Any restraint procedure that interferes with such movement will quickly produce suffocation.

Other causes of hypoxia include regurgitation with inhalation of ingesta, bloat, and a concurrent respiratory disease such as pneumonia or emphysema. Wild animals are capable of masking signs of severe respiratory disease until the condition is almost terminal. In a number of instances animals have quickly suffocated and died during restraint. Necropsy revealed a functional lung capacity of approximately 10% of normal.

Pulmonary edema is a special problem seen when unconditioned domestic or captive wild animals are forced to exercise. A female bison dropped after five trips around a large pen to escape roping. She died of pulmonary edema. Her free-ranging counterpart could probably have run for miles without harm.

CLINICAL SIGNS. Minimal hypoxia causes dyspnea, cyanotic mucous membranes, and accelerated pulse. As hypoxia deepens, cerebral anoxia produces unconsciousness. An animal will likely begin to struggle vigorously at this point or even convulse. To a casual observer, this may convey the impression that the animal is struggling against restraint.

If cerebral and cardiac anoxia are prolonged for more than 4–5 minutes, damage is irreparable and death ensues.

THERAPY. The mechanism causing hypoxia should be corrected and supplemental oxygen supplied. When dealing with wild animals, it is wise to have emergency oxygen available at all times.

If the animal is breathing, insert a tube into the nostril for oxygen insufflation. A color change in the mucous membranes should be noted quickly. If respiration has ceased, the trachea must be intubated. If suitable tubes and specula are available, oral intubation is sufficient. If not, an emergency tracheotomy must be performed and oxygen supplied under pressure.

Hypocalcemia (eclampsia, puerperal tetany, milk fever)

DEFINITION. Hypocalcemia is decreased concentration of calcium ions in the blood.

ETIOLOGY. Calcium is required for numerous chemical reactions in the body, including those of normal nerve and muscle function. Decreased circulating calcium produces many systemic manifestations.

Critical serum calcium levels are normally maintained through calcium ingestion. If the calcium level in the diet is inadequate, the deficiency is made up by drawing on bone stores.

Malnutrition predisposes restrained animals to hypocalcemia. Wild animals in captivity, particularly those in private ownership, are frequently not supplied with a diet providing sufficient levels of calcium, vitamin D, and phosphorus in the required ratio. Bone decalcification is the initial response. Eventually serum calcium drops to such a low level that the clinical syndrome of hypocalcemia appears.

Hypocalcemic tetany may be induced during restraint by either hypoxia or respiratory alkalosis brought on by hyperventilation. Alkalosis increases the quantity of calcium bound to protein, thus reducing ionized calcium.[22] Forced hyperventilation during anesthesia may also produce alkalosis.

CLINICAL SIGNS. Hypocalcemia results in hyperirritability of nerves and muscles, causing muscle cramping, muscle twitching, laryngeal spasm, carpopedal spasm, stridor, and generalized convulsions.

Caged birds are frequent victims of hypocalcemia. Clinical signs include wing fluttering, falling from perches, and tetanic convulsive seizures on the floor of the cage. A lizard exhibiting signs of hypocalcemia falls into extensor rigidity with the limbs extending backward along the body. In mammals, the nictitating membrane may extend over the eye because the ocular muscles contract, pulling the bulb back into the orbital socket. Respiration may be inhibited by spasms of respiratory muscles.

Milk fever in the cow and puerperal tetany in the bitch and the mare are also manifestations of hypocalcemia. Cattle are unique: instead of tetany, paresis results from hypocalcemia. In the mare and bitch, classical signs of tetany are more prominent.

In the bitch, signs noted are nervousness and anxiety, frequent whining, and difficult locomotion. The animal may stagger and walk stiffly. Usually, increased muscular activity results in an elevated body temperature. Ultimately the animal collapses and falls to the floor. The legs and neck are rigidly extended. Twitching may develop, followed by periods of relaxation. The convulsive seizures may progress to severe tetanic spasms and ultimate death.

THERAPY. Treat acute hypocalcemia with an intravenous solution of calcium gluconate (Table 9.1). In small species, or if no vein can be raised, the intramuscular route can be used.

Intravenous solutions of calcium salts must be administered carefully. Monitor the heart rate. If tachycardia develops, slow the infusion.

Hypoglycemia (hypoglycemic shock, insulin shock)

DEFINITION. Hypoglycemia is abnormal decrease of glucose levels in the blood.

ETIOLOGY. Captive wild animals, particularly those kept as pets, may be malnourished, with depleted glycogen reserves. Energy needs increase at the time of restraint. With no reserves for the body to call upon, glucose levels drop. Hypoglycemic shock may ensue.

Many animals enter a state of torpidity, characterized by decreased metabolic activity, when exposed to extremes of environmental temperature or when food becomes unavailable. Such animals are capable of maintaining themselves for an extended period in the torpid state; however, they are particularly prone to develop hypoglycemic shock if they are disturbed and called upon to quickly mobilize energy reserves. Hibernators must be handled carefully when torpid. Alligators

TABLE 9.1.   Parenteral dosage of calcium gluconate for acute hypocalcemia

	Percent Calcium Gluconate Solution	Dose Actual Calcium Gluconate	Dose Actual Calcium Gluconate	Ml Solution per kg B.W.	Ml Solution per lb B.W.
Large animals (cow, antelope)	20 (200 mg/ml)	100–200 mg/kg	50–100 mg/lb	0.5–1	0.25–0.5
Medium-sized animals (dog, cat)	10* (100 mg/ml)	100–200 mg/kg	50–100 mg/lb	1–2	0.5–1
Small birds and reptiles	1† (10 mg/ml)	0.1–0.2 mg/g	. . .	0.01–0.02 ml/g	. . .

*1 ml 20% calcium gluconate in 1 ml water = 10% solution calcium gluconate.
†0.5 ml 20% calcium gluconate in 9.5 ml water = 1% solution calcium gluconate.

and other crocodilians become seasonally torpid. Handling them during this time is hazardous.

CLINICAL SIGNS. Hypoglycemia deprives the brain of the nutritive substrate upon which it is dependent for oxidative metabolism. Thus hypoglycemia results in anoxia of the neurons in the central nervous system.

Hypoglycemia is characterized by tetany varying from slight, transient tremors to incoordination, twitching, and convulsions. Signs of autonomic nervous system malfunction include copious salivation, tachycardia, and profuse sweating. Prolonged cerebral anoxia causes irreversible brain damage.[7] Hypoglycemic convulsions may be controlled by sedation, but sedation does not prevent brain damage from anoxia. When conducting a differential diagnosis, hypoglycemia must be considered, and ruled out, before sedation is administered to a convulsing animal. Failure to correctly diagnose and treat a hypoglycemic animal may result in mental retardation, partial paralysis, ataxia, epilepsy, or death.

THERAPY. Administer a 10–50% dextrose solution intravenously. Response should be immediate. If intravenous injection is impossible, inject the solution intramuscularly.

Table 9.2 lists the daily basal metabolic caloric requirements of animals ranging in weight from 0.05 to 2,000 kg, using the formula: $70 \times (\text{B.W. in kg})^{0.75} = \text{kcal}/24 \text{ hr}$.

One ml of 50% dextrose yields 2 kcal. One ml of 5% dextrose yields 0.2 kcal. A 10-kg animal requires 379 kcal/24 hr or 190 ml of 5% dextrose to supply the needed calories. In a 10-kg animal, 50 ml of 5% dextrose is not likely to alleviate hypoglycemia for more than a few minutes.

Epinephrine, 1:1000, injected subcutaneously, produces an immediate gluconeogenic effect and is helpful in relieving acute hypoglycemia. Give a large animal 0.5–1 ml/50 kg of a 1:1000 solution. Give a small animal 1 ml/10 kg. Dilute the 1:1000 solution 1:10 before administering.

Long-term therapy consists of providing adequate nutrition and making certain the animal consumes it. Comprehensive and long-term therapy should be instituted following emergency treatment.

Dehydration

DEFINITION. Dehydration is excessive loss of body fluids. The mammalian body is composed of 60–80% water. Higher amounts of body fat decrease the percentage of water. Except for desert animals, adult mammals require water consumption in amounts of approximately 40 ml/kg of body weight daily to maintain normal water balance in a basal metabolic state. This is equivalent to the fluid lost in urine and feces and through insensible evaporation via skin and lungs.

Fluid requirements vary with the size of the animal and its ability to conserve moisture. Desert-adapted species are superbly capable of minimizing fluid loss. An animal such as the kangaroo rat, *Dipodomys* spp., from the deserts of the western United States, may live out its life without drinking water because it is able to utilize metabolic water maximally and does not allow itself to become hyperthermic.

The dromedary camel, *Camelus dromedarius*, is legendary for its ability to go without water. The camel is able to concentrate urine, desiccate fecal excretions, and utilize a unique diurnal variation in body temperature.[19] During the heat of the day, the camel's body temperature may elevate to 40°C, without harm. The excess heat is dissipated during the cool desert night, when its temperature may drop to 35°C. Thus the animal avoids the necessity of evaporating moisture to cool the body. A dromedary may also lose 25% of its body weight

TABLE 9.2. Energy requirements for animals

	A. Mammal Energy Requirements (kcals/day)					
Body Weight (kg)	Placental Mammals (K = 70)	Placental Maintenance (BMR × 1.5)	Placental Maintenance (+2×)	Marsupial Mammals (K 49)	Marsupial Maintenance (BMR × 1.5)	Marsupial Maintenance (+2×)
0.05	7.4	11	33	5.4	8	24
0.5	41.6	62	186	29.4	44	132
1	70	105	315	49	74	222
2	117.7	177	531	82.3	123	363
4	198.9	298	894	138.7	193	579
6	268.4	403	1209	187.7	282	846
8	333.0	500	1500	233.2	350	1050
10	393.6	590	1770	275.4	413	1239
20	662.0	993	2979	463.5	695	2085
30	897.3	1346	4038	628.2	942	2826
40	1113.4	1670	010	779.6	1168	3504
50	1316.2	1974	5922	921.1	1382	4146
60	1509.1	2264	6792	1056.4	1585	4755
70	1694.0	2541	7623	1185.8	1779	5337
80	1872.5	2809	8427	1310.7	1966	5898
90	2045.4	3068	9204	1431.8	2148	6444
100	2213.6	3320	9960	1549.4	2324	6972
200	3722.8	5584	16752			
500	7401.6	11102	33306			
800	10529.4	15794	47382			
1000	12448.0	18672	56016			
1500	16872.0	25308	75924			
2000	20934.9	31402	94206			

[a]BMR or MEC = basal metabolic rate or minimum energy cost = K × body weight$_{kg}^{0.75}$.

TABLE 9.2. Continued

B.–Avian Energy Requirements (kcals/day)					
Body Weight (kg)	Passerine Birds BMR (K = 129)	Passerine Maintenance (×1.5)	Passerine Maintenance (+1×)	Passerine Maintenance (+2×)	Passerine Maintenance (+3×)
0.05	14.2	21.3	43	64	85
0.06	15.5	23	46	69	92
0.08	19.4	29	58	87	116
0.10	23.2	35	70	105	140
Body Weight (kg)	Non-passerine Birds BMR (K = 78)	Non-passerine Maintenance (×1.5)	Non-passerine Maintenance (+1×)	Non-passerine Maintenance (+2×)	Non-passerine Maintenance (+3×)
0.05	8.6	13	17	27	36
0.07	10.9	16.4	33	49	66
0.09	12.5	18.8	38	56	75
0.1	14.1	21.0	42	63	84
0.3	31.9	47.9	96	144	192
0.5	46.0	69	138	207	276
1	78	117	234	351	468
2	131	197	394	591	788
4	220.7	331	662	993	1 324
6	298.7	448	896	1 344	1 792
8	371.3	557	1114	1 671	2 228
10	438.4	658	1316	1 974	2 632
20	737.9	1107	2214	3 321	4 428
30	999.9	1500	3000	4 500	6 000
40	1241.0	1862	3724	5 586	7 448
50	1466.4	2200	4400	6 600	8 800
60	1681.7	2523	5046	7 569	1 092
70	1887.6	2831	5662	8 493	11 324
80	2086.5	5130	260	9 390	12 520
90	2279.2	3419	6838	10 257	13 676
140	2826.7	4240	8480	12 720	16 960

C.–Reptile Energy Requirements (kcals/day)			
Body Weight (kg)	BMW (K = 10)	Maintenance (BMR × 1.5)	Maintenance (+1)
0.05	1.1	2	4
0.5	6.0	9	18
1	10.0	15	30
2	16.8	25	50
4	28.3	42	84
6	38.4	58	116
8	47.6	71	142
10	56.2	84	168
20	94.6	142	284
30	128.2	192	384
40	159.1	239	478
50	188	282	564
60	215.6	323	646
70	242	363	726
80	267.5	400	800
90	292.2	438	876
100	316.2	474	948

[a] Basal metabolic rate or minimum energy cost (MEC).

through temporary fluid loss without ill effects and is able to rehydrate with a single intake of large amounts of water.[19]

ETIOLOGY. Dehydration may be caused by water deprivation prior to restraint, failure of a newly acquired animal to recognize the water source, a frozen water source, failure to use automatic waterers, failure to provide sufficient water during hot weather, overheating, prolonged chase for capture, severe diarrhea, persistent vomiting, hemorrhage, or loss of fluid as a result of burns.

CLINICAL SIGNS. Early signs of mild dehydration (3% B.W. loss) in nondesert-adapted species are low urine output, dryness of the mouth, and some loss of skin elasticity. Feces become dry and hard. Fluid is lost first from interstitial fluid compartments. Homeostatic mechanisms function to keep plasma volume constant as long as possible.[11]

Moderate dehydration (5% B.W. loss) is accompanied by marked loss of skin elasticity. The eyes are sunken. Blood pressure may fall as a result of decreased plasma volume. Weakness, fever, and weak pulse may be observed.

Marked dehydration (10% B.W. loss) involves circulatory failure from decreased plasma volume. Signs of shock and coma are evident.

Severe dehydration (12–15% B.W. loss) results in renal failure, marked by uremia and acidosis. At this point severe kidney damage may preclude recovery even though fluid is supplied.

Death usually follows a fluid loss of 20–25% body weight. Laboratory examination shows elevation of packed cell volume (PCV), hemoglobin, and plasma proteins, but blood test results of dehydrated anemic animals may show normal values.[18] Desert-adapted species can cope with dehydration levels incompatible with life in other species.

THERAPY.   Provide fluids orally. If the animal cannot drink, gastric intubation is indicated. Fluid is absorbed rapidly if circulation is functioning. Because fluid is also readily absorbed from the colon, plain water enemas are effective in rehydration, especially if vomiting animals are unable to retain ingested liquids.

In acute dehydration stress, intravenous fluids must be given. Veins are often collapsed, making it necessary to expose the vein (via a skin incision) to effect administration.

Physiological saline solutions or 5% dextrose solutions are satisfactory for intravenous treatment of dehydration. Do not use hypertonic solution. Tap water or saline-dextrose solution can be given orally or rectally. A customary mistake is to underestimate the volume of fluid required. A resting animal's basal fluid requirement is 40 ml/kg body weight daily. As much as three to five times that amount may be required to make up the deficit of marked dehydration. A 240-kg animal may require as much as 48 L of water to restore fluid balance.

Adrenocortical Insufficiency (Addison's disease, adrenal failure)

DEFINITION.   Adrenal insufficiency is failure of the adrenal cortex to produce sufficient corticosteroids to maintain homeostasis.

ETIOLOGY.   Responses to prolonged, intense stress may exhaust the adrenal cortex, resulting in adrenocortical atrophy. Prolonged glucocorticoid (cortisone) therapy causes iatrogenic atrophy of the adrenal cortex. Sudden withdrawal of cortisone causes acute insufficiency.

CLINICAL SIGNS.   Acute adrenocortical insufficiency is a rapidly fatal shock syndrome. Increased serum potassium levels lead to bradycardia and heart block. Other electrolytic changes cause hypotension, vasomotor collapse, renal failure, and uremia. Hypoglycemic shock may also be involved.

Chronic adrenal insufficiency in the dog is characterized by progressive weakness, weight loss, lethargy, chronic inter-mittent gastrointestinal upsets (vomiting, diarrhea), dehydration, polyuria, and polydipsia.

Some signs of insufficiency in the dog reflect a deficiency of mineralocorticoids (aldosterone) and glucocorticoids (cortisol). Adrenal exhaustion from stress may or may not affect aldosterone production. The clinical picture of chronic adrenal exhaustion in most animals has not yet been delineated.

Laboratory procedures may assist in diagnosis. Lymphocytosis, eosinophilia, slight to moderate hypoglycemia, hyperkalemia, hyponatremia and hypochloremia, increases in blood urea nitrogen, and hemoconcentration may be defined in laboratory tests.[5]

Animals with chronic adrenocortical insufficiency cannot tolerate exercise or any other stress. Restraint is likely to precipitate acute collapse.

THERAPY.   Begin intensive shock therapy at once. However, if adrenal insufficiency is suspected, do not use solutions containing potassium (lactated Ringers). Therapy should begin by administering 5% dextrose in physiological saline. Prednisolone (solu-delta-cortef) in doses of 50% mg/kg intravenously are used in the dog. This can be added to the intravenous fluids.[18]

If bradycardia is pronounced—suggesting aldosterone deficiency—give desoxycorticosterone acetate (DOCA) at a rate of 0.1 mg/kg intramuscularly.[5]

It is imperative to carefully monitor the patient and institute appropriate remedial measures if complications arise.

Shock

DEFINITION.   Shock is a clinical condition characterized by signs and symptoms arising when cardiac output fails to fill the arterial tree with blood under sufficient pressure to provide organs and tissues with an adequate blood flow.

With reduced tissue perfusion, oxygen available to the tissues diminishes. Oxygen deficit causes deterioration of the heart and circulatory system, compounding the problem. Irreversible shock occurs when deterioration proceeds to the point that tissue cannot be rejuvenated.

ETIOLOGY.   Shock results from severe physical and psychological insult. Shock is often the terminal manifestation of traumatic or metabolic disorders that develop during restraint (Table 9.3).

CLINICAL SIGNS.   Typical signs of shock include decreased blood pressure, pale mucous membranes, depression, cool-

TABLE 9.3.   Shock classification, important in restraint

Cardiogenic—failure of the heart as a pump, ventricular fibrillation, catecholamine response, cardiac standstill, cholinergic response, cardiac tamponade (pressure on the heart)
Hypovolemic (actual)—decrease in blood volume, hemorrhage (whole blood loss), plasma extravasation (contusions, burns), dehydration (exercise, hyperthermia)
Hypovolemic (relative)—change in vascular bed, increasing its relative capacity
Neurogenic response—pain, fear, anger
Endotoxins—concomitant enteric infections
Toxins—drugs

ness of the skin, muscular weakness, coma, rapid breathing, rapid and weak pulse, dilated pupils, and decreased body temperature.

Laboratory tests may be helpful in establishing a diagnosis. Shock is characterized by hemoconcentration; increased levels of nonprotein nitrogen, glucose, and potassium; decreased levels of alkali reserves, chloride, and PO; and inhibited blood coagulation.

The lesions of shock are nonspecific. A definitive diagnosis cannot be made at necropsy because of species variation in the lesions of affected organs. Necropsy may, however, show suggestive lesions including hyperemia or petechial hemorrhage of the liver, kidney, and mucosa of the gastrointestinal tract, lungs, and serous membranes; empty and bloodless spleen; effusions into the serous cavities; ischemia of peripheral muscles; and intravascular coagulation of blood.

Psychogenic or neurogenic shock is produced when an animal is subjected to pain or experiences intense emotions such as fear or anger. The pathogenesis of neurogenic shock is not known; however, it is mediated through interference with the balance of vasodilators and vasoconstrictors of the arterioles and venules. It may be closely related to the cholinergic bradycardia syndrome but usually produces less serious consequences.

In neurogenic shock, the blood volume is sufficient but vascular muscle tone is lessened, allowing increased reservoir capacity in both arterioles and venules. Pooling in these vessels effects a decrease in venous return to the right side of the heart, subsequently reducing cardiac output. This syndrome may be seen after or accompanying acute gastric dilatation.

The signs of neurogenic shock differ slightly from those of typical hypovolemic shock in that the pulse rate is usually slow, accompanied by decreased blood pressure. The skin is characteristically warm and may be flushed.

THERAPY. The crucial triad of therapeutic measures to treat shock consists of (1) eliminating the cause of the shock, (2) providing supplemental oxygen, and (3) restoring circulating blood volumes to normal levels.[5]

Establish a patent airway and provide supplemental oxygen. If possible, intubate with a cuffed endotracheal tube to allow assisted or controlled ventilation. Intubation may be impossible when dealing with certain nondomestic species because of the extremely small size of the trachea and inaccessibility to the glottis through the oral cavity of these species. If endotracheal intubation is not possible, a face mask, nasal catheter, transtracheal catheter, pediatric incubator, oxygen tent (enclose a cage with a plastic bag), or a special oxygen cage may be used to achieve ventilation. Tracheotomy and insertion of an endotracheal tube may be indicated if airways of the nasal or oral cavities are obstructed.

Use the most expedient method to supply oxygen to an unconscious animal. If the animal is conscious, select the least stressful method available. Applying severe physical restraint to place a nasal catheter may do more harm than good. It is unwise to utilize chemical restraint or sedation to supply supplemental oxygen.

Begin intravenous fluid therapy simultaneously with providing a patent airway. Lactated Ringers solution or physiological saline are suitable solutions. A minimum volume that can be given in a few hours is 88 ml/kg. Implement careful monitoring of cardiovascular function to determine if additional fluids are required.

Glucocorticosteroid therapy is somewhat controversial but is generally recognized as beneficial. Dosages have been established for dogs. Hydrocortisone sodium succinate is given intravenously at the rate of 50 mg/kg.[18] Dexamethasone (Azium) is given concurrently (also intravenously). The dosage is 4 mg/kg, repeated every 4 hours.

The development of metabolic acidosis is inevitable in cases of shock. If blood-gas analysis is available, the precise amount of sodium bicarbonate needed to counteract acidosis can be calculated, using the formula: $NaHCO_3$ required = base deficit in mEq/L $\times$ 0.03 $\times$ B.W. in kg.

Without blood-gas analysis, give an initial dose of 4.5–5.6 mEq of sodium bicarbonate per kg of body weight slowly, intravenously, and add a similar amount to intravenous fluid administered over the next several hours.[18]

Ischemia of the liver parenchyma and the intestinal epithelium predispose these tissues to necrosis. Bacterial invasion of the body is common during and following shock. Broad-spectrum antibiotic therapy is essential to prevent septicemia. Use a high dosage and continue therapy for 5 days.

In a hospital situation, with laboratory backup and availability of monitoring equipment, additional therapeutic measures may be instituted. The use of diuretics, ionotropic agents, sedatives, and anticoagulants may be indicated in specific situations. To alleviate disrupted thermoregulation, keep the patient warm and monitor the body temperature.

Cholinergic Bradycardia (syncope, fatal syncope, fainting, vagal reflex, vagal bradycardia)

DEFINITION. Cholinergic bradycardia is the slowing of the heart rate produced when vagal stimulation overrides the usual adrenergic response of alarm.

ETIOLOGY. Usually during restraint the typical adrenergic alarm response is initiated, characterized by vasoconstriction and hypertension. Centers in the hypothalamus normally stimulate the sympathetic system. However, similar centers in the hypothalamus can also stimulate the parasympathetic system.

Under intense stimulation—in some animals—the cholinergic response overpowers the adrenergic, resulting in a precipitous fall in blood pressure and slowing of the heart rate. Unconsciousness may result.

Syncope (fainting) is an ordinary phenomenon in humans. Cerebral ischemia brought about by rapid carotid hypotension causes unconsciousness. In humans, this effect is usually transitory. As soon as the person lies flat, normal pressure is restored and consciousness returns.

Why do animals die? The answer is not known. It is known that animals may slip from syncope into irreversible hypovolemic shock. If syncope occurs in an animal in hand, death may be prevented by permitting it to lie out flat, giving it a chance to recover.

Fatal syncope may also occur in humans if the upright position is maintained. Crucifixion causes death through a form of recurrent syncope, brought about in this manner. Some fainting individuals wedged in an upright position in a panic-stricken crowd have suffered similar mortality.[20] The diving reflex of marine mammals is a normal cholinergic bradycardia. The response may be initiated in a seal by grasping the muzzle and clamping the nostrils shut.[17]

Other reflexes that may initiate cholinergic bradycardia are triggered by ocular pressure, carotid sinus pressure, and increased abdominal pressure (valsalva maneuver—forced expiration against a closed glottis).[20] It is important for the animal restrainer to be aware of these reflexes because any of the pressures mentioned may be applied during restraint.

In humans, actions initiating a vagal response are cold water on the face, tilting the head downward, elevating the feet, or standing in water. Convulsive seizures may result in syncope because of carotid sinus pressure. Individuals vary in their susceptibility to this phenomenon.

Aspirated vomitus in the trachea or acute pleural irritation such as may occur from trauma to the thoracic wall may initiate reflex vagal stimulation and bradycardia.[10]

When an animal senses the futility of struggling to extricate itself from a hopeless situation, it may die. The precise mechanism of such death is not known, but bradycardia is a prominent clinical sign. The zebra or gnu that is finally dragged down by a lion usually gives up without additional fighting although physically capable of further struggle. Perhaps at this point, bradycardia and cerebral anoxia deaden the pain of the inevitable outcome.

Physicians have recorded many unexplained deaths of persons faced with either a real or imaginary hopeless situation. Imprisonment as a prisoner of war, loss of a loved one, confinement in a nursing home, physical incapacitation, and voodoo curses have led to death. Such persons simply give up and resign themselves to death. This type of fatality is called submissive death or the helplessness syndrome.[20]

Animal experimentation has documented that some rats, monkeys, chickens, dogs, and even cockroaches die when faced with circumstances over which they have no control. Instead of responding with the usual adrenergic stimulation, a cholinergic response takes place.

When wild Norway rats were physically restrained until they had ceased struggling and were then placed in a tank of warm water, some immediately sank to the bottom and drowned. Bradycardia was documented via electrocardiographic monitoring. Cage mates placed in the water without prior physical restraint began to swim.[20] Researchers could condition animals to tolerate more restraint by subjecting them to intermittent periods of physical restraint. The animals learned that the situation was not hopeless.

Submissive death may explain the high mortality of newly captured wild animals. Placing such an animal in a confining crate and shipping it to a strange environment is ample cause for an animal to give up. Successful wild animal capture and shipping can be accomplished by slow conditioning.

In Africa, professional collectors go to great lengths to capture animals quickly and move them without delay to a conditioning center, where they are released into a large cage or pen. The pen is constructed to be as compatible as possible with the animal's previous environment. Human interference is minimized.

Related to submissive death, but of less intensity (nonfatal), is the response of an animal that feigns death when grasped. This catatonic response (frozen posture) is known by many names: animal hypnosis, tonic immobility, death feint, playing possum, catalepsy, and mesmerism.

A small caiman (<1 m) placed on its back and held for 15 seconds will struggle briefly and relax. Although released, it will remain immobile in that position for several minutes.

Chickens are easily mesmerized, and some rabbits become catatonic each time they are handled. This reaction can be beneficial if restraint for therapy is desired. However, diagnostic examination of a catatonic animal yields little of value.

Professional collectors capitalize on mesmerism to handle newly captured dangerous animals. A zebra or giraffe can be manually handled and crated immediately after a chase with little danger. Approaching the same animal in a catch pen during the conditioning period would be foolhardy.

Cholinergic bradycardia is more likely to affect an animal weakened from malnutrition, parasitism, or a variety of other subclinical illnesses, but an otherwise healthy animal that has resigned itself to helplessness will rapidly deteriorate. Anorexia is common. Such animals are more susceptible to infection from viral and bacterial agents.

CLINICAL SIGNS. Cholinergic bradycardia is characterized by slowing of pulse and heart rate, heart stoppage, unconsciousness, and death. Lesions of cholinergic heart stoppage are minimal. The heart is usually engorged with blood, indicative of a gradual but steady decrease in the heart rate.

THERAPY AND PREVENTION. It is not likely that cholinergic bradycardia will be detected clinically in time to allow treatment. However, atropine sulfate, 0.04 mg/kg, given intravenously will block the cholinergic (vagal) response. No experimental work has been done to determine the prophylactic efficacy of administering atropine to wild animals prior to restraint.

Prevention primarily consists of using the least amount of restraint possible to minimize the feeling of helplessness. Restraint procedures should be completed quickly and external stimuli diminished to decrease stressor effects.

Cardiac Tamponade

DEFINITION. Cardiac tamponade is cardiac failure as a result of the inability of the heart to expand sufficiently to fill with blood.

ETIOLOGY. External pressure on the heart from pericardial or pleural effusion causes cardiac tamponade. Heart-based tumors and excessive external thoracic pressure may simulate such conditions. Gloves reduce tactile discrimination and frequently result in the handler squeezing tighter than necessary to restrain an animal. Tiny species can be easily injured in this manner.

CLINICAL SIGNS. Cardiac failure results in shock and rapid death. If the syndrome is recognized and the etiology can be quickly reversed, the animal may live.

THERAPY. Correct the cause and supply oxygen.

Ventricular Fibrillation (heart flutter)

DEFINITION. Ventricular fibrillation is uncoordinated rapid contraction of the ventricular cardiac muscles.

ETIOLOGY. This phenomenon is caused by many conditions but the primary cause during restraint is elevated levels of catecholamines (epinephrine and norepinephrine). During the alarm response, a normal tachycardia develops under catecholamine stimulation. If, however, the cardiac muscle has been previously sensitized to catecholamines by acidosis or hypoxia, or both, such stimulation may lead to ventricular fibrillation.

CLINICAL SIGNS. In ventricular fibrillation, agonal struggling may simulate normal resistance to restraint. The ventricles can neither fill nor pump blood normally. Circulatory failure is followed quickly by unconsciousness and death. No pulse can be palpated nor can the heartbeat be picked up by auscultation. An electrocardiogram would provide a definitive diagnosis, but the animal will die before such diagnostic techniques can be employed.

THERAPY. The prognosis for ventricular fibrillation is grave. Electrical stimulation with a defibrillator is the only effective therapy. This hospital procedure is not likely to be available to the animal restrainer in the field. Preventive medicine involves minimizing conditions causing acidosis or hypoxia.

Exertional Stress (capture myopathy, stress myopathy, overstraining disease, muscular dystrophy, capture disease, degenerative polymyopathy, idiopathic muscle necrosis, white muscle stress syndrome)[2,10,14]

DEFINITION. Exertional stress, associated with capture and restraint, is a complex alteration of metabolic processes that may cause peracute lethal acid-base and electrolyte imbalances or acutely produce necrosis of cardiac and striated muscles. The syndrome is primarily observed in wild ruminants, but it may occur in primates, seals, horses, cattle, sheep, dogs, and birds.[23]

ETIOLOGY. Various investigators classify exertional stress into three or four different phases (capture shock, muscle necrosis, ruptured muscle, delayed effects), but all are part of a basic physiopathologic process. An animal responds to a restraint episode by releasing catecholamines, which in turn initiates a complex of neurohormonal responses. Muscular activity generates heat, and anaerobic muscle metabolism produces lactic acid. Muscle ischemia caused by hypoxia or restraint practices compounds the problem. The mechanism is protective initially, but if the stimulus becomes prolonged or is too intense, destructive factors enter the picture. Acidosis, electrolyte imbalance, hypoxia, hyperthermia, pulmonary edema, and muscle necrosis may develop depending on the time frame from the exertional episode.

CLINICAL SIGNS

Capture shock. Shock may occur in as short a time as 15 minutes or as long as 6 hours following a capture or restraint episode. Signs include depression, shallow rapid breathing, hyperthermia, tachycardia, hypotension, circulatory collapse, and death.

Muscle necrosis (ataxic myoglobinuria). This form of the syndrome usually occurs in 3–6 hours or may not appear until several days later, depending upon the degree of muscle necrosis. Signs include ataxia, torticollis, paresis, paralysis, myoglobinuria, elevated serum enzymes (aspartate aminotransferase [AST], also called glutamic-oxaloacetic transaminase [GOT]; creatinine phosphokinase [CPK]; lactate dehydrogenase [LDH]). Secondarily, trauma of the exposed surfaces of the limbs may be brought about through the animal's struggles to stand. If heart muscle becomes necrosed, acute death may ensue.

Ruptured muscle syndrome. Muscle rupture (usually the gastrocnemius) may occur 24–48 hours following severe, prolonged muscular exertion. Signs include hyperflexion of the hock and a drop in the hindquarters. Signs may be obscured if the animal is recumbent for other reasons.

Delayed effects. An animal may appear normal following capture or restraint, but mild necrosis of cardiac or skeletal muscle may have resulted. If animals are disturbed or subjected to another restraint episode (even a minimal one) within a few days, major muscle necrosis may occur, including cardiac muscle.

NECROPSY. In the shock form, lesions may be minimal, because the process is biochemical. However, pulmonary congestion and edema may be present. Hemorrhages may appear on serosal surfaces. In the muscle necrosis form, light grayish streaks are observed in affected muscles. Hemorrhages are evident. Histologically, cellular degeneration—with or without hemorrhage—is seen. Fibrosis is present in protracted cases. Muscle separation is noted in the gastrocnemius muscle mass in the muscle rupture form.

THERAPY.   Prevention must be paramount. Use a well-trained restraint team and work quickly to minimize muscular exertion. Employ chemical restraint when appropriate. Avoid capture and restraint procedures during hot humid weather. Avoid sympathetic autonomic nervous system stimulation.

In the initial stages with hyperthermia and potential shock present, administer fluids intravenously and correct acidosis. When blood pH determinations are not available, begin with a dose of 4.0–6.0 mEq of sodium bicarbonate per kg body weight, and repeat this dose if signs indicate a need. Monitor body temperature and cool hyperthermic animals quickly. Supplemental oxygen insufflation is desirable.

Once muscle necrosis has occurred, general nursing care, plus hot packs to the affected muscles, may provide some relief, but the prognosis is unfavorable.

Regurgitation

DEFINITION.   Regurgitation is the forceful expulsion of the contents of stomach or rumen backward through the esophagus and the mouth or nose. Usually the ingesta is cast out of the mouth with no untoward effects. Ruminant species normally cast a bolus of ingesta (the cud) back up the esophagus into the mouth for rechewing. This is not regurgitation.

Camelids (camels, llamas, alpacas) may spew foul-smelling ingesta on persons attempting to restrain them. Although unpleasant for the person involved, this type of regurgitation is harmless to the camelid.

ETIOLOGY.   Regurgitation is a sign of many diseases and is a serious consequence of both physical and chemical restraint. A recently fed excited animal may regurgitate the meal. Physical restraint may inhibit normal evacuation of vomitus through the mouth, causing inhalation of food particles into the trachea and lungs.

Reflex response to stimulation of the tracheal mucosa by inhalation of food particles may initiate cholinergic bradycardia and fatal syncope. If sufficient food is inhaled, airways are obstructed and strangulation occurs. Gangrenous pneumonia is the universally fatal consequence of inhaling a quantity of ingesta.

The cardiac sphincter of the stomach may relax in a chemically restrained animal. Improper positioning of the body may place too much pressure on the abdomen of such animals and force ingesta up through the esophagus.

Regurgitation is more common in ruminants that must remain recumbent for prolonged procedures. To prevent regurgitation, maintain ruminant species in the sternal position with the shoulders higher than the hindquarters. If lateral recumbency is necessary, it is even more important to keep the shoulders and head elevated.

Regurgitation in the horse and other equids is a grave sign because the elongated palate directs regurgitated ingesta through the nose instead of the mouth, facilitating inhalation of ingesta.

CLINICAL SIGNS.   Stomach contents issuing from the nostrils or mouth is diagnostic. Gagging or retching may momentarily precede evacuation. Regurgitation of an animal under chemical restraint is usually passive, with ingesta flowing out of the mouth or nose. The odor of the stomach or rumen contents is fetid and may be a clue to the presence of ruminal ingesta in the mouth.

Inhalation of ingesta may produce coughing spasms, dyspnea, strangulation, and immediate death. Gangrenous pneumonia and death in 3–7 days may follow an inhalation episode.

PREVENTION AND THERAPY.   Once inhalation of a quantity of ingesta has occurred, death is certain. To help prevent inhalation, avoid prolonged immobilization in lateral recumbency. The sternal position is safest in all species. The cardiac sphincter of the stomach is in the most natural position in sternal recumbency. If possible, keep head, neck, and shoulders slightly higher than the rest of the body to aid in preventing bloat and regurgitation. Avoid pressure on the abdomen of a restrained animal. Do not restrain animals that have recently fed except as a last resort.

If retching or regurgitation begins, lower the head and neck quickly to allow regurgitated material to exit through the mouth easily and completely. The hazard of regurgitation can be eliminated in anesthetized animals by intubation of the trachea with an inflatable cuff.

Bloat (tympany, gastric dilatation, hoven)

DEFINITION.   Bloat is overdistension of the stomach or intestines, usually of ruminants. Bloat is a frequent cause of mortality in species such as the impala and other antelopes, giraffe, and African buffalo kept restrained in lateral recumbency.[2]

ETIOLOGY.   Restraint procedures are seldom carried out on animals subjected to prior fasting. Thus the rumen and stomach may contain ingesta undergoing fermentation and digestion. Bloat may be caused by excessive gas formation, but is more likely a result of the inability of the animal to eructate normally.

It is dangerous to keep ruminants in lateral recumbency for extended periods. In this position, ruminal fluid covers the esophageal opening, preventing the escape of gases.

Some drugs such as succinyl chloride and curare-like drugs may contribute to bloat production by relaxing the voluntary muscles of the esophagus. The voluntary control of regurgitation and eructation is subject to wide species variation.

A starved animal given unlimited access to food may engorge itself. This is particularly dangerous when dry food is provided. Water taken into a stomach already full of dry food produces marked swelling, with classic signs of bloat, and such pressure can kill.

CLINICAL SIGNS. If given the opportunity, the animal shows evidence of colic by frequently lying down and getting up, kicking at the abdomen, and rolling.

Rumen motility is increased initially, but as bloat progresses the rumen becomes atonic. Tympanitic sounds are heard on percussion. Dyspnea is marked, accompanied by cyanosis and rapid pulse. Pressure on abdominal vessels prevents adequate circulation. Electrolyte changes and shock ensue. Regurgitation is a common sequel, with potential for inhalation of ingesta and, consequently, the development of gangrenous pneumonia.

THERAPY. In ruminal or stomach distension, slowly reduce intraluminal pressure by means of a stomach tube. Internal pressure on the cardia may impede the passage of a stomach tube, but gentle pressure will usually overcome the obstruction. It may be necessary to manipulate the tube in order to locate and release all the gas pockets within the rumen. Alternatively, a large needle (12 gauge) or a trocar and cannula may be used to deflate the rumen. Penetrate the rumen through the skin in the left paralumbar fossa. If time permits, prepare the area surgically, but if the patient is in critical condition, immediate penetration is imperative.

If gaseous intestinal distension is detected early, rapid evacuation is permissible. If distension has been prolonged, a gradual release of gas is essential. All the veins will have collapsed. Capillary permeability will have increased. Too rapid reduction of intraabdominal pressure will cause venous distension, splanchnic pooling, and possibly shock.

Intestinal distension is less prevalent than bloat during restraint. If it does occur, it is likely to be as a result of bowel obstruction caused by a twisted loop of bowel or by drug paralysis.

Therapy for bowel obstruction is more complicated than for gaseous distention. More definitive diagnostic techniques must be used to determine the etiology. Medical and/or surgical intervention may be required to relieve the condition.

NECROPSY. Bloat associated with restraint is usually acute and readily diagnosed antemortem. In some cases the animal may bloat and die after release from restraint. Differentiation between bloat—which killed the animal—and postmortem gaseous distention is not easy. Pressure ischemia of the abdominal viscera—especially of the liver—present in bloat, may be a key to such differentiation.

Death from bloat is caused by anoxia. The blood is dark and does not clot. Dyspnea prior to death is indicated by petechial hemorrhage of the tracheal mucosa and congestion or hemorrhage of lymph nodes draining the upper respiratory tract.

POST-RESTRAINT COMPLICATIONS

Reduced resistance to disease is an ill-defined consequence of restraint stress. (See Chapter 7.) Disruption of the integrity of skin and mucous membranes may allow opportunistic microorganisms to gain entrance and cause infection. Pneumonia, general sepsis, wound infection, and enteric infection are frequent sequelae to restraint procedures.

When working with wild species, one cannot discount the accumulative effects of the chronic stress syndrome. Animals suffering from chronic stress may develop adrenal exhaustion and hypoadrenal shock during any subsequent stressful period such as inclement weather, introduction of new animals, or reduced food intake.

Handling may initiate a period of anorexia. Snakes commonly refuse to feed for weeks to months after being pinned. Mammals and birds may be similarly affected, especially if roughly handled. Agalactia may be induced in a lactating female, causing the infant to become hypoglycemic.

Capture myopathy has been known to develop as long as 30 days following a capture operation. Continued tonic muscle activity or metabolic changes can precipitate ischemia and necrosis.

SPECIAL PROBLEMS

Infant animals are subject to special problems during restraint procedures. Youngsters are much more liable to trauma because of their size and inexperience. Infants are easily crushed, gored, trampled on, and bitten by pen mates or cage mates or even by the dam, who may be excited by capture operations.

Wild species under stress may exhibit drastic behavioral changes. The mother's protective behavior may become so aggressive that she kills the infant. It is wise to separate young animals from larger specimens before attempting to capture either.

Young animals are more susceptible to heat and cold stress than are adults. Intense excitement places added burdens on the young. An infant prevented from nursing the mother for an extended period may develop hypoglycemia. Furthermore, a drugged or excited mother may suffer temporary or even permanent agalactia, causing the infant to suffer from malnutrition subsequent to the restraint procedure.

If at all possible, postpone shipping until after weaning so that young and their larger dams may be crated separately.

HUMAN INJURY DURING RESTRAINT

Trauma to restrainer or assistant is common during restraint procedures. Be prepared to administer first aid.

Lacerations, contusions, abrasions, fractures, concussions, bite wounds, and kicks are all consequences of failure to adequately prepare for a restraint procedure.[4] In almost every instance, a human mistake precedes an injury.

As with the animal, the most important first aid measures for a person include stopping hemorrhage and maintaining adequate air exchange. All individuals working around animals should know rescue breathing techniques (mouth-to-mouth, etc.).

Traumatic shock occurs more frequently in persons than in animals. Be prepared to alleviate shock by having the patient lie down, lowering the head, and providing warmth.

The most effective therapy for many traumatic cases is to apply ice packs. Crush ice and put it into a plastic bag. Do not add salt or any other foreign substance to the ice so the bag can be placed directly against the skin without freezing the tissue. The patient may experience transient pain while the skin is cooling. A thin towel can be placed between the skin and the ice for sensitive individuals.

Coolness minimizes extravasation of plasma and induces vascular constriction with resultant decreased hemorrhage, lessening swelling and pain. Function of the injured tissue returns sooner than if the inflammatory process is allowed to run its course. Standard first aid should be carried out until a physician can be consulted.

The person in charge of a restraint procedure is legally obligated to protect those participating, including the animal's owner, who may be assisting. It is incumbent on the person in charge to select an appropriate restraint procedure and to instruct all concerned as to how the technique should be safely carried out.

Veterinarians who deal with restraint procedures daily must be certain that assistants are capable of carrying out a given procedure. Do not assume that a person's general knowledge extends to handling animals in unusual situations or rely on someone's "common sense." There is no such thing as common sense. Common sense is only the result of direct or vicarious experience. One person may be experienced in the handling of cattle but ill equipped to deal with dogs or wild animals. Do not assume that everyone knows that anteaters have strong recurved claws that are dangerous weapons.

Warn assistants of the tremendous strength possessed by animals, particularly by wild species. Prescribe safe distances from hoofs, claws, horns, and antlers. Emphasize the incredi-ble quickness with which even large species such as the rhinoceros and elephant can move.

Assistants, particularly owners of animals, are reluctant to "hurt" the animal and frequently fail to grasp it firmly. The struggling animal escapes and in the process injures the handler. Even customarily affectionate pets may injure their owners when under restraint tension.

Animal protein allergies may cause problems for some individuals. A person may be sensitive either to general animal dust or be species specific. One of my colleagues is extremely sensitive to black buck and bush buck antelope (cutaneous and respiratory signs develop moments after contact with these species) but not to other antelope species.

The owner of the animal or other assistants may faint during restraint procedures. Critical problems may be created if the person who is holding the animal faints. The suddenly freed, excited animal may injure anyone nearby. The fainting person usually recovers quickly, following momentary recumbency.

If an individual who fears an animal is pressed into assisting with animal restraint, there is danger for all concerned. Such a person cannot be relied on to properly respond to directions. It is extremely dangerous to permit a person with ophidiophobia (fear of snakes) to handle poisonous species.

CONCLUSIONS

Numerous medical problems may develop during restraint procedures. Table 9.4 tabulates signs that can be observed and lists a group of potential etiologies for each sign. A differential diagnosis can be made utilizing information presented in this chapter.

REFERENCES

1. Adams, H.R. Ed. 1995. Veterinary Pharmacology and Therapeutics, 7th ed. Ames: Iowa State Univ. Press.
2. Basson, P.A., and Hofmeyr, J.M. 1973. Mortalities associated with wildlife capture operations. In: E. Young, Ed. Capture and

TABLE 9.4.   Possible etiology of signs observed during restraint

Convulsions (seizures)—Anoxia, hypocalcemia, hypoglycemia, hyperthermia, hypoxia, pneumonia, struggling, cardiac failure, brain contusion, catatonia (drug reaction), epilepsy, fracture of cervical vertebrae and acidosis.
Tetany—Hypocalcemia, hypoglycemia, hypothermia (shivering).
Rapid breathing—Hyperthermia, hypoxia, acidosis.
Elevated body temperature—Latent infection, increased muscle activity, drug effects on central thermoregulation, restraint practices that prevent heat dissipation, catatonia, convulsive disorders.
Decreased body temperature—Drug effects on central thermoregulation, failure to provide proper environment, prolonged anesthesia.
Pale mucous membranes—Anemia, shock, hemorrhage.
Dark mucous membranes—Normal pigmentation of mucosa in that species, hypoxia (strangulation, pneumonia, pulmonary edema).
Bloat (stomach or intestines)—Improper positioning of body during restraint, twisted intestine, ileus, drug-induced ileus.
Loose stool—Fright, previous enteric disease, response to drugs.
Regurgitation—Pressure on thorax or abdomen, improper positioning of body during restraint, relaxation of cardia by drug action, excitement.
Carrying a limb—Fracture of a bone, severe sprain, contusion to hoof or claw.
Unable to stand on leg—Nerve damage, ruptured tendon or ligaments, capture myopathy, fracture.
Unable to use hindquarters—Fracture of thoracic or lumbar vertebrae, fracture of pelvis, thrombus in an iliac vessel.
Inability to use all four limbs—Fracture of cervical vertebrae, brain contusion, hypoglycemia.
Urination and frequent defecation—Fright, response to drugs.

Care of Wild Animals, pp. 151–71. Capetown, South Africa: Human and Rousseau.

3. Calnek, B.W., Barnes, H.J., Beard, C.W., Reid, W.M., and Yoder, H.W., Jr., Eds. 1991. Diseases of Poultry, 9th ed. Ames: Iowa State Univ. Press.

4. Douglas, L.G. 1975. Bite wounds. Am Fam Physician 11:93–99.

5. Ettinger, S.J., and Feldman, E., Eds. 2005. Textbook of Veterinary Internal Medicine: Diseases of the Dog and Cat, 5th ed., vols. 1, 2. St. Louis, Elsevier/Saunders.

6. Feldman, B.F., Zinkl, J.G., and Jain, N.C. 2000. Schalm's Veterinary Hematology, 5th Ed. Philadelphia, Lippincott Williams and Wilkins.

7. Goodman, L.S., and Gilman, A. 1990. The Pharmacological Basis of Therapeutics, 8th ed. New York: Macmillan.

8. Harthoorn, A. 1974. A relationship between acid base balance and capture myopathy in zebra (Equus burchelli) and an apparent therapy. Vet Rec 94:337–41.

9. Jones, D.R., and Johansen, K. 1972. The blood vascular system of birds. In: D.S. Farner, and King, J.R., Eds. Avian Biology, vol. 2, p. 159. New York: Academic Press.

10. Jubb, K.V.F., and Kennedy, P.C. 1985. Pathology of Domestic Animals, 3rd ed., vol. 3, p. 15. New York: Academic Press.

11. Kirk, R. W., and Bistner, S.I. 1990. Handbook of Veterinary Procedures and Emergency Treatment, 5th ed. Philadelphia: W.B. Saunders.

12. Leman, A.D., Straw, B.E., Mengeling, W.L., D'Allaire, S., and Taylor, D.J., Eds. 1996. Diseases of Swine, 7th ed. Ames: Iowa State Univ. Press.

13. Linford, R.L. 2002. Laminitis. In: Smith, B.P., Ed. 2002. Large Animal Internal Medicine. 3rd Ed. St. Louis, Mosby/Elsevier, pp. 1116–24.

14. Munday, B.L. 1972. Myonecrosis in free-living and recently-captured macropods. J. Wildl. Dis. 8:191–92.

15. Pugh, D.G. Ed. 2002. Sheep and Goat Medicine. St. Louis, Saunders/Elsevier.

16. Radostits, O.M., Gay, C.C., Blood, D.C., and Hionchcliff, K.W. 2000. Veterinary Medicine. Philadelphia, W.B. Saunders, pp. 1805–10.

17. Ridgway, S., Ed. 1972. Homeostasis in the aquatic environment. In: Mammals of the Sea, pp. 597. Springfield: Charles C. Thomas.

18. Ross, J.N., Jr. 1975. Heart failure and shock. In: S.J. Ettinger, Ed. Textbook of Veterinary Medicine, pp. 825–64. Philadelphia: W.B. Saunders.

19. Schmidt-Neilson, K. 1975. Animal Physiology, Adaptation and Environment, p. 255. London: Cambridge Univ. Press.

20. Seligman, M. 1974. Giving up on life. Psychol. Today (May): 80–85.

21. Smith, B.P., Ed. 2002. Large Animal Internal Medicine. 3rd Ed. St. Louis, Mosby/Elsevier.

22. Sodeman, W.A., and Sodeman, W.A., Jr. 1979. Pathologic Physiology, Mechanisms of Diseases, 6th ed. Philadelphia: W.B. Saunders.

23. Spraker, T.R. 1993. Stress and capture myopathy in artiodactylids. In: Fowler, M.E., Ed. Zoo and Wild Animal Medicine, Current Therapy 3, pp. 481–88. Philadelphia: W.B. Saunders.

24. Yagil, R., Etzion, Z., and Berlyne, G.M. 1975. Acid base parameters in the dehydrated camel. Tijdschr. Diergeneeskd. 100:1105–07.

PART 2

Domestic Animals

Horses, Donkeys, Mules

CLASSIFICATION

Order Perissodactyla
    Family Equidae: horse, pony, ass, burro, donkey, mule, hinny

Although horses are no longer used extensively as primary draft animals, there are more horses in the United States at the present time than existed at the zenith of the horse's use for power. Racing and general recreation account for the phenomenal increase in numbers.

Horses are seen in all shapes and sizes, from tiny ponies less than 1 m (39 in.) tall and weighing less than 45 kg (100 lb) to large draft horses, 160 cm (68 in.) tall and weighing 1,364 kg (3,000 lb).

Donkeys and mules are intermediate in size and share many characteristics with the horse. Restraint practices are essentially the same.

See Table 10.1 for the names of gender used in the equine.

TABLE 10.1. Names of gender of equine

Animal	Adult			Immature		
	Male	Female	Neutered	Newborn	Male	Female
Horse, pony	Stallion, stud	Mare	Gelding	Foal	Colt	Filly <4 years
Donkey, ass, burro	Jack	Jenny	Gelding	Foal		
Mule*	Mule	Mare	Gelding	Foal		

*(male donkey + female horse = hybrid).

DANGER POTENTIAL

Horses can kick, strike, bite, and press persons against walls. Even a foal or a pony can injure a handler's foot by stepping on it. The bite of a horse is serious. A large stallion is capable of grasping a person by an arm or shoulder and lifting him/her off the ground. Once the horse has grasped a person, the jaw remains closed and the tissue is pulled through the teeth. Serious contusion results (Fig. 10.1).

Horses usually kick directly backward with either or both hind feet. A few horses are adept at kicking forward and outward (cow-kicking) and can reach up to their front legs.

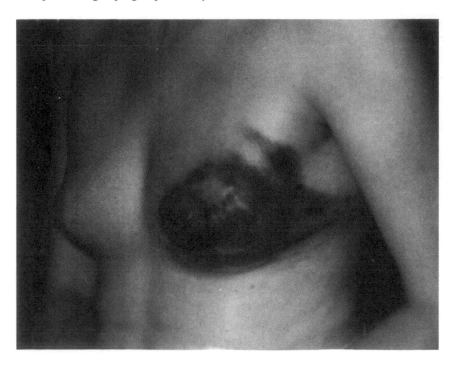

FIG. 10.1. Woman's breast 2 days after being bitten by a pony stallion.

Mules and donkeys are experts at this. Handlers may be kicked in the head and killed as they bend over to work on the legs of such a horse. It is wise when working around a horse's legs to keep your head above the knee or the hock at all times.

Horses may strike with one foreleg from a standing position, or they may rear and strike with both legs. Striking often occurs when an attempt is made to apply a twitch. A horse may also hit the handler with its head as it swings it to avoid capture. The safest place to stand is next to the left foreleg, close to the body, to prevent kicking, striking, and biting.

PHYSICAL RESTRAINT[1,2,5,10,11]

Horses are startled by quick movements and loud noises but usually respond to voice commands. Speak firmly, but do not shout. Voice and other mannerisms betray fear, quickly detected by a horse. If you lack confidence, remain silent.

Horses enjoy being stroked, and this is soothing during handling procedures. The wise handler continually speaks to the horse and maintains physical contact by stroking. Since horses may be ticklish, stroking must be firm, avoiding such sensitive areas as the flanks or around the ears and eyes.

Mules and donkeys may be more stubborn than horses and require more patience and perseverance.

Horses are usually handled with a halter and lead shank. Permanent halters are constructed of leather or nylon webbing (Fig. 10.2), or cotton and nylon rope (Fig. 10.3). Temporary halters may be constructed of rope (Fig. 3.37).

Leather halters are usually the weakest unless triple-stitched and made of heavy straps. Haltering is accomplished as illustrated in Figure 10.4. The horse will stand more quietly for haltering if a rope is placed around its neck first. The lead

shank may be a simple rope tied to the halter ring. Most shanks use a snap for easier attachment to the ring. Frequently the snap is the weakest link and may break at an inopportune time.

The snap-chain shank is popular. The chain may be attached to a rope or leather strap. The snap may attach

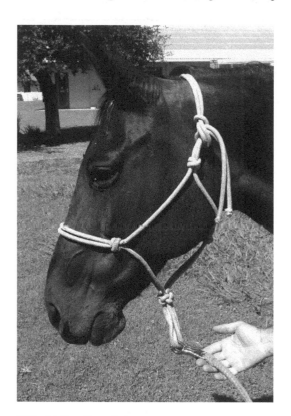

FIG. 10.3. Rope halter.

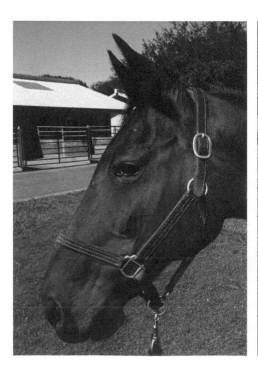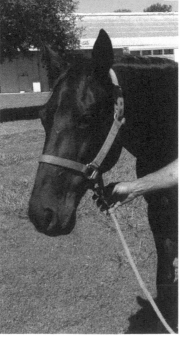

FIG. 10.2. Triple-stitched leather halter, left; nylon web halter, right.

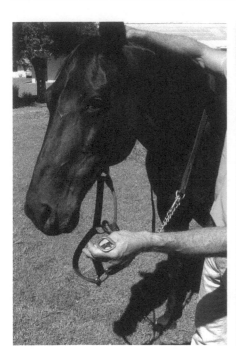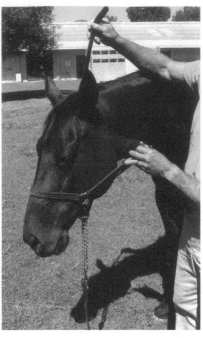

FIG. 10.4. Haltering a horse.

directly to the halter ring or be threaded through the ring and snapped to itself, adding strength to the snap and making it possible to grasp the shank closer to the head of the horse without having to grab the chain.

The chain shank is frequently used for further restraint. The chain may be placed through the mouth and attached to the cheek ring on the opposite side, serving as a bit or bridle (Fig. 10.5). If the mouth is jerked or otherwise injured by the chain, the animal will thereafter resist any bit. The chain may also be placed over the bridge of the nose (Fig.10.6 left). By

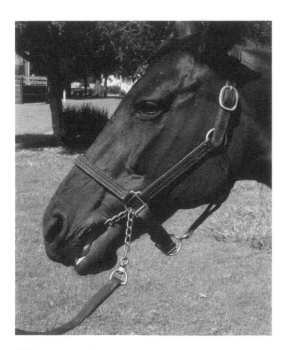

FIG. 10.5. Chain shank through the mouth.

gently tugging the shank, one can divert the animal's attention. The pressure exerted tends to pull the nose down.

If the chain is placed under the chin instead of over the bridge of the nose, this is mechanically a mistake. When the chain is pulled, the horse naturally throws its head up to relieve pressure underneath the chin, making the horse unmanageable instead of controlling it.

Keep the lead rope high and short when tying a horse (Fig. 10.7) to prevent it from entangling its feet. A horse will fight to extricate itself from such a predicament, and serious rope burns and injury to the cervical vertebrae may occur in the ensuing struggle.

The twitch is the most important manual tool used in equine restraint. The principle is based on reaction to pressure applied to the sensitive lip. Endorphins are released that cause lowering of the heart rate and an increased tolerance for discomfort associated with procedures performed elsewhere on the limbs or body. Used injudiciously, serious damage can be done to the lip. For example, a judo expert assisting in a procedure nearly tore the lip off his horse because he twisted the twitch too tightly.

The most satisfactory twitch consists of a short length of chain attached to a hardwood handle approximately 2 feet long. A rope loop may also be used. A pick handle with two holes drilled at the sides to admit the rope to pass through is a satisfactory base.

The rope twitch is gentler but is slower to twist up. Another disadvantage is that if the horse pulls loose from the handler, the loop is slow to untwist. In such a situation the horse usually swings its head, flailing the twitch handle around, endangering both horse and handler. A chain twitch in the same situation drops off quickly.

To use a twitch, grasp the twitch and the cheek piece of the halter with the right hand. Place the fingers of the left hand

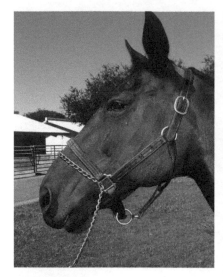

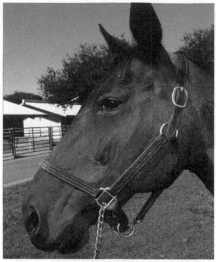

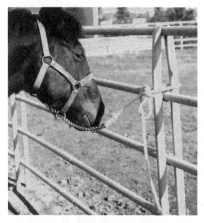

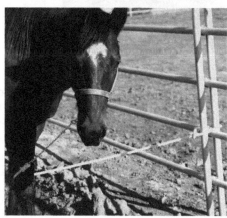

FIG. 10.6.   Use of the chain shank. Over the nose provides excellent mild restraint. Under the chin may cause head tossing and is not recommended.

FIG. 10.7.   Horse tied properly, high and short, left; and tied improperly allowing a leg to be entangled in the rope, right.

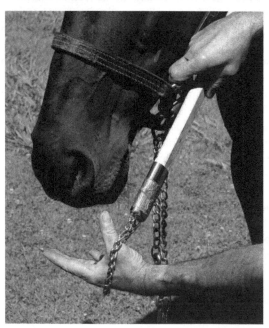

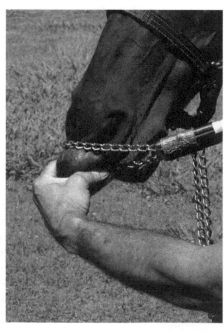

FIG. 10.8.   Applying twitch.

partially through the loop of the twitch (Fig. 10.8). Do not insert the whole hand to the wrist, as this complicates placement of the twitch. Bring the left hand over the bridge of the nose and gently move it to the upper lip. Once the operator is prepared to grab the lip, it should be done firmly to prevent the horse from pulling away. The more times the horse successfully escapes the operator, the more difficult it will be to place the twitch. Once the fingers have a firm grasp of the nose, the rope or chain is brought over the lip and the right hand begins to twist the loop. Twist firmly to maintain a grip, but not so tightly that severe pain is felt, or the horse will resist by pulling away or even striking. It is important for the operator to maintain a grip on the handle with both hands or the handle may be pulled away. The halter shank should be used to pull the head toward the left side. Do not use the twitch as a lever. The pressure on the lip should be a twist, not a pull.

When twitching, pull the head to the left so that the operator is not exposed to the front legs if the horse should strike. The handler should stand close to the shoulder (Fig. 10.9). Never stand in front of the horse.

Once the twitch is in place, do not maintain a constant pressure or the lip will become numb and fail to provide the necessary restraint. It is more desirable to carry out a rocking motion with the handle so the twist is released and tensed periodically. If the animal shows signs of fidgeting or failing to respond to the twitch, shake the nose more vigorously. Jerking the nose or twisting too hard will cause permanent damage to the lip. It is not likely that a twitch left in place for more than 15 minutes will remain effective. A horse may appear to go to sleep, but then may explode. Periodic rest is necessary for prolonged procedures.

Removing the twitch requires as much care as placing it on the nose. The moment of release seems to be a stimulus

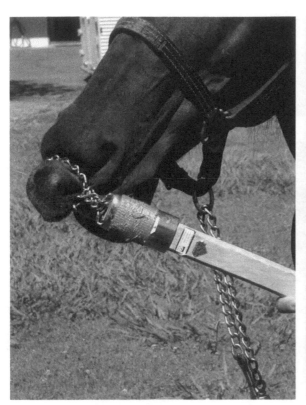
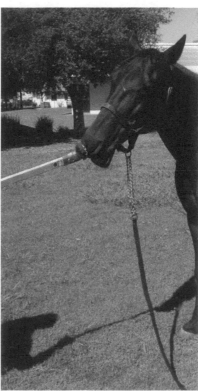

FIG. 10.9. Proper, left, and improper, right, positions for holding a twitch.

for the horse to pull away and perhaps even to strike. Remove the twitch quickly to prevent the horse from jerking it out of your hand and swinging it around. After twitching, it may be desirable to massage the lip to restore circulation. The twitch can be used repeatedly if the horse is not injured by rough handling during the procedure.

The hand may be used as a mild twitch (Fig. 10.10 upper). The lone operator may use a self-retaining twitch (Fig. 10.11). Placing a twitch on the ear is hazardous, as the ear may be permanently damaged.

A horse's attention may be diverted by grasping a fold of skin at the shoulder (Fig. 10.12). The lip chain utilizes the chain shank and is placed as illustrated in Figure 10.13. Tension must be constantly applied or it will slip off. Use caution, because the rough chain can severely traumatize the mucous membrane of the lip and premaxilla.

Some horses will fight a twitch but can be restrained by applying pressure to one or both ears. To do it, stand in front of the shoulder alongside the neck. To ear a horse, lay the right hand on the top of the poll with the palm down, the fingers together, and the thumb extended (Fig. 10.14, left). Push the hand forward to the base of the ear so the web between the thumb and the forefinger is tight against the base. Then bring the fingers and thumb together and squeeze the ear. The closure of the hand tends to lift the ear from the top of the head (Fig. 10.14, right). Grasp the left ear with the right hand. The left hand grasps the halter or is placed over the bridge of the horse's nose. Pull the horse's head toward its left side to keep the animal slightly off balance. As soon as the animal feels pressure on the ear, it will pull away toward the right.

Even if the horse pulls the operator toward the right, the grip should be maintained. The horse is not apt to strike in

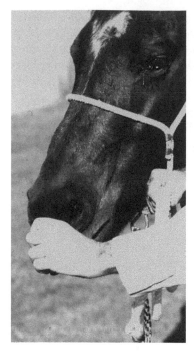
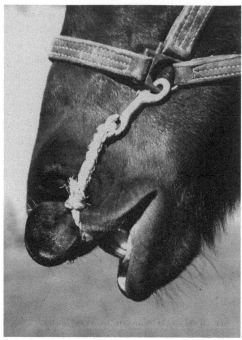

FIG. 10.10.   Using the hand as a twitch, left. Self-retaining twitch, right.

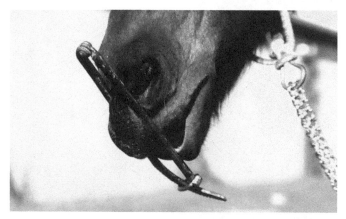

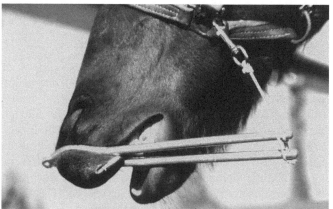

FIG. 10.11.   Self-retaining twitches.

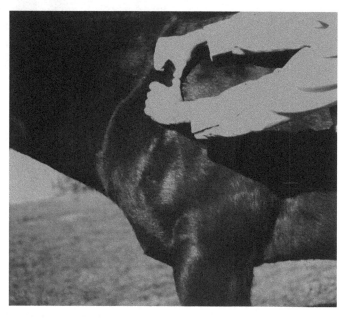

FIG. 10.12.   Mild restraint may be obtained by lifting a fold of skin at the shoulder.

this position, being more concerned with trying to pull away from the pressure on the ear. The tension on the ear can be relaxed and increased by simply opening and closing the hand. At no time should the ear be twisted or the pinna bent and cramped since these actions are likely to injure the pinna, causing the horse to become head shy.

An alternate method of earing the horse may be carried out using both hands. One person must hold the halter. Another approaches the horse in the same manner as previously described, on the left side, only in this instance the right arm is draped over the neck and both hands brought up as before. The right hand is placed on the right ear and the left hand on the left ear. In this position the handler can control the head and neck. The animal is less able to rear because of the added weight of the handler on the neck.

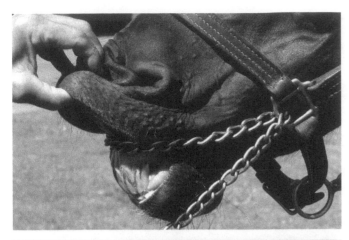

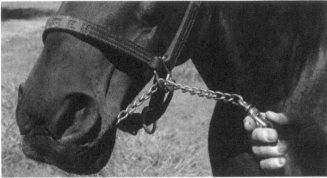

FIG. 10.13. Applying lip chain.

Manipulating Feet and Legs

The foreleg may be lifted by a rear or front approach. With the rear approach on a left foreleg, place the right shoulder against the horse's left chest. Press the right forearm forward against the back of the knee and run the hand down the leg to grasp the pastern or cannon bone. When approaching from the front, pull the knee forward to make the horse lift its leg (Fig. 10.15).

Examine the foot while holding it with one hand, or by straddling the leg and supporting the foot with the knees (Fig. 10.16). The most comfortable position for the handler is with the knee slightly flexed. The feet should be about 12 in. apart with the toes turned in, driving the knees together. Once the limb is lifted, it is important that the handler maintain the grip and not allow the horse to set its foot down again until desired. If the horse is permitted to pull its foot away and place it on the ground, it will attempt to do this again and again. Fortunately most horses that have experienced some handling are content to lift the leg, providing it is not pulled into an abnormal position and the animal is allowed to balance on the other three legs. Holding one leg up is an excellent way to minimize kicking while someone works elsewhere on the horse. Do not underestimate a horse's ability to balance, however. Some can kick even while balancing on two legs.

The left hind leg is lifted as follows: Face the back of the horse, place the left hand on the point of the hip, and move the right hand over the rump of the horse and down its hind

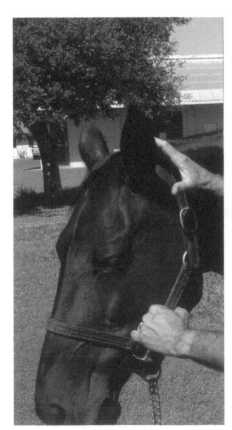

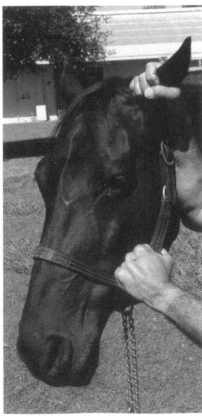

FIG. 10.14. Earing a horse.

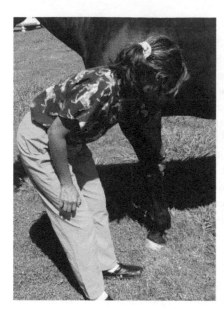

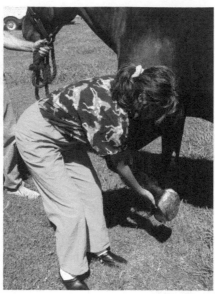

FIG. 10.15. Lifting a foreleg from the front approach.

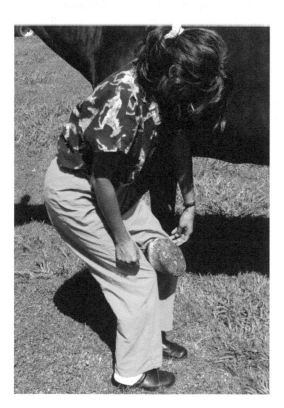

FIG. 10.16. Holding a foreleg.

leg (Fig. 10.17). This manipulation alerts the horse that you are going to be working on that hind leg. If it is inclined to kick, it will probably indicate this as well. Do not tickle the flank area. The right hand is brought down over the thigh and hock, ultimately resting on the midtarsal region. Pull the leg forward and upward (Fig. 10.17). Some horses may kick, but a person in the proper position will not be injured. Next place the left hand over the hock and step back under the leg. Finally, the leg is supported by the legs and body of the

handler (Fig. 10.18), leaving both hands free to examine and manipulate the foot.

A foal does not usually respond well to a halter or to being led. Instead of placing a halter on the head of a foal, the halter may be strapped around the thorax, acting as a harness, like those used on dogs and cats. If a detailed examination must be given, grasp the foal by the tail and hold under the neck (Fig. 10.19). Older foals and small yearlings can also be held in this manner by individuals with adequate strength or by two people. Rarely, a foal will reach around and bite when grabbed like this. A word of caution: If the grip on the tail is held tight for too long, the foal will attempt to sit down.

Sometimes a foal is difficult to catch. The mare may be placed against a wall so that the foal will wedge between her and the wall (Fig. 10.20). If the mare is not a kicker, the handler can step in behind and tail the foal. The mare handler must prevent the foal from escaping forward.

Never stand directly facing the hind legs. Stand sideways, to prevent receiving a kick in the abdomen or groin.

A foal can be taught to be led by placing a rope over the rump and through a halter (Fig. 10.21). More pressure is placed on the butt rope. A foal can be cast quite simply by pulling the tail between the hind legs and maintaining pressure. Soon the foal will begin to relax and slump to the ground (Figs. 10.22 and 10.23). Maintain the cast position by pulling the tail up in front of the stifle and placing pressure on the neck (Fig. 10.24). Another technique, especially applicable to neonates, is to stand on one side, twist the head and neck rearward on the opposite side, and place pressure over the rump. The foal will sit down.[7]

A foal is extremely curious. In a pasture it is sometimes possible to catch a foal by simply squatting down and allowing it to come up and investigate. As it approaches the handler, it can be grasped in the manner previously described.

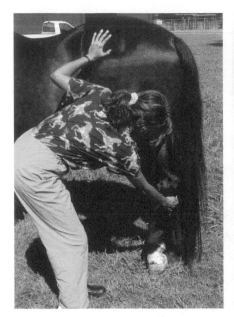 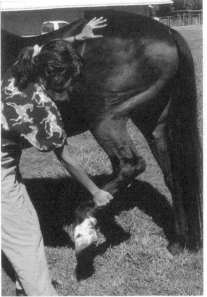

FIG. 10.17. Approach to lifting a hind leg.

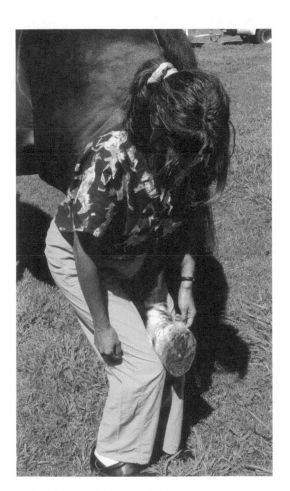

FIG. 10.18. Holding a hind leg.

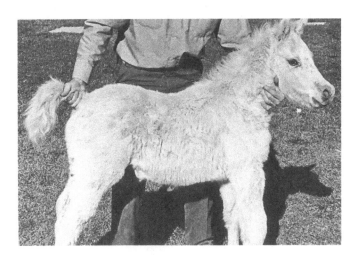

FIG. 10.19. Proper way to hold a young foal.

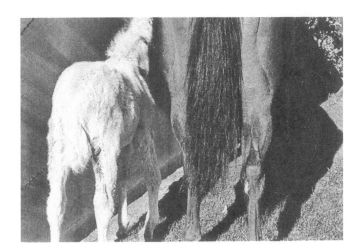

FIG. 10.20. Capturing a foal by holding the mare against a wall.

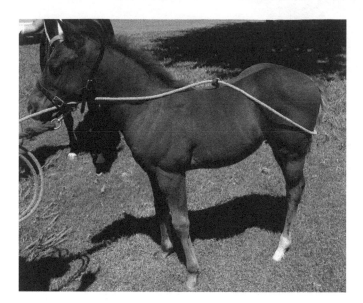

FIG. 10.21. Use of a rump rope to lead a foal.

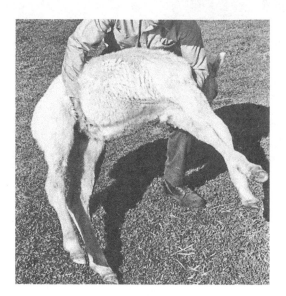

FIG. 10.23. Foal relaxing and slumping to the ground.

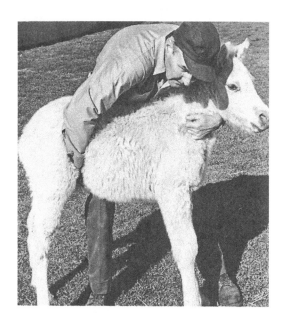

FIG. 10.22. Casting a foal by pulling tail between the hind legs.

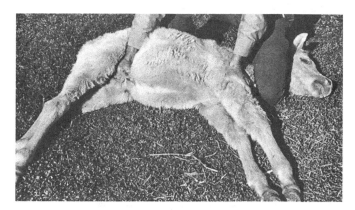

FIG. 10.24. Holding foal down by maintaining grip on tail and pressure on stifle.

This procedure sometimes works with wild animals, too. A partially tranquilized elk calf walked up to me when I was squatted down.

Casting Harness (Hobble)

It is frequently necessary to restrain the horse on the ground in a recumbent position. A casting harness is rarely employed for equine restraint in North America and Europe, but should it be necessary the technique is described fully in *Restraint and Handling of Wild and Domestic Animals*, Second Edition. Immobilizing agents and anesthesia are routinely used instead of physically overpowering the horse.

A sideline is used to prevent a horse from kicking backward when an operator has to work at the rear, for example, when conducting pregnancy examinations or genital examinations for infertility. The sideline is placed by tying a large bowline loop around the neck. The running end is brought over the side of the shoulder and around the hind pastern. The rope is brought back up to the neck rope and secured by a halter tie (Fig. 10.25).

The danger of rope burns may be obviated by wrapping the pastern with cotton first. However, if the horse is a kicker, wrapping may be hazardous. Hobbles are safer and can be constructed of leather, webbing, or a roll of burlap (Figs. 10.26, 10.27).

Breeding hobbles are commonly used to prevent injury to valuable stallions (Fig. 10.28). The simplest, safest, and most effective hobble consists of a system of straps and ropes. One strap encircles the neck. Another strap is attached to a ring on the neck strap and goes between the front legs. This strap ends in the ring, which is the focal point of the hobble.

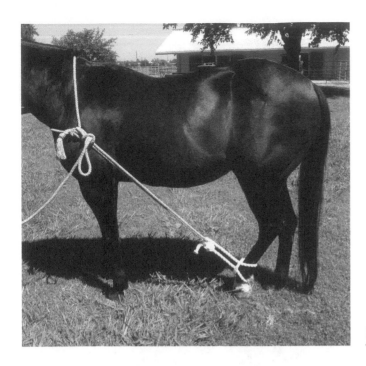

FIG. 10.25. Sideline using hobble.

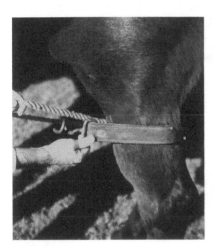 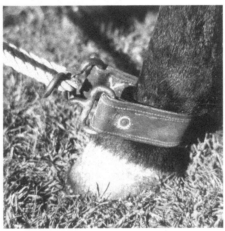

FIG. 10.26. Leather hobble with corkscrew ring for rapid attachment.

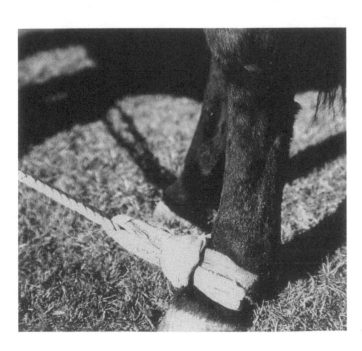

FIG. 10.27. Burlap loop used as pastern hobble.

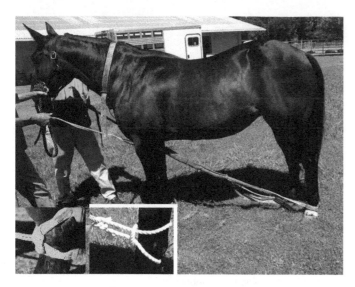

FIG. 10.28. Breeding hobble. Figure eight hock hobbles can be constructed of leather or webbing.

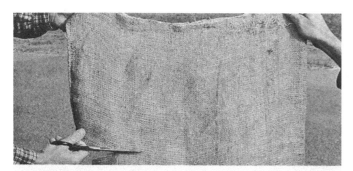

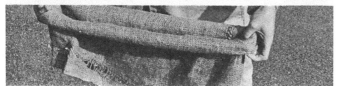

FIG. 10.29. Construction of a burlap hobble.

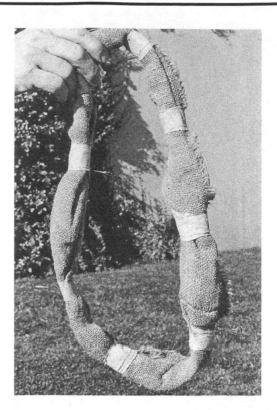

FIG. 10.30. Burlap hobble.

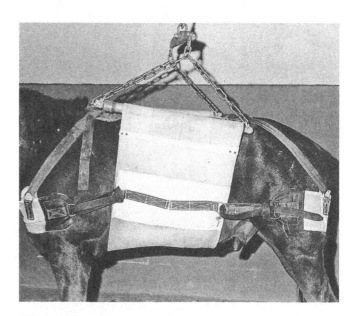

FIG. 10.31. Canvas sling.

Figure eight hobbles are applied to the hocks. A length of nylon rope with a strong snap on one end is attached to one hobble. The rope is threaded through the ring and tied at the other hock. A burlap roll may be used in lieu of web or leather hock hobbles (Figs. 10.29, 10.30).

Slings are used to provide partial and temporary support for a weak or injured horse. A horse cannot hang free in a sling for more than a few minutes, so it must be conscious and capable of some degree of self-support. An excellent heavy-duty sling is illustrated in Figure 10.31. Chest and butt straps prevent the horse from slipping forward or back. The belly band should be spread with a single-tree or a similar device. The horse must be lifted with a block and tackle. Refer to Chapter 3 for a consideration of the size of rope and type of blocks necessary. The head is tied to prevent the horse from swiveling around the block and tackle.

A rope sling (Figs. 10.32 to 10.34) may be used to lift a horse to its feet or to extricate it from a predicament such as falling into a ditch. Continual support with a rope sling will compromise circulation. A multipurpose sling, designed by Dr. John Madigan, Davis, California, has become a prototype for biologically sound slings (Figs. 10.35, 10.36). It has been used to support hospitalized horses and to evacuate injured horses from remote wilderness areas by helicopter. A new

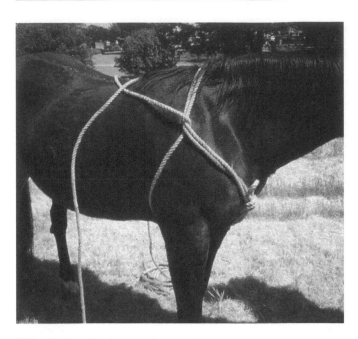

FIG. 10.32. Beginning of a rope sling.

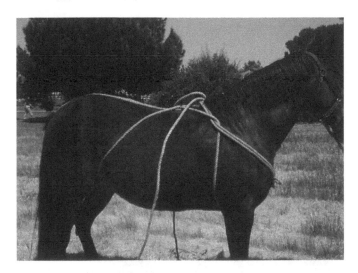

FIG. 10.33. Further construction of a rope sling.

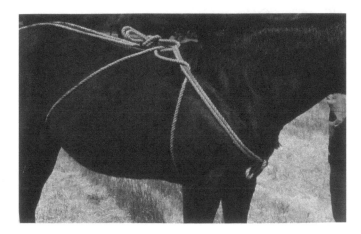

FIG. 10.34. Rope sling completed.

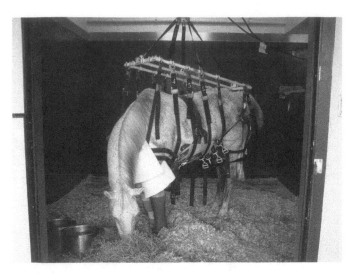

FIG. 10.35. Madigan-designed sling. Head free (Manufactured by Anderson Sling, P.O. Box 53, Potter Valley, CA 95469. Courtesy, Dr. John Madigan).

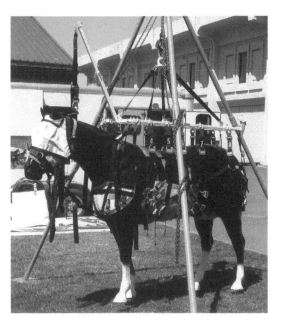

FIG. 10.36. Madigan designed sling. Head supported.

Madigan design called a large animal lift is easier to apply and will support a horse for a short time (Fig. 10.37).

Blindfolding usually has a calming effect on most horses. Special blinders are available for trailering horses. Towels may also be used (Fig. 10.38). Blindfolded horses must be watched to prevent them from stepping off tailgates or getting into other predicaments. Occasionally a horse becomes terrified when blindfolded and is unmanageable. These horses cannot be blindfolded, and other techniques must be used to control them.

Cradles are used to prevent a horse from chewing on bandages or surgical sites. A simple one constructed of rope and doweling is illustrated in Figure 10.39.

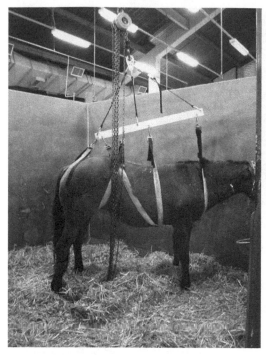

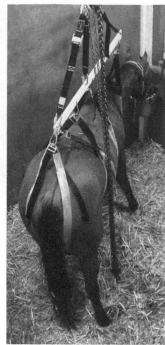

FIG. 10.37. The large animal lift sling.

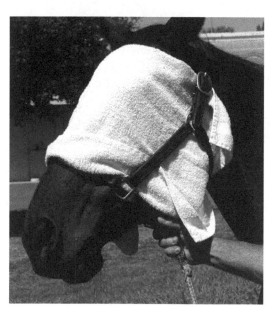

FIG. 10.38. Blindfolded horse.

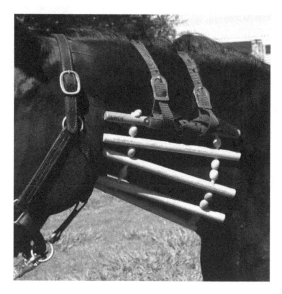

FIG. 10.39. Cradle.

A horse in a trailer or in a tie stall must be approached with caution. Such horses are easily excited; unless you know the horse, you cannot determine whether or not it may kick. Some horses are prone to squeeze, as well, if you walk alongside them. The most serious complication occurs if the horse shies and pulls back as its head is approached. Then if it finds itself restrained by a rope, it may jump forward. Unless there is adequate room to move away, you may be pawed or crushed by the horse. If possible, approach the horse from the front.

A cross tie is useful to control the head and prevent whirling. Place ropes between any contiguous structures such as doorways, corners of stalls, alleyways, or stocks (Fig. 10.40). Tie from the check rings and anchor the ropes or chains high enough to prevent the horse from rearing and entangling its foot in the rope.

TRANSPORT

Horses are moved extensively by truck and trailer. They can and should be trained to load easily and ride without stepping on themselves or getting excited. Many hazards are associated with trailering. These can be minimized by making certain the trailer is properly constructed and repairs made promptly.

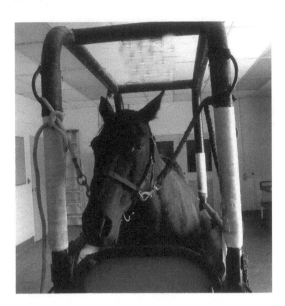

FIG. 10.40. Cross tie.

Protruding objects of any kind are dangerous. Even blunt objects become dangerous when a 1,000-lb horse jams against them. Nuts should always be secured away from areas in which the horse will stand or walk. On dividers, all nuts and bolt heads should be countersunk.

The floor must be given special attention. Most trailers have wood surfaces. Some have no subflooring. Constant wearing by the standing horse plus urine and feces may weaken the wood. It was necessary to euthanize a horse that had broken through a floor while being trailered.

Few commercial trailers are now constructed without a cover. Some rental trailers may have just a high front end and no cover. Horses' eyes suffer severely from wind, insects, and dirt. If a horse must be trailered in an open unit, drive less than 40 MPH or put goggles on the horse. High-speed travel in open trailers also makes breathing difficult.

Be particularly mindful of obstructions on the roof of the trailer. Joints or seams with downward projecting flanges are dangerous. Head tossers are particularly liable to cut their scalps. Do not trailer tall horses in low trailers. Simple balancing when stopping and starting can result in head injuries in a trailer with no headroom.

Wire manger dividers in two-horse trailers may become dangerous. If a strand breaks, the eyes and face of the horse may be lacerated.

Some horses are poor travelers. In most cases it is the result of bad experiences. Careful schooling and patience will overcome a few of these. Boots or wraps must be put on the feet of some horses to protect against injury if the horse walks all over itself. If a horse comes out of a trailer lame, examine the pastern and fetlock carefully to see if the horse has stepped on itself while trying to regain its balance. Application of cold water or ice for an hour or so will reduce pain and swelling. If the skin is cut, further first aid is required. Bruises may occur even though boots are put on the horse.

It is wise to put wraps on the lower legs of even the best trailer-mannered horse. A sudden swerve may throw any horse off balance. Be certain that wraps are snug, but not too tight, and that the bandage is applied with uniform tension up and down the leg. On long trips, wraps have the added advantage of minimizing "stocking" of the legs.

"Tail rubbers" are a special problem. A tail wrap should be used; however, some horses will work these off. Most trailers have a chain that is supposed to prevent rubbing, but in some cases a special tailboard must be constructed. Train the horse to allow a rope to sit under the tail. Some horses have gotten their tails over a chain and then clamped down. Some start kicking. Some react like a foal that is "tailed up"; they relax and sit down. One horse broke its tail by sitting on it in a trailer.

The point of the hock may be bruised easily in a trailer. If the driver starts or stops too quickly, capped hocks will occur sooner or later. The kicker presents a more difficult problem. Hock pads are useful but difficult to keep in place. A pad can be placed behind the horse once it is loaded.

A great hazard occurs at the moment the hind feet step into or out of a step-up trailer. These trailers are low slung, but a horse can always slip a foot under the floor of the trailer. If it moves forward without pulling the foot backward, a severe laceration or even a fracture of the cannon bone may result. Be cautious about shoving a horse into this type of trailer.

The first experience of trailering is the most critical for a horse. It may occur soon after birth or at any time through adulthood. Most foals will follow their mothers into a trailer or a truck. It helps to have a quiet mare to show the way. Keep the foal close to the mare as you approach the trailer. It is better if the foal is broken to lead, although not essential. Crowd the foal into the trailer as soon as the mare is settled.

Dividers present special problems for a mare and foal. High pipe dividers are dangerous, as small foals will duck under them and even crawl under the mare. The divider may be removed with a quiet mare and a careful driver but, generally speaking, it is dangerous to do so. Even a well-behaved mare may be forced to sidestep for balance and inadvertently injure the much smaller foal. A nervous mare would be almost certain to do so. A solid plywood or metal partition is best. This allows a mare and foal to nuzzle each other and at the same time protects them from accidents. Although solid dividers are best to separate a mare and foal, solid partitions between narrow standing areas make it difficult for a horse to spread its legs to maintain balance when a vehicle turns around a corner. Full-length bars provide better side-stepping areas.

A young foal should not be tied in the trailer. Injuries to the neck vertebrae and subsequent development of "wobbler syndrome" are all too common in the foal that hauls back on a tie rope.

Be sure the foal cannot jump out over the tailgate. Usually it is best to string ropes over the top of the tailgate to dissuade jumping in the event the foal turns around.

Teach the horse to stand in the trailer until given a command to back. Never open a trailer door or, more especially, unsnap the chain or drop the butt board without first being certain the horse is untied. Any horse may spook, and it is natural for them to pull back. When nothing pushes from behind, they pull harder and then may suddenly jump forward into the manger.

When a horse jumps forward, anyone in the front of the trailer may be severely injured. Do not stand in front of the manger with either the tailgate closed or the horse tied. If you can walk through, or if there is an escape door, or you can walk on the other side of the divider, the horse can be led in. To walk into a closed trailer and squeeze out alongside the horse is foolhardy. Teach the horse to enter by itself or take a longer lead rope up through the front.

Walk alongside the horse, using a short shank, when entering a walk-through trailer. Move slightly ahead of the horse, and keep looking forward. Do not try to drag the horse into the trailer; lead it in. Watch out for the horse that jumps into the trailer, since it may step on your heels.

Loading is only part of the experience. Driving style is critical to successful trailering. Quick starts and stops throw a foal around much more than an adult horse. It will remember the trailer as an unpleasant place and will be harder to load the next time.

Yearlings that have never been in a trailer are a special problem, especially if they haven't been handled constantly. They are big enough to do a lot of damage but have not yet learned to accept discipline readily. If time permits, one of the best methods of accustoming the uninitiated horse to a trailer is to park the trailer in the corral. Solidly block it so that it cannot move, and feed the horse in the trailer. When the horse is in the trailer, close the door or snap a chain across it quietly. Continue to talk to the horse as you stroke it. Then unsnap the chain or open the door, walk away, and let the horse come out at will.

How does one load a spoiled horse into a trailer? No one trick will work on every horse. People push, pull, curse, and whip, and in the end sometimes sit down and cry when the horse is victorious. Study the horse to figure out the best approach. Once the horse is overexcited, wait until both you and the horse cool off. Then, take a different tack.

Never tranquilize a horse that is spooked and excited by exhausting attempts to load it into a trailer. The drug may have an adverse reaction and excite the horse even further. If a horse is a known bad trailerer, give the tranquilizer to the calm horse an hour before loading. Over-tranquilization is undesirable since it depresses the horse and may upset its equilibrium in the trailer.

If a horse does not go into the trailer after a few attempts, try one of the following:

1. If at least three people are available, put one on the shank and the other two alongside the horse, facing the tail. They can reach around the rump and lock hands or arms, then turn and push forward. They must stay in close to the horse to control sidestepping. The person on the lead shank only directs the horse but does not pull. The two in the rear begin pushing the horse slowly forward, giving it a chance to smell the trailer and get acquainted with it. The pushers keep up steady pressure until the butt chain is snapped.

    Be cautious in using this technique with step-up trailers, since the hind legs may slip under the floorboards. This technique is also somewhat hazardous with a kicker, but unless the horse is a bad "cow-kicker," it will work. It requires two people who are physically capable of staying with the horse and pushing it in. Surprisingly, most horses will respond to light pressure. This is generally the most effective way of putting a horse into a trailer.

2. If alone, place a rope over the rump and through the halter and apply gentle, steady pressure (Fig. 10.41).

3. Another technique is to tie a rope on each side of the trailer. Two people cross them behind the horse

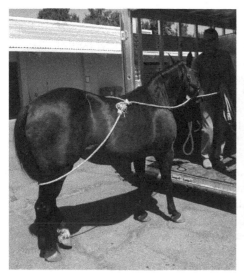
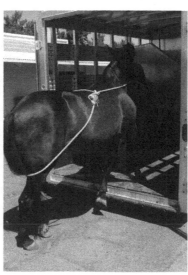

FIG. 10.41. Loading horse into trailer with a rump rope.

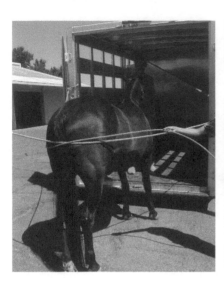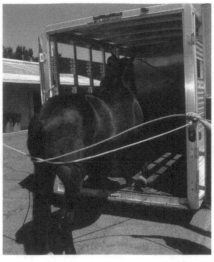

FIG. 10.42.   Loading technique using two ropes.

and apply pressure (Fig. 10.42). This procedure is safer for the horse because the assistants can drop the ropes on command.

4. Preventing a horse from jumping to the side is both desirable and difficult to manage. A narrow alley or loading chute may help. Alternatively, pull the trailer up to the side of a building and eliminate one side of the problem.

5. A whip is usually ineffective and tends to aggravate rather than help a difficult situation. A swat with a house broom or the flat of a scoop shovel works well in encouraging a horse to move into a trailer. The noise is more effective than inflicting pain.

A horse should be tied in the trailer with a quick-release knot or a snap that will release while under pressure (Fig. 10.43). Every horseman or horsewoman should be able to tie the halter tie blindfolded. It is the only acceptable knot for tying a horse in a trailer. If a neck rope is used, it should be secured with a bowline knot.

Hobbles may be useful for restricting movement (Fig. 10.44). However, some individuals may learn to gallop, keeping both front legs moving together. It may then be necessary to hobble three legs together.

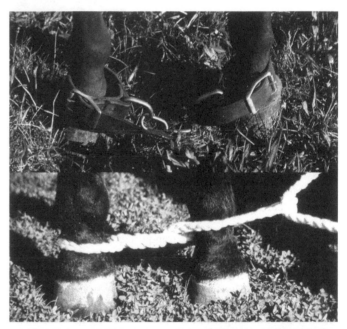
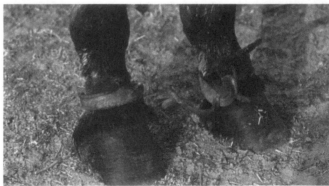

FIG. 10.44.   Various types of hobbles (leather, rope, rawhide).

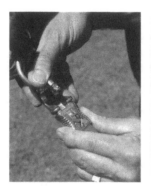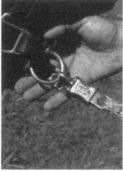

FIG. 10.43.   Quick release snap.

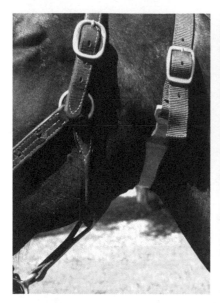
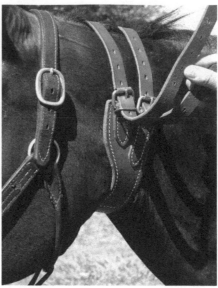

FIG. 10.45. Cribbing straps used to minimize cribbing.

Special devices have been constructed to minimize vices such as cribbing (Fig. 10.45).

CHEMICAL RESTRAINT[3,4,6,8,10,12]

The chemical restraint agents and combinations mentioned in this chapter represent those used by experienced veterinarians with detailed knowledge of horses. Other protocols have been used and no claim is made for including all possible drugs and combinations. For more detailed information, particularly for anesthesia, consult Hubbell[4] or Tranquilli.

The principles of equine tranquilization, chemical immobilization, and anesthesia are well known and documented. No attempt will be made to describe all the techniques and agents in current use. Rather, techniques used to sedate or immobilize fractious horses that cannot be approached or caught without danger to the operator will be described here. See Tables 10.2 and 10.3 for drugs used in sedation and immobilization, respectively.

Trained horses can usually be given intravenous medication, which will facilitate the speed of the restraint procedure. Some horses or mules may be tied or snubbed to a ring, post, or beam for administration of intravenous medication. Horses that are vicious or fractious to the point of preventing haltering or tying must be given oral medication or intramuscular injections. Tranquilization and sedation should be planned in advance to avoid medicating an excited or angry horse. Catecholamine release and other alarm responses may negate the effects of the tranquilizer and/or may cause adverse responses.

Until the 1970s, chloral hydrate was used as a component of equine anesthetic mixtures. Now chloral hydrate has little application, except as a last resort as an oral sedative for an unapproachable horse. Chloral hydrate has a bitter taste and normally a horse will not consume water containing the drug. If a horse cannot be approached otherwise, remove the

TABLE 10.2. Chemical restraint agents for standing sedation in horses, mules, donkeys

Agent	Oral (mg/kg)	Intamuscular (mg/kg)	Intravenous (mg/kg)
Acepromazine	No	0.04–0.1	0.02–0.04
Promazine	Granular form, 3.0–7.0 gms/kg, which is = to 1.0–2.0 mg/kg of the active promazine		
Chloral hydrate	110.0		
Xylazine	No	0.5	0.25–0.45
Detomidine	No	0.02	0.009
Diazepam	No		0.02
Butorphanol	No	0.1	0.1

TABLE 10.3. Chemical restraint agents used for immobilization of horses, mules, donkeys

Agent/combination	Intramuscular dose (mg/kg)	Intravenous dose (mg/kg)
Xylazine/ketamine	1.1/2.2	1.1/2.2
Detomidine/ketamine	No	0.2/2.2
Medetomidine/ketamine	0.02–0.04/2.2	0.02–0.04/2.2
Tiletamine/zolazepam	0.5–1.1	0.02–0.5

water source for 24 hours. Then offer 3.0–4.0 L of water containing the appropriate dose of chloral hydrate. They usually will drink it. Within 30–60 minutes the horse will be sufficiently tractable to allow handling.

A horse free in a pasture, and which defies capture, presents a difficult problem. Chloral hydrate in the drinking water may be used if it is possible to remove all other water sources from the pasture. Alternatively, the projectile syringe may be used. Agents used in such capture operations have included succinylcholine chloride (0.65–1.0 mg/kg), xylazine (1.0–2.0 mg/kg), acepromazine maleate (0.1–0.2 mg/kg), and etorphine (0.04–0.08 mg/kg).

Succinylcholine chloride is a muscle relaxant and has no anesthetic, analgesic, or tranquilizing effect. (See Chapter 20 for more details.) It is an effective chemical immobilizing agent when administered to a horse intravenously, but because the horse is fully conscious, it can feel pain and experience the alarm reaction; therefore, this drug should not be used in place of more appropriate anesthetics or sedatives.

At one time, succinylcholine was the only immobilizing agent approved by the Bureau of Land Management (United States Department of Agriculture) for handling feral horses on western ranges. A dose of 0.65 mg/kg administered intramuscularly produced immobilization in approximately 2 minutes.

Table 10.2 lists drugs used for equine standing sedation. Immobilizing combinations are listed in Table 10.3.

A horse under the effects of xylazine may appear lethargic with the head held low and drooping of the eyelids, but is fully capable of kicking when the limbs are touched.

Phenothiazine type tranquilizers (acepromazine) may cause hypotension in horses. Be cautious about sedating horses with severe blood loss or dehydration. Furthermore, acepromazine will cause relaxation of the retractor penis muscles of male horse with prolapse of the penis from the sheath. Although uncommon, persistent penile paralysis may occur necessitating support for the penis to avoid trauma when lying down or arising.

Succinylcholine chloride has a broad therapeutic dose range in horses. Nonetheless, fatalities have occurred following its use, possibly from complications of hypertension. It should not be used on animals that have been wormed or treated in any way with an organic phosphate anthelmintic or insecticide within the previous 2 weeks.

If tranquilizers can be injected into a horse before it becomes excited, calming may result, which will allow handling. When tranquilizers are injected intramuscularly, allow 30–60 minutes before attempting to handle the horse. Early stimulation may negate the tranquilizing effect.

REFERENCES

1. Anderson, R.S., and Edney, A.T.B., Eds. 1991. Practical Animal Handling, 1st ed. Oxford, U.K. Pergamon Press, 198 pages.
2. Beard, W.L. 1991. Physical restraint of the horse. In: Muir, W.W., and Hubbell, J.A.E., Eds. Equine Anesthesia Monitoring and Emergency Therapy, St. Louis, Mosby Yearbook, pp. 127–39.
3. Geiser, D.R. 1990. Chemical restraint and analgesia in the horse. Vet Clin North Am, Equine Pract 6(3):495–509.
4. Hubbel, J.A.E. 2007. Horses. In: Tranquilli, W.J., Thurman, J.C., and Grimm, K.A., Eds. 2007. Lumb and Jones' Veterinary Anesthesia and Analgesia, 4th Ed. Ames, Iowa, Wiley-Blackwell Publishing, pp. 717–30.
5. Leahy, J.R., and Barrow, P. 1954. Restraint in Animals, 2nd ed. Ithaca, N.Y., Cornell Campus Store.
6. LeBlanc, P.H. 1991. Chemical restraint for surgery in the standing horse. Vet Clin North Am, Equine Pract 7(3):521–31.
7. Madigan, J. 2007. Personal communication. College of Veterinary Medicine, University of California, Davis.
8. Matthews, N.S., and Hartsfield, S.M. 1993. Using injectable anesthetic drugs safely in horses. Vet Med North Am, Equine Pract 88(2):154–59.
9. Muir, W.W., 3rd, Hubbell, J.A.E., and Gabel, A.A. 1991. Overview of equine chemical restraint. In: Muir, W.W., 3rd, and Hubbell, J.A.E., Eds. Equine Anesthesia Monitoring and Emergency Therapy, St. Louis, Mosby Yearbook, pp. 1–6.
10. Sheldon, C.C., Sonsthagen, T., and Topel, J.A. Animal Restraint for the Veterinary Professional. 2006. St. Louis, Mosby/Elsevier, 239 pages.
11. Sonsthagen, T.F. 1991. Restraint of Domestic Animals. Goleta, California, American Veterinary Publications, 149 pages.

CHAPTER 11

Cattle and Other Domestic Bovids

CLASSIFICATION

Order Artiodactyla
Suborder Ruminantia Family Bovidae
Subfamily: Bovinae
Tribe Bovini: European cattle, zebu, yak, kouprey, water buffalo, banteng, gayal

The domestication of wild bovids was a major step forward in the process of civilization. A number of species have wild counterpart populations spread throughout tropical, subtropical, and temperate regions of the world (Table 11.1). Domestic bovids are usually gentle and all can be handled and restrained in much the same manner. Differences in handling are dictated by culture.

More than 1.3 billion cattle of numerous breeds provide milk, meat, and leather[2,6] (Table 11.2). In some cultures, cattle carry the loads, plow the fields, and pull the wagons. Names of gender are given in Table 11.3. In the United States the cattle are of European descent *Bos taurus* (Jersey, hereford, zebu [Fig. 11.1]). Much cross breeding has taken place resulting in some uniquely North American breeds such as the Santa Gertrudis.

Asiatic (water) buffalo (Fig. 11.2) are second only to cattle in worldwide numbers and economic importance. An estimated 150 million tame water buffalo exist[1]: 50 million in India and Pakistan, 20 million in East and Southeast Asia, and the remainder spread throughout numerous countries, including Japan, Hawaii, Central and South America, and the United States.

Just as there are many breeds of domestic cattle, there are many breeds of water buffalo. Some are adapted for a semiaquatic habitat; others thrive without an intimate water relationship. In general, buffalo are handled in the same manner as domestic cattle. Nose rings, nasal septum thongs, and halters are used to control work animals. Stocks are used to restrict movement while giving injections or carrying out minor surgery.[3] Water buffalo bulls are usually more docile than cattle bulls. Some can be handled without nose rings.

The yak is adapted to the cold and bleak existence of the Tibetan steppes (Fig. 11.3). It replaces cattle and buffalo in Nepal, Tibet, and parts of Mongolia at elevations over 2,000 m. Other domestic bovids are of lesser economic importance.

There are more than 1,000 breeds and types of cattle.[4] They may differ markedly in their reactions to manipulation.[6]

TABLE 11.2. Weights of domestic bovids

Animal Cattle	Bull (kg)	Bull (lb)	Cow (kg)	Cow (lb)
Holstein-Friesian	998–1,089	2,200–2,400	681	1,500
Jersey	545–817	1,200–1,800	363–545	800–1,200
Brown Swiss	817–1,180	1,800–2,600	590–817	1,300–1,800
Guernsey	568–1,022	1,250–2,250	363–726	800–1,600
Ayrshire	863	1,900	545–681	1,200–1,500
Hereford	817–908	1,800–2,000	545	1,200
Angus	908	2,000	636	1,400
Charolaise	908–1,135	2,000–2,500+	565–908	1,250–2,000
Shorthorn	908	2,000	681	1,500
Santa Gertrudis	908–999	2,000–2,200	636	1,400
Brahman (Zebu)	817	1,800	545	1,200
Water Buffalo	<1,350	<2,970	>150	>330
Yak	<900	1,980	350	770

TABLE 11.3. Names of genders of cattle

Gender	Adult	Newborn	Immature
Male	Bull	Calf	Bullock, bull calf
Female	Cow	Calf	Heifer
Castrated male	Steer, ox, bullock	. . .	Steer, bullock

TABLE 11.1. Domestic bovids[2,3,6]

Name	Wild counterpart	Countries where used as a domestic animal	Countries where wild populations exist or had existed in recent times
European cattle	Auroch	Worldwide	Europe
Zebu	Auroch	Worldwide	Asia, Africa
Yak	Wild yak	Bhutan, Nepal, Tibet, Mongolia	Northern Tibet
Asiatic (water) buffalo	Water buffalo	Southeast Asia, but also worldwide	India, Southeast Asia, China
Banteng (Bali Cattle)	Banteng	Bali, Indonesia	Java, Borneo, Burma
Gayal	Gaur	India, Burma	India, Burma, Malaysia

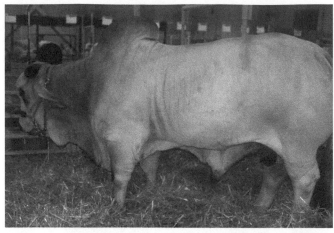

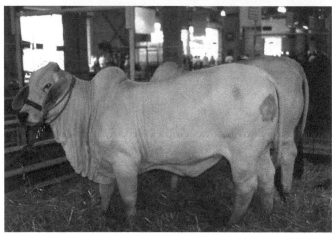

FIG. 11.1. Zebu bull and cow Bos taurus.

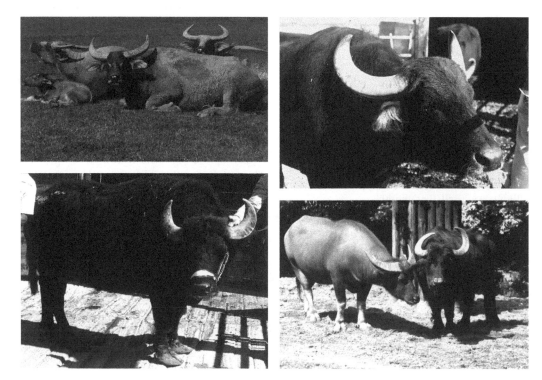

FIG. 11.2. Asiatic (water) buffalo *Bubalus bubalis*.

118

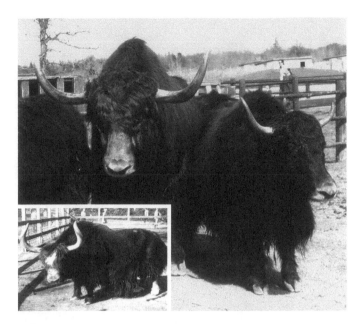

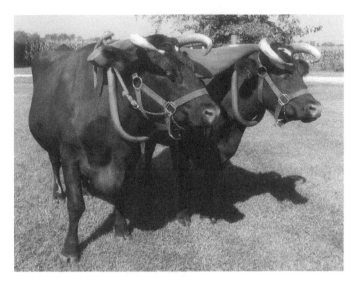

FIG. 11.4. Oxen (milking shorthorns) *Bos taurus.*

FIG. 11.3. Yak *Bos grunniens.*

Dairy cows are usually accustomed to being handled by milkers and handlers and, as a result, are likely to be more docile than other breeds. However, the dairy cow can become extremely nervous and may vigorously resist handling if she is not soothed and treated gently.

Cattle having little association with people are easily frightened; techniques used to handle them must involve chutes and stocks where movement can be restricted before they are approached. Beef cattle are usually grazed in pastures, thus handled less, and frequently exhibit flighty reactions.

Although the dairy cow is often easily handled, the same is not true of the adult dairy bull. Dairy bulls are extremely dangerous, and special restraint practices must be observed when working with them. Contrarily, the beef bull is generally as easily handled as the female. Nevertheless, all cattle are capable of injuring a careless handler.

Oxen are the castrated males of any breed of domestic cattle that are used for work (Fig. 11.4). Other species and breeds of cattle may be popular attractions in zoos and on private farms including Watusi (ankole) gayal and banteng (Fig. 11.5).

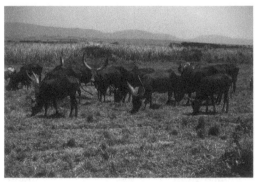

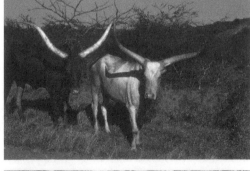

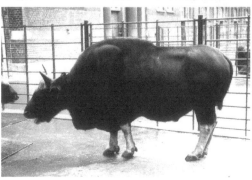

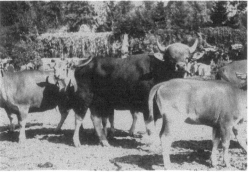

FIG. 11.5. Exotic cattle—Ankole cattle, top; gayal (domestic form of gaur *Bos gaurus*), bottom left; and banteng *Bos javanicus*, bottom right.

DANGER POTENTIAL

Cattle resist restraint by various actions. The horned animal is capable of quick thrusts sideways and forward and may fatally gore the unwary individual. A handler working around the head of a horned animal must be continually conscious of the swinging arc of the head and the extent of reach of the horns.

Both polled and horned animals may butt. They may rush at people and knock them down or crush them against fences or walls. Cattle may also push against people with their bodies, squeezing persons against walls, fences, or other animals.

Cattle seldom use the front feet as weapons, though they may paw the ground to display anger and threaten. However, being stepped on is a minor hazard of working with cattle; even small calves can inflict pain if they step on a toe, and heavier animals may severely bruise or fracture the toes and feet.

Cattle are adept at kicking with the hind feet. The kick is usually forward and out to the side in an arc reaching some distance. Cattle are less likely to kick directly backward, though able to do so. Usually only one leg kicks at a time, as contrasted with the equine species where both hind feet habitually kick simultaneously. Probably the safest place to stand is right at the shoulder, but remember that a cow can kick forward past her shoulder with the hind leg.

The tail is used to swat flies and switches in response to any touch on the skin. The tail may be a source of annoyance during restraint procedures and may also contaminate a prepared surgical field. Furthermore, it may inflict personal injury if the hair of the tail flicks the eyes. The tail becomes an awesome weapon when it is filled with foreign bodies such as burrs or grass awns. These can be removed most easily by immersing the tail in mineral oil and slipping the burrs out. If this proves unsuccessful, a matted entanglement of burrs in the hair of the tail necessitates clipping off the switch and allowing the hair to regrow. Bovine tails are fragile and therefore must be tied or attached only to the animal's own body when restriction of tail switching is required.

Cattle rarely bite. They lack upper incisors.

PHYSICAL RESTRAINT[1,3,7,8]

The temperament of each cow must be considered before approaching her for examination or to apply severely restrictive restraint devices. With beef cattle, it is likely that the animal must be roped or put into a chute or stock to halter it or approach closely enough to conduct an examination. Dairy animals usually may be readily approached if confined in a stanchion or tied to a fence (Fig. 11.6).

When working with any species, the handler must alert the animal to prospective movements. Quick motions usually startle animals, so firm, slow, deliberate actions should be the rule. Speaking to animals lets them locate your position and avoids startling them with an unexpected touch. Do not

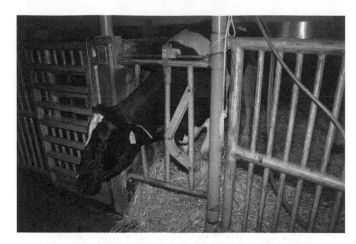

FIG. 11.6.   A solid adjustable stanchion.

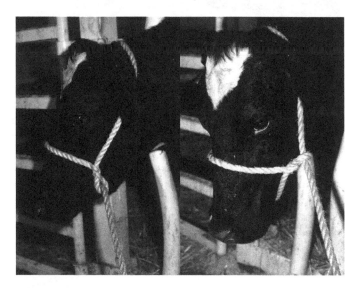

FIG. 11.7.   Rope halter properly placed, with the free end exiting beneath the mandible, left. Rope halter improperly placed with free end exiting from over the poll, right.

approach any animal directly from the front unless it is secured in a stock. It is natural for an animal to charge forward and butt anyone who makes such an approach. It is most desirable to approach the animal from either the left or right shoulder area. Placing a firm hand on the shoulder lets it know that you are there and that you are confident. Then, if necessary, the approach to the head may take place.

A rope halter is the basic tool of restraint for working with cattle and many other species (Fig. 11.7). Commercial halters are also available and the temporary rope halters described in Chapter 3 are satisfactory. It is important to place the halter correctly. Frequently a halter is put on upside down (Fig. 11.7, right) or improperly placed with the rope behind the horns but not behind the ears. This results in the rope crossing over or near the eye, endangering the eye.

Placing the halter on an animal in a chute or stanchion offers no particular challenge. An animal loose in a box stall may present some difficulty. However, if the nose loop is made slightly larger than the poll loop, one can often flip it over the nose and then over the poll and behind the ears very easily. If it is impossible to approach the animal in this manner, it may be necessary to first place a rope around its neck. Use the shank of the halter or rope the animal first with a honda loop and place the halter on after the animal is subdued.

Once haltered, the animal may be tied to a post, a ring, or any other secure object to carry out additional procedures. It is usually necessary to fix the head by pulling it tightly to the side or upward, or both, and snubbing it to the post with the halter tie (Fig. 11.8). It is somewhat difficult to remove all the slack from the rope when completing the halter tie. Practice is necessary to form the loops closely around the object. Many procedures such as withdrawing blood, giving injections, or examining the teeth and various other body areas can be carried out by controlling the head in this manner. If the halter is to be left on an unattended animal, be certain that it is the type that will not slip and become a noose around the neck.

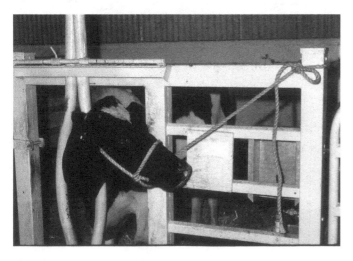

FIG. 11.8. The head is properly secured with rope halter tied for quick release.

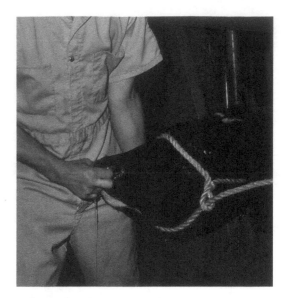

FIG. 11.9. Using thumb and finger as a temporary nose tong.

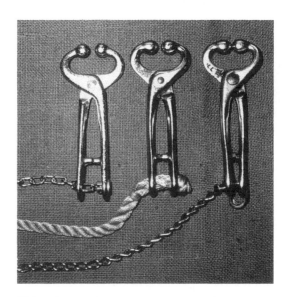

FIG. 11.10. Cattle nose tongs: Undesirable tong with no space between the clamps, right. Tong with rope lead, middle. Chain and rope lead, left.

Cattle have an unusually sensitive nasal septum. A routine restraint practice is to grasp the nasal septum between thumb and finger via the nostrils, forming a nose tong (Fig. 11.9). A large animal is difficult to hold by hand because one cannot maintain sufficient pressure to restrain the animal for more than a few seconds.

For more permanent, more secure restraint, mechanical devices acting on the septum are available. By applying a clamp in the form of a nose tong, one can severely restrict activity. When fully closed, a space of approximately 3.5 mm (1/8 in.) should remain between the two metal balls of the nose lead (Fig. 11.10), to prevent necrosis of the nasal cartilage. Furthermore, one should be certain that the surface of

the balls is smooth to avoid scrapes or lacerations. Poor quality nose leads may be die cast. The break in the cast usually leaves a rough edge in the middle of the ball. A file or emery cloth should be used to smooth out such edges or any other roughness on the ball surface.

Placement of the nose tong is not always easy, particularly if an animal has experienced the device previously. The animal frequently darts its head about in an attempt to prevent placement. If the animal is in a squeeze chute or stock, grasp the head or nose of the animal in the manner shown in Figure 11.11. Do not try to push a tong straight into the nose. The nose tong should be placed in the nostrils with a rotating

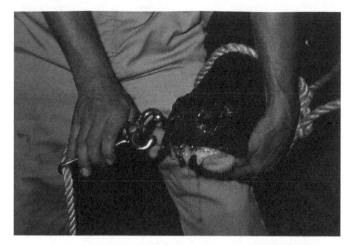

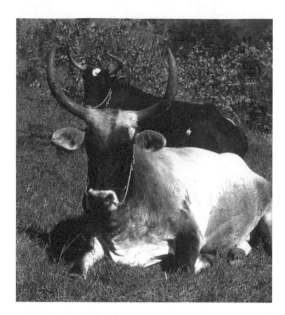

FIG. 11.12. Halter consisting of a rope thong tied around the head and through a hole in the nasal septum.

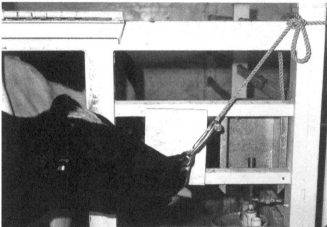

FIG. 11.11. Use of a nose tong: To apply nose tong, first insert one prong, then with a quick rotation insert the other, top . Cow secured with a nose tong, bottom.

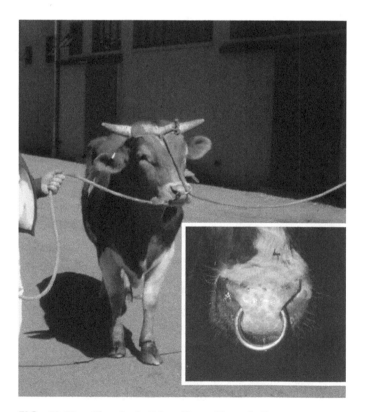

FIG. 11.13. Use of a bullring. Controlling a bull with two ropes. Detail of bullring, inset.

motion. Insert one side of the tong, rotating across the nasal septum to apply the other, as shown. Then quickly close the tong and move away.

To keep the tong in place, tension must be maintained. An assistant must hold the tong, or the rope may be tied above and to the side of the stanchion or chute. Do not leave the animal unattended. Use the halter tie for quick release in case the animal should fall or otherwise get into a predicament. It is not desirable, nor is it humane, to proceed with significantly painful procedures on an animal restrained by a nose tong. Painful procedures require sedation or anesthesia.

Water buffalo and oxen in countries other than the United States are usually handled with some variation of the rope thong (Fig. 11.12).

Adult dairy bulls should never be trusted. Do not approach such animals closely unless they are confined in special chutes or stocks. A dairy bull usually has a ring in the nose and may be controlled by two rope leads attached to the nose ring (Fig. 11.13), or a bull staff (Fig. 11.14).

The eyelids of bovine species are firm and difficult to evert for proper examination. Rotation of the head exposes much of the scleral surface and some of the conjunctival surface. To do this, with the head in a chute or stanchion, approach the animal from the right side, grasp the nose with

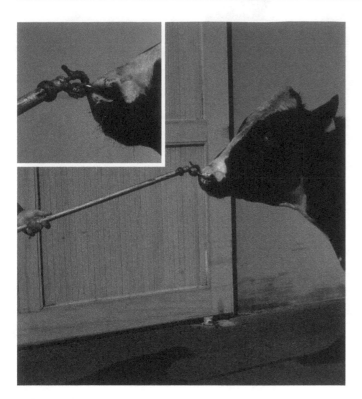

FIG. 11.14. Use of a bull staff. Detail of the hook and ring, inset.

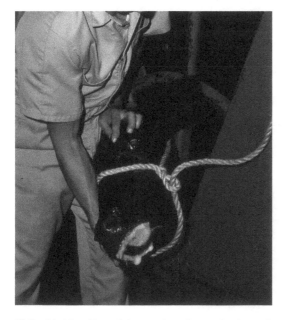

FIG. 11.15. Examining conjunctiva and sclera of the eye by rotating the head.

the right hand, and press on the horns or grab an ear and press down (Fig. 11.15). This rotates the poll toward the right and pulls the muzzle up. The eye rotates accordingly. Reverse the rotation to expose the lower sclera and conjunctiva. It may be necessary for one person to manipulate the animal while another person examines the eye. Repeat both maneuvers from the left side to examine the opposite eye.

Complete physical examination of a bovid usually involves an oral and/or pharyngeal examination. The techniques and special devices used for these examinations are illustrated in Figures 11.16 to 11.20. Insertion of a stomach tube may be performed by one person (Fig. 11.21) or requires two people (Figs. 11.22, 11.23). Medicating with a balling gun is performed as illustrated in Figure 11.24, being sure to go past the base of the tongue.

Dairy cattle may require hobbles to prevent them from kicking; they usually tolerate the hobbles quite well. Chain hobbles (Fig. 11.25) or rope hobbles (Fig. 11.26) are suitable.

The tension is adjustable. Be certain the animal retains the ability to separate its legs widely enough to maintain stability.

Carefully observe an animal being hobbled for the first time to avoid serious and possibly permanent injury. I have seen a frightened cow cast itself and severely lacerate the muscles and tendons on the anterior aspect of the hock while struggling against hobbles. Chain hobbles should not be left on an unattended animal.

Placement of a rope hobble may be hazardous if the animal is a kicker. To avoid being kicked, a longer rope and two persons are required to apply the hobble. The rope must be long enough for a person to stand out of reach of the kick on either side of the animal.

Another device to minimize kicking is a short length of rope tied around the flank of the animal (Fig. 11.27 left) or a special "can't kick" clamp may be placed over the top of the loin and cranked tight in the flank area (Fig. 11.27, right). Pressure in the flank area inhibits kicking but does not provide absolute control; the animal still may kick, but the intensity of the kick is usually diminished. Use caution when applying this type of restraint on a milking cow or a breeding bull, since the pressure of the rope is exerted directly over the udder of the cow or the prepuce of the bull. Temporary flank restraint may be applied by lifting the flank on the side in which protection is desired (Fig. 11.28 left). The knee can also be used to apply pressure in front of the stifle (Fig. 11.28 right). The animal then cannot reach forward. The animal may, however, graze the leg of the individual carrying out the restraint.

Manipulating the feet and legs of domestic cattle is not as simple as handling those of horses. Dairy cattle that are handled continually may allow a manipulator to pick up the foot and examine the bottom for evidence of foot rot or foreign bodies (Fig. 11.29), but other cattle will probably not permit this.

Most techniques for examining the hind feet or trimming the hoofs require casting the animal in lateral recumbency or holding the limb up with ropes. A strong manila or nylon rope with a honda (preferably a quick-release honda) is used to lift the hind leg (Fig. 11.30). Leave approximately 1 foot of the rope free at the honda end and tie a clove hitch around the leg above the hock. Slip the running end of the rope through the ring on a beam clamp and back through the honda end of the rope. It is easier to thread the rope through a quick-release

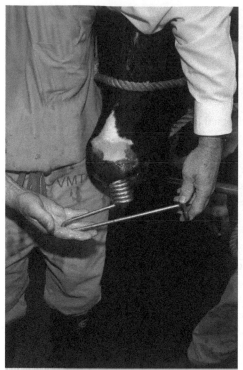
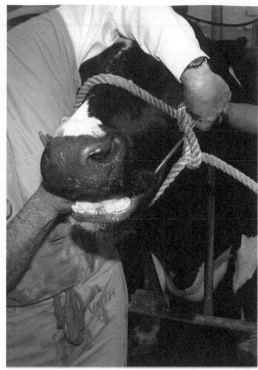

FIG. 11.16.   A type of dental wedge.

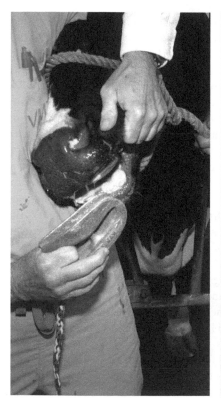
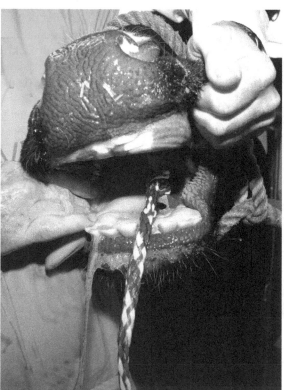

FIG. 11.17.   A dental wedge that opens the mouth wider.

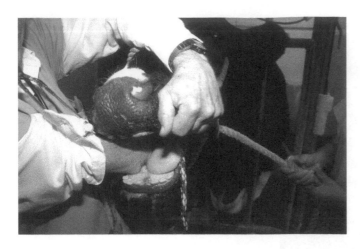

FIG. 11.18. Manual examination of the pharynx using a wedge.

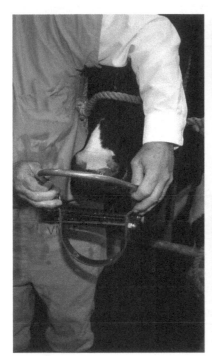
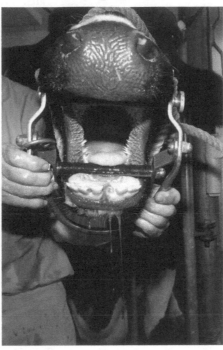

FIG. 11.19. Hauptner dental speculum.

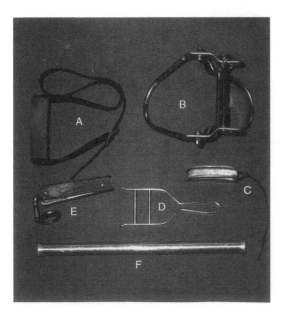

FIG. 11.20. Dental speculae: **A.** Wooden block, **B.** Hauptner speculum, **C.** wedges, **D.** calf speculum, and **E.** Frick speculum.

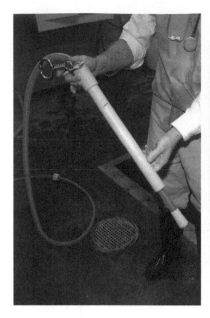
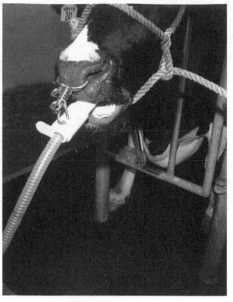

FIG. 11.21. Special speculum and stomach tube to allow a single person to complete the procedure.

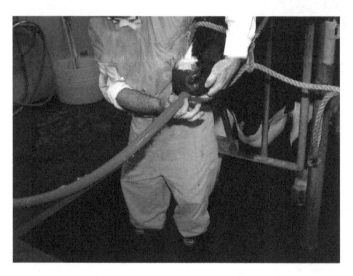

FIG. 11.22. Passage of a large (Kingman) stomach tube.

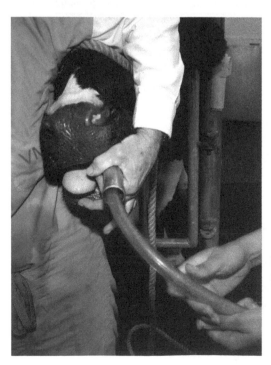
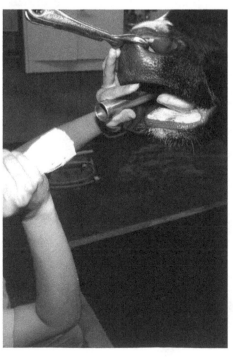

FIG. 11.23. Using a Frick speculum to pass a stomach tube or to perform an oropharyngeal examination.

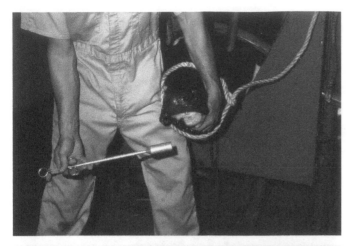

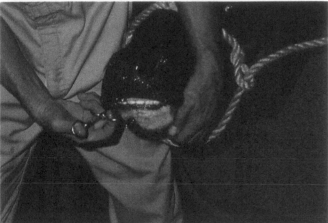

FIG. 11.24. Procedure for administering a medication via a balling gun.

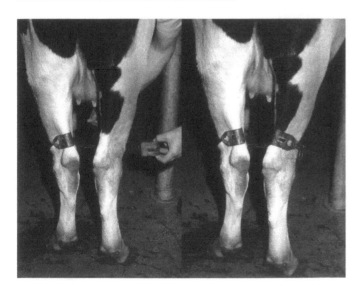

FIG. 11.25. Chain hobbles for dairy cows.

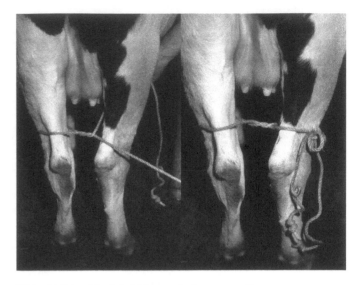

FIG. 11.26. Hock hobbles made from a small rope. Secure with a bowknot for quick release.

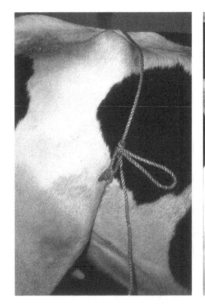

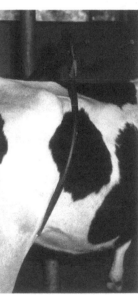

FIG. 11.27. Flank restraint: Use of flank rope, left. Commercial flank clamp, right.

honda. The leg is then lifted from the ground by pulling upward on the running end. The mechanical advantage gained by running the rope through a clamp allows exertion of greater pressure than is achieved by manually lifting the foot. Once the limb is elevated to the desired position, a loop hitch prevents the rope from loosening. With the foot in this position, the limb is extremely mobile. Caution should be exercised when approaching the foot because the animal can kick either from side to side or forward and back. The device only prevents the animal from placing the foot back on the ground.

A technique for immobilizing the limb further utilizes either the beam clamp or any other site within the shed or barn where a hitch can be taken. It may also be used with an animal confined in a chute (Fig. 11.31). A loop is placed around the pastern. The rope is extended upward and backward around a ring, a pole, a pipe, or any other sturdy object in front of the animal to pull the limb upward and backward.

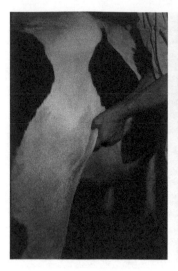
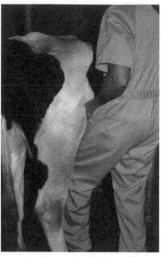

FIG. 11.28. Flank restraint: Grasping flank with hands, left. Using hands and inserting knee in flank, right.

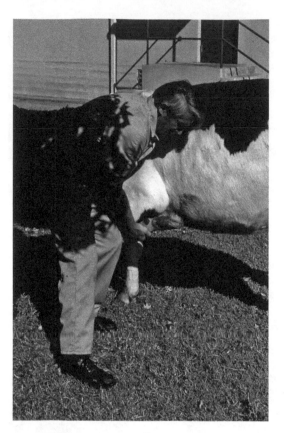

FIG. 11.29. Lifting foreleg of a cow.

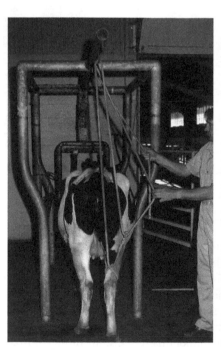
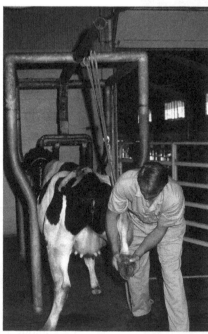

FIG. 11.30. Raising a hind leg. The pull is directly upward, thus there is little fixation of the leg in a forward and backward direction.

At the same time, slack is removed from all of the ropes. The limb is held extended to the rear and anchored to the front. The rope around the tendon above the hock also serves to partially paralyze or immobilize the animal, permitting any desired manipulation.

In barns or sheds built with exposed overhead beams, special clamps may be used to provide a fulcrum from which

to lift a leg. The clamp should be attached to a beam directly above the limb (Fig. 11.32).

Special stocks have been made to assist in trimming the feet of large bulls. A heavy beam is attached to upright braces about a foot above the ground. Holes are drilled through the beam at suitable locations. The beam should extend past the upright braces. The animal is led into the stock and stan-

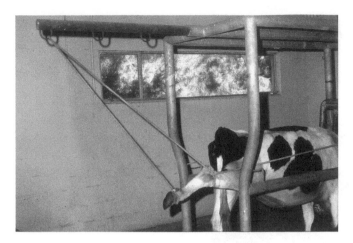

FIG. 11.31. Alternate method for raising and fixing a hind leg. Ropes are anchored forward, upward, and backward.

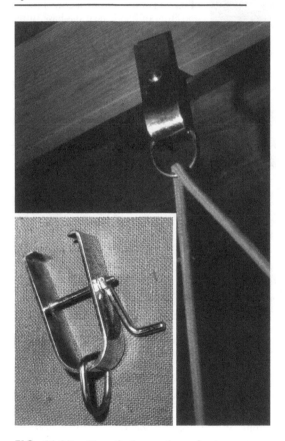

FIG. 11.32. Use of a beam clamp for temporary attachment of ropes and pulleys. Ice tongs can also be used.

chioned. A small rope with a loop is placed on the foot, the foot is lifted manually, and the running end of the rope is put through the hole in the beam to anchor the foot.

None of these techniques are entirely suitable for use on extremely wild range cattle. Many range animals struggle sufficiently against restraint devices to seriously injure themselves. To examine or treat the feet or trim the hoofs of such animals, use chemical immobilization or manually restrain the animal into lateral recumbency.

Manipulation of the tail can be an excellent method of restraint. It is primarily applied to the dairy cow that is accustomed to being handled. However, it can be used for beef animals and other species of tailed bovids if they are restricted in lateral movement. Although an excellent restraint, one must be cautious that pressures are properly applied, otherwise the tail may be fractured and permanently disfigured.

When tailing, tie the animal up or put it in a stanchion and stand directly behind it. Lift the tail with one hand, reaching under and grasping the tail at the base with the other hand. Then grasp it close to the base with both hands, pressing the tail upward, straight over the back (Fig. 11.33). When this technique is carried out properly, pressure will not break the tail, yet will pinch the vertebrae and the caudal nerves sufficiently to make the animal relax and ignore manipulation elsewhere. Once the animal has settled down, the pressure can be released, to be reapplied only when a particular procedure requires the animal to stand quietly. It is important for the pressure to be exerted at the base of the tail, not further along it. The tail of the bovine is not as strong as that of the equine, and improper manipulations may fracture the coccygeal vertebrae.

If restriction of the tail's activity is required, tie the tail to some part of the animal's body (Fig. 11.34), not to a stock or a chute. Unlike equines, bovines cannot support the body weight hanging from the tail.

A technique used to control tame cattle in countries other than the United States is to place a rope on either a foreleg or hind leg (Fig. 11.35).

Calf Restraint

The newborn calf is easily held by placing one arm underneath and around the neck to the opposite shoulder while holding the other hand over the tail or around the hindquarters (Fig. 11.36).

Calves up to 90 kg (200 lb) may be placed in lateral recumbency either by flanking (Fig. 11.37) or by lifting a foreleg (Fig. 11.38). To flank a calf, hold it by the head either with a halter or a honda loop around the neck. Flanking can be carried out on either side. Place the left hand over the neck and almost immediately grasp the animal over the back with the right hand in the right flank. The right knee is in the left flank of the animal (Fig. 11.37). As the calf struggles or jumps, take advantage of the movement by quickly lifting it slightly off its feet, bending your knees to push the left side underneath the animal and quickly pressing the animal onto its left side.

The novice may feel this is extremely laborious and requires lifting too heavy an animal. Obviously this technique is impractical for an animal over 90 kg but is effective with smaller animals. The secret of successful manipulation is to take advantage of the animal's jumps to push and pull it off balance.

An alternate technique for casting both small and large calves is legging. A skilled person can throw a 160-kg (350-lb) calf to the ground using this technique. With the head secured by a lariat or halter, approach the animal on the right

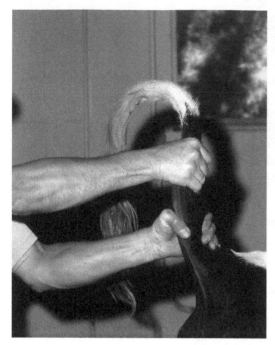

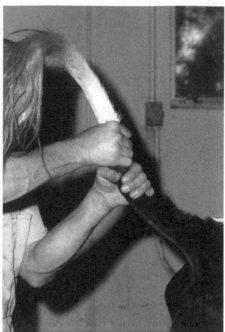

FIG. 11.33. Tailing a cow: Proper position of hands near the base of the tail, left. Improper positioning of hands (too far from base), right.

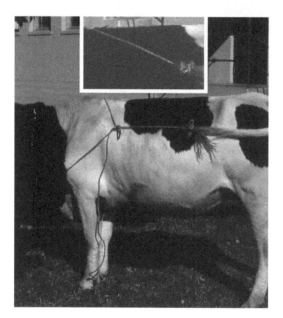

FIG. 11.34. Tail tie on cow: To the neck on the same side, lower. Over the back to the opposite front leg, upper.

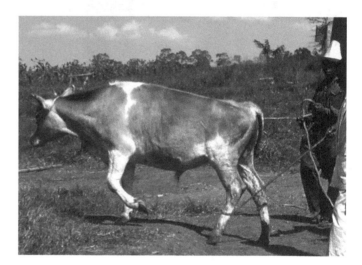

FIG. 11.35. Controlling a steer by a foot rope.

side. Going down the neck, grab the right front leg. Grasp the cannon bone and pull the leg out, forward, and upward with one motion (Fig. 11.38, top). Keep the leg straight. Use the leg as a battering ram, driving it against the rib cage (Fig. 11.38, bottom). This pushes the animal off balance so that it will fall on its left side. All these techniques require practice to achieve proficiency in utilizing the movements of the animal to create the subtle imbalances necessary to tip the animal over.

As the animal goes down, quickly step across the thorax of the animal, grasp the right leg, and apply a loop of a short

length of 64-mm (4-in.) rope (called a piggin string) over the upper metacarpal area (Fig. 11.39, top). Then toss the rope across the animal. While holding the right foreleg with the left hand, reach back with the right hand and pick up both hind legs above the point of the hock (Fig. 11.39, bottom). Then sit down over the buttocks of the animal. Your right knee is behind the hocks of the calf (Fig. 11.39 bottom). In this position the calf cannot kick you in the groin. The knee is used to press the hind legs forward. Place the hind legs on top of the right foreleg in a crisscross position. Then grasp the rope and wrap it around all three legs in the metacarpal and metatarsal region. The first wrap must be tight or the animal will be able to struggle free. Two or three wraps should be used to anchor the leg firmly. Draw the end of the rope through the last loop to secure the tie.

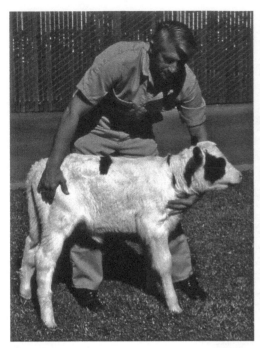
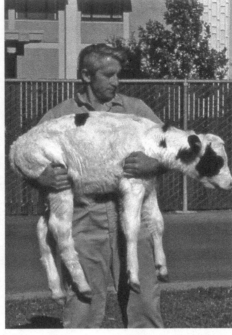

FIG. 11.36.   Handling a calf: Restricting, left. Lifting, right.

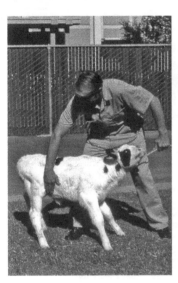
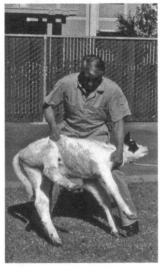

FIG. 11.37.   Flanking a calf: Grasp calf by the opposite flank and over the neck, left. Lift with both hands, simultaneously pushing knee into the flank, right.

If the rope has been properly placed, the animal cannot struggle loose for some time. In the event that any one limb is not available to be incorporated into the rope, any three limbs may be tied or all four limbs may be included in the wrap. Tying four legs of a thick-bodied beef animal is not suitable because bringing both front legs close together is not only difficult but also may interfere with respiration.

If a calf is to be held in lateral recumbency without tying the legs, have one person hold the upper foreleg flexed at the knee. The calf may reach forward and lash out with a hind leg, but this reaction is unusual; in contrast, a wild animal, such as a deer, under similar circumstances would kick

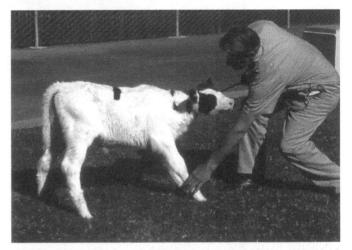

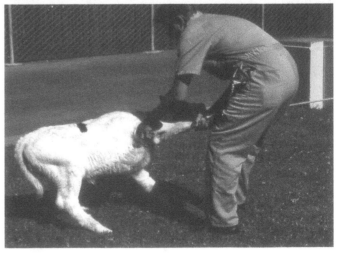

FIG. 11.38.   Legging a calf: Grasp front leg and begin to lift, top. Lift the leg higher and drive it against the body, pushing the calf over, bottom.

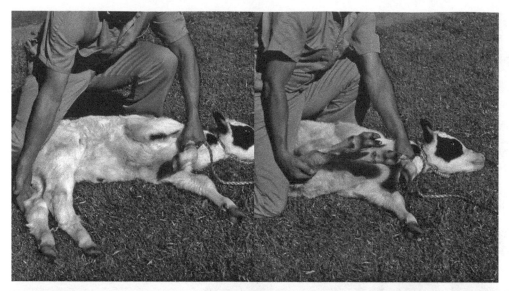

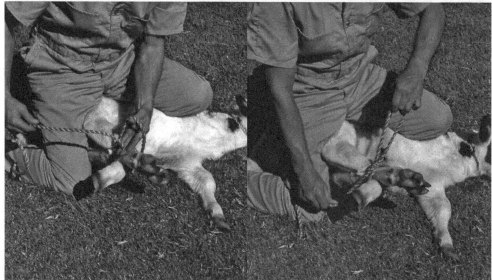

FIG. 11.39.   Three-leg calf tie.

viciously to free itself. To control the hind legs more securely, grasp the upper leg and stretch it back while pushing the lower leg forward with the heel over the point of the hock (Fig. 11.40).

Casting Cattle

Small animals may be cast by placing a lark's head hitch around the thorax and abdomen (Fig. 11.41). Pressure is applied by pulling up on the rope.

Large cattle, including bulls, may be cast with ropes.

Suitable methods for placing these animals in lateral or dorsal recumbency include various techniques for applying pressure to the thorax and abdomen. The physiologic mechanism by which this pressure produces weakness and paresis is unknown. Nonetheless it is an effective method of persuading the animal to lie down. With patience and suitable strength, the technique works on large bulls or oxen as well as on cows.

The half-hitch method is accomplished as follows (Figs. 11.42 to 11.44): Tie a loose bowline around the neck of the

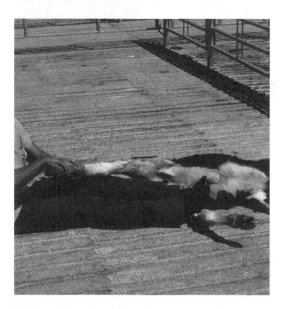

FIG. 11.40.   Stretching a calf.

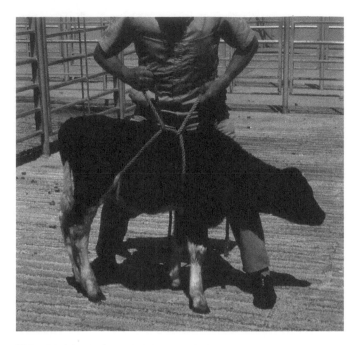

FIG. 11.41. Using a lark's head hitch to cast a calf.

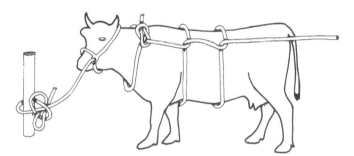

FIG. 11.42. Diagram of the half-hitch method of casting.

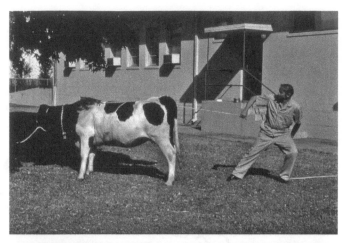

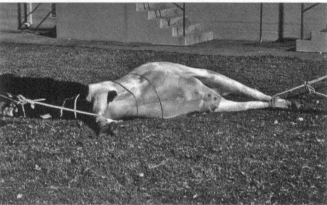

FIG. 11.43. Half-hitch method for casting cattle.

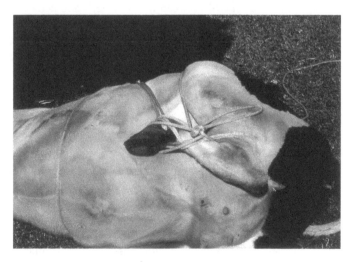

FIG. 11.44. Securing the upper hind leg in half-hitch casting.

animal. Some prefer to tie the rope around the neck between the front legs, but this is unnecessary in most cases. A half hitch is then placed behind the shoulders over the thorax. Another loop is placed just over the caudal portion of the rib cage. In large animals, a third loop may be placed in the flank area, but when handling milking dairy cows and bulls, one must be aware of potential injury to the subcutaneous abdominal milk vein or to the penis when pulling on the rope.

I have seen heavy bulls, particularly beef breeds, set their legs in a sawhorse stance and refuse to go down. In these

The animal's head must be securely tied—preferably low to the ground—so that when the animal falls, it will not hang from the head. Remove all slack from the hitches. Steady pressure is placed on the rope by pulling backward. Some animals fall immediately; others resist and even jump forward or sideways to rid themselves of the inconvenience, but if the pressure is consistently maintained, the animal will ultimately sink to its knees and lie over on its side.

instances, a rope hobble which keeps the limbs together, particularly the hind limbs, forces the animal to fall down when pressure is applied. Once the animal is in lateral recumbency, maintaining the pressure may assist in keeping the animal down, but some will continue to struggle until they can get up. Usually, to maintain recumbency, the animal must be

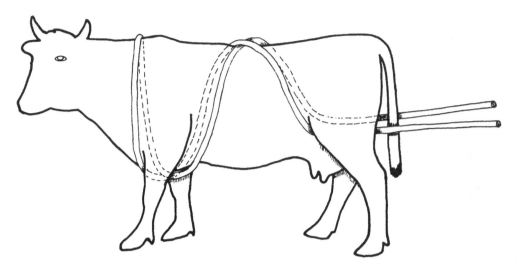

FIG. 11.45. Diagram of the criss-cross method of casting.

secured by stretching fore and aft with ropes tied to the front and hind legs. For details of the foot wrap, see Figure 3.25. Alternatively, the hind limb may be secured as in Figure 11.44. The crisscross is an alternative technique (Figs. 11.45, 11.46). Two people are required to apply the ropes. A rope approximately 12-m (40-ft) long is divided in half with each half coiled to the center. Place the center of the rope over the neck and pass each coil between the front legs and across to the opposite side. A person must stand on each side to manipulate the ropes. This technique is safest with an animal that does not kick, but it may also be used on a kicker by throwing (instead of passing) the rope between the legs. The ropes are then crossed over the top of the thorax to the side. The two persons then exchange ropes and pass them between the hind legs. All slack is removed from the ropes and pressure applied by pulling the ropes from the rear. Either one or both persons can exert the pressure necessary to pull the animal down. The advantage of using this method is that since no ropes cross the abdomen, there is no danger of injury to the milk vein or the penis.

Slinging

Adapted commercial or custom-made slings, similar to those used for horses, are used for cattle. A rope sling may be used to lift an animal to its feet or extract it from a predicament. (See Figs. 3.47 and 3.48.) A special hip lifter has been designed to lift a dairy animal with prominent tuber coxae (Fig. 11.47). The device is adjustable to fit various sizes of cattle. This device must not be left in place for more than a few minutes at a time lest necrosis occur as a result of pressure on the muscles below the tuber coxae. Additional padding such as sponge rubber may be inserted, but no amount of padding will prevent pressure on the bones, cutting off the

blood supply to the muscles. For a weak animal, reluctant to get up, this help in arising may be all that is necessary. No sling should be used to support a cow for extended periods. A cow, capable of standing on her own, may refuse to do so while hanging in a sling. If the sling is lowered abruptly, the cow may be startled into bracing herself and stand.

Flotation

Recently, flotation in water has been used to encourage downer (recumbent) cattle to stand (Fig. 11.48).[3] A square tub (tank) with removable opposite ends is required. The recumbent cow is placed on a rubber mat, sized to fit the tub. The mat is dragged into the tub and the ends attached. Water at 37°C (100°F) is run into the tub. The animal's head must be supported as the tub fills.

A cow in lateral recumbency will usually roll to the sternal position when the water rises to a depth of 45–60 cm (18–24 in.). Most cows will float up and eventually stand. A cow may be left in the tub for 6–10 hours, and the process may be repeated the following day if necessary.

Chutes

Many stocks or chutes have been designed to restrain cattle. These vary from crudely constructed pole chutes (Figs. 11.49, 11.50) to sophisticated commercial models (Figs. 11.51 to 11.53). A chute may have to be custom built for special cattle such as the Watusi (Fig. 11.54). Commercial chutes are also designed for use with calves or young stock (Figs. 11.55 and 11.56).

The use of a chute is not without risk to the animal. The design of the chute determines the overall safety as well as the efficiency and ease of manipulation. Items of concern are:

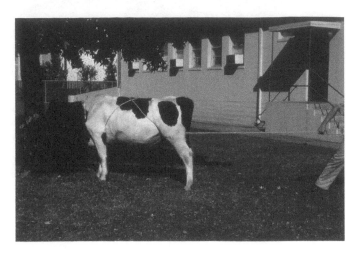

FIG. 11.46. Criss-cross method for casting cattle.

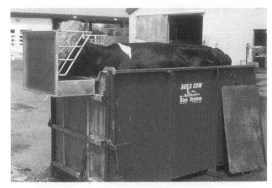

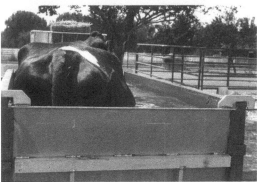

FIG. 11.48. Flotation tank for recumbent cattle.

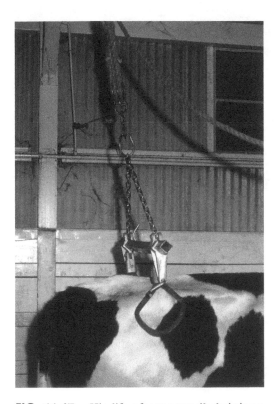

FIG. 11.47. Hip lifter for temporarily hoisting a cow.

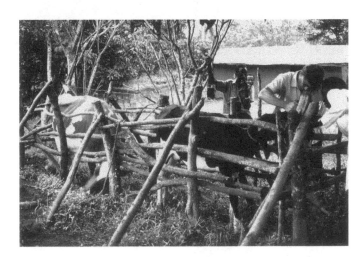

FIG. 11.49. Improvised stock chute made with poles.

1. The danger of securing the head in such a manner that respiratory passages are obstructed. Suffocation may result if the animal twists, if it falls onto a bar across the base of the neck, or if the head is improperly held in the chute.
2. Openings in the sides and front of the chute, large enough to allow an animal to catch a foot or put a foot through, provide leverage by which an animal may easily fracture a limb. Access ports are necessary in order to utilize the chute to examine or work on the body, but the best chutes have access ports that remain closed until the animal is in the chute and fully restrained.
3. The ease with which the animal can be released following conclusion of the procedure, or if the animal becomes distressed, is important. A chute is dangerous if it does not permit an animal to arise after it falls down in the chute. Some chutes come apart at the sides so that a downed animal can be pulled out. With others, the head must be released back into the

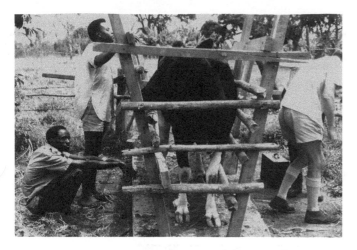

FIG. 11.50. Wooden chute.

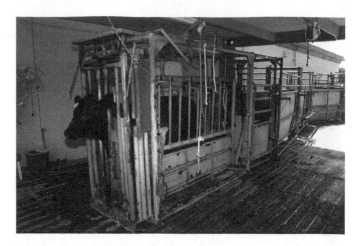

FIG. 11.52. Another commercial cattle chute.

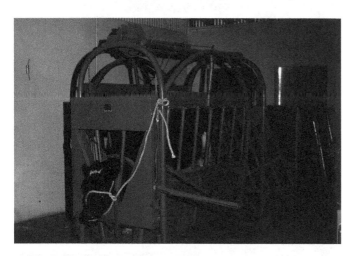

FIG. 11.51. Commercial cattle chute.

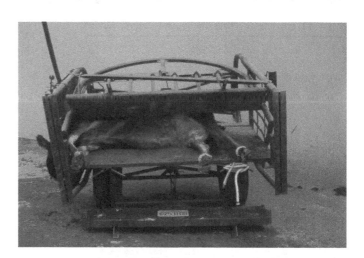

FIG. 11.53. Tip chute for cattle.

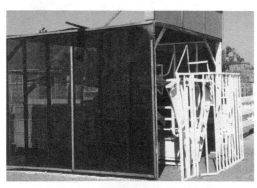

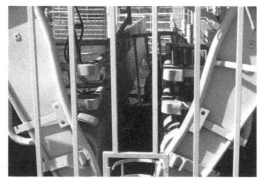

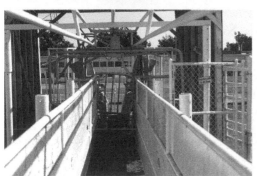

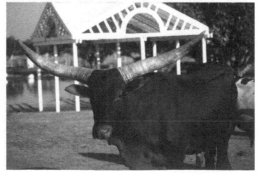

FIG. 11.54. Custom built chute for handling Watusi cattle.

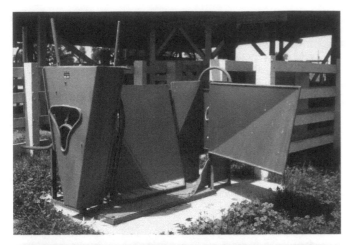

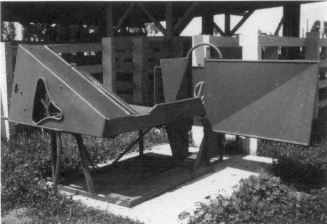

FIG. 11.55. Calf chute.

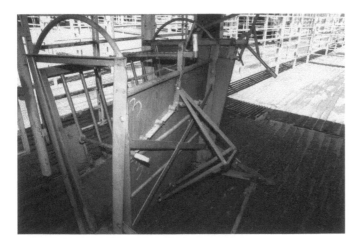

FIG. 11.56. Alternate calf chute.

chute before the front gate can be opened. These are more dangerous and thus less satisfactory than those opening to the side.

4. Sharp protrusions on the inside or outside of the chute provide sources of injury to the animal and to those working the chute. Eliminate any projections.

Elaborate or simple arrangements may be designed to funnel cattle into a chute. Special circular lanes or cutting gates can be constructed to sort animals or to remove calves from their dams.

TRANSPORT

Cattle are easily transported. They can be herded into trucks, trains, or trailers. Intercontinental air or sea craft routinely carry bovines in crates designed for one or more individuals.

Group cattle, placed in close quarters for shipping, according to size. To protect calves from injury by the cows, separate them by partitions within crates or ship in different crates.

CHEMICAL RESTRAINT[5]

The chemical restraint agents and combinations mentioned in this chapter represent those used by experienced veterinarians with detailed knowledge of cattle. Other protocols have been used, and no claim is made for including all possible drugs and combinations. For more detailed information, particularly for anesthesia, consult Riebold.[5] The use of sedatives and tranquilizers is not as common in cattle as it is in horses. Chemical immobilization is rarely necessary, but if employed, adult cattle should be fasted for 36–48 hours and water withheld for 24 hours before proceeding, to minimize the danger of bloat and regurgitation.

Xylazine is the most widely used tranquilizer for cattle, even though it has not been cleared for use in cattle by the U.S. Federal Food and Drug Administration. It has, however, been given extensive field trials. See Table 11.4 for dosages.

TABLE 11.4   Chemical restraint agents used for sedation and immobilization of cattle

Drug/combinations	Intramuscular (mg/kg) or as indicated	Intravenous (mg/kg)
Standing sedation		
Xylazine	0.015–0.025	0.015–0.025
Detomidine		0.0025–0.01
Immobilization		
Xylazine/ketamine	0.1–0.2	
Xylazine/telazol	0.1/4.0	0.05/1.0
Tiletamine/zolazepam		4.0
Diazepam/ketamine		0.1/4.5

Acepromazine maleate may be used in cattle at a dosage of 0.1 mg/kg (IM or IV).

For chemical immobilization, use the high doses of xylazine (Table 11.4), or preferably, combinations. If cattle must be immobilized, they should be fasted as indicated above. Xylazine may be given intravenously at approximately one-fourth the intramuscular dose to animals already in hand.

Succinylcholine chloride is contraindicated for cattle. Apnea will occur and persist for 30 minutes, even with minimum doses. Assisted respiration may be required to keep a distressed animal alive.

All of the standard intravenous and inhalation anesthetic agents are used in cattle.

REFERENCES

1. Anderson, R.S., and Edney, A.T.B., Eds. 1991. Practical Animal Handling, 1st ed. Oxford, U.K. Pergamon Press, 198 pages.
2. Briggs, H.M. 1969. Modern Breeds of Livestock, 3rd ed. New York: Macmillan.
3. Cockrill, W.R. 1974. Husbandry and Health of the Domestic Buffalo, p. 281. Rome: Food and Agriculture Organization.
4. Porter, V. 2002. Mason's World Dictionary of Livestock Breeds, Types and Varieties, New York, CABI Publishing.
5. Riebold, T. 2007. Ruminants. In: Tranquilli, W.J., Thurman, J.C., and Grimm, K.A., Eds. 2007. Lumb and Jones' Veterinary Anesthesia and Analgesia, 4th Ed. Ames, Iowa, Wiley-Blackwell Publishing, pp. 731–47.
6. Sambraus, H.H. 1992. A Colour Atlas of Livestock Breeds, Germany, Wolfe.
7. Sheldon, C.C., Sonsthagen, T., and Topel, J.A. 2006. St. Louis, Mosby/Elsevier, 239 pages.
8. Sonsthagen, T.F. 1991. Restraint of Domestic Animals. Goleta, California, American Veterinary Publications, 149 pages.

CHAPTER 12
Sheep and Goats

CLASSIFICATION

Order Artiodactyla
    Family Bovidae
        Subfamily Caprinae
            Tribe Caprini: domestic sheep, domestic goat

Sheep and goats provide meat, milk, and fiber to vast numbers of people throughout the world. Many different breeds have been developed to suit the needs of a given culture. Sheep and goats are classified by gender in Table 12.1. The size range of various breeds is listed in Table 12.2.

TABLE 12.1. Names of gender of sheep and goats

Name	Mature Male	Mature Female	Newborn and Young
Sheep	Ram, buck	Ewe	Lamb
Goat	Buck, billy	Doe, nanny	Kid

TABLE 12.2. Weights of sheep and goats

	Male		Female	
Breed	(kg)	(lb)	(kg)	(lb)
Sheep				
Rambouillet	115–135	250–300+	65–100	150–225
Southdown	85–90	185–200	60–70	135–155
Hampshire	115	275	80–90	180–200
Dorset	100	225	80	175
Suffolk	125	275	90	200
Columbia	100–135	225–300	55–90	125–200
Karakul	75–90	170–200	60–70	130–160
Goats				
Angora	80–102	180–225	30–100	70–110
French alpine	75	170	60	135
Saanen	85	185	60	135
Nubian	80	175	60	135
Toggenburg	75	160	55	120

SHEEP
Danger Potential

Sheep are one of the easiest of large domestic animals to handle. Sheep do not bite, strike, or kick. The only danger of injury they offer is from the use of the head as a battering ram. A large horned ram may weigh over 136 kg (300 lb) and may seriously injure a careless handler. Mature rams often show aggression when being fed by butting the feeder from behind.

Ewes and large lambs may occasionally jump with considerable force at a sorting-gate operator, hitting them at about chest level. This may also occur when a handler enters a chute containing sheep.

Behavior and Physiology

Most sheep have strong flocking instincts and normally move in a group. It is difficult to separate one individual from the group. If one animal can be enticed to pass through a gate, the rest usually follow.

Sheep can be easily guided with panels, either wire or wood. Most sheep will not jump over a 1.2-m barrier. Range-raised sheep may be exceptions and may jump or scramble over a 2-m fence, particularly if separated from a group. The minimum group size for predictable behavioral responses is three to four. Sheep should never be housed alone, for this is a most stressful event for a sheep.

In hot weather, be cautious when handling sheep, especially those that are heavily fleeced. The normal body temperature of sheep is high, 39.5°C (103°F). Because of this characteristic, plus the insulating layer of wool, any struggle in hot weather may result in the rapid development of hyperthermia.

Physical Restraint[1,4,5]

The most valuable aid in handling sheep is a well-trained dog (Fig. 12.1) directed by an able shepherd. Many breeds of dogs have been specifically developed for this task.

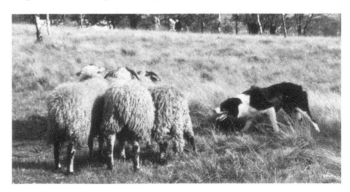

FIG. 12.1. Border collie working sheep.

Whenever possible, sheep should be crowded into alleyways or narrow chutes for mass medication, examination, and vaccinations (Fig. 12.2). A single sheep is easier to capture if left with the flock. Alone in a large enclosure, a sheep may panic and attempt to escape, but if allowed to stay with the flock it can be approached and grasped quite easily.

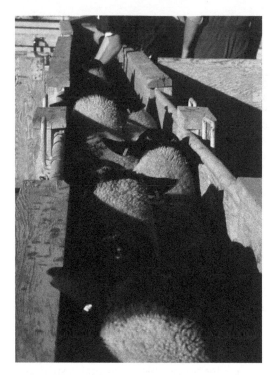

FIG. 12.2.   Sheep squeezed into a narrow chute.

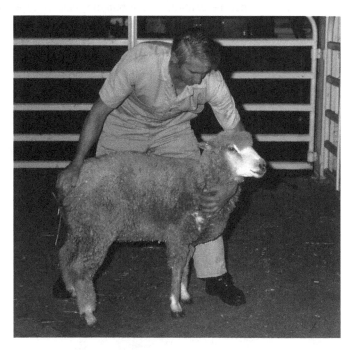

FIG. 12.3.   Holding a sheep.

Approach the animal quietly with deliberate movements; reach down and place one hand under the chin or breast, stopping its forward motion (Fig. 12.3). With one hand around its chest and the other holding its dock, even the largest sheep can be guided into any desired position. The sheep usually remains upright and able to walk.

Never grab the wool of a sheep when attempting to catch the animal because this damages delicate wool fibers and causes the wool to decrease in quality, or it pulls out. Furthermore, pulling the wool causes subcutaneous hemorrhages that would downgrade a market lamb carcass. If the wool requires examination, one individual should hold the animal and another should carefully part the wool with the fingers or hands. One person may hold a gentle sheep as shown in Figure 12.4.

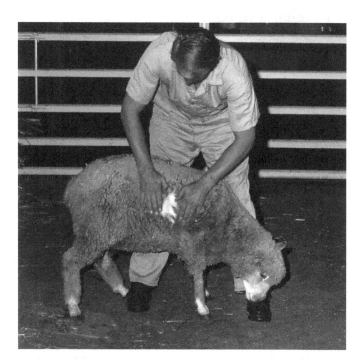

FIG. 12.4.   Parting wool.

The largest ram can be set up on its haunches by application of the proper mechanical principles. The approach described is from the left side; however, one can cast the animal just as easily in the opposite direction. Start from the basic holding position. Place the right knee in the left flank and move the right hand from the dock to the right flank. Change the left hand from encircling the chest to grasp the animal by the lower jaw. Twist the head to the right with the left hand (Fig. 12.5). At the same time, press in on the right flank and whirl the animal. The quick coordinated movement forces the animal to sit down on its left hip and the twirling motion sets the sheep up on its rump.

The handler's legs should be spread slightly to cradle the sheep's back. The animal should be sitting at approximately 60 degrees to the vertical. If the animal is too perpendicular it will struggle to free itself and perhaps will be able to gain enough balance to throw itself forward and escape. If the animal is too horizontal, too much pressure is exerted on the handler's legs and the animal is less accessible for examination and treatment.

If the sheep is properly balanced, both arms of the handler will be free to examine the feet, trim hoofs (Fig. 12.6), and

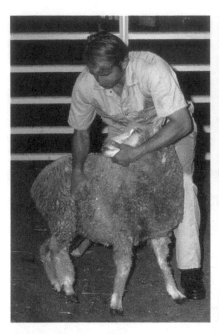 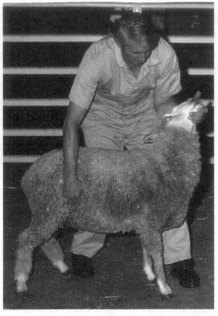

FIG. 12.5. Setting up a sheep: Proper position for holding the head, left. Improper position, right. Do not lift the head up over the back.

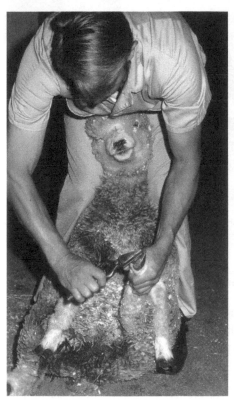 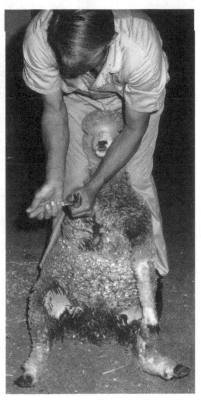

FIG. 12.6. Hoof trimming from set-up position.

examine the mouth (Fig. 12.7), mammary glands, prepuce, or testicles. Occasionally, an animal may flail its front legs; care should be taken to protect one's face from such action. Be aware of the relative positions of the head and feet of the sheep at all times.

Rams weighing over 136 kg (300 lb) may seem too large to set up in this manner; some animals set their chins down on the ground, seeming almost to defy a handler to lift and twist the head to the side. Nonetheless, grasping the animal's chin firmly and lifting and twisting it up to the side will enable the handler to set up the largest animal. It is important to twist the head to the side, not just pull it up dorsally (over the back). It is unnecessary and undesirable to lift the animal off the ground. Simply twist it, using mechanical advantage to position the animal.

A device known as a Gambel humane sheep restrainer may be placed over the neck of a sheep, and the front legs placed in reversed "U" bends in the device (Figs. 12.8, 12.9). The sheep lies down and is tranquil without being medicated or overly restrained, allowing transport or treatment of a

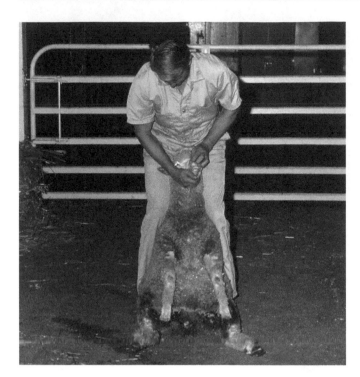

FIG. 12.7.   Oral examination from set-up position.

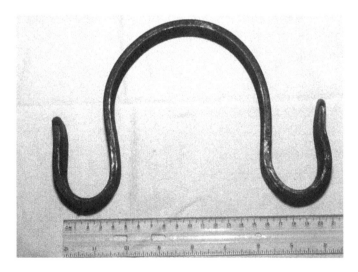

FIG. 12.8.   A Gambel sheep restrainer.

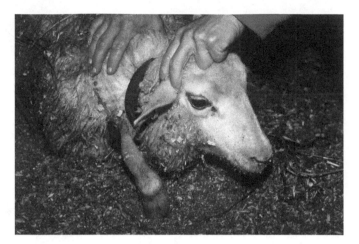

FIG. 12.9.   A Gambel sheep restrainer in use.

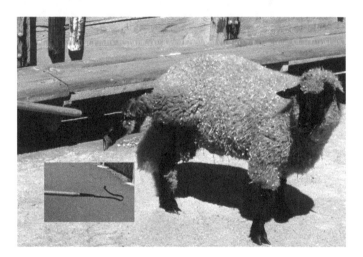

FIG. 12.10.   Shepherd's crook.

single animal, especially one with dystocia or prolapsed vagina.

The crisscross rope casting technique used with cattle is used on sheep in lieu of a net or snare.

A shepherd's crook allows the catching of a sheep without violating its flight distance (Fig. 12.10). Avoid twisting the limb with the crook to minimize the risk of rupturing the ligaments of the stifle. Lamb crooks are used to grasp the lower neck.

Lambs are easily handled. Support the body underneath the chest (Fig. 12.11). The lamb can be held for castration or

docking in the manner illustrated in Figure 12.12. The forelegs and hind legs are held together.

Halters may be used on sheep, but the nose is short so take care that the halter does not slide off or pull down over the nostrils, restricting air movement.

Various drenching techniques are used to medicate sheep. Large flocks are easily handled by crowding the animals into a narrow chute or corner (Fig. 12.13). The person conducting the drenching can then walk through the animals and insert the dose syringe nozzle into each mouth without resorting to additional restraint. The presence of the other animals keeps each patient secure for the treatment.

Straddle the sheep, walk up alongside it, or reach over and lift its head slightly by placing a hand under the chin. Insert the dose syringe in the commissure of the mouth, over the base of the tongue, and immediately clasp the mouth and nostrils closed while quickly injecting the medication into the pharynx. Automatic drenching guns have been designed for mass medication. Automatic vaccination guns are currently

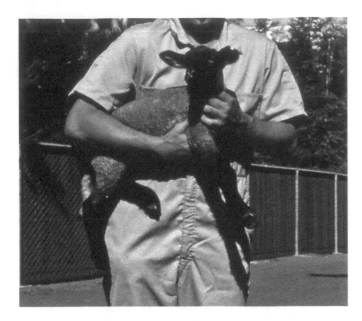

FIG. 12.11. Holding a lamb.

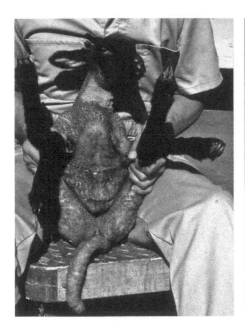

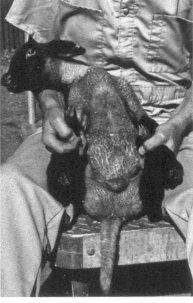

FIG. 12.12. Methods of holding a lamb for castration or docking.

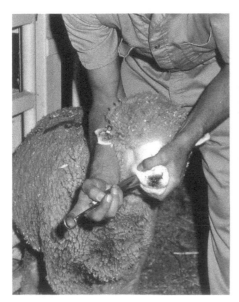

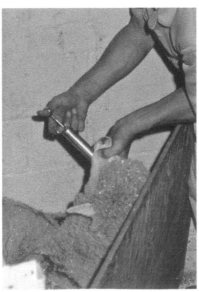

FIG. 12.13. Medicating a sheep with a drench syringe.

the primary means of mass medication, because most medications are formulated for subcutaneous administration.

Solid medication in bolus or tablet form is given with a balling gun (Fig. 12.14). Insert the tip of the gun through the interdental space.

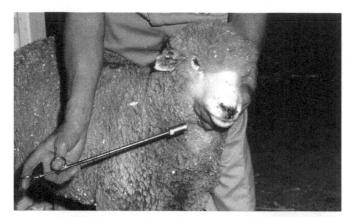

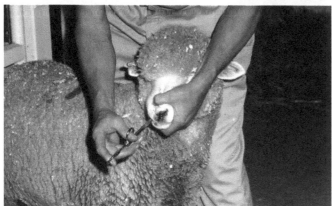

FIG. 12.14. Medicating a sheep with a balling gun.

GOATS

Although goats have the reputation of being able to withstand heavy stresses, in reality they are quite delicate. Their bones are small and easily broken. Usually, rough handling is not necessary. When accustomed to being handled, goats are docile and easily managed by a child (Fig. 12.15). Most respond to gentle treatment. Figure 12.16 shows a goat being held by an adult, and the inset shows a goat snapped to a post via a neck chain.

Uncastrated males have scent glands that produce a secretion with a very disagreeable odor. The secretion of the odoriferous material is under the control of androgens; hence, the glands are not active in castrated males. It is difficult to prevent the odor from impregnating the clothing of anyone handling a buck. Furthermore, the mature male is prone to urinate on its legs, neck, and body. The resulting pungent scent is of significance in breeding behavior.

The scent glands of the male are diffused in the area around the base of the horn. When a young buck is dehorned,

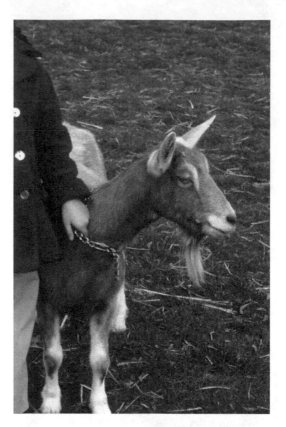

FIG. 12.15.   Female goat handled by a child.

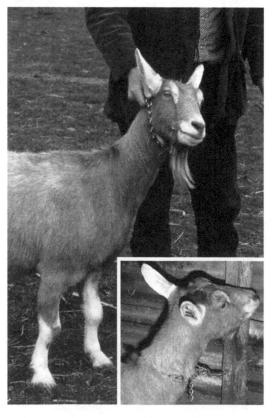

FIG. 12.16.   Goat being held by an adult. Goat snapped to a post via a neck chain, inset.

if 13 mm (1/2 in.) of skin is taken around the base of the horn, the gland is excised also. It is important that all males in a breeding group be descented if any are so treated. Otherwise, the females will prefer the scented males over the descented males.

Danger Potential

Goats do not strike or kick but usually fuss more than sheep. They vocalize and they may stamp their feet in obvious threat, but once they are grabbed, they do not strike. They do, however, use their heads for butting. Species having horns may use them as battering rams. The buck (male) is frequently adorned with heavy horns that may inflict serious injury on the unwary. A male goat is much more likely to initiate an attack than is a male sheep. Most dairy goats in the United States are dehorned as kids or are naturally polled, which lessens the hazard of butting. Nevertheless, even a hornless animal can cause injury.

A buck goat may show aggression when does are removed from a pen or when the handler steps between him and his does. Goats will bite if the handler over-restrains them, inflicts pain, or makes them angry.

Physical Restraint

The initial approach to handling a goat is similar to that for sheep in that one arm is placed around the goat's chest as the other hand grasps the dock (tail) area. The similarity ceases here, because goats cannot be "set up" like sheep. Goats are far more agile and less prone to accept such restraint. If placed in the set-up position, a goat will lash out with both forefeet and hind feet in a purposeful attack on the face and hands of the handler.

A group of goats can be herded into a chute or corner to single out or capture an individual. Approach a cornered buck with caution. He may attack. Threats are characterized by vocalization and stamping of the feet.

Angora goats kept in range flocks must be confined to sheds or chutes to capture them. Goats are much better jumpers than sheep, so chutes or pen fences must be 2 m (6 ft) or higher. Highly excited goats have been known to attempt to jump over a handler. Sometimes all four feet will be planted on the chest or head of the person who gets in the way. Angora goats are also highly sensitive to heat stress and may die from hyperthermia under conditions that sheep and other goat breeds easily tolerate. Shade must be available to these goats.

Goats may be roped, but the roper must be skilled. Goats, because of their speed and dodging abilities, are frequently used to sharpen the skills of rodeo calf ropers. Ropers must be prepared to jerk the loop tight quickly if fortunate enough to catch a goat.

Most dairy goats wear a neck chain or collar. Chains are preferred because pen-mates cannot chew them off. The size of most adult goats makes the chain convenient to hold the goat or lead it. If present, the horns may be used to grasp the goat in lieu of a chain. Although the horns may be used for

initial capture, goats dislike being held by the horns or ears. To hold a goat without a collar or a halter, place the open hands on each side of the lower jaw beneath the ears. The beard may be grasped to assist in immobilizing the head (Fig. 12.17). A small goat may be restrained by holding one leg (Fig. 12.18).

Small halters may be put on temporarily since many goats have been taught to stand quietly when haltered. Halters

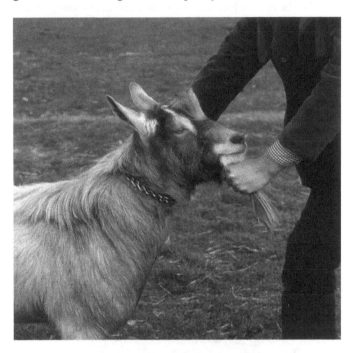

FIG. 12.17. Goat restraint by holding a buck by the beard.

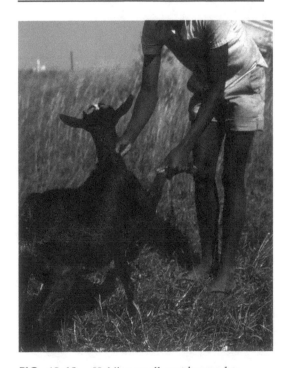

FIG. 12.18. Holding small goat by one leg.

that are left on will be chewed up. If haltered goats are left unattended, they may either chew the rope or loosen the knot. Some goats become very proficient at escaping from any restriction. Some learn how to unlatch gates; others are prone to climbing over walls, fences, and other restricting devices.

Dairy goats are likely to be accustomed to being snapped to a post or wall ring for milking, hoof trimming, or examination. Some goats can be milked from a small platform (Figs. 12.19, 12.20). The head is locked in a stanchion. Hoof trimming, examination or treatment of mastitis, and other procedures can be carried out while goats are restrained in this position.

The feet and legs of a goat may be picked up as are those of a horse. Usually one person holds the hind leg while another manipulates the feet. One person can hold the goat if necessary (Fig. 12.21), but the goat is more likely to struggle with one handler than with two.

An adult goat may be placed in lateral recumbency by flanking it (method is similar to that used for casting a calf). Kids are as easily handled as lambs (Figs. 12.22, 12.23). The horns of immature goats should not be used as handles for restraint, because the horns are easily fractured (Fig. 12.24).

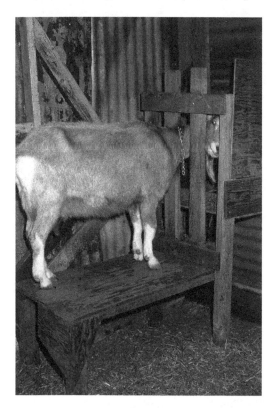

FIG. 12.19. Goat on milking platform.

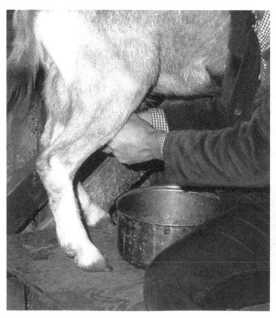
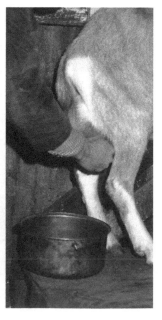

FIG. 12.20. Milking from behind, right, with goat on platform. Milking from the side, left.

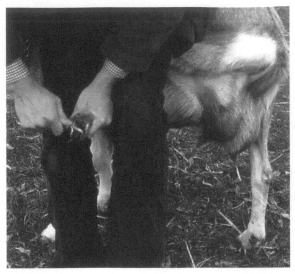
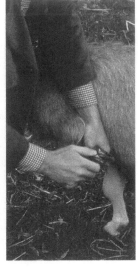

FIG. 12.21. Trimming the feet.

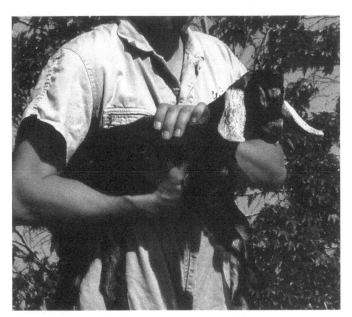

FIG. 12.22. Holding a kid.

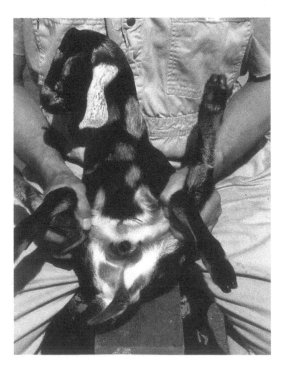

FIG. 12.23. Holding a kid for castration.

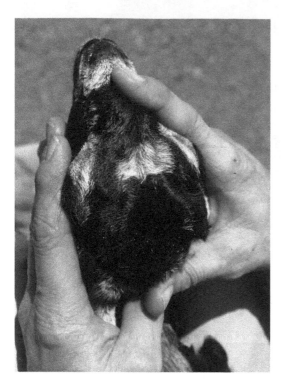

FIG. 12.24. Holding the head for dehorning.

TRANSPORT

Sheep and goats are easily transported in trucks, trailers, trains, and ships. They tolerate being closely confined.

The wool insulation layer of sheep predisposes them to hyperthermia, so arrangements must be made to keep sheep cool.

CHEMICAL RESTRAINT[2,3]

Domestic sheep and goats are so easily handled that chemical immobilization is rarely practiced. If sedation for minor surgery is required, xylazine (0.1–0.6 mg/kg), intramuscularly, or tiletamine/zolazepam (Telazol) (2.5 mg/kg), intramuscularly, are suitable agents. For more detailed information on sedation and immobilization, see Lin[2] and Reibold[3]. Monitor sedated animals closely for evidence of hyperthermia.

REFERENCES

1. Anderson, R.S., and Edney, A.T.B., Eds. 1991. Practical Animal Handling, 1st ed. Oxford, U.K. Pergamon Press, 198 pages, hardback.
2. Lin, H.-C., and Pugh, D.G. 2002. Anesthetic management. In: Pugh, D.G., Ed. Sheep and Goat Medicine. St. Louis, Elsevier, pp. 405–20.
3. Riebold, T. 2007. Ruminants. In: Tranquilli, W.J., Thurman, J.C., and Grimm, K.A., Eds. 2007. Lumb and Jones' Veterinary Anesthesia and Analgesia, 4th Ed. Ames, Iowa, Wiley-Blackwell Publishing, pp. 731–47.
4. Sheldon, C.C., Sonsthagen, T., and Topel, J.A. 2006. St. Louis, Mosby/Elsevier, 239 pages.
5. Sonsthagen, T.F. 1991. Restraint of Domestic Animals. Goleta, California, American Veterinary Publications, 149 pages, paperback.

CHAPTER 13

Swine

CLASSIFICATION

Order Artiodactyla
    Suborder Suiformes
        Family Suidae: swine

Swine are short-necked, short-legged, heavy-bodied descendants of the wild European boar. They are used for meat in tropical, subtropical, and temperate areas of the world. Names of the genders of swine are listed in Table 13.1. Weights of different breeds are listed in Table 13.2.

TABLE 13.1. Names of gender of swine

| | | Male | | | | |
Mature male	Mature female	Castrated before maturity	Castrated after maturity	Young female	Young of either sex	Newborn
Boar	Sow	Barrow	Stag	Gilt	Shoat	Piglet

TABLE 13.2. Weights of selected breeds of swine

| | Male | | Female | |
	(kg)	(lb)	(kg)	(lb)
Berkshire	410	900	365	800
Hampshire	410	900	320	700
Poland China	445	975	385	850
Duroc	430	950	340	750
Chester white	420	925	330	725
Yorkshire	320	700	370	600

DANGER POTENTIAL

The principal weapon of the pig is the teeth. Baby pigs have sharp, needlelike deciduous teeth, which inflict nasty wounds that are without exception septic and may be serious. Adult swine tear flesh easily. They have extremely strong jaws capable of crushing bones. Boars also develop elongated canine teeth called tusks, which are fearsome weapons capable of disemboweling a horse and certainly a person. The sow with a litter is a formidable, menacing animal and should be approached with caution.

Pigs do not usually behave as a "herd," but when handling an individual pig in the company of other pigs, be watchful for the development of a mob reaction. On one occasion I attempted to catch a small pig of approximately 18 kg (40 lb) in a large enclosure. The pig was roped around the body and picked up. As soon as the rope was in place, the animal began to squeal. Immediately all of the other pigs in the pen crowded around, grunting and threatening to attack. I was forced to drop the pig and move out of the area as quickly as possible.

ANATOMY, PHYSIOLOGY, AND BEHAVIOR

Swine behavior sets them apart from other domestic animals. They have little banding or herding instinct and are stubborn and contrary, resisting all efforts to drive them in a given direction or move them from one place to another. Never enter an enclosure with adult swine without taking safety precautions. Always make note of a quick escape route.

Pigs are unpredictable and frequently become aggressive with little warning. This is particularly true of sows with litters or adult boars. Rely on the caretaker for information about the general behavior of an individual animal.

Pigs naturally pull back when pressure is applied around the upper jaw. This peculiarity makes it possible to manipulate many swine that otherwise could not be handled.

Swine conformation allows a pig to run through underbrush easily. The body is streamlined, the head usually pointed, and separation between the head and body is not well demarcated. The lack of a definite separation at the head and neck prevents the use of halters or ropes around the neck to restrain pigs.

Because of their slick, smooth bodies, it is impossible to handle wet pigs. To successfully work with a pig, it should be clean and confined in a dry enclosure with absorbent bedding.

The strong neck muscles developed by rooting enable swine to lift with considerable force. Any panels on fences used to contain swine must be firmly attached to the ground; otherwise the animal may put its snout underneath and throw the panel over its head to escape or attack.

PHYSICAL RESTRAINT[1–7]

It is virtually impossible to capture or handle an adult pig in a large enclosure. Move the pig into a small pen by driving, or entice it into the small enclosure with feed. Pigs can be driven into a smaller pen either individually or as a group.

If a group of swine of mixed sizes must be handled, sort them out by size first to prevent large animals from trampling smaller individuals.

Unfortunately swine frequently have the habit of moving in the opposite direction to that desired by the handler. Thus an individual pig may be difficult to move. A snout rope utilizes the natural propensity to pull back against pressure on the upper jaw to enable a handler to point the animal's rump in the desired direction and back the pig into an enclosure.

A bucket or blindfold over the head of the animal triggers the same idiosyncrasy (Fig. 13.1). The pig will move in a negative direction to escape the bucket, and by continuing to hold the bucket over the pig's head, it can be directed as is a ship by its rudder.

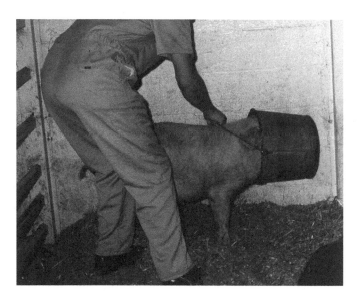

FIG. 13.1.   Directing pig backward with a bucket.

A cane or a narrow flat stick is excellent for directing a pig (Fig. 13.2). The stick or cane is not used to inflict pain, but is merely tapped on the side of the head to indicate to the animal the desired direction.

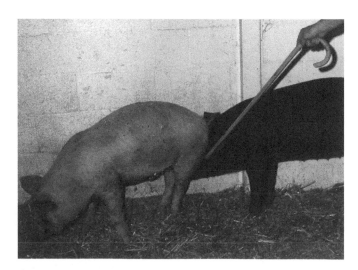

FIG. 13.2.   Cane is used to indicate direction.

A broad leather or canvas strap attached to a short wooden handle is effective in moving swine because it makes a loud noise when slapped against the body.

When directing pigs into a pen or through a gate, use either a broad shovel (Fig. 13.3) or wire paneling or solid plywood shields (Fig. 13.4). A shield is also a safe structure to work behind when dealing with a dangerous animal. Recognize that a large boar or an extremely aggressive sow could manage to work its snout under the shield and attack, but usually this can be prevented by tilting the top of the board back toward the handler or by slapping at the snout.

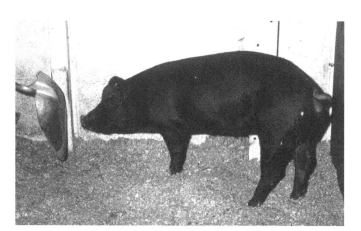

FIG. 13.3.   Directing a pig with a broad shovel.

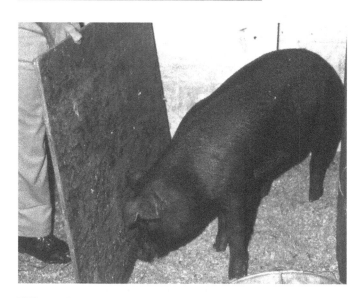

FIG. 13.4.   Moving a pig using a shield.

The snout, although used for rooting in the ground, is not callused but is an extremely sensitive organ. One can slow a pig down or even change its direction by tapping on the snout. Do not hit the snout hard, since inflicting severe pain may result in a negative response. The animal then becomes more aggressive rather than subdued, and the handler must then deal with an awesome opponent. A slap on the snout with a board or a cane may stop the rush of the animal, giving the handler time to escape. Kicking the snout may also work, but it is an extremely dangerous practice, because a pig can move its head swiftly and can bite through the shoe, injuring the foot severely.

Swine chased excessively, particularly during hot weather, become exhausted. The deep layer of insulating fat does not allow efficient conduction of heat, and these animals overheat rapidly if harassed too long during manipulative procedures. Any pig that must be restrained for any length of time and which struggles during that period should be examined frequently with a rectal thermometer to determine whether the body temperature is elevated. Temperatures above 40°–40.5°C (104°–105°F) require that immediate steps be taken to cool the animal with cold water enemas or sprays. Proceed with caution when the animal is under heat stress.

Although more stringent restraint practices may be required, it is often possible to work on adult sows and even boars by speaking to them in a kind, gentle manner, particularly if this is done by the usual caretaker. A sow lying down comfortably can be talked to, scratched on the body (Fig. 13.5), and calmed sufficiently to take her temperature without causing her to jump up. This method should always be attempted first, especially when performing simple procedures. Keep in mind, however, that these animals can turn and bite swiftly. Take precautions to assure that the animal does not twirl and bite the hand.

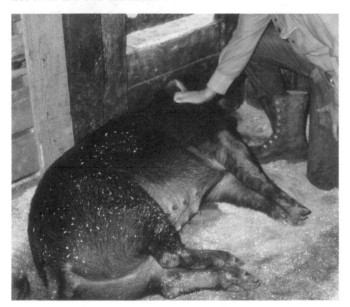

FIG. 13.5.   Calming recumbent sow by gentle stroking and using a soft voice.

Ropes are rarely used to capture swine. It is virtually impossible to rope a pig and prevent it from pulling its head back out of the loop because it has no neck. However, the animal can be put into a harness. Place a loop over the head and tighten it gently (Fig. 13.6). Form a half hitch, throw it over the head, and allow the animal to walk through it until the loop is past the front legs (Fig. 13.7). Then pull it up tight (Fig. 13.8).

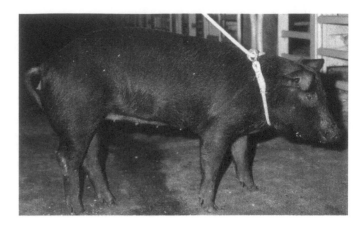

FIG. 13.6.   Applying rope harness to a pig. Loop is placed over the head and gently tightened from behind.

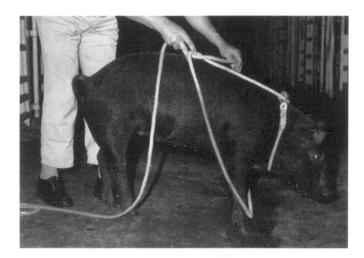

FIG. 13.7.   The pig is allowed to walk through a half-hitch loop.

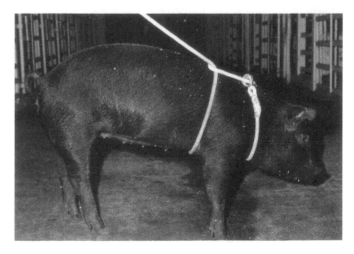

FIG. 13.8.   The second loop is tightened behind the forelegs.

The snout rope and cable snare are the prime restraint tools for swine. They are used in a variety of procedures requiring the moving or holding of swine. The size of rope used to form a snout loop varies with the size of the animal. To pull down snugly over the upper jaw, ropes sized from 3.2-mm (1/8-in.) manila to 13-mm (1/2-in.) nylon may be used. A small honda should be formed and the running end pulled through the honda to form a loop. The honda should be small enough so that it covers no more than one-third of the arch over the top of the nasal bones. For an adult boar or sow, a 6.5–10-mm (1/4–3/8-in.) nylon rope is suitable as a snout rope.

The technique for applying the snout rope varies with the location of the animal. Ideally, if the pig is restricted in a chute or panel arrangement, one can approach from the side and rear. The enlarged loop is worked over the top of the snout until it rests in the mouth (Fig. 13.9). The rope is then pulled back into the mouth with a sawing action. It is usually not difficult to pull the rope between the lips. The animal may try to go forward or back up, and the operator must be free to move with the animal. Once the rope is placed in the mouth, pull the loop tight (Fig. 13.10). When the loop is tightened around the upper jaw, the animal characteristically pulls back. Thus if the end of the rope is tied to a suitable post or ring in front of the pig, it pulls back, maintaining tension on the loop (Fig. 13.11).

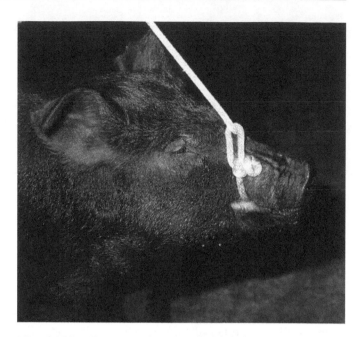

FIG. 13.10.   Snout rope loop is pulled tight from behind.

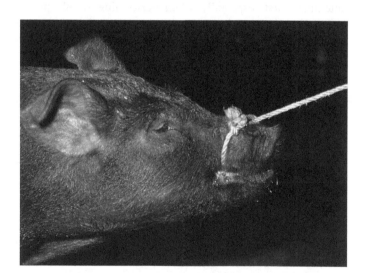

FIG. 13.11.   Free end of rope is brought forward to anchor the animal.

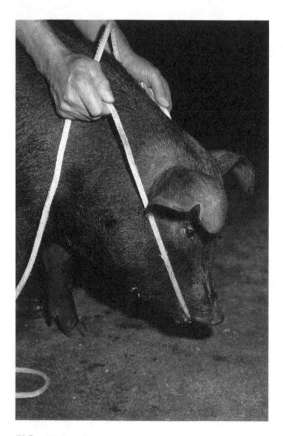

FIG. 13.9.   Snout rope placement: Loop is pulled into the mouth.

If the animal is not confined in a chute but is quiet, it may be approached from the rear and to the side with the loop extended.

It may be difficult to apply such a rope to a dangerous boar or a sow with piglets. Stay in close to the head to prevent the animal from turning to the side and raking the hand or the leg. It is sometimes difficult to thread the rope loop over the enlarged tusks of a big boar, but it is essential that the rope be placed behind the tusks since this serves as the anchor point for a large animal.

The cable snare is commonly used to capture swine and is safer and easier to manipulate than the snout rope. Usually the snare is formed on the end of a pipe or hollow tube. The handle that pulls the snare closed is on the opposite end, which is grasped by the handler. The cable maintains a previously formed loop, making it unnecessary for the hand to approach the head of the animal. Maneuver the snare over the top of the pig's head and into its mouth, sawing it back and forth until it is in place behind the incisors. The snare is closed by clamping the handle. The animal is held in the same manner as with the snout rope (Figs. 13.12, 13.13, 13.14, 13.15).

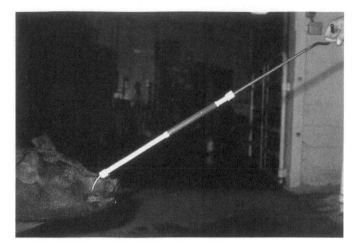

FIG. 13.14. An obstetrical snare used as a hog snare.

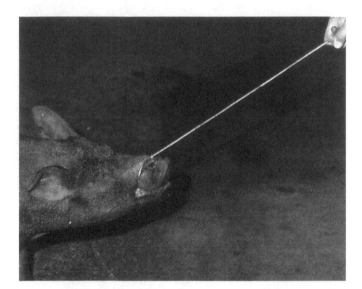

FIG. 13.12. Hog snare 1.

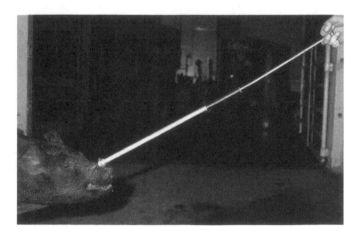

FIG. 13.13. Hog snare 2.

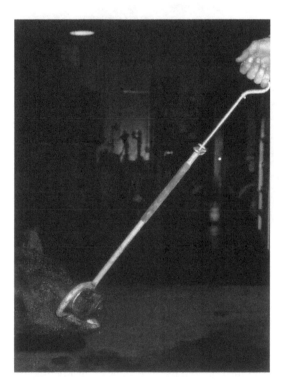

FIG. 13.15. A special guard to keep the loop open until it is in the mouth.

Once the snout rope or cable snare is in place, constant pressure must be applied forward lest the animal shake the loop from the upper jaw. Making use of the natural tendency of the animal to pull backward, the rope may either be held manually or secured to a post or ring. The snout rope or snare serves the same purpose for swine as the halter does for other species.

Other devices, based on the same principle, are used to hold swine (Fig. 13.16). Hog holders are essentially cable snares. Some have elaborate catches and quick releases. The cable obstetrical snare, designed to deliver a fetus, may be satisfactory for use on swine if made with a firm cable so that the loop stays open while being manipulated onto the upper jaw.

Do not leave a pig tied with a snout rope or cable snare for more than 15–20 minutes. A pig will pull back with sufficient force to produce a tourniquet effect around the upper jaw. In addition, the animal may chew through a rope and free itself. Baby pigs do not respond well to this technique and are likely to refuse to pull back if such a snout rope is applied. A

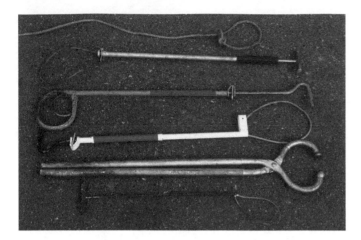

FIG. 13.16. Snares and tongs.

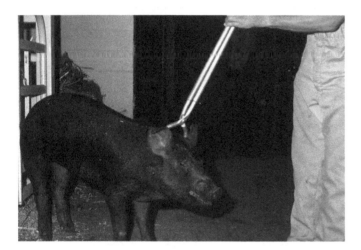

FIG. 13.17. Hog tongs placed behind ears of a pig will temporarily immobilize the animal.

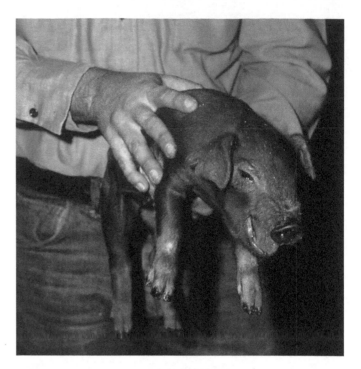

FIG. 13.18. Handling baby pigs: When lifting, the hands should be under and over the body.

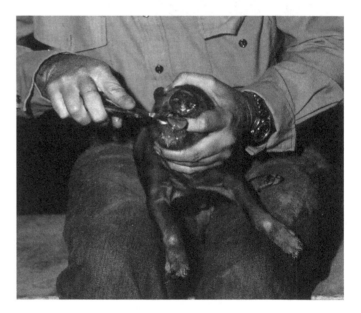

FIG. 13.19. Restraint for clipping "needle" teeth.

pig will become wary after a snare has been used repeatedly; placement of the snare will become difficult.

Long-handled neck tongs may be employed to grasp a pig in order to place the snout rope (Fig. 13.17). The pig is approached from the rear and the tongs placed just behind the ears. The pig automatically pulls back and squeals, allowing the loop to be inserted in the mouth; if the animal is in a relatively confined position, the tongs fix the head, making it easier to place the snout rope or snare. The tongs are then removed. Tongs are used for medium-sized swine up to approximately 40 kg (90 lb).

Although even a tiny pig is capable of inflicting a severe bite, most newborn piglets do not resist handling if grasped gently. It is important to remember that a small pig squeals when taken from its mother. The squealing elicits a dramatic response from the sow, and if she can reach the handler she is likely to inflict serious injury. Therefore piglets should be separated from the sow prior to being picked up and handled. This is most easily accomplished by driving the sow into a farrowing chute where the piglets are free to move away from

the sow because the fence does not reach to the ground. The sow is confined to the chute and cannot attack a handler picking up the small pigs. To minimize the sow's agitation and distress, move the piglets out of her hearing before manipulating them. Larger piglets are handled by supporting the body under the chest (Fig.13.18). Figure 13.19 shows how to restrain a piglet for clipping "needle" teeth.

Pigs less than 28 kg (60 lb) should be confined to a small pen or alleyway before individual handling is attempted

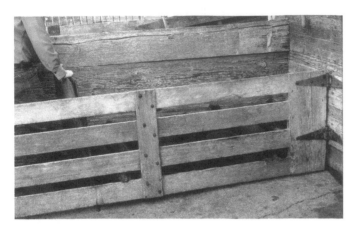

FIG. 13.20. Squeezing pigs into small area with a panel gate.

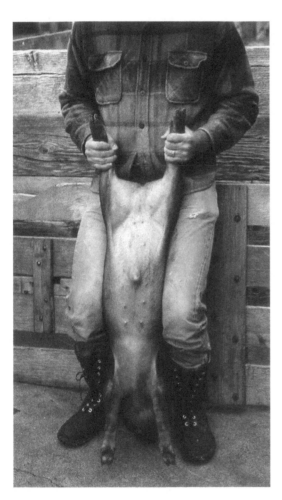

FIG. 13.21. Holding a medium-sized pig.

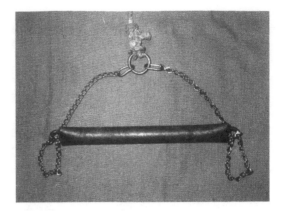

FIG. 13.22. Hog shackle.

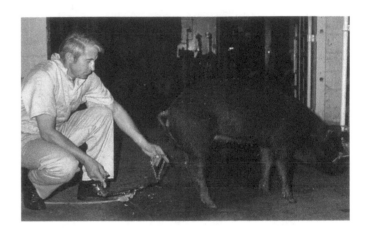

FIG. 13.23. Casting technique using a shackle. Form loops at ends of shackle. Lift each foot, and place a loop around a leg.

(Fig. 13.20). Pick up a pig by grasping above the hock and lifting the pig off its feet (Fig. 13.21). Be careful not to twist the leg as this may dislocate the hip joint. The pig may be held with the head up as well. This is a suitable position for minor surgical procedures such as castration or vaccinations. The handler should keep in mind that a pig held in this way

is able to bite. However, if the animal's head is confined by the handler's legs, this is not an undue hazard.

Larger pigs (45–56 kg; 100–125 lb) may be handled in a similar manner, except that it requires two people, each grabbing one of the hind legs, to lift it off the ground and hold it for a short time. Pigs over 68 kg (150 lb) are usually not captured or held in this manner. They should be placed in a small enclosure and handled with a snout rope or snare. If it is necessary to cast a pig or place it in lateral recumbency, one of the following techniques may be used. All require securing the pig with a snout rope before beginning.

1. The first technique utilizes a shackle. The shackle can be temporarily constructed of rope and a 50 × 100 mm (2 × 4 in.) board. A permanent shackle can be made by welding rings to an iron pipe through which loops of chain attached to the shackle are threaded (Fig. 13.22). Place the loops on the hind limbs, above the hocks if possible. Each hind leg is lifted in turn and placed through the loops (Figs. 13.23, 13.24). It is not difficult to lift the leg of even a large boar for a sufficient length of time to do this.

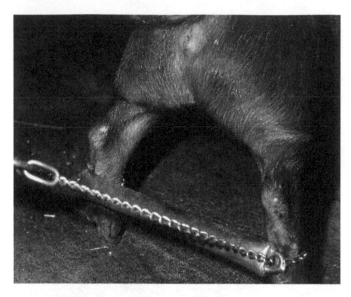

FIG. 13.24. Loops in place.

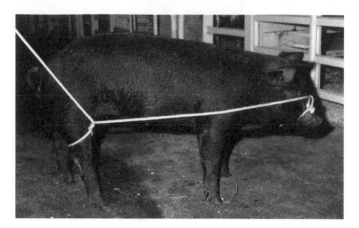

FIG. 13.26. Casting procedure utilizing snout rope and half hitch above the hock.

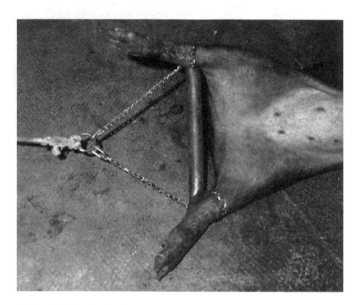

FIG. 13.25. Animal cast and stretched, secure with a trucker's hitch.

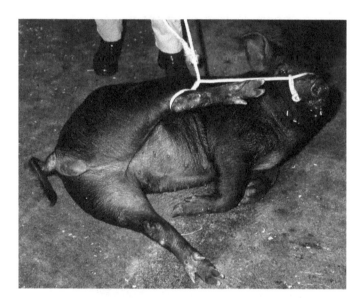

FIG. 13.27. Casting procedure completed.

When both loops are in place, attach another rope to the center pull and stretch the animal. The pig will roll over on its side and can be maintained in either lateral or dorsal recumbency by applying tension (Fig. 13.25). A trucker's hitch is suitable to maintain tension. Once the animal is down, the legs can be maintained in the stretch position for minor surgery such as castration or repair of umbilical hernias.

2. A large pig can be cast by placing a snout rope and a hitch around the hock or using a hock hobble. Maintaining tension, bring the snout rope around through the hock loop and pull the hind leg up to the snout. The snout rope may be used to surround the hock as well (Figs. 13.26, 13.27). The operator stands on the side opposite to the hobble and by pulling on the snout rope forces the animal to lie on its side. This is suitable restraint and positioning for castrating a boar.

3. For the third casting technique, place a short rope on both foreleg and hind leg on the side of the animal upon which you wish it to lie when cast. Take the ropes beneath the body of the animal, up the opposite side, and over the back (Fig. 13.28). The handler stands on the side of the animal to which the ropes are secured and pulls on the rope over the top of the body. This procedure pulls the legs out from under the pig. The animal lies on its side but is otherwise relatively free and must be further secured (Fig. 13.29). An animal can be held by placing a knee on the neck. Use a local anesthetic

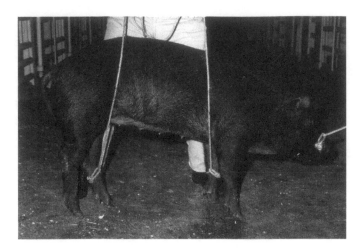

FIG. 13.28. Casting procedure for large swine: Secure with snout rope. Then place leg ropes.

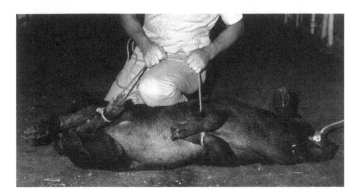

FIG. 13.29. Casting large swine. Pull legs out from under the animal and roll it onto its side.

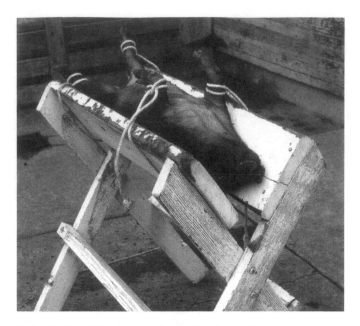

FIG. 13.30. Wooden trough restraint for small pigs.

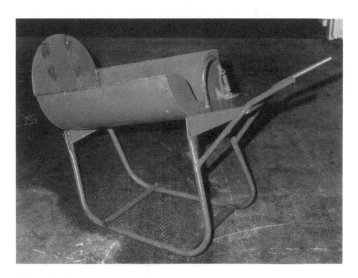

FIG. 13.31. Metal trough for restraint of small pigs.

for painful procedures. For prolonged operations, the legs must be secured and stretched to prevent them from flailing and injuring people.

Various types of troughs or cradles are used to restrain pigs in dorsal recumbency (Figs. 13.30, 13.31). A bar or rope may be placed over the snout to keep the head down; the hind limbs are secured by a short length of sash cord. This method of restraint, coupled with either local or general anesthesia, is suitable for abdominal surgery in swine. The animal can also be bled from the anterior vena cava while in this position. If the animal is to be maintained in ventral recumbency, a home-made network of nylon or cloth strips may be constructed. The legs protrude through the network (Fig. 13.32).

Commercial squeezes are available for handling swine. Pressure may be exerted on the neck, body, and buttocks to keep swine in the squeeze (Fig. 13.33). These devices are useful when working with adult or market swine that must be bled either from the ear or from the anterior vena cava.

Examining the mouth of the adult pig is difficult. Place a snout rope on the animal and allow the pig to pull back against it. Open the mouth with a speculum and examine the mouth with a flashlight.

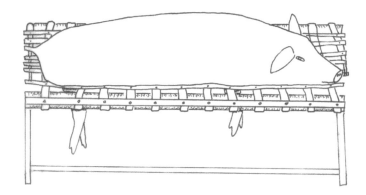

FIG. 13.32. Network for restraining swine.

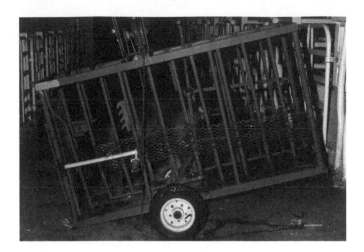

FIG. 13.33. Portable squeeze chute for swine.

Miniature Pigs (Pot-bellied pigs)

Pot-bellied pigs require special consideration (Fig. 13.34). Owners usually have no background in livestock care and will not tolerate many of the physical restraint practices routinely employed when handling swine reared for food. Miniature pigs are usually docile and much can be accomplished with minimal physical restraint. If blood collection or other diagnostic procedures necessitate immobilization, the administration of isoflurane via a mask is the preferred method (Table 13.3).

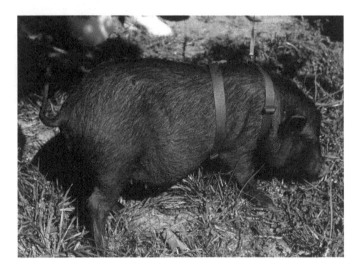

FIG. 13.34. Pot-bellied pig.

TABLE 13.3. Sedatives and immobilizing agents for pot-bellied pigs

Agent	Dose mg/kg, Route
Diazepam	0.5–1.0, IM
Azaperone	0.23–1.0, IM
Tiletamine/zolazepam	0.5–1.0 IM
Ketamine/diazepam	10.0–18.0/1.2–2.0, IM
Xylazine/tiletamine/zolazepam	2.2/1.0, IM
Isoflurane	3% induction, 2.5% maintenance, Face mask

Blood Collection[1]

Techniques for collecting blood samples from swine depend upon the skill and experience of the operator, the age and docility of the animal, and the means of restraint. The latter is likely the key to obtaining samples from a number of locations, including the cranial vena cava, jugular vein, caudal auricular vein, cephalic and saphenous veins, tail vein, femoral vein, and the orbital sinus.

The cranial vena cava is the preferred site for the collection of large volumes of blood. Anatomic relationships are similar in all suids and tayassuids (peccaries). The cranial vena cava is formed by the confluence of the subclavian vein cranial to the first rib, and the external and internal jugular veins dorsal to the manubrium sternum but ventral to the trachea (Figs. 13.35, 13.36).

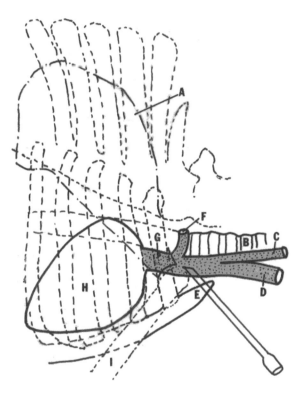

FIG. 13.35. Diagram of the major veins near the thoracic inlet, lateral view. **A.** Scapula, **B.** trachea, **C.** internal jugular vein, **D.** external jugular vein, **E.** manubrium of the sternum, **F.** subclavian vein, **G.** cranial vena cava, **H.** heart, and **I.** humerus. (Photo used by permission, W.B. Saunders, Philadelphia.)

In adult domestic pigs, a snare may be placed on the upper jaw, caudal to the tusks. The head is then extended and lifted up to expose the site. A thumb is placed in the right jugular groove and slipped along caudally to the termination of the groove. The needle is directed slightly caudally and dorsally toward the left distal scapula (upper shoulder). Smaller swine, weighing less than 20 kg, may be placed in dorsal recumbency with the head extended in a V-shaped trough.

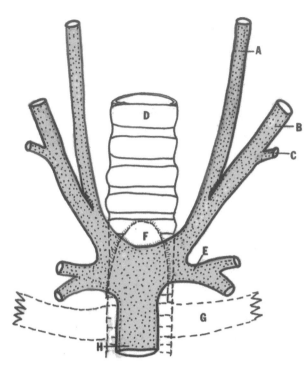

FIG. 13.36. Diagram of the major veins near the thoracic inlet, dorsoventral view. **A.** Internal jugular vein, **B.** external jugular vein, **C.** cephalic vein, **D.** trachea, **E.** subclavian vein, **F.** manubrium of the sternum, **G.** first rib, and **H.** cranial vena cava. (Photo used by permission, W.B. Saunders, Philadelphia.)

TRANSPORT

Swine are easily transported in crates, trailers, trucks, and trains. Hyperthermia is a constant threat.

CHEMICAL RESTRAINT[2–7]

Many procedures can be carried out on swine under physical restraint. Sometimes blood collection, radiography, or other diagnostic procedures may stimulate minimal struggling, necessitating sedation or chemical immobilization. The special challenges associated with sedation and chemical immobilization of domestic swine include the difficulty of ensuring an intramuscular injection because of heavy subcu-

TABLE 13.4. Sedatives used in swine

Agent	Dose (mg/kg), route
Azaperone	2.0, IM
Diazepam	0.2–0.5
Midazolam	0.1–0.5, IM

TABLE 13.5. Selected chemical restraint agents for swine

Agent	Dose mg/kg, route
Tiletamine/zolazepam	0.5–1.0 IM
Xylazine/ketamine	2.0–3.0/10.0–12.0, IM
	1.0–2.0/10.0–12.0, IV
Xylazine/Tiletamine/zolazepam	1.1–3.0/1.0, IV

taneous fat or the cannulation of a vein for intravenous administration. Drugs used in other livestock species may be less effective when used in swine. (See Tables 13.3–13.5.)

The chemical restraint agents and combinations mentioned in this chapter represent those used by experienced veterinarians with detailed knowledge of swine. Other protocols have been used, and no claim is made for including all possible drugs and combinations. For more detailed information, particularly for anesthesia, consult Thurmon.[8]

REFERENCES

1. Anderson, R.S., and Edney, A.T.B., Eds. 1991. Practical Animal Handling, 1st ed. Oxford, England, Pergamon Press, 198 pages.
2. Fowler, M.E. 1993. Wild swine and peccaries. In: Fowler, M.E., Ed. Zoo and Wild Animal Medicine, 3rd Ed. Philadelphia, W.B. Saunders, pp. 513–22.
3. Fowler, M.E. 1996. Husbandry and diseases of captive wild swine and peccaries. Revue Scientifique et Technique 15(1):141–54.
4. Lehman, A.D., Straw, B.E., Mengeling, W.L., D'Allaire, S., and Taylor, D.J., Eds. 1992. Diseases of Swine, 7th ed. Ames, Iowa State University Press.
5. Morris, P.J., and Shima, A.L. 2003. Suidae and Tayassuidae (wild pigs and peccaries). In: Fowler, M.E., and Miller, R.E., Eds. 2003. St. Louis, Saunders/Elsevier, pp. 586–602.
6. Sheldon, C.C., Sonsthagen, T., and Topel, J.A. 2006. St. Louis, Mosby/Elsevier, 239 pages.
7. Sonsthagen, T.F. 1991. Restraint of Domestic Animals. Goleta, California, American Veterinary Publications, 149 pages.
8. Thurman, J.C., and Smith, G.W. 2007. Swine. In: Tranquilli, W.J., Thurman, J.C., and Grimm, K.A., Eds. 2007. Lumb and Jones' Veterinary Anesthesia and Analgesia, 4th Ed. Ames, Iowa, Wiley-Blackwell Publishing, pp. 747–64.

CHAPTER 14
Camelids

Suborder Tylopoda
> Family Camelidae: Old World and New World camelids
> Old World
>> *Camelus bactrianus*: Bactrian camel
>> *Camelus dromedarius*: dromedary camel
> New World
>> Species *Lama glama*: llama
>>> *Lama pacos*: alpaca
>>> *Lama guanicoe*: guanaco
>>> *Vicugna vicugna*: vicuña

Old World camels and New World llamas and alpacas are domestic animals that have been important contributors to the culture and economies of their native countries for thousands of years. When accustomed to being handled, they are tractable, but like any other domestic animal, they must be tamed and trained.[12-15] Camelids are commonly kept in zoos, and if the zoo's policy is a no-hands-on relationship with the keeper, a different type of restraint may be necessary. Guanacos and vicuñas are wild animals and may be difficult to handle. However, guanacos may be tamed and handled similarly to llamas if procedures are carried out slowly and quietly.

DANGER POTENTIAL

Camel males have large canine teeth employed in intraspecific aggression with other males vying for a female, as shown in Figure 14.1. Bites from Old World camels may be fatal to humans. Where the camel is used by native people, instances have been reported of a camel grasping a child by the head and shaking it. The child's neck may be fractured and possibly the calvarium penetrated.

Llama males have saber-sharp canines (Figs. 14.2, 14.3), but they are rarely employed against humans, except by behaviorally maladjusted males (too much human attention during early development). Mature males have one lower and two upper canine teeth on each side of the mouth. Unless blunted or cut short, these teeth are formidable. The canines of females and early-castrated males are usually small or may even be absent. Normal breeding llama males may be safely handled by children in contrast to the males of most domestic ungulates. Biting is usually reserved for aggression between intact males.

One must be continually alert when working around even tame camels. A young camel was restrained in a chute to be

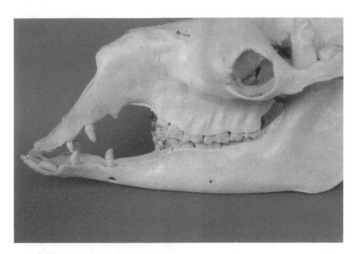

FIG. 14.1. Dental morphology of a male camel. Note the five pairs of canine teeth.

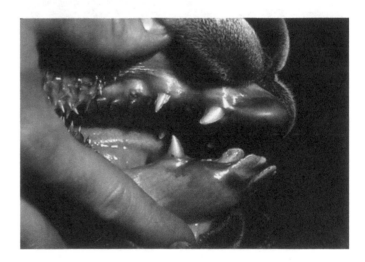

FIG. 14.2. Canine teeth of a mature male llama.

weighed and medicated (Fig. 14.4). The camel pushed one foot out through the bars, and as an assistant bent down to assist the animal in releasing the foot, the camel reached around and grasped him by the back of the neck. An immediate hard slap on the muzzle of the animal by a helper caused it to release its grip; another few seconds might have meant a fractured neck as the animal shook the assistant.

Offensively, male llamas bite, charge, chest butt, and rear up and strike down on another male. Properly reared and

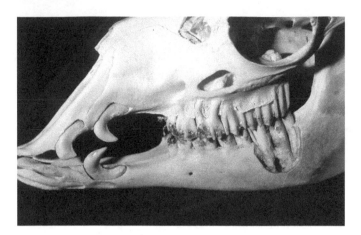

FIG. 14.3. Canine and cheek teeth of mature male llama sculpted to visualize the roots of the teeth.

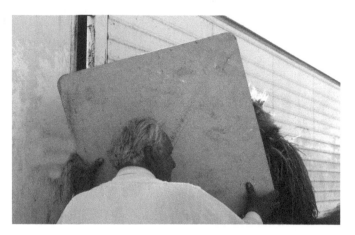

FIG. 14.5. Shield used to deflect stomach contents spewed by a Bactrian camel.

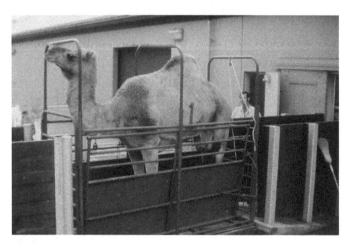

FIG. 14.4. Obtaining accurate body weight is important for determining medication dosage.

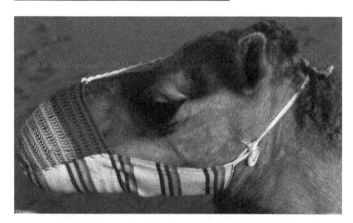

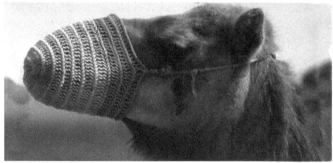

FIG. 14.6. Muzzles on a camel to prevent spitting, biting, and eating.

trained, male llamas are as safe and as easy to handle by humans as female llamas. Imprinted (rogue) males are a different matter. Camelids generally "cow-kick" by arching a rear limb forward and outward. However, they also kick with a quick jab directly backward. The padded foot mitigates the sharpness of a kick, but the potential for injury from a large llama should not be underestimated. Alpacas tend to kick with less provocation than do llamas; suri alpacas may be more prone to kick than huacayas. Fortunately, SACs (South American camelids or New World camelids) are not as agile kickers as their Old World cousins, the camels. The safest place to stand when handling an SAC is near the shoulder. Not so for camels, since they can reach far forward of the shoulder to strike a handler. Adult llamas rarely strike with a front limb. They may rear to escape an unpleasant situation, but usually without directed striking.

Camels may kick in any direction, and a camel is able to reach up and scratch its head with a hind foot. A Bactrian camel kicked and broke a 10×10 cm (4×4 in.) post. South American camelids may also kick, usually in a sweeping

forward and outward motion, as a cow kicks. Llamas and alpacas may also kick with a quick jab backward. Alpacas are more prone to kick than llamas. The padded foot mitigates the sharpness of a kick, but the potential for injury from a large llama should not be underestimated.

Llamas may swing the head and hit a person in the face when an attempt is made to halter them. The author is aware of two individuals who sustained fractured nasal bones as a result of such head flinging.

The most common human injury caused by an alpaca is a bloody nose or thick lip, produced when the alpaca raises the head explosively, striking the handler in the face. The

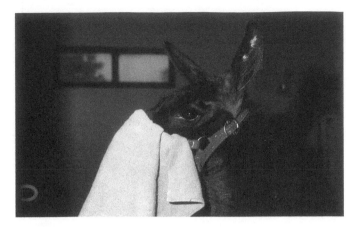

FIG. 14.7. A towel attached to halter to prevent spewing of stomach contents onto handlers.

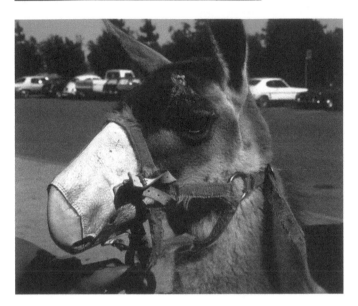

FIG. 14.8. Muzzling a llama to prevent biting.

alpaca is not purposefully trying to injure the handler, but this is a normal reflex. When being approached in a group, animals may have their heads down, as if to hide, get behind another animal, or go under a fence. When a handler grabs an alpaca its normal response is to lift the head quickly.

BEHAVIOR

Effective restraint requires understanding of camelid behavior. See Chapter 5.[6–8,16] All camelid species are social animals, which may be an advantage when driving the animals into a smaller enclosure for close observation or capture. Alpacas are more herd or flock oriented than llamas and llamas more than camels.

Camelids may vocalize during restraint procedures. Camels emit a grumbling sound. Llamas may scream during restraint even if undergoing non-pain-inflicting diagnostic procedures; however, this behavior is much more common in alpacas. The extremely angry llama may actually screech, but

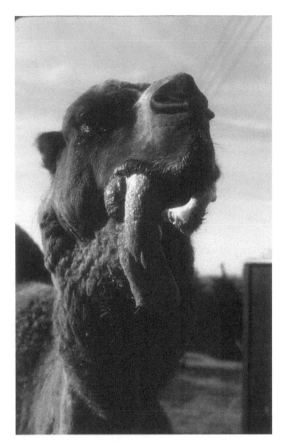

FIG. 14.9. Dhula (gulah) of a dromedary camel. This is an inflatable diverticulum off the soft palate.

this type of vocalization usually occurs when males are fighting one another.

Camelids use so-called "spitting" (actually regurgitated stomach contents) as an offensive and defensive behavior. Usually, the animals spit at each other in hierarchical or defensive situations, but if an animal becomes agitated with a human, it may employ this behavior. The observant restrainer may anticipate an approaching episode. The ears are laid back against the neck prior to the onset of defensive action (Fig. 5.4). A gulping or gurgling sound will be heard in the throat region, and a bolus of ingesta will be regurgitated from compartment one of the stomach. Ingesta is spewed out of the mouth in a diffuse pattern and may spray as far as 1 or 2 m. The unfortunate recipient will find that the obnoxious odor persists until after a shower and shampoo.

In llamas and alpacas, the material is directed forward and the head need only be pointed away from handlers to prevent being showered. Camels, however, have a propensity to spit out of the corner of the mouth, making it difficult to find a safe location to stand, unless a shield is used (Fig. 14.5). Camelids may be muzzled (Fig. 14.6) or a "spit rag" may be attached to the halter to avoid the spray (Fig. 14.7). Muzzles are also employed to prevent biting (Fig. 14.8).

Dromedary camel males have an inflatable pouch, a diverticulum off the ventral soft palate (dhula, gulah) (Fig. 14.9). When agitated or in rut, the animal may inflate the pouch, which will protrude out of the mouth and emit a gurgling vocalization, a sight that may be quite alarming to the neophyte camel handler.

PHYSICAL RESTRAINT

There is a distinct handling difference between camels, llamas, and alpacas.[2,4,5] The optimal area for initial capture is to drive camelids into a small catch pen or enclosure where animals are usually fed, hence accustomed to entering (Fig. 14.10).

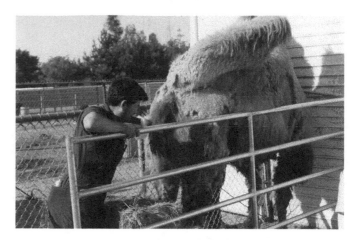

FIG. 14.12. Improvised chute for a camel. A pipe gate is secured near a corner of a barn and chain-link fence. Bales of straw are placed behind the camel to protect the operator from being kicked.

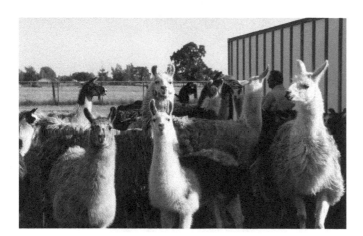

FIG. 14.10. Llamas moved into a catch pen.

Camels[17]

Camels may be restricted by placing them in a chute. Several chutes are illustrated in Figures 14.11–14.17.

Camels accustomed to being handled may be haltered and led into stocks used for horses (Fig. 14.11). Keep in mind the potential sweep of the legs.

Camels may be roped and snubbed to a tree or post or moved to a more contained area to be haltered. An improvised

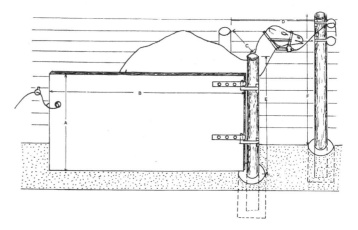

FIG. 14.13. Simple camelid chute, side view.

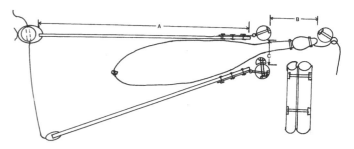

FIG. 14.14. Simple camelid chute, top view.

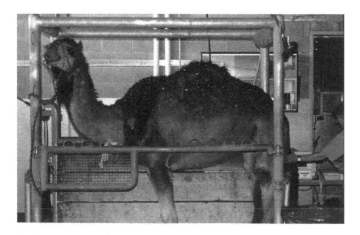

FIG. 14.11. Camel in an equine stock.

chute may be constructed alongside a barn or fence (Fig. 14.12). Wilder or more aggressive camels may require sedation before they can be safely handled.

Camels have been physically restrained in the sternal recumbent position (kushed) for centuries in camel-using countries. Either a leather strap or rope is used to place a loop or figure 8 around the front limb when the leg is flexed at the

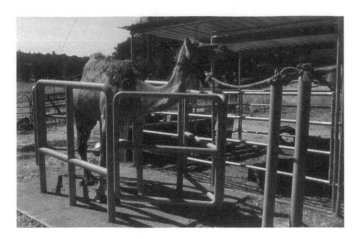

FIG. 14.15. Home constructed camel chute.

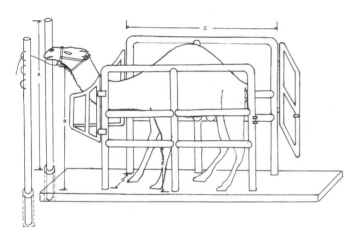

FIG. 14.16. Diagram of a home constructed camel chute.

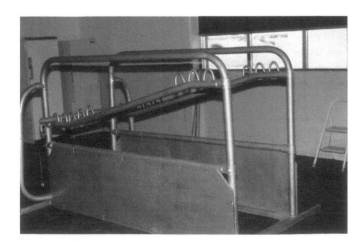

FIG. 14.17. Camel chute used for artificial insemination in the Middle East.

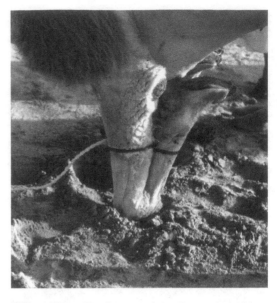

FIG. 14.18. Foreleg restraint to keep a camel in sternal recumbency (kushed).

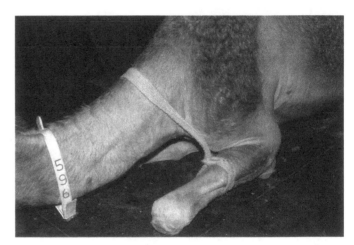

FIG. 14.19. Forelimbs linked by rope or strap over the neck.

carpus (Fig. 14.18). Alternatively, both front limbs may be linked together by a rope or strap over the neck (Fig. 14.19). The camel can only rise to its knees.

Rear limb restraint is accomplished as depicted in Figures 14.20 and 14.21. A soft cotton rope is brought up behind the hind limbs as the camel is being directed to kush (lie down); optimally, the rope should be below the fetlock. Once recumbent, the rope is placed medial to the stifles and tied tightly over the back behind the hump, as shown in Figure 14.21. The camel accustomed to this procedure will allow physical examination (rectal, genital tract, digestive tract).

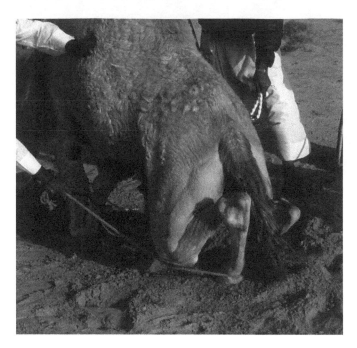

FIG. 14.20. Applying soft rope to assist a camel into sternal recumbency.

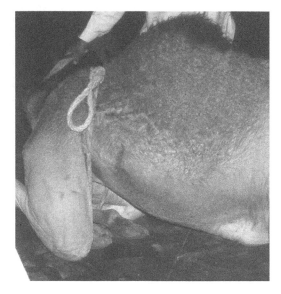

FIG. 14.21. Tying the rope over the back to prevent the camel from rising.

Llamas

The author is well aware that many techniques are used for taming and training llamas.[12–15] The person who must work with a llama that is strange to them, should inquire about the type of training the animal has had and the owner's feelings as to how restraint should be carried out. Well-trained animals do not require some of the techniques that follow. Use the least amount of restraint necessary to perform a task.

Llamas may be herded into a catch pen, narrow alleyway, or chute, like camels (Fig. 14.22). Llamas may also be

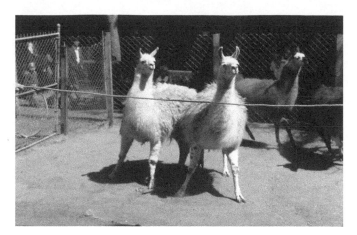

FIG. 14.22. Llamas moved into a catch pen.

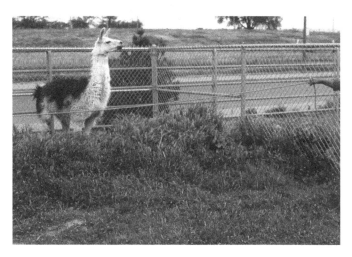

FIG. 14.23. Using a rope to contain llamas to a corner.

herded into a corner with ropes (Fig. 14.23). Only one person should signal the team to move forward or retreat.

Two people may hold a rope (minimum length of 6 m) taut between them, 1 m above the ground. Most farmed llamas will not challenge the rope. Occasionally, an individual will run under the rope or try to charge through it. This technique is not recommended for zoo animals unaccustomed to being handled. One end of the rope may be tied to a fence to free a handler to move among the llamas to place a rope or halter on the one(s) selected.

In a large pasture, with more help, two ropes may be used in a crisscross pattern, which allows a llama group to be restricted along a fencerow instead of into a corner. A modification of this technique employs long bamboo poles or plastic pipes, each carried by a single individual in the manner of a tightrope walker (Fig. 14.24). Two or more of the poles are used to herd and contain the llamas.

The method used by "llameros" (handlers) in the Andes to load packs is as follows: pack llamas are driven into a group, and llameros surround the group with llama fiber ropes

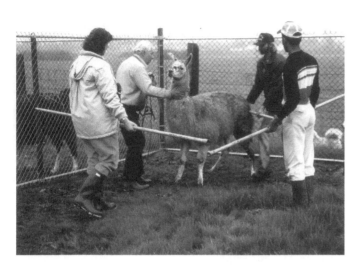

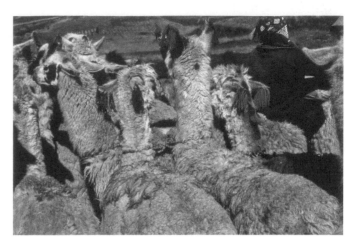

FIG. 14.26. Three pack llamas tied together with a rope around their necks.

FIG. 14.24. Using poles to extend the arms to restrict movement of llamas.

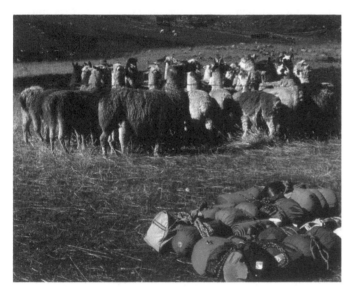

FIG. 14.25. Pack llamas in the Andes contained in a group with a rope surrounding them.

(Fig. 14.25). While the rope ring is in place, other llameros work their way into the herd and with a shorter rope tie three animals together by their necks (Fig. 14.26). The rope is looped around the neck of the first llama, the ends given one or two twists, then looped around another and twisted, and finally a third llama is included before the ends are tied together. Once all the triads are roped up, the perimeter rope is dropped. Since three llamas tied together will not all go in the same direction, they stand still. Packs may then be placed on their backs.

Mother-reared male llamas are usually no more difficult to handle than females, in contrast to bulls, stallions, and rams. Bottle-fed orphan males or neonates given too much

human attention may imprint on humans and develop a dangerous behavioral pattern. Essentially, an imprinted male treats a human as if he or she is another male llama.

This behavior may be anticipated in the male youngster that approaches and pushes its nose into a person's face or gallops up and pushes the owner around with its neck or chest. Peculiarly, overt aggression may not manifest itself until maturity, and then a particular person may bear the brunt of the aggression. A number of people have been severely injured by vicious attacks of males that are otherwise able to be handled.

In a full attack, the ears will be laid back against the llama's neck. He will charge and attempt to knock a person down by butting with his chest. If this fails, he may rear up and slam down on the person. A person who falls will be trampled with the llama's forefeet and bitten. A victim who remains standing may be bitten at the neck, knees, or any other spot within reach. When male llamas fight with other males, they bite the neck, hind limbs, and scrotum.

Several anatomic adaptations in male SACs protect against fatal injuries during such encounters. (See Blood Collection in this chapter.) The skin of the upper cervical region is as much as 1 cm thick. Instead of lying superficially in a jugular furrow, the camelid jugular vein lies deep, in juxtaposition to the carotid artery. Finally, a ventral projection of the transverse process of the cervical vertebrae forms an inverted U channel that protects vital cervical structures.

Aggressive males are ferocious, uttering loud vocalizations and attempting to climb fences to get at intended victims. One male alpaca attempted to climb up on to the seat of a tractor to reach a young driver. Once this behavior has been exhibited, contact with that llama is no longer safe for any person. A few individual animals have been deconditioned with negative stimulation, but usually safety has been achieved only for the individual deconditioning them. Others remain at risk.

Not all imprinted males develop aberrant behavior, and some may become obnoxious but not dangerous. It is also possible to hand raise an orphaned male llama without it becoming imprinted, if no loving attention is given while it is nursing and it is returned to the herd after feeding to be socialized as a llama. Hand-reared females may also develop aggressive tendencies, but it is less common than in males.

Castration of adult males is not effective in changing abnormal behavior, as it is in bulls and stallions. It is recommended that orphaned males that have been given extensive human attention be castrated by 2 months of age or, at the latest, before weaning.

A handler may not be able to enter an enclosure housing an aggressive imprinted male. It may be necessary to rope such an animal to gain initial contact, but llamas quickly learn how to dodge the loop and are elusive to all but the expert roper. Once caught, a halter may be placed or a temporary rope halter fashioned from a loop around the neck. (See Chapter 5.) Alternatively, the animal may be sedated.

Llamas generally dislike having their heads touched or scratched, unless gentle desensitization has been carried out. Trainers usually state that llamas are sensitive about the head, because every time someone touches them, something less than pleasant happens. To place a halter, the llama should be approached from the left side at the withers. The right arm should reach over the neck while the halter's poll strap is pushed under the neck to be grasped with the right hand. The nose loop should be slowly moved up and positioned over the nose. The llama may try to dodge this action. With the nose loop in place, the poll strap can be buckled or snapped to the cheek ring. If placed correctly, the nose loop should not slip down over the bridge of the nose if the llama pulls back against the restraint.

Halters used on llamas resemble pony-sized horse halters. Most llama owners prefer not to leave a halter on a llama when it is free in a corral or pasture for fear a strap may catch on something and the llama be injured. Some llama owners leave a leather or fiber neck band in place to facilitate capture.

In a restricted area the llama may be slowly approached and one arm placed around the chest and neck while the opposite hand grasps the tail. This is similar to the way a sheep is handled. It may be difficult to hold a llama weighing over 150 kg in this manner unless it can be quickly pushed against a wall or fence.

A llama responds to "earing" as does a horse. Always ask the owner if this is an acceptable means of restraint. If this hold is applied correctly (gently, but firmly), the llama will not become "ear shy" or be more difficult to capture another time.

The procedure for earing a llama is similar to that for earing a horse.[5] The handler should stand on the left side of the withers, place the right arm over the neck, and work the opened palm of the hand up the neck to surround the base of the ear (Fig. 14.27). The handler should squeeze firmly, because the llama may try to pull free at this point. Frequently, the llama will jerk its head toward the left and the handler to escape pressure on the right ear, using its head as a battering

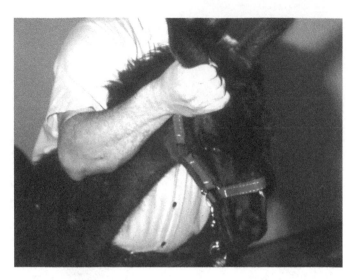

FIG. 14.27. Earing a llama.

ram. One handler suffered a broken nose when an obstreperous llama slammed its head into her face. The left ear may be grasped as well for additional restraint.

An individual llama in a herd can be restrained for quick procedures by one handler grasping the ears and another grasping the tail. Greater restraint is achieved by pushing the llama against a fence or wall. Care should be taken to assure that the llama does not put a foot or leg through a net fence or under or through a wooden fence or wall.

Optimal veterinary care of camelids requires suitable restraint facilities. Chutes and/or stocks should be provided so that work on the animals may be done safely and efficiently, such as for blood collection and diagnostic examination.[4,11] Reproductive tract examination necessitates a chute or some degree of sedation. Many homemade chutes function admirably, and commercially available chutes are also being used in the llama industry. Some provide more flexibility than others, and there is wide variation in cost and ease of construction. Several designs are illustrated in Figures 14.28 through 14.32 and described below:

Fowler Design.[4] This chute may be constructed against the solid wall of a barn, or both sides may be left free to swing on hinges at the post(s) (Figs. 14.28, 14.29, 14.30). A 10- to 15.2-cm (4- to 6-inch) post is set approximately 25.4 cm (10 in.) from the wall or another post. A sheet of plywood, 2.54 cm (1 in.) × 1.22 m (4 ft) × 2.44 m (8 ft), is hung on heavy-duty hinges from the post. This chute allows the head and neck to protrude and to be pulled forward and upward. The plywood is used to squeeze the llama against the wall.

Ebel Design.[4] This is an excellent, versatile chute that has been modified over the years and is now the most popular commercially available chute, and may be constructed of metal rather than completely of wood (Figs. 14.31, 14.32).

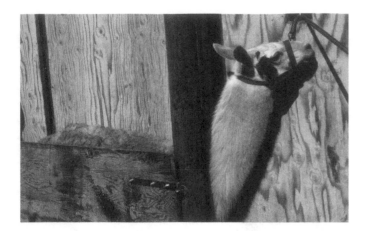

FIG. 14.28. A simple restraint chute (Fowler design).

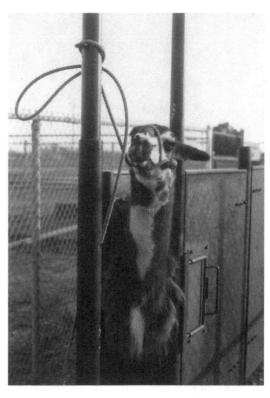

FIG. 14.30. Simple chute, free-standing, front view.

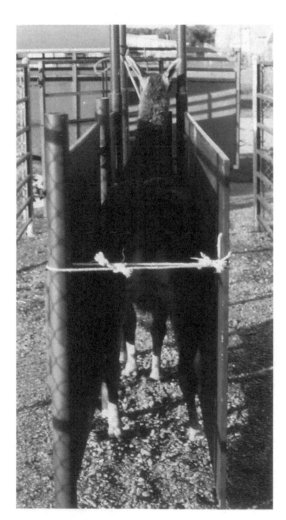

FIG. 14.29. Simple chute, free-standing, rear view.

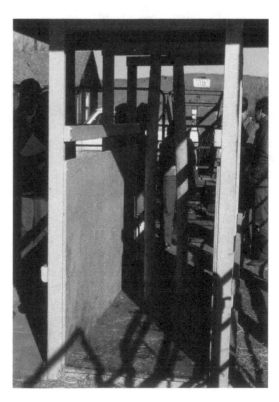

FIG. 14.31. An excellent chute (Ebel design) for restricting llama activity, rear view.

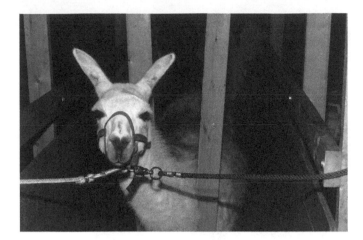

FIG. 14.32. Ebel design wooden chute, front view.

Alpacas

Alpacas are the most social of the camelids, and a herd should be handled as a unit until selected individuals are grasped. Many alpacas have been taught to accept a halter and be led, but others may be physically restrained by holding them as a sheep or a foal would be held. Place an arm around the chest and grasp the base of the tail with the other hand, as shown in Figure 14.33 or alternatively as illustrated in Figure 14.34.

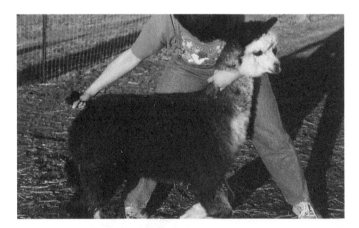

FIG. 14.33. Holding an alpaca by neck and tail.

Alpacas may be held in the kushed position by a process called chukkering. A loop of soft cotton rope with approximately 15 cm (6 in.) of slack is tied around the body just cranial to the pelvis, as shown in Figure 14.35. The handler reaches across the back and lifts the opposite rear leg and places the foot in the loop under the abdomen. Then the handler lifts the other foot and places it in the loop. This causes the alpaca to sit down, and eventually, kush (Figs. 14.36, 14.37). The front legs may be restricted by placing a loop over the flexed carpus, as with the camel. Alpacas have been carried in the cabin of a private small airplane using this form of restraint.

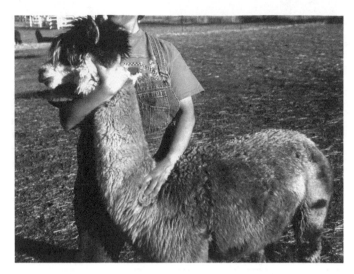

FIG. 14.34. Alternate method of holding an alpaca.

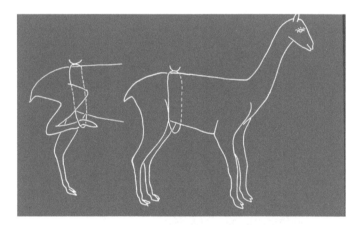

FIG. 14.35. Diagram of chukkering.

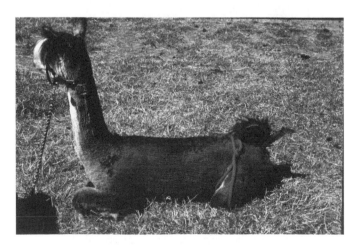

FIG. 14.36. Chukkering.

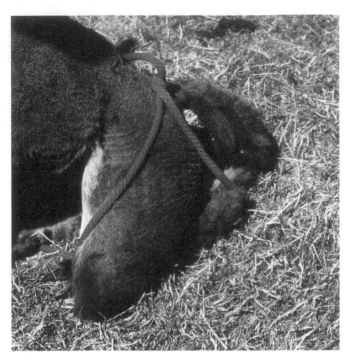

FIG. 14.37. Chukkering, details.

Guanacos and Vicuña

Guanacos respond to human handling and training as do llamas, but zoo animals usually must be handled by chemical immobilization, particularly aggressive males. Guanacos and vicuñas are more easily frightened and excited than are llamas and will fight more vigorously if unaccustomed to being haltered or placed in a chute. The author has worked with handlers of vicuñas in Peru that were roped and then grasped as one would a sheep or goat (Figs. 14.38, 14.39).

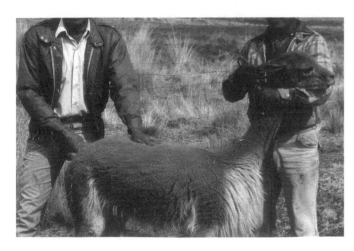

FIG. 14.38. Restraint of a vicuña.

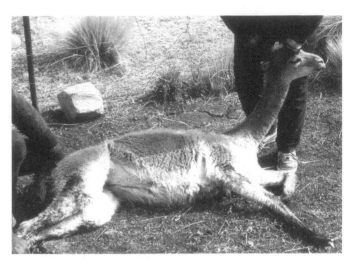

FIG. 14.39. Restraint of a vicuña in lateral recumbency.

SPECIAL HANDLING
Neonates and Juveniles

All camelid neonates may be handled by methods similar to those used for a foal or calf. One arm should be placed around the chest while the base of the tail is grasped with the opposite hand (Fig. 14.40). Prolonged pressure on the tail will cause a neonate to slump to the ground. A juvenile up to 20 kg (45 lb) may be lifted with one arm around the chest and the other behind the rear legs (Fig. 14.41). Larger animals may

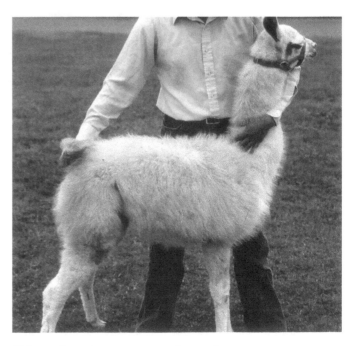

FIG. 14.40. Correct restraint of a standing juvenile llama.

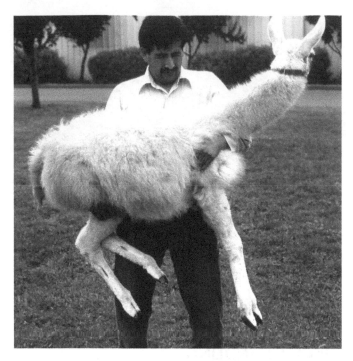

FIG. 14.41. Method of lifting a juvenile llama.

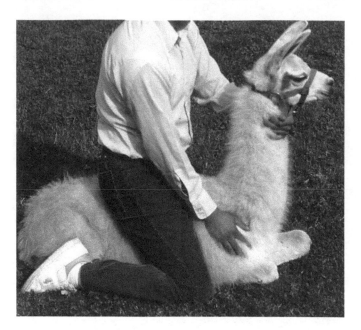

FIG. 14.43. A single person may straddle a juvenile llama.

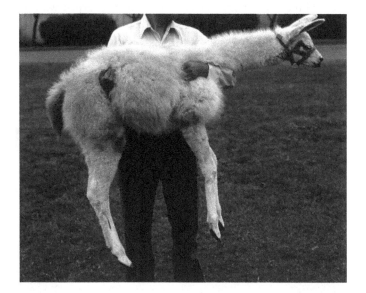

FIG. 14.42. Alternate method of lifting a juvenile llama.

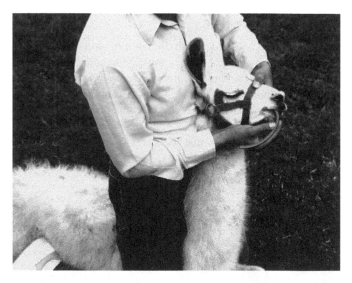

FIG. 14.44. Passing a stomach tube or collecting a blood sample.

struggle and push themselves from the handler's arms. An arm in front of the rear legs (Fig. 14.42) has a natural calming influence on the animal and reduces struggling.

A single person may pass an orogastric tube, perform venipuncture, or give an enema by straddling the neonate while it is in a kushed position. Fold the forelimbs and while the animal goes down, straddle the body and gently force the neonate into the kushed position (Figs. 14.43, 14.44). The handier does not sit on the animal, but rather straddles it. A larger cria may be placed in lateral recumbency and then allowed to rise to the kushed position underneath a straddled person.

To cast the animal into lateral recumbency, reach over the back and grasp both limbs on the approach side. Lift slightly with the knees and go down with the animal. The arm holding the forelimb should lie over the neck to hold it down. The person holding the animal must maintain the hold and therefore is unable to perform any other task (Fig. 14.45). An alternative way to cast is illustrated in Figure 14.46, but the handler should still lift slightly with the knees and go down with the animal.

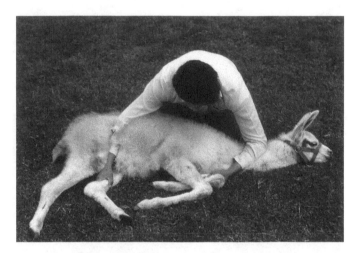

FIG. 14.45. Holding a juvenile llama in lateral recumbency by pressing on the neck while holding both lower limbs.

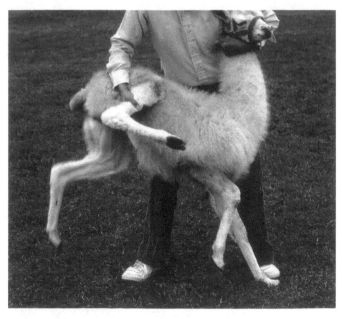

FIG. 14.46. Initial holding of a juvenile llama that will be placed in lateral recumbency. Lift the animal slightly to take it off its feet, then lower it to the ground.

Weanlings and Older Juveniles

These age groups are the most difficult to restrain for blood collection, general examination, passing an orogastric tube, or other diagnostic or therapeutic procedures. These animals are too large to force into sternal recumbency, as described for neonates, and too small to be put into one of the described chutes. Many animals of these age groups have not been halter trained and may struggle excessively if tied for the first time. Some llamas have sustained neck injuries while "fishtailing" on the end of a lead rope. The most satisfactory method is to hold the youngster with one arm under the chest and grasp the base of the tail with the other hand. Even with this mild restraint, animals of this age are inclined to jump.

It is surprising how quickly an untrained llama may learn to be led. In the beginning, it is helpful for a second person to walk behind, encouraging forward progression. A single person may encourage the llama to lead by pulling forward on a loop over the rump, a technique often used to teach a foal to lead (Fig. 14.47).

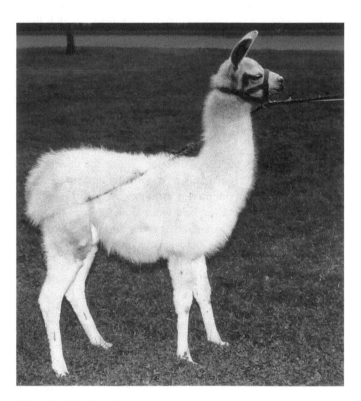

FIG. 14.47. Teaching to lead.

TRANSPORTING[1,3,9,10]

Llamas and alpacas are moved in every imaginable vehicle from Volkswagen "bugs" to Mercedes sedans; however, vans and small trucks or trailers are most commonly

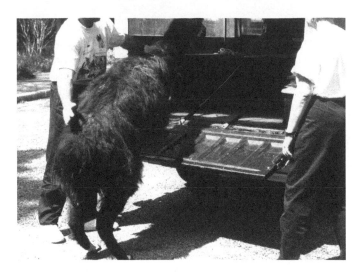

FIG. 14.48.   A llama jumping into a pickup truck.

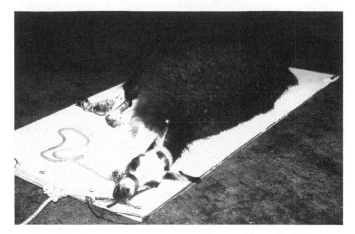

FIG. 14.49.   Plywood sheet used as a skid to move a large llama.

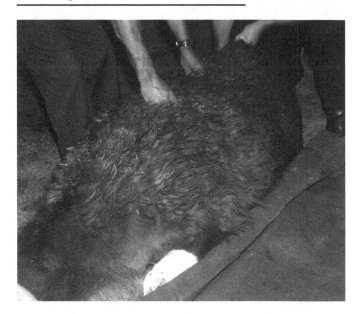

FIG. 14.50.   Using a tarp to move a llama. Roll up one half of the tarp and lay it close to the llama in sternal recumbency.

used. Llamas may be trained to jump into and out of high-level trailers and even pickup trucks (Fig. 14.48). Some caution is necessary, particularly if transporting a sick llama to a clinic, since it may not have normal coordination. Even healthy llamas have fallen as they have jumped out of a truck bed. Llamas and alpacas travel well. The majority lie down soon after the beginning of a journey and remain recumbent while moving. It is unwise to travel with the animal tied with a lead rope; some fatal accidents have occurred.

Special consideration must be given to traveling during weather extremes. In cold weather, the floor of the trailer should be heavily bedded with straw. Since the underside of the llama is relatively hairless, a recumbent llama may become chilled from cold penetrating an unprotected floor. Similar precautions must be exercised when traveling in hot, humid weather because llamas and alpacas are particularly susceptible to heat stress. It may be necessary to travel at night. It is essential to make certain there is adequate airflow. Air-conditioned vehicles or trailers are used by owners in some sections of the United States.

A mother and baby may be transported together, but it is dangerous to move llamas in large groups, unsegregated by size. Infants may easily be crushed by larger animals during a quick stop.

Camels are usually moved in horse trailers or trucks. In the Middle East, pickup trucks are often selected.

Moving a recumbent or immobilized camelid presents a challenge. South American camelids, in fact all small- to medium-sized ungulates, may be moved in one of three ways. A sheet of plywood may be used (Fig. 14.49). This procedure may also be employed when moving an adult camel, but the power required to move or lift the heavy animal necessitates a tractor or front-end bucket loader.

A plastic or canvas tarp that is longer than the length of the animal is rolled up on one side and placed next to the animal that is moved into sternal recumbency (Fig. 14.50). Do not roll the animal on its back onto the tarp; it may cause regurgitation and possibly inhalation pneumonia. Allow the animal to resume lateral recumbency so that the tarp may be unrolled beneath the animal (Fig. 14.51). Then both sides of the tarp are rolled up to form a handhold for those who will lift and carry the animal (Fig. 14.52). The number of persons required to lift and carry is determined by the size of the animal. The head and forequarters should be kept higher than the rear-quarters to avoid passive regurgitation.

The third method is to fashion a travois (Figs. 14.53 to 14.55). The equipment required includes a plastic or canvas tarp and two heavy wooden poles or pipes that are long enough to extend 0.5–1.0 m beyond the tarp.

Two people can carry an alpaca, as shown in Figure 14.56.

An improvised sling for a llama or alpaca my be constructed from a large bath towel or piece of canvas. A small stone is inserted into each corner of the towel, as illustrated in Figures 14.57 and 14.58. The cords are then tied to the sides of a chute or a transport vehicle.

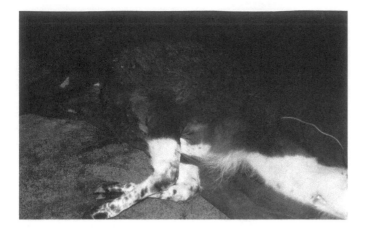

FIG. 14.51. Allow the llama to go to lateral recumbency on the tarp, then unroll the tarp under the legs.

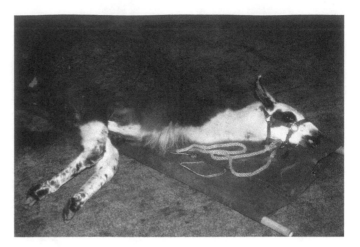

FIG. 14.54. A stretcher may be improvised by folding the tarp into thirds over two pipes or strong poles. (This is similar to the technique taught in human first aid courses.)

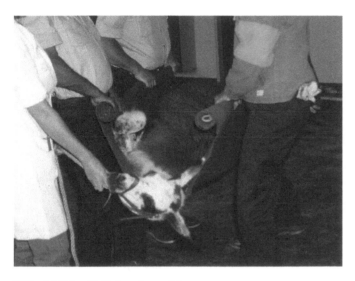

FIG. 14.52. Roll the edges of the tarp to serve as hand holds.

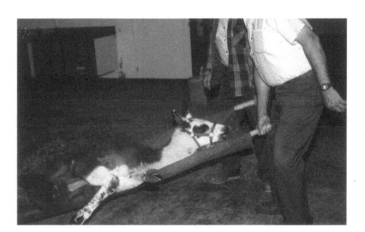

FIG. 14.55. The animal may be carried in a stretcher fashion or drug as a travois.

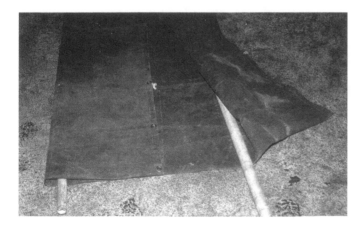

FIG. 14.53. Constructing a stretcher.

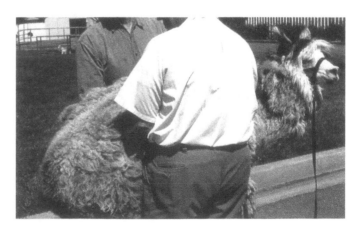

FIG. 14.56. Two-person carry.

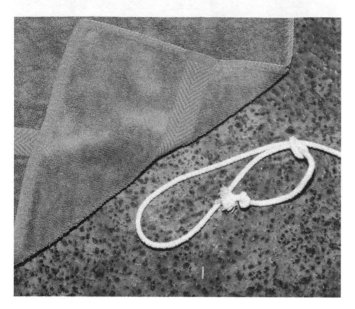

FIG. 14.57. The corner of the towel is folded over a small stone.

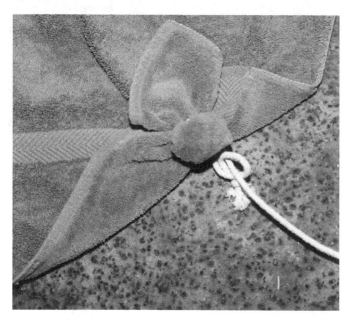

FIG. 14.58. A slip knot is used to secure a cord to each corner.

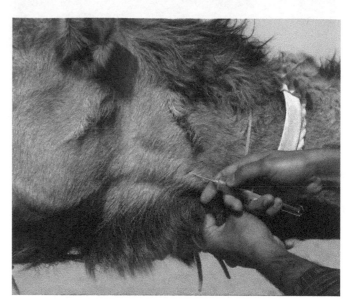

FIG. 14.59. Bleeding a camel from the jugular vein.

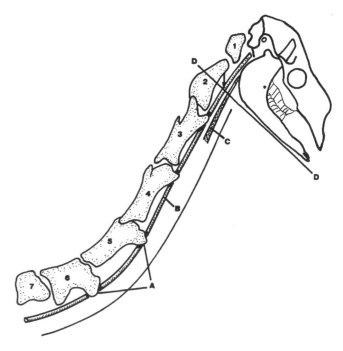

FIG. 14.60. Diagram of sites for blood sample collection in a llama. **A.** low neck site, **B.** jugular vein, **C.** tendon of sterno-mandibularis muscle, **D.** line along lower border of mandible. *Arrow*, site for high neck blood collection.

BLOOD COLLECTION

A blood sample may be obtained from the jugular vein of a camel (Fig. 14.59). In llamas and alpacas, samples may be collected from the jugular vein, ear veins, or tail vein (Figs. 14.59 to 14.65).

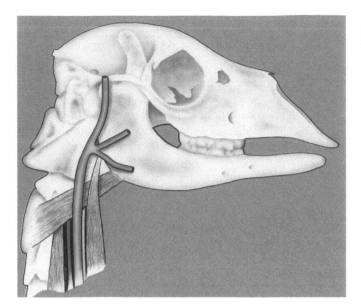

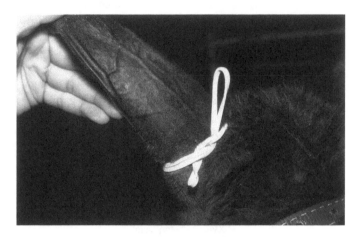

FIG. 14.61. A drawing of the relationship of the jugular vein to other structures of the neck.

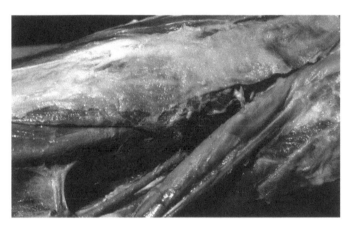

FIG. 14.62. Anatomical dissection of the neck.

FIG. 14.64. Blood vessels on the caudal surface of the ear.

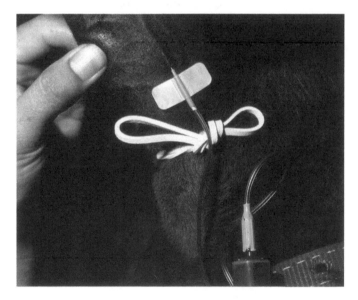

FIG. 14.65. Using a butterfly catheter to collect blood.

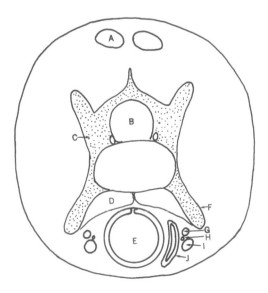

FIG. 14.63. Diagram of a cross-section of the upper neck from the front. **A.** Ligtamentum nuchae, **B.** neural canal, **C.** body of the vertebra, **D.** muscle, **E.** trachea, **F.** ventral projection of the transverse process of the vertebra, **G.** carotid artery, **H.** vagospmpathetic trucnk, **I.** jugular vein, **J.** esophagus.

177

SEDATION AND CHEMICAL IMMOBILIZATION[4,5]

The chemical restraint agents and combinations mentioned in this chapter represent those used by the author or by and experienced veterinarian with detailed knowledge of camelids. Other protocols have been used, and no claim is made for including all possible drugs and combinations. For more detailed information, particularly for anesthesia, consult Mama.[11]

A number of drugs or drug combinations are currently being used to quiet excitable camelids or immobilize fractious animals (Table 14.1). If possible, camelids should be fasted 24–36 hours before being chemically immobilized to minimize the risk of passive regurgitation and inhalation of ingesta. Animals should be kept in sternal recumbency if possible.

The clinical signs of xylazine sedation include the drooping of the lower lips, salivation, relaxation of the eyelids, and lacrimation.

Chemical immobilization is often used to immobilize a camelid prior to inhalation general anesthesia. See Chapter 20, Chemical Agents, for the procedure for endotracheal intubation in camelids. Figures 14.66 and 14.67 illustrate inserting a catheter into the trachea and threading an endotracheal

Table 14.1. Chemical restraint agents for camelidae[4,5]

Agent	Standing sedation (mg/kg)	Immobilization (mg/kg)*·**
Xylazine	0.1–0.2 IV	Not suitable for immobilization by itself
Butorphanol	0.02–0.1 IV	
Detomidine	0.02	
Diazepam	0.1–0.5	
Xylazine/butorphanol	0.1/0.05–0.1	
Xylazine/ketamine		0.4/5.0 IM
		0.25/3.0–5.0 IV
Ketamine/xylazine/butorphanol		2.0–3.0/0.1/0.05–0.1
Ketamine/diazepam		5.0–8.0/0.2–0.3 IM
		3.5–5.0/0.1–0.2 IV
Ketamine/medetomidine		2.0–4.0/0.06–0.08
Ketamine/detomidine		2.0–4.0/0.02–0.04
Tiletamine/zolazepam		4.0–6.0, free-ranging guanaco
		2.0–3.0 captive llama

* Keep the animal sternal, if possible, to avoid regurgitation and inhalation.
** For reversal agents, see Chapter 20, Chemical Restraint.

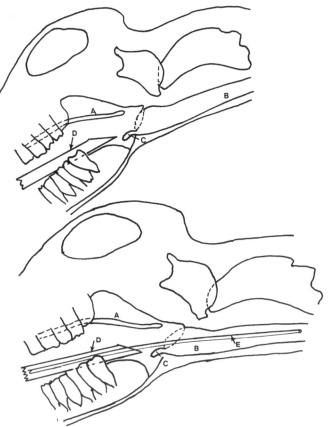

FIG. 14.66. Visualizing the glottis, top. Inserting a catheter into the trachea, bottom. **A.** Elongated soft palate, **B.** trachea, **C.** epiglottal cartilage, **D.** blade of the laryngoscope, **E.** catheter.

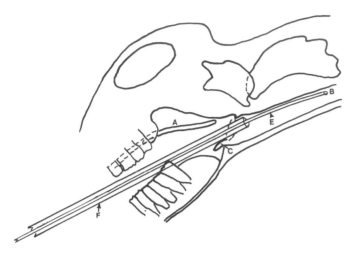

FIG. 14.67. Threading an endotracheal tube over the catheter. **A.** Elongated soft palate, **B.** trachea, **C.** epiglottal cartilage, **D.** endotracheal tube, **E.** catheter.

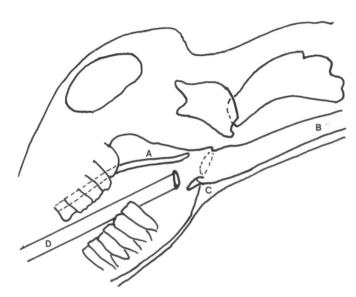

FIG. 14.68. Using a plastic tube as the laryngoscope **A.** Elongated soft palate, **B.** trachea, **C.** epiglottal cartilage, **D.** Plastic tube used for a laryngoscope.

tube over the catheter. Figure 14.68 illustrates using a plastic tube as a laryngoscope.

REFERENCES

1. Anonymous. 2007. Live Animal Regulations, 34th Ed., International Air Transport Association, 2000 Peel St., Montreal, Quebec, CANADA, H3A 2R4. pp. 102–03. Telephone +1 (514) 844 6311.
2. Bravo, P.W., and Fowler, M.E. 2001. Order Artiodactyla, Family Camelidae. In: Fowler, M.E., and Cubas, Z.S. 2001. Biology, Medicine and Surgery of South American Wild Animals. Ames, Iowa State University Press, pp. 392–401.
3. Faiks, J., and Faiks, J. 1993. Flying alpacas. Alpacas, Summer pp. 18–21.
4. Fowler, M.E. 1998. Anesthesia. In: Fowler, M.E., Medicine and Surgery of South American Camelids, 2nd Ed. Ames, Iowa State University Press, pp. 91–97.
5. Fowler, M.E. 2003. Camelidae. In: Fowler, M.E., and Miller, R.E., Eds. Zoo and Wild Animal Medicine. 5th Ed. St. Louis, Saunders/Elsevier. pp. 614–15.
6. Fowler, M.E. 2008. Behavioral clues for detection of illness in wild animals: Models in camelids and elephants. In: Fowler, M.E., and Miller, R.E. 2007. Zoo and Wild Animal Medicine, Current Therapy, 6th Ed. St. Louis, Saunders/Elsevier, pp. 33–59.
7. Franklin, W.L. 1982. Llama language. Llama World 1(2):6–11.
8. Franklin, W.L., and Johnson, W.E. 1994. Hand capture of newborn open-habitat ungulates: the South American guanaco. Wildlife Society Bulletin 22(2):253–59.
9. Greth-Peto, F. 1990. A comprehensive look at the transportation industry. Llamas 4(3):93–96.
10. Mallon, J. 1991. Headin' down the road. Llamas 5(7):109–11.
11. Mama, K.R. 2007. Camelids. In: West, G., Heard, D., and Caulkett, N. 2007. Ames, Iowa, Blackwell Publishing, pp. 159–96.
12. Johnson, L. 1987. Llama restraining chutes. Llamas 11(5):30–32.
13. McGee, M. 1994. Llama handling and training. In: Johnson, L.W., Ed. Update on Llama Medicine, Veterinary Clinics of North America, Food Animal Section 10(2):421–34.
14. McGee, M. 1992. The TTEAM approach to herd management (a Video tape). Dundee, NY, Zephyr Farm and Videosyncracies.
15. McGee, M. 1992. Llama Handling and Training—the TTEAM approach. Dundee, NY, Zephyr Farm Press.
16. Pollard, J.C., and Littlejohn, R.P. 1995. Effects of social isolation and restraint on heart rate and behavior of alpacas. Applied Animal Behaviour Science 45(1/2):165–74.
17. Ramadan, R.O. 1994. Sedation and general anesthesia. In: Ramadan, R.O. 1994. Surgery and Radiology of the Dromedary Camel, Saudi Arabia, Al-Jawad Printing Press, pp. 48–59.

CHAPTER 15

Dogs

CLASSIFICATION

Order Carnivora
    Family Canidae: dog

Possibly the dog has been domesticated longer than any other animal.[3] We have manipulated the gene pool of this species until greater physical and behavioral variations exist from breed to breed than in any other species of animal (Table 15.1). The male dog is called a dog, the female is called a bitch, and the newborn and young are called a pup or puppy.

TABLE 15.1. Weights of selected breeds of dogs

Breed	Male (kg)	Male (lb)	Female (kg)	Female (lb)
Toy				
Pekingese	3.2–5	7–11	3.6–5.4	8–12
Toy poodle	<2.3	<5	<2.3	<5
Pug	6.3–8.2	14–18	6.3–8.2	14–18
Chihuahua	<2.3	<5	<2.3	<5
Pomeranian	1.8–3.2	4–7	1.4–2.7	3–6
Dachshund	5	11	5	11
Medium				
German shorthair pointer	25–32	55–70	23–30	50–65
Springer spaniel	22–25	49–55	20–23	45–50
Afghan	27	60	23	50
Labrador retriever	27–34	60–75	25–32	55–70
Greyhound	30–32	65–70	27–32	60–70
German shepherd	36–57	80–125	<45	<100
Pointer	25–34	55–75	20–30	45–65
Giant				
Irish wolfhound	>54	>120	48	>105
St. Bernard	68–90	150–200	<80	<175
Great Pyrenees	45–57	100–125	40–52	90–115
Great Dane	>54	>120	45	>100

DANGER POTENTIAL

A dog's only weapons are its large canine teeth and to a lesser extent the toenails. Scratches from a dog are usually not serious, but a bite from a large Alsatian or St. Bernard can both disfigure and disable. Every precaution should be taken to prevent injury. Approach any strange dog with caution.

If a dog attacks, protect the face with a hand or an arm. Some dogs have trained offense responses (guard dogs). These animals should be handled only by competent personnel. Certain breeds are thought to be more aggressive, but training is the most important factor in the behavior of these dogs.

BEHAVIORAL CHARACTERISTICS

The behavior of a dog is determined by breed, training, previous disagreeable experiences, and degree of human association.

Canids have been studied in depth by animal behaviorists; numerous texts elucidate various aspects of canine behavior.[4,5] Adverse behavioral patterns usually develop as the result of abuse or lack of understanding on the part of a dog owner.

In this book dogs are classified in the following categories for restraint purposes:

1. The stray or free-roaming dog that has little association with people except, perhaps, when fed. If owned, the owner may be afraid of the dog. These dogs must be handled as if they are wild canids because they are liable to bite with the slightest provocation.
2. The well-cared-for pet or working dog. Fortunately most dogs are in this category. They are docile and respond to a low-pitched soothing voice and slow, deliberate handling.
3. The extremely nervous, frightened dog. This dog can be recognized by an anxious expression, rapid movements of the head, and constant pricking of the ears in response to every sound or movement. The head will likely be ducked and the animal may cower in a corner. The lips may be pulled back in a grimace. These animals may also be boisterous and attempt to nip at the handler. Above all, they can be expected to bite in response to almost any type of approach. All these signs telegraph "beware!" to a perceptive handler.

   There is little question that there are neurotic and even psychotic dogs that are unpredictable, to say the least.
4. The vicious, aggressive dog. Many of these dogs are large, are capable of inflicting serious injury, and will bite with little or no provocation. These dogs do not always exhibit aggressiveness in an obvious manner, but signs of potential viciousness can be seen. The head is held low, and these dogs will not look directly at you. They may attack without warning.

Rough handling may provoke adverse responses in the most amiable of dogs. Gentleness is wisest when dealing with any dog. Confidence and calmness are necessary for successful control.

It should be recognized that the temperament of a dog may change drastically when it is sick or injured. Such a dog is far more apt to bite than a healthy dog.

Kennel owners and others who must handle a variety of dogs day in and day out learn to understand dog behavior. They become adept at performing many procedures with no more restraint than talking to and soothing a dog into a relaxed state. The casual or infrequent dog handler will find it more difficult to carry out manipulative procedures and may have to resort to more stringent restraint practices.

A technique used by some veterinarians is to stand between the client or owner and the dog during an examination. The dog is not as likely to try to move away, but will tend to attempt to get closer to the owner and thus be moving toward the veterinarian.

Keep in mind the fact that dog owners often resent anyone who handles an animal in what appears to them a rough manner, but many owners are incapable of holding a pet in such a manner that it cannot bite the person attempting to examine or treat it. Furthermore, some pet owners cannot be led to believe that a usually docile pet may respond to a strange or frightening situation by biting someone. Pet owners are seldom satisfactory assistants to the handler. A veterinarian may be liable if a dog bites its owner during an examination.

PHYSICAL RESTRAINT[1,6,7]

The leash is an important device. The leather and chain leashes used by owners when they walk their dogs are rarely suitable for restraint. The light leather strap can be bitten through by a frightened or angry dog, and the swivel attachments are usually flimsy.

Collars vary greatly in design. Their function is to carry identification plates or tags, kill fleas, or look pretty (Fig. 15.1). It is virtually impossible to place a collar tightly enough around the neck to preclude a determined dog from slipping out of it. A nylon cord 3 mm (1/8 in.) in diameter may serve both as a collar and a leash.

The collar and leash are used in many restraint situations. If a small dog is cowering in the back of a cage, a loop tossed over its head may be used to pull the dog off balance and to hold the head away from the handler while the dog is grasped. The aggressive, vicious dog may be subdued to administer a sedative by threading the leash through an eye bolt embedded in the wall and pulling the head up tight. Another person grabs the tail or a hind leg and makes a quick intramuscular injection. Do not wrap the leash around a table or chair leg; a medium-sized or large dog can easily upset a table. If an eye bolt is not available, the leash may be slipped through a partially opened door, which is then lightly closed on the leash (Fig. 15.2). The dog is pulled up tightly to the door, which is

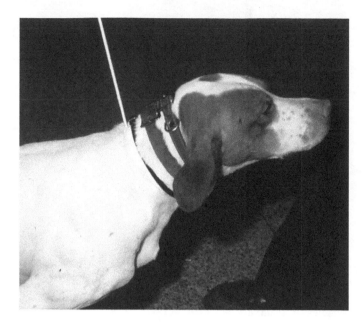

FIG. 15.1.   Various collars for dogs.

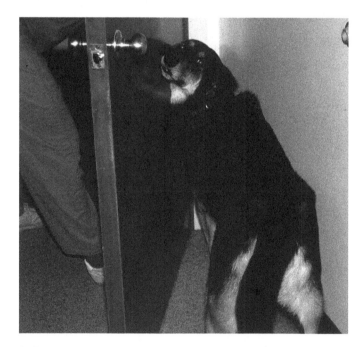

FIG. 15.2.   Leash threaded through a hinged door to safely administer a sedative to a vicious or aggressive dog.

held shut by the handler outside the door while the second person administers the sedative. Intravenous injections into the saphenous vein can be made with the dog held in this position.

Small dogs may be fitted with leather harnesses that surround both neck and thorax. While a harness is effective for an owner taking a dog for a walk, it is not a good restraint device because there is no control of the head.

Puppies of any breed may be handled with ease. Place one hand under the abdomen and chest to give support). In almost all instances puppies respond quietly, offering no resistance. If the puppy squirms to free itself, place a hand over its back and bring it in close to your body for additional comfort and support.

Always talk to a dog as you approach it to pick it up. Approach from the side rather than directly from the front. Pick up small and middle-sized adult dogs as you would a puppy (Fig. 15.3). The leash may be helpful if an assistant can pull the head away from the lifter.

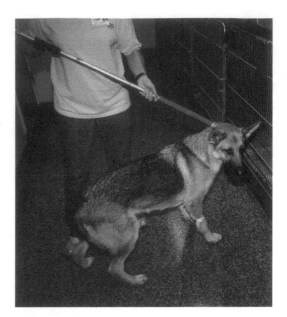

FIG. 15.4. Snare used to remove a dangerous dog from a cage.

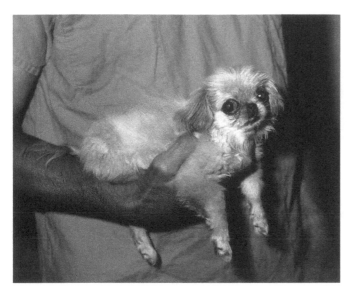

FIG. 15.3. Proper way to lift and carry a puppy or small dog.

Removal of a dog from a cage is an art. The cage is its familiar territory, even if only temporarily. One should not take chances with a vicious dog. Snare or net the dog to pull it out of the cage, where a muzzle may be applied or a sedative given (Fig. 15.4).

The frightened or nervous dog is another matter. One should distract or confuse the dog to divert its intentions to bite. Do not reach out with a hand on first approach. Sit down close to the dog. The size of your body may intimidate it. You may then be able to soothe and calm the dog by speaking to it. Some handlers approach a small, nervous dog without looking directly at it. This confuses the dog. Another technique is to use the leash as described previously. One may also apply a muzzle or place a towel over the dog to partially blind it (Fig. 15.5).

To lift a medium-sized to large dog from the floor, squat next to the dog and place one arm around the dog's chest in front of the forelimbs. The other arm is placed under the abdomen. Pull the dog toward your body to shift the weight nearer to your legs. Then stand up (Fig. 15.6). If the dog struggles, pull it tightly against your chest or set the animal down on a table (Fig. 15.7). Reverse the process when releasing the dog; do not drop it or let it jump from the table. If

there is abdominal trauma or distention of the abdomen for any reason, it is better to lift from behind the rear limbs, instead of against the abdomen. The dog may be held in lateral recumbency as illustrated in Figure 15.8.

Vicious dogs cannot be handled in this manner lest the handler be bitten. The owner or the customary handler of the animal may be able to muzzle it. If not, leash the animal before attempting to place the muzzle. A muzzle can be constructed from a piece of 5-cm (2-in.) gauze bandage or a small cord. Form a loop large enough to drape over the mouth of the animal, keeping the hand some distance away (Figs. 15.9, 15.10). The leash prevents the dog from backing away when approached.

Dogs that are muzzled repeatedly may learn the trick of blowing on the light gauze loop as one attempts to place it over the jaws. Counter this by wetting the gauze. Additional weight, to keep the loop open, may be produced by tying a knot in the gauze and fashioning the loop to place the knot at the bottom of the loop.

With the muzzle properly in place, the dog cannot bite. Snug the knot sufficiently tight to preclude partial opening of the mouth. If the loop is anchored too close to the nostrils, the dog may paw the loop off or the nostrils may be clamped shut. Tie the muzzle at the back of the neck with a quick-release bowknot. A dog may struggle to the point of collapse from hypoxia or it may vomit. Both necessitate prompt release from a muzzle.

Remember that cooling mechanisms of the canid species involve panting and lolling of the tongue. Muzzling prevents both. Therefore do not work with a muzzled dog in a hot environment for prolonged periods.

Leather muzzles available commercially should be fitted precisely to an individual dog (Fig. 15.11). In most cases,

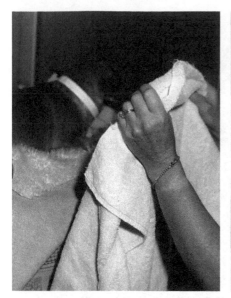

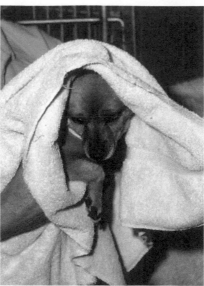

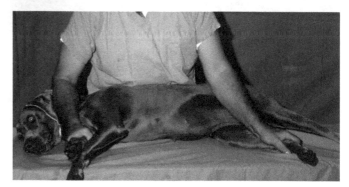

FIG. 15.5. Nervous or frightened dog may be calmed by placing a towel over it.

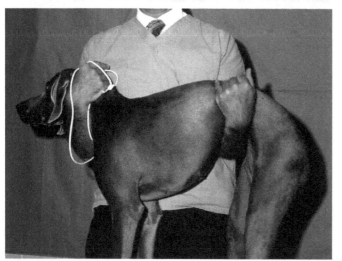

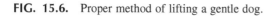

FIG. 15.6. Proper method of lifting a gentle dog.

FIG. 15.8. Holding a dog in lateral recumbency.

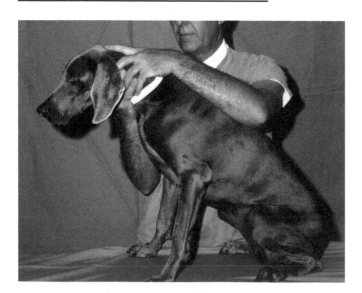

FIG. 15.7. Dog restrained on a table.

there is enough play in the muzzle to allow partial opening of the mouth, and thus pinch biting. The wire muzzles used on racing greyhounds are suitable.

If a muzzle is unavailable and the manipulative procedure is short, the dog can be hand muzzled. Long-nosed breeds of dogs are easily handled in this manner. Brachycephalic or pug-nosed breeds are more difficult to grasp. Place the thumb over the bridge of the nose with the hand cupped around the lower jaw (Fig. 15.12, left). The middle finger is flexed and inserted between the rami of the mandible (Fig. 15.12, right). With the hand firmly placed, the finger between the rami forms an additional securing lock that prevents the head from pulling free. If this technique is prolonged or harshly administered, the dog may resist as though it were being strangled. Use it judiciously.

To prevent the dog with a short muzzle from biting, surround the whole head with the hands. Be cautious not to cover the nares and inhibit breathing.

The dog's mouth can be easily opened for examination or medication. Place a hand over the bridge of the nose and

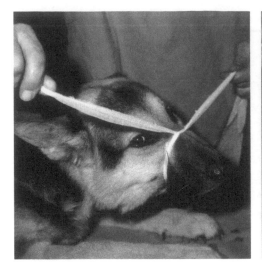
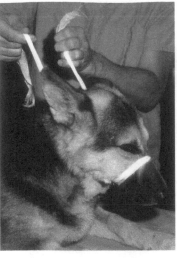

FIG. 15.9. Muzzling a dog with gauze bandage.

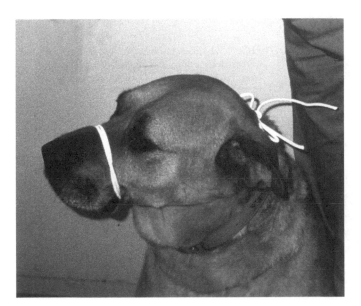

FIG. 15.10. Completed muzzle.

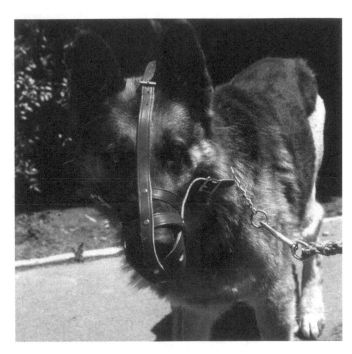

FIG. 15.11. Leather muzzle on a dog.

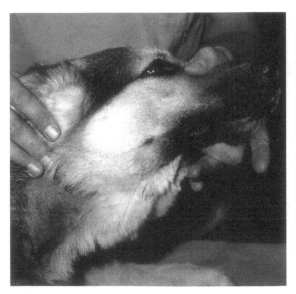
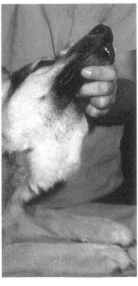

FIG. 15.12. Hand-muzzle control: Thumb over bridge of the nose and fingers beneath the jaw, left. Finger inserted between rami of the mandible, right.

185

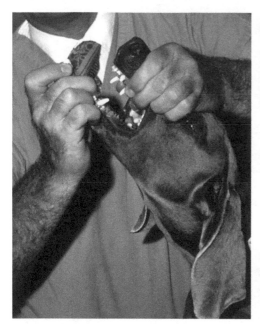

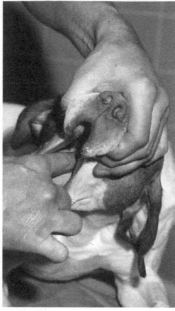

FIG. 15.13. Administering tablet medication correctly to a dog, left. Improper method of examining the mouth or pilling, right.

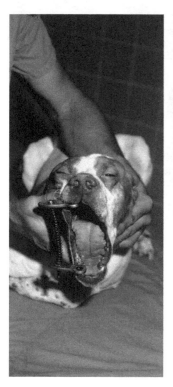

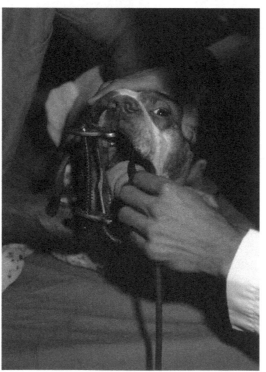

FIG. 15.14. Canine mouth speculum in place for oral examination and insertion of a stomach tube.

pull the upper lip upward (Fig. 15.13). The head should be tilted up, which minimizes the dog's ability to bite. The other hand pulls the lower jaw open. If a tablet or capsule is to be given, it can be dropped at the base of the tongue. Gravity will aid in proper placement. A quick thrust with the index finger will push the tablet over the tongue and initiates the swallowing reflex. Pull the fingers out quickly and release the hold on the jaws. If the dog swallows the tablet, the tongue will flick out between the teeth and lips as a flag that the

mission is accomplished. If this does not occur, rest assured that the tablet will be spit out later.

A word of caution. Do not press the dog's lips over its teeth with your fingers. The dog may bite its own lips and your fingers at the same time. Keep your fingers free of those crushing molars.

If it is necessary to keep the mouth open for an extended period, a special dental speculum (Fig. 15.14) or dowel speculum (Fig. 15.15) may be used. If a dental speculum is used

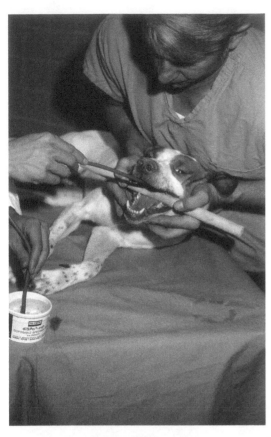

FIG. 15.15. Dowel speculum holding the mouth open for passage of a stomach tube.

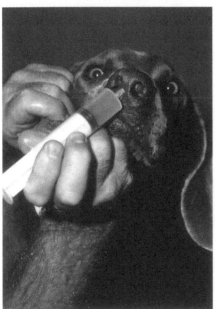 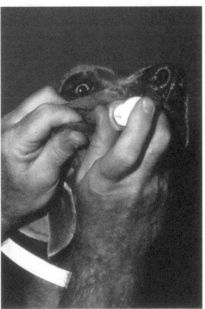

FIG. 15.16. Administering liquid medication to a dog: Form a pouch with the lips, right. Deposit small amount and wait for tongue to flick. If dog will not swallow, place a drop on the nose, left.

on an un-sedated dog, the speculum may pop out of the mouth and hit the handlers or bystanders.

Liquid medication may be given by depositing the fluid inside the lips at the commissure of the mouth (Fig. 15.16. Tilt the head back slightly and form a pouch with the cheek. Deposit a small quantity of the medication to initiate licking and swallowing. This is signaled by the tongue flicking out of the mouth. If the dog fails to swallow, deposit some of the medication on the tip of the nose (Fig. 15.16). Only

after the dog is swallowing should a large quantity be deposited.

Elizabethan collars prevent self-mutilation (Fig. 15.17). These can be placed on the animal in either normal or reverse position. Similar collars can be improvised from sheets of plastic, large bottles, or buckets.

Blood samples may be obtained from the cephalic vein (Figs. 15.18, 15.19), the jugular vein (Figs. 15.20, 15.21), or the saphenous vein.

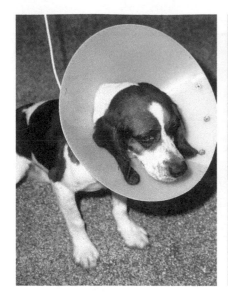 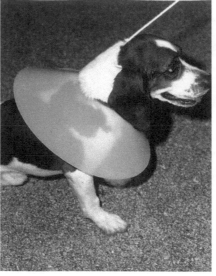

FIG. 15.17. Elizabethan collars.

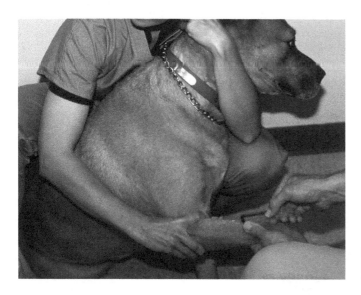

FIG. 15.18. Method for holding a dog for cephalic intravenous injections.

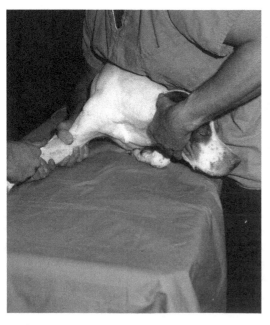

FIG. 15.19. Alternate method of holding for cephalic venipuncture.

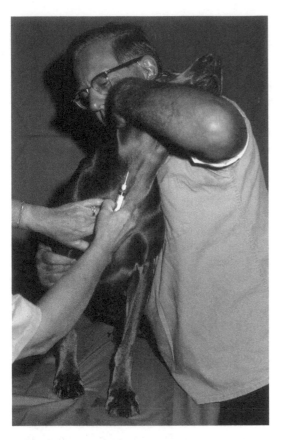

FIG. 15.20. Dog being restrained for collecting sample from the jugular vein.

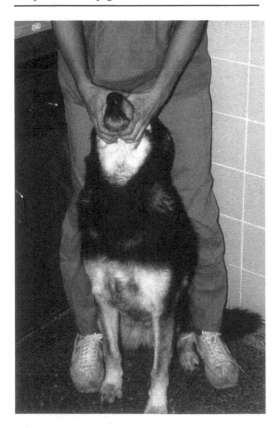

FIG. 15.21. An alternate method of holding a large dog for jugular venipuncture.

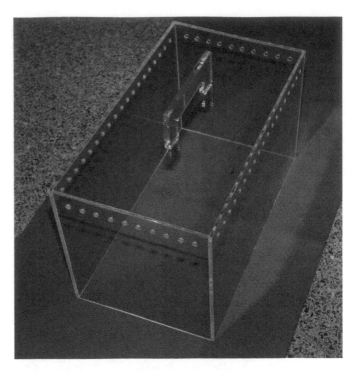

FIG. 15.22. A plastic open-ended box to restrict movement of a small dog.

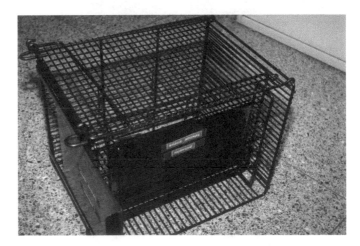

FIG. 15.23. Squeeze cage for a small dog or cat.

Miscellaneous Procedures

A clear plastic box with no bottom and a handle on top may be used to contain a small dog in an area of the cage while cleaning (Fig. 15.22). Small, portable squeeze cages are also available commercially (Fig. 15.23). Plastic shields may be constructed to fend off an aggressive dog (Fig. 15.24).

Dogs vary tremendously in size. Accurate weight determination is necessary before medications are administered. Small dogs may be held and weighed on a bathroom scale (subtract your own weight). Larger dogs must be placed on a platform scale. Small to medium-sized dogs can be suspended and weighed from a hanging scale (Fig. 15.25).

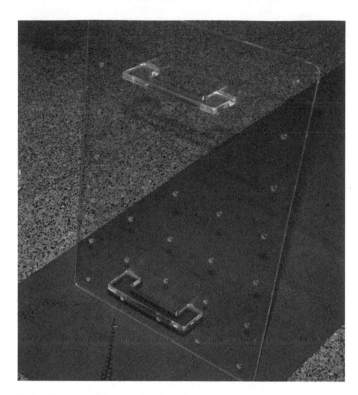

FIG. 15.24.   Shield for fending of an aggressive dog.

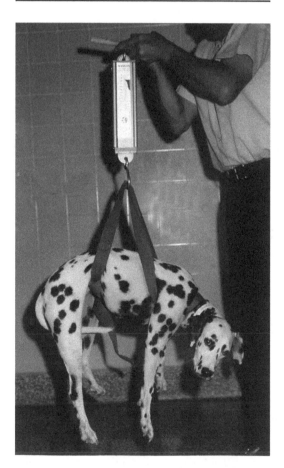

FIG. 15.25.   Weighing a dog with a hanging scale.

Cradles of various types are used to support the dog or to keep it in different positions to facilitate surgical procedures.

Unfortunately dogs are frequently traumatized in automobile accidents. Be cautious when attempting to render first aid. The most docile dog is liable to bite when dazed or in shock. Try to leash the dog first, perhaps with a belt. A muzzle can be improvised from a necktie or shoelace. Try to ease the dog onto a coat or blanket to lift the dog into a vehicle.

TRANSPORT

Dogs are usually amenable to any type of transport. They customarily ride free in automobiles but must be confined in carrying crates for air shipment. Some dogs are susceptible to motion sickness. Acepromazine hydrochloride (0.4 mg/kg) is an appropriate preventive medication to be given prior to shipment.

CHEMICAL RESTRAINT

The chemical restraint agents and combinations mentioned in this chapter represent those used by an experienced veterinarian with detailed knowledge of dogs (Table 15.2). Other protocols have been used, and no claim is made for including all possible drugs and combinations. For more detailed information, particularly for anesthesia, consult Bednarski[2] or Tranquilli et al.[8]

TABLE 15.2.   Chemical restraint agents used for sedation and immobilization in dogs

Agent	Sedation dose (mg/kg)	Immobilization dose (mg/kg)
Acepromazine	0.05–0.22	
Butorphanol	0.05 IV	
	0.4 SC, IM	
Midazolam	0.05–0.1, usually combined with opioid	
Diazepam	0.2–0.5, usually combined with opioid	
Ketamine/Xylazine		6.6–10.0/1.25–2.0
Ketamine/medetomidine		2.5/0.08
Ketamine/acepromazine		10.0/0.1
Tiletamine/zolazepam (Telazol)		3.0–5.0

Many tranquilizers are available to quiet the nervous or vicious dog. Each clinician establishes a usage pattern suitable to the type of dogs most often seen (Table 15.2). When immobilization or induction for inhalation anesthesia is indicated, drug combinations are usually recommended to decrease the dosage of each agent and to minimize untoward actions (Table 15.2). Reversal agents are listed in Table 15.3.

An anesthesia chamber, as shown in Figure 15.26, is used. Once anesthetized, the dog is secured to an operating table as illustrated in Figure 15.27. Short pieces of sash cord are placed over the limb above the knee and above the hock if possible. A half hitch placed over the limb below the loop

TABLE 15.3. **Reversal agents used for immobilization of dogs**

Reversal Agent	Immobilizing Agent	Dosage (mg/kg), IV
Yohimbine	Xylazine	0.1
Atipamezole	Xylazine, medetomidine	0.04–0.5
Flumazenil	Diazepam, midazolam, zolazepam	0.2–3.0

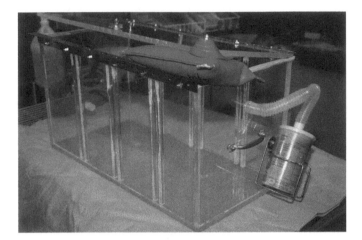

FIG. 15.26. Anesthetic chamber for a small animal.

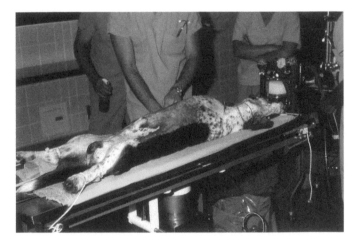

FIG. 15.27. Dog restrained preparatory to abdominal surgery.

secures the animal. This technique does not exert a tourniquet effect on the limb. Stretch the legs into the position desired. Keep in mind that an anesthetized animal may be twisted into positions jeopardizing circulation of the limb or which overstrain joints and ligaments. Make the stretching as comfortable as possible. Deep-bodied animals may be secured more easily by placing sand bags on either side to prevent them from twisting over.

The stray or feral dog presents a difficult handling problem. Animal control personnel are faced with a dilemma. They may not be able to approach such dogs closely enough to net them, yet chemical restraint drugs are either unsafe or are restricted to use by licensed veterinarians or trained animal handlers only. Popular literature and television have promulgated the idea that all one needs to do is point a tranquilizer gun at an animal and it is safely in hand. This is not true. Two suitable drugs are now available for remote restraint: xylazine hydrochloride (2.2 mg/kg) and a combination of tiletamine hydrochloride and zolazepam (Telazol) (5.0–10.0 mg/kg). Accurate weight estimation is essential for safe usage of these drugs. Both are restricted to use only by licensed veterinarians.

I recommend that animal control program administrators limit the usage of chemical restraint to trained key personnel. These individuals could use one of the above drugs under the supervision of or in consultation with a veterinarian. Training programs in the use of these drugs are not currently readily available but may be set up by veterinary schools, professional associations, or humane societies.

REFERENCES

1. Anderson, R.S., and Edney, A.T.B., Eds. 1991. Practical Animal Handling, 1st ed. Oxford, U.K. Pergamon Press, 198 pages.
2. Bednarski, R.M. 1996. Dogs and cats. In: Thurmon, J.C., Tranquilli, W.J., and Benson, G.J., Eds. 1996. Lumb and Jones' Veterinary Anesthesia. 3rd Ed. Philadelphia, Lippincott Williams and Wilkens, pp. 591–596.
3. Dangerfield, S., and Howell, E., Eds. 1971. The International Encyclopedia of Dogs. New York, McGraw-Hill.
4. Fox, M.W. 1965. Canine Behavior. Springfield, Ill.: Charles C. Thomas.
5. Fox, M.W., Ed. 1968. Abnormal Behavior in Animals. Philadelphia, W. B. Saunders.
6. Sheldon, C.C., Sonsthagen, T., and Topel, J.A. 2006. St. Louis, Mosby/Elsevier, 239 pages.
7. Sonsthagen, T.F. 1991. Restraint of Domestic Animals. Goleta, California, American Veterinary Publications, 149 pages.
8. Tranquilli, W.J., Thurman, J.C., and Grimm, K.A., Eds. 2007. Lumb and Jones' Veterinary Anesthesia and Analgesia, 4th Ed. Ames, Iowa, Wiley-Blackwell Publishing.

C H A P T E R 1 6

Cats

CLASSIFICATION

Order Carnivora
    Family Felidae: cat

Although domesticated for thousands of years, the cat has never completely subjected itself to people.[5] Despite many examples of affectionate relationships between persons and cats, in most instances the cat retains a certain aloofness. Weights and names of gender are listed in Table 16.1.

TABLE 16.1. Weights and names of gender of cats

	Name	Weight
Adult male	Tom	Average: 3.0 kg
		Range: 1.4–5.4 kg
Adult female	Queen	Average: 2.6 kg
		Range: 1.4–3.6 kg
Newborn	Kitten	100.0 gm
Castrated male	Male	May weigh >9.0 kg

DANGER POTENTIAL

Of all domestic animals, the cat is one of the most difficult to handle. The cat defends itself by biting and clawing. Cats are well equipped with needle sharp canine teeth capable of inflicting serious wounds; retractable claws become formidable weapons in an excited and/or angry cat. Both forefeet and hind feet must be reckoned with when restraining a cat.

ANATOMY, PHYSIOLOGY, AND BEHAVIOR

Cats are agile and seldom tolerate manipulation without response. They are individualistic and vary widely in response to handling. Cats tend to be less amenable to manipulation than dogs. Behaviorally, they are less inclined than dogs to develop extremely close relationships with their owners.

Cats often exhibit territorial characteristics. Territoriality may cause a cat to resent being picked up from its own cage as an invasion of territory. The same animal, in strange surroundings, may not be aggressive when approached.

Most domestic cats will allow handling by the owner and usually will permit a stranger to approach if quietly reassured that no danger is present. To reassure a cat, talk soothingly but confidently to the animal. Some handlers blow gently into the cat's face or stroke it beneath the chin or beside the ears. Some cats enjoy a firm stroke over the back, always moving

from head to tail. Recognize that each cat is an individual and that it will take some time before a cat will accept handling by a new person. Some cats will never tolerate manipulation by a stranger. The handler must work quickly. A cat will tolerate manipulation just so long. When the cat's patience is exhausted, it is virtually impossible to proceed. Use as mild restraint as possible.

Cats are unpredictable, demonstrating quicksilver changes in behavior. They are sometimes rather timid and apprehensive and may show evidence of depression when placed in strange situations such as a new cage or unusual surroundings. The depressed state may quickly give way to a hostile state if the animal is roughly handled at this point. A ferocious cat, confined in a strange cage for several hours, may become more docile, especially if it can be convinced that ferociousness will not be rewarded in an acceptable manner. Even when apparently docile, if such an animal is picked up and subjected to painful manipulations, it may revert to aggressive hostility. If the manipulation is particularly unpleasant, the animal's behavior may rapidly deteriorate into a fit of rage, and one must cope with a snarling, clawing, biting buzz saw. In such a fracas, attempts to pin or control the animal usually end with an injured cat, the result of application of excessive pressure. It is wise to back off from an enraged cat, let the animal relax until it is calm, and begin anew with a less stressful method of restraint.

Cats with impaired breathing often resist handling, and struggling may compound the oxygen deficit.

PHYSICAL RESTRAINT[1,6,7]

Neophyte cat handlers often apply more force than is necessary, causing the cat to resist. If a cat struggles, relaxing the grip may end resistance.

When a cat in a cage is approached, it quickly gives evidence as to whether or not it is friendly. An unfriendly cat hisses and spits at the person nearing the cage. If closer contact is attempted, the cat will strike out with a paw or attempt to bite an encroaching hand. The person must then either assume the cat is bluffing and risk picking it up or, preferably, take steps to divert the cat's attention while capturing it.

A cat permitted to come out of a cage into strange surroundings (strange territory) is usually intimidated and seldom exhibits hostile behavior. Often, if such a cat is approached in a calm manner, restraint will not provoke undesirable behavior.

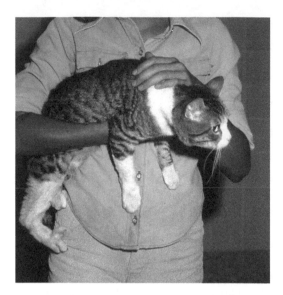

FIG. 16.1.   Method for carrying a gentle cat.

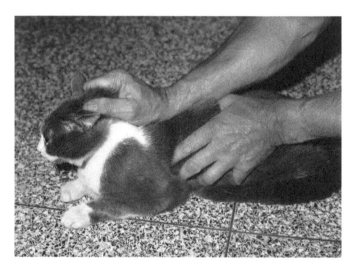

FIG. 16.2.   Natural handhold for grasping a cat. Pick up skin close to the ears so head can be tilted up if cat begins to scratch.

Pick up the cat by placing a hand over the top of the animal and around to the opposite side, with the palm of the hand supporting the sternum or chest area (Fig. 16.1).

Alternatively, grasp the cat by the loose skin over the back of the neck close to the head (Fig. 16.2). This is a natural handhold for lifting a cat. If the cat becomes unruly, the head can be tilted backward, which unbalances the cat and lessens the inclination to bite and scratch.[2] Most cats do not resent this, but some may strike out to claw with the front feet and may, if extremely excited, attempt to scratch with the hind feet as well.

Grabbing a cat by the loose fold of skin on the neck makes use of a phenomenon retained from kittenhood. When the queen picks up her kitten by the scruff of the neck to carry it, the kitten becomes limp, curling up the paws and tail, until

it is released. This behavioral response prevents possible injury caused by the mother having to bite tightly or by the kitten twisting its neck in struggling. This response occurs in all species of domestic and wild felidae and can be utilized successfully to restrain kittens up to weaning age. Kittens grasped in this manner completely relax, and nonpainful manipulations can easily be carried out with this technique. If a cat becomes unmanageable during any restraint procedure, grasp it by the nape and hold it away from your body (Fig. 16.3). An obstreperous cat can be picked up and moved using both hands (Fig. 16.4).

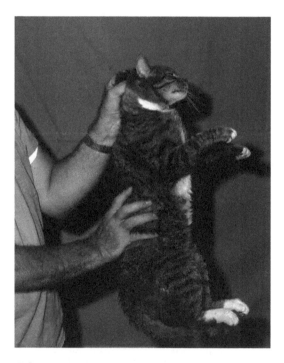

FIG. 16.3.   Obstreperous cat can be grasped by the nape and pushed away from handler.

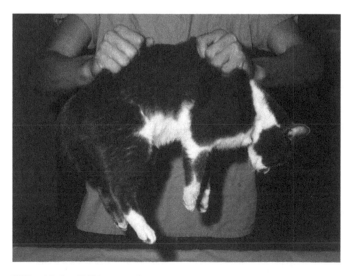

FIG. 16.4.   Lifting an obstreperous cat.

It is seldom wise to wear gloves when handling cats, although gloves may minimize scratch injuries. One cannot rely on gloves to prevent penetration by the canine teeth; even a small cat can bite through heavy leather. Furthermore, wearing heavy gloves requires a harder squeeze to maintain the same degree of immobilization as can be achieved with a light grip of the bare hand. Squeezing hard may injure small cats. The danger is intensified because gloves reduce tactile discrimination, making it difficult to determine the degree of pressure applied. The pressure may be much greater than supposed and greater than necessary to maintain control. When examining a cat in a veterinary hospital, have the animal placed on a smooth, slick table. The cat is distracted by the effort required to maintain stability and is less likely to use a paw for scratching. To carry out general examination and manipulation, gently hold the animal on the table with the hands cupped over the back. If the animal must be held more firmly, grasp the loose skin over the back of the neck, pressing the cat onto the table with both hands, one over the neck and one over the loins (Fig. 16.5). This prevents the cat from lashing out with either front or back paws.

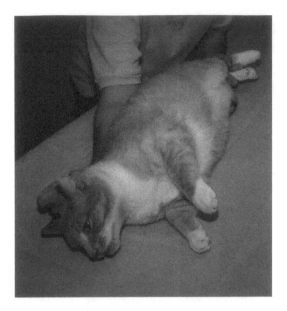

FIG. 16.6. Stretching a cat while in lateral recumbency.

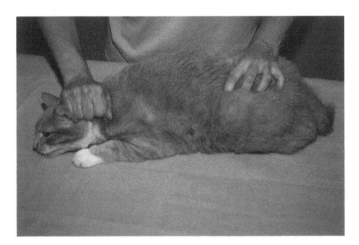

FIG. 16.5. Restraining obstreperous cat by pressing it onto a table.

If more restricted activity is required, the cat can be held in lateral recumbency (Fig. 16.6). The paws are held immobile by the hands, and the head is restrained by placing the forearm over the neck. It is necessary for an assistant to secure the head of an obstreperous cat during this procedure.

If a procedure requires some time to complete, yet is not painful, the limbs may be immobilized by taping the front feet together and the hind feet together. The head can be easily controlled with one hand.

The mouth of the cat can be opened in the same manner as the dog's. If the front paws are not held by an assistant, the handler may be clawed. It is difficult to administer solid medication to a cat orally. Some prefer to use forceps to place a pill into the pharynx.

Intravenous cannulation of the cephalic vein for obtaining blood samples or injecting medication may be performed

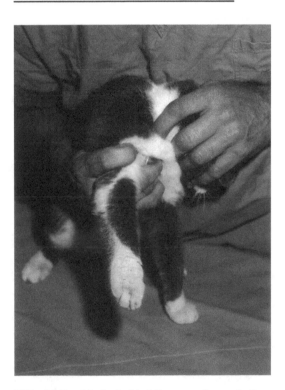

FIG. 16.7. Method of holding a cat for cephalic venipuncture.

while holding the cat by a method similar to that used for holding a dog (Fig. 16.7). The saphenous or jugular vein may also be used.

The jugular vein may be cannulated with the cat's head held vertically (Fig. 16.8) or with the cat lying on its back (Fig. 16.9). Both methods should be practiced, because some cats accept one placement more readily than the other, with the majority being more comfortable on the back. If difficulty

A cat can be controlled by rolling it in a towel or alternatively wrapping the towel around the cat's neck (Figs. 16.10, 16.11). The extended claws entangle in the towel, keeping the paws within the wrap. A single limb may be withdrawn for examination or for exposure of a vein to administer intravenous medication or to withdraw blood for a laboratory sample. The head is controlled equally well and may be exposed for examination or treatment in the same manner as the legs.

A cat bag is an excellent tool for restraining a cat for semi-uncomfortable manipulations (Fig. 16.12, 16.13). Pick the cat up by the nape to place it into the bag. Once the cat is inside the bag, either the head or any limb may be left outside for various manipulative procedures while the other limbs or the head are contained in the bag and cannot interfere. Cat bags can be obtained commercially, or they can be improvised.

A net is another satisfactory tool for handling extremely nervous or unruly cats. The net may be introduced through a partially open door and placed over a cat in a small enclosure; a larger enclosure may be entered to place the net. Many manipulative procedures can be carried out on a cat in a net. Almost any part of the body may be examined or a limb may be withdrawn through the mesh. The animal usually entangles its claws in the mesh, so scratching is not a hazard. The head can be restrained by grabbing the cat behind the back of the head with one hand.

It may be necessary to use a snare to handle extremely vicious cats. The snare is a less desirable tool because of the

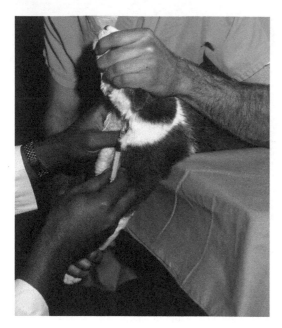

FIG. 16.8. Holding a cat for jugular venipuncture.

is encountered with one method of jugular bleeding, the other may be successful. Restraint for jugular cannulation may be stressful for a dyspneic cat. Try other methods first.

The medial saphenous vein may be cannulated. The vein is prone to roll away from a needle injection, so sharp needles should be used.

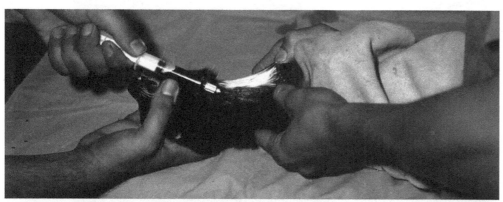

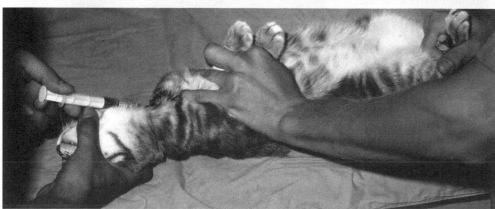

FIG. 16.9. Jugular venipuncture with cat on its back: Handheld, lower. In restraining bag, upper.

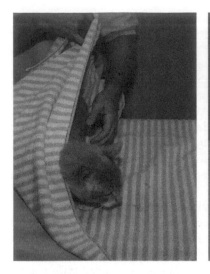
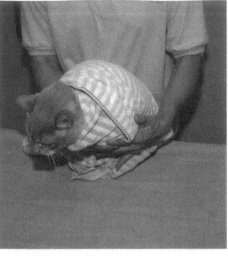

FIG. 16.10. Wrapping cat in a towel: Place cat in center of the towel. Lift one end over the top of the cat, then quickly roll the cat.

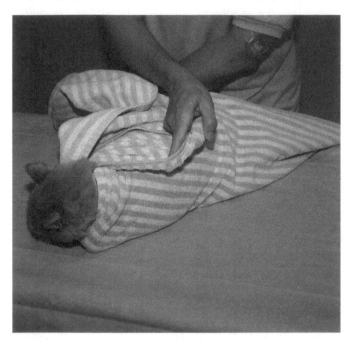

FIG. 16.11. Wrapping the towel around the neck of the cat.

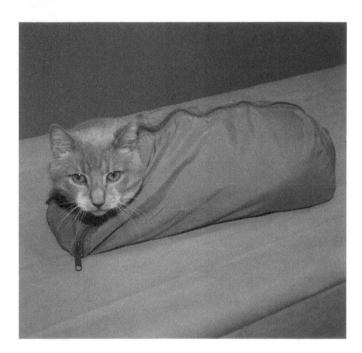

FIG. 16.12. Adjustable cat bag is a valuable tool for working with cats and many other small mammals.

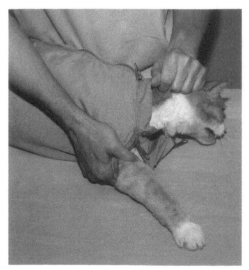
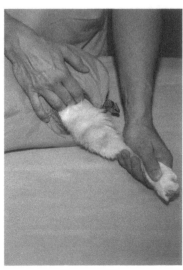

FIG. 16.13. Modern bags provide options for limb manipulation and exposure to other areas of the body. Forelimb, left, and hind limb, right.

possibility of injuring the cat. Nevertheless, no one should be subjected to being bitten or scratched by an ill-mannered animal. It is not prudent to take excessive chances with any animal.

Experience in handling cats allows some individuals to approach seemingly vicious cats without difficulty. The inexperienced individual frequently must use special restraint techniques to minimize the chances of being scratched and bitten.

TRANSPORT

Cats are commonly carried or shipped to shows in small individual cages. Cats may vocalize loudly when confined.

CHEMICAL RESTRAINT

Various tranquilizers have been administered to domestic cats for sedation (Table 16.2). When it became necessary

to immobilize domestic cats for diagnostic or therapeutic procedures, ketamine was the drug of choice for many years. Ketamine may also be sprayed into the mouth of a ferocious cat (20.0–30.0 mg/kg). Although ketamine is still effective, newer chemical immobilizing agents and/or combinations are more effective and produce fewer side effects (Table 16.2). Immobilization or induction of inhalation anesthesia may be accomplished using an anesthetic chamber as illustrated in Chapter 15, Dogs.

The chemical restraint agents and combinations mentioned in this chapter represent those used by experienced veterinarians with detailed knowledge of cats. Other protocols have been used, and no claim is made for including all possible drugs and combinations. For more detailed information, particularly for anesthesia, consult Bednarski[2] or Tranquilli.[8]

TABLE 16.2.   Selected chemical restraint agents for domestic cats

Agent	Dose, sedation (mg/kg), route	Dose, immobilizing (mg/kg), route
Diazepam, usually combined with opioid	0.2. IV	
Midazolam, usually combined with opioid	0.1–0.2, IV	
Medetomidine*	0.05–0.12, IM, IV	
Ketamine		2.0–10.0, IM, IV
Ketamine/xylazine*		5.0–10.0/0.7–1.0, IM, IV
Tiletamine/zolazepam (Telazol)		2.0–3.0, IM, IV
Telazol/butorphanol		3.0/0.2
Telazol/Butorphanol/ medetomidine**		3.0/0.15/0.015

* Reversal with atipamezole 0.075 mg/kg IV.
** Ko[3].

REFERENCES

1. Anderson, R.S., and Edney, A.T.B., Eds. 1991. Practical Animal Handling, 1st ed. Oxford, U.K, Pergamon Press, 198 pages.
2. Bednarski, R.M. 1996. Dogs and Cats. In: Thurmon, J.C., Tranquilli, W.J., and Benson, G.J., Eds. 1996. Lumb and Jones' Veterinary Anesthesia. 3rd Ed. Philadelphia, Lippincott Williams and Wilkens, pp. 591–596.
3. Ko, J.C.H., Abbo, L.A., Weil, A.B., Johnson, B.M., and Payton, M. 2007. A comparison of anesthetic and cardiorespiratory effects of tiletamine-zolazepam-butorphanol and tiletamine-zolazepam-butorphanol-medetomidine in cats. Veterinary Therapeutics 8(3):164–176.
4. Necker, C. 1970. The Natural History of Cats. New York, A.S. Barnes.
5. Pond, G., Ed. 1972. The Complete Cat Encyclopedia. New York, Crown.
6. Sheldon, C.C., Sonsthagen, T., and Topel, J.A. 2006. St. Louis, Mosby/Elsevier, 239 pages.
7. Sonsthagen, T.F. 1991. Restraint of Domestic Animals. Goleta, California, American Veterinary Publications, 149 pages.
8. Tranquilli, W.J., Thurman, J.C., and Grimm, K.A., Eds. 2007. Lumb and Jones' Veterinary Anesthesia and Analgesia, 4th Ed. Ames, Iowa, Wiley-Blackwell Publishing.

CHAPTER 17

Laboratory Rodents and Rabbits

CLASSIFICATION

Hundreds of species of domestic and wild animals that are maintained in facilities for investigational purposes may require handling. This chapter is devoted to traditional pet and laboratory rodents and rabbits only. Other species are dealt with in separate chapters.

Order Lagomorpha
    Family Leporidae: rabbit
Order Rodentia
    Family Muridae: rat, mouse
    Family Cricetidae: golden hamster, Chinese hamster
    Family Cavidae: guinea pig

No special names are given to male or female rodents. The young are called offspring, youngsters, or pups (mice and rats). The male rabbit is a buck, and the female a doe. Newborn rabbits are kits or youngsters. Weights are listed in Table 17.1.

TABLE 17.1. Weights of laboratory animals

Animal	Male	Female	Newborn	Weanling
Guinea pig	1–1.2 kg	850–900	90	250
Rat	200–400	250–300	5–6	40–50
Mouse	20–40	25–90	1.5	7–15
Golden hamster	90–120	95–140	2	35
Gerbil	46–131	53–133	3	. . .
Rabbit				
New Zealand	4–5 kg	4.5–5.5 kg	60	
Flemish giant	4.5–6.4 kg			
Dwarf	0.9 kg			

Note: Weight is in grams unless otherwise indicated.

DANGER POTENTIAL

All laboratory rodents and rabbits have large incisor teeth adapted for gnawing. All are capable of inflicting significant bite wounds, although the propensity to do so varies from species to species. Rabbits may scratch a handler with the hind feet.

BEHAVIOR

Domestic laboratory animals are generally docile and easily handled unless previously subjected to unpleasant manipulation. Rats can easily climb up their own tails when suspended, but mice are less agile and cannot.

Free-ranging rodents and rabbits thermoregulate by escaping the heat through burrowing or nocturnal behavior. Domestic species will suffer from heat stress unless kept in a temperature-controlled environment. Domestic laboratory animals are easily tamed and frequently kept as children's pets.

PHYSICAL RESTRAINT

Hundreds of devices have been developed to restrain various species of laboratory animals for certain specialized procedures. It is not my intent to describe or review all available techniques and equipment. The reader is referred to voluminous literature on this subject.[2–9] General techniques suitable for the pet, zoo animal, or laboratory animal will be described and illustrated.

Rabbits

Rabbits are usually kept in small cages or a hutch. A domestic rabbit may be grasped by the loose skin over the shoulders (scruff) (Fig. 17.1). Cradling the hindquarters with the other hand provides added support (Fig. 17.2) and may prevent the rabbit from kicking backward and possibly fracturing its spine in the lumbosacral region as it is lifted. Small rabbits can be picked up in the same manner as puppies and kittens, by the scruff without supporting the hindquarters. Do not pick up a rabbit by the ears since this inflicts needless pain and causes the animal to struggle violently to free itself, even to the point of fracturing its neck.

Most rabbits may be carried with their head tucked under the handler's upper arm and their body lightly supported by the hand and forearm (Fig. 17.3, bottom and top). When returning a rabbit to a cage, set the rear quarters down first, with the head facing the door.

To examine the abdomen, genital organs, or vent, hold the legs together (Fig. 17.4).

Rabbits easily enter the torpid state (hypnotized, mesmerized) if placed and held on their backs for a few seconds (Fig. 17.5). Blindfolding may prolong the effect. A tap on the table is usually sufficient to reverse the trance. Occasionally, a rabbit sitting upright will go limp while being examined.

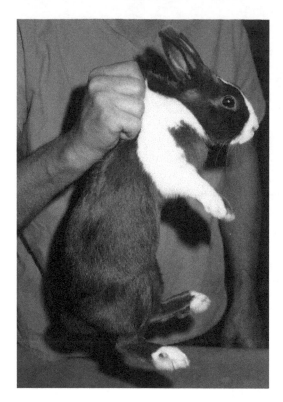

FIG. 17.1. Lifting rabbit by the loose skin over the back and neck.

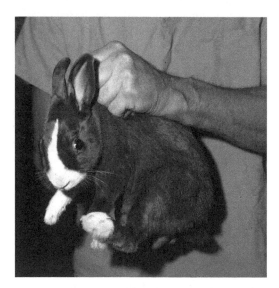

FIG. 17.2. Lifting rabbit by grasping neck skin while supporting the hindquarters.

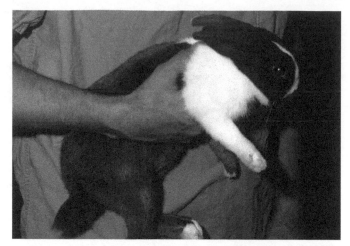

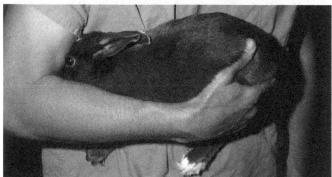

FIG. 17.3. Proper way to carry a docile rabbit.

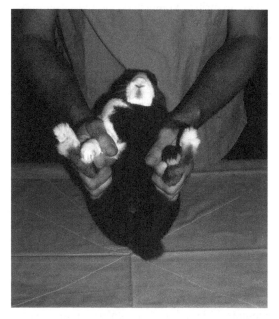

FIG. 17.4. Restraint for examination of abdomen and perineal area.

This eliminates the need for restraint, but the torpidity interferes with accurate clinical evaluation of a diseased rabbit.

When employing any special restraint device, be certain that the rear legs are controlled to protect the back from inadvertent fracture. A rabbit wrapped in a towel cannot scratch the handler (Fig. 17.6). More effective restraint is achieved by placing the rabbit in a cat bag (Fig. 17.7) or a stainless steel adjustable container (Fig. 17.8).

Small volumes of blood (0.1–3.0 ml) are usually obtained from the prominent marginal ear veins (Fig. 17.9). The vein is raised by applying pressure either digitally or with a tourniquet (string or paper clip) or padded clamp proximal to the

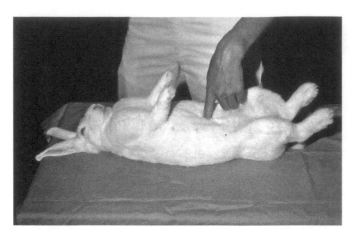

FIG. 17.5. Mesmerizing a rabbit.

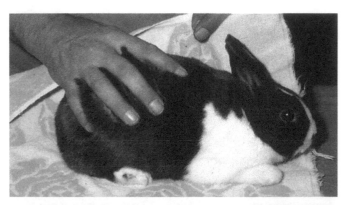

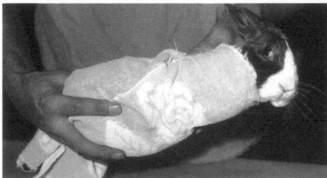

FIG. 17.6. Wrapping rabbit in a towel.

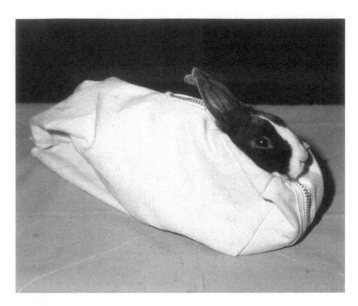

FIG. 17.7. Rabbit in a cat bag.

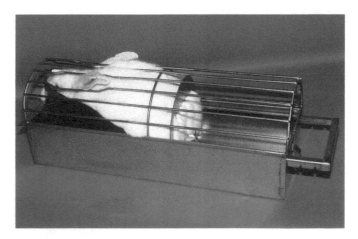

FIG. 17.8. Stainless steel adjustable rabbit restraint container.

venipuncture site. Larger volumes of blood (3.0–50.0 ml) may be collected from the central ear artery. The lateral saphenous vein, which runs along the lateral aspect of the rear leg, may be similarly used for venipuncture.

Mouse

The ease of handling mice varies greatly with the individual. The pet mouse, used to being handled by a child, may be picked up and held in a cupped hand. It will seldom jump from the hand or bite, but care should still be taken to prevent jumping and falling by blocking the view of the mouse with the other hand. Some pets, although willing to accept manipu-

lation by the owner, may not allow the same degree of familiarity by a stranger, particularly a veterinarian who is examining the animal.

Mice kept in laboratory colonies are usually accustomed to being restrained with devices or techniques developed for handling large numbers of animals. Mice are frequently picked up by the base of the tail and removed from a cage. This may be done with the bare hand by simply grasping the tail close to the body with a finger and thumb (Fig. 17.10). Rubber-covered tongs may be used if a sterile handling technique is required, as it is in some specific pathogen-free mouse colonies.

If more restrictive restraint is necessary, grasp the base of the tail, allow the animal to crawl away slowly on a rough surface that allows the animal to grip and pull away from you, then reach quickly with thumb and finger alongside the neck to grasp a skin fold encompassing the scruff (Figs. 17.10,

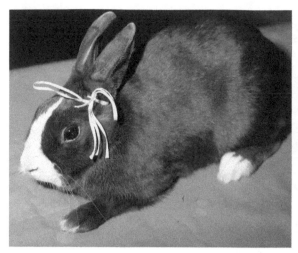

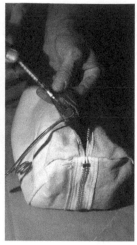

FIG. 17.9. Using umbilical tape, a string, or towel clamp to raise vein.

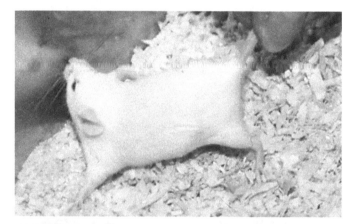

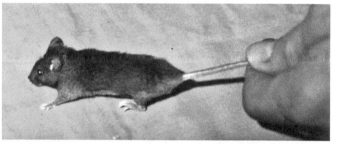

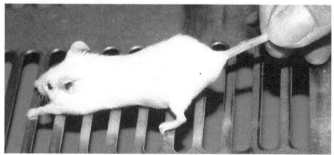

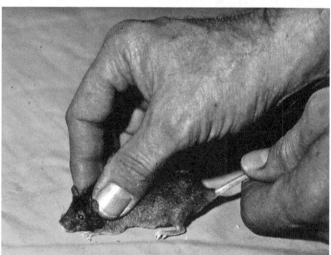

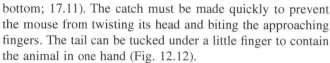

FIG. 17.10. Picking up a mouse near the base of the tail.

FIG. 17.11. Holding a mouse.

bottom; 17.11). The catch must be made quickly to prevent the mouse from twisting its head and biting the approaching fingers. The tail can be tucked under a little finger to contain the animal in one hand (Fig. 12.12).

Wild mice (i.e., Peromyscus spp.) are jumpers. Place a holding cage in a tall garbage can before removing the top. Oral medication may be given to a mouse with a feeding needle (Fig. 17.13). The needle should be 18 or 20 gauge, 4.0 cm, straight or curved, and modified by soldering a ball to the tip to prevent damage to the esophagus. Insert the needle gently through the esophagus into the stomach. If such a needle is unavailable, pass a small plastic or rubber stomach tube. A plastic container for disposable needles, special forceps, or a small dowel drilled with a hole may serve as a speculum to aid in passing the tube and to prevent the mouse from biting off and swallowing the tube.

Obtaining blood samples from small laboratory rodents is challenging. Postorbital sinus or plexus bleeding under anesthesia is widely accepted as a satisfactory technique for use in mice, hamsters, and rats, but it is most successful in mice and hamsters.[10] The mouse has an orbital sinus that completely surrounds the globe. The sinus in hamsters is on the dorsal, caudal, and ventral aspect of the orbit.[10]

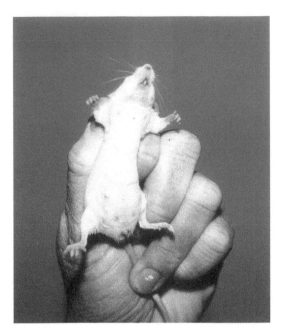

FIG. 17.12. Holding a mouse by the scruff of the neck and the tail.

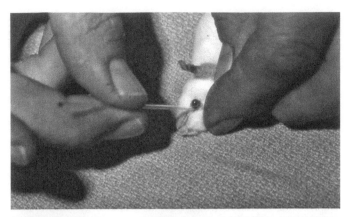

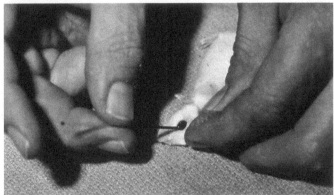

FIG. 17.14. Bleeding a mouse with capillary tube inserted retrobulbarly.

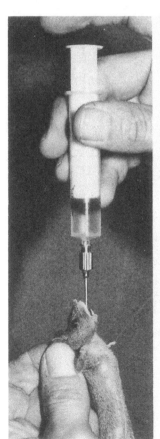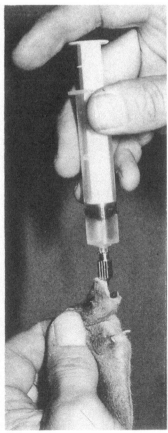

FIG. 17.13. Esophageal intubation with a 16-gauge, 5-cm needle with a ball soldered to the tip. Head and neck must be held straight.

The animal is anesthetized with injectable or inhalant anesthesia. When anesthetized, grasp it, fixing the head firmly. Proptose the eyeball slightly by stretching the upper eyelid. Insert a suitable capillary tube slightly dorsal to the medial canthus of the eye with a slight twist (Fig. 17.14). Direct the tube toward the medial side of the bony orbit. Blood may well up in the tube during insertion. If not, once the bone is touched, withdraw the tube slightly to fill it. Rodents have been repeatedly bled by this method without producing ill effects; 0.1 ml of blood may be safely withdrawn from a 50-g mouse and 0.5 ml from a 200-g rat. These quantities are sufficient for a complete hemogram and blood chemistry if micro-techniques are employed. Slight hemorrhage may occur following removal of the tube. This is not cause for concern; however, it would be inadvisable to use this technique to bleed a pet in front of an anxious owner. Alternatively, blood may be collected from the lateral tail veins or ventral tail artery.

Rats

Immature rats are handled similarly to mice. However, recall that a rat is capable of climbing up its own tail, so take care when lifting a rat from a cage by the tail base, barehanded (Fig. 17.15). Quickly shift the rat to a sleeved arm (Fig. 17.16) and then grasp the rat around the neck cranial to the forelimbs with the index and middle finger and grasp with the thumb

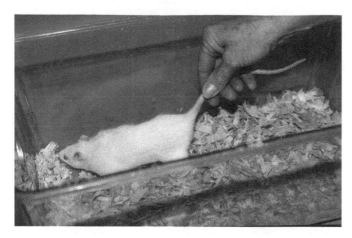

FIG. 17.15. Lifting a rat by grasping near base of tail.

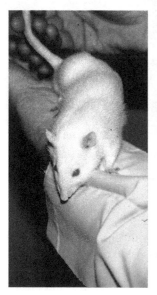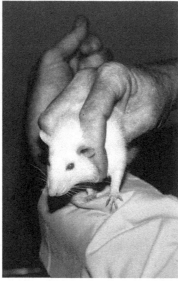

FIG. 17.16. Allowing the rat to cling to a sleeved arm, left. Grasping rat with fingers around the neck and behind the forelimbs, right.

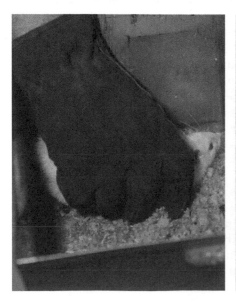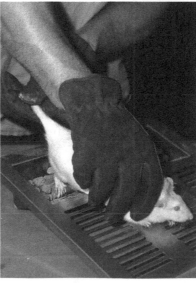

and other fingers around the body (Fig. 17.16, right). It may be preferable to catch unfamiliar rats with a gloved hand (Figs. 17.17, 17.18).

Both rats and mice may be placed in adjustable plastic tubes for bleeding from the tail or inhalant anesthesia induction (Fig. 17.19). A rat may be wrapped in a towel or restrained in a cake decorator's plastic cone (Fig. 17.20) or in appropriate-sized tubes (Fig. 17.21).

Esophageal intubation by means of needle gavage tubes (16–20 gauge, 4.0–7.5 cm) may also be used for medicating rats.

Guinea Pigs

Pet guinea pigs are usually handled frequently and may ordinarily be picked up and examined with ease. Laboratory animals are more excitable and may resist being picked up. Guinea pigs should be approached slowly and with minimum fuss, to prevent frantic stampeding and possible leg or foot injury. Guinea pigs seem to bite only out of curiosity, so

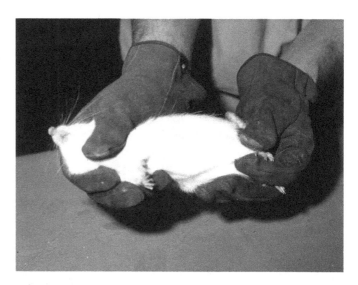

FIG. 17.18. Rat held with gloved hands.

FIG. 17.17. Rat manually controlled with a gloved hand.

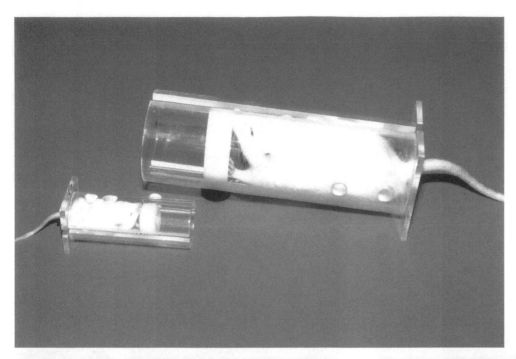

FIG. 17.19.   Rat and mouse placed in adjustable plastic tubes for venipuncture or inhalant anesthesia induction.

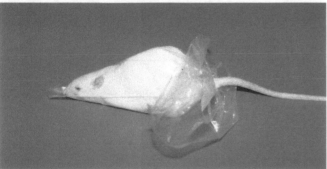

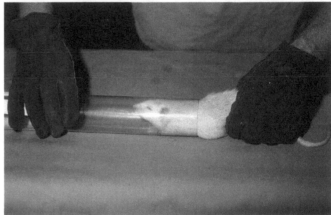

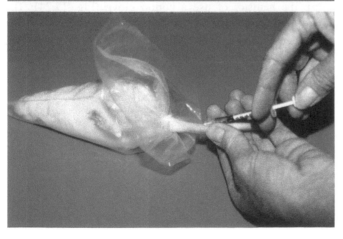

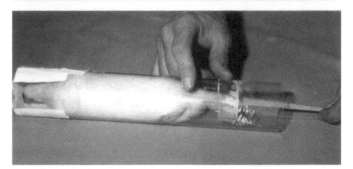

FIG. 17.20.   Rat placed in cake decorator's plastic cone.

FIG. 17.21.   Rat in a tube.

gloves may not be indicated. Guinea pigs can best be restrained by using both hands, one to support the upper body and one to support the lower body (Fig. 17.22). Guinea pigs are easily wrapped in a towel (Fig. 17.23).

Dental problems (incisor malocclusion, cheek teeth malocclusion) are common to all laboratory rodents, especially guinea pigs. The mouth should be examined only with the

animal under sedation. A special speculum may be constructed or improvised to hold the mouth open and expand the cheeks to visualize the teeth and oral cavity. (See Fig. 22.34, Chapter 22.) Cheek teeth malocclusion is common in guinea pigs so a thorough oral examination is important. Oral medication may be administered by inserting a plastic eyedropper or syringe tip through the commissure of the mouth and dropping fluid into the pocket. Gavage tubes are not recommended in guinea pigs due to the anatomy of the soft palate.

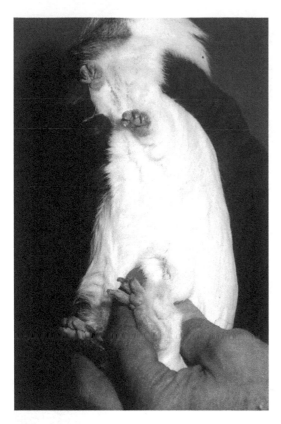

FIG. 17.22. Proper restraint and support of a guinea pig.

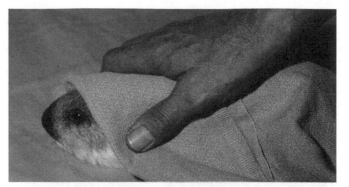

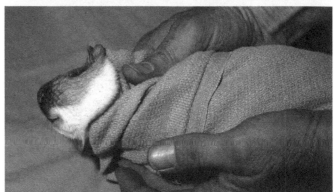

FIG. 17.23. Wrapping guinea pig in a towel.

Hamsters

Hamsters are more nervous and more difficult to handle than mice or rats. In the hands of pet owners, hamsters are usually quite gentle, but if strangers try to grasp them, they are easily frightened and may be difficult to capture. Hamsters are definitely prone to biting. They also do not respond well

if one tries to pick them up while they are sleeping or just awakening. An animal may roll over on its back in a submissive posture, but will bite anyway. Hamsters are fast and agile, and they lack a tail to grasp. To capture a hamster from a cage, use a 30-cm (12-in.) square sheet from a roll of cotton and grasp the hamster or use a cotton glove (Fig. 17.24). The mouth may be opened with a dowel or forceps (Fig. 17.25). Some handlers pick up hamsters as they would rats; however,

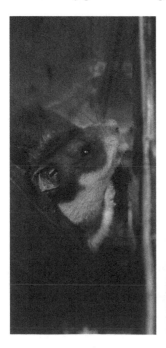

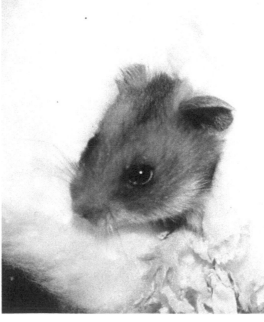

FIG. 17.24. Grasping a hamster using a gloved hand, left, or a sheet of cotton, right.

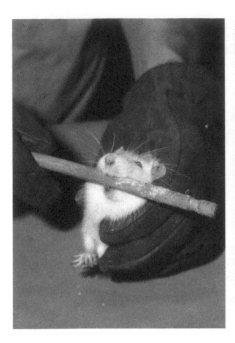
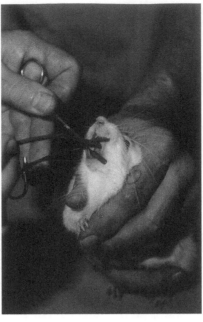

FIG. 17.25. Holding the mouth of a rat open with a dowel or a forceps.

grasping hamsters by the scruff tends to be a more secure method to restrain them. The handler must grasp sufficient skin as they can wiggle around in the loose skin and escape the grasp during prolonged restraint.

Miscellaneous Species

Many other species of rodents are kept as pets or laboratory animals. The general principles covering restraint and handling of these rodents are similar to those mentioned above. Any unique problems will be discussed in Chapter 22.

TRANSPORT

Laboratory animals are transported more frequently than any other group of animals. Special cages have been designed for air and truck shipment. Shippers must strictly adhere to the International Air Transport Association specifications for caging, feeding, and watering.[1]

Pets may be moved in their own cages or in special shipping boxes. Rodents must not be left in cardboard containers because they may quickly gnaw their way out.

CHEMICAL RESTRAINT

Small rodents and rabbits are commonly used for laboratory investigations. Every conceivable drug and drug combination has been employed in laboratory animals to sedate, immobilize, ameliorate pain, and anesthetize them. It is not possible to review the literature or even summarize the use of restraint agents used in laboratory animals. Rather selected procedures that may be used for pet rodents and rabbits will be tabulated (Table 17.2). Further information on this subject may be found in standard textbooks and references on laboratory animal medicine and veterinary anesthesia.

TABLE 17.2. Selected immobilizing agents used in pet rodents and rabbits[6]

Agent	Dosage (mg/kg), route
Mice	
Ketamine	80.0–100.0, IM
Xylazine	2.5, IM
Tiletamine/zolazepam	20.0–40.0
Rats	
Ketamine	50.0–100.0, IM
Ketamine/medetomidine	60–75/0.25–0.5, SQ
Ketamine/xylazine	40.0–87.0/5.0–13.0, IM
Tiletamine/zolazepam	20.0, IM
Guinea pigs	
Diazepam	2.5–5.0, IP
Xylazine	5.0–40.0, IP
Ketamine	40.0, IM
Ketamine/xylazine	30.0–40.0/0.1–4.0, IM
Tiletamine/zolazepam	10.0–18.0, IM
Hamsters	
Ketamine	40.0–80.0, IM
Tiletamine/zolazepam	20.0–40.0
Rabbits	
Diazepam	2.0–5.0, IM
Midazolam	2.0, IV
Ketamine	20.0–60.0, IM
Ketamine/xylazine	10.0/3.0, IV
Ketamine/diazepam	60.0–80.0/5.0–10.0, IM
Tiletamine/zolazepam	32.0–64.0, IM

It is not the author's intent to discuss laboratory animal anesthesia, but rather sedation and chemical restraint for the purpose of physical examination, diagnostic procedures, and collection of laboratory samples.

Numerous drugs and combinations are used to sedate laboratory animals. Immobilization may be induced with isoflurane in oxygen administered via a mask or anesthetic chamber from a calibrated vaporizer.

Intramuscular sedatives and restraint agents are useful in some species but not in others. Rabbits are relatively refractory to many restraint agents. Table 17.2 provides a list of drugs and dosages that are currently being used.[4–6] Although tiletamine/zolazepam (Telazol) has been a satisfactory chemical restraint agent in many mammals, it has not been as useful in laboratory rodents, and may even be contraindicated in rabbits.[4]

REFERENCES

1. Anonymous. 1992. Live Animal Regulations, 19th Ed., pp. 100–101. Montreal, Can.: International Air Transport Association.
2. Carpenter, J.W., Mashima, T.Y., and Rupiper, D.J. 2001. Exotic Animal Formulary, 2nd Ed., St. Louis, MO, W.B. Saunders/Elsevier.
3. Carpenter, J.W. 2003. Lagomorpha (Pikas, rabbits, hares). In: Fowler, M.E., and Miller, R.E., Eds. Zoo and Wild Animal Medicine. 5th Ed. St. Louis, Saunders/Elsevier. pp. 410–412.
4. Eisele, P.H. 1990. Anesthesia for laboratory animals: Practical considerations and techniques. In: B.E. Rollin, and M.L. Kesel, Eds. The Experimental Animal in Biomedical Research, Vol. I, pp. 275–317. Boca Raton, Fla.: CRC Press.
5. Flecknell, P.A. 1987. Laboratory Animal Anesthesia. New York: Academic Press.
6. Flecknell, P.A., Richardson, C.A., and Papovic, A. 2007. Laboratory Animals. In: Tranquilli, W.J., Thurman, J.C., and Grimm, K.A., Eds. 2007. Lumb and Jones' Veterinary Anesthesia and Analgesia, 4th Ed. Ames, Iowa, Wiley-Blackwell Publishing, pp. 765–784.
7. Harkness, J.E., and Wagner, J.E. 1989. The Biology and Medicine of Rabbits and Rodents, 3rd Ed. Philadelphia: Lea and Febiger.
8. Kesel, M.L. 1990. Handling, restraint, and common sampling and administration techniques in laboratory species. In: B.E. Rollin, and M.L. Kesel, Eds. The Experimental Animal in Biomedical Research, Vol. I, pp. 333–352. Boca Raton, Fla.: CRC Press.
9. Sainsbury, A. 2003. Rodentia (rodents). In: Fowler, M.E., and Miller, R.E., Eds. Zoo and Wild Animal Medicine. 5th Ed. St. Louis, Saunders/Elsevier. pp. 420–426.
10. Timm, K.I. 1980. Peri-orbital bleeding technique for the mouse, hamster, and rat-anatomical consideration. Synapse 13 (1):14–16.

C H A P T E R   1 8
Poultry and Waterfowl

CLASSIFICATION

Order Galliformes
    Family Phasianidae: chicken
    Family Meleagrididae: turkey
Order Anseriformes
    Family Anatidae: Pekin duck, Muscovy duck, goose,
        Canada goose, mute swan

Chickens, turkeys, ducks, and geese are frequently kept as pets or in small home flocks as well as in large commercial operations. Techniques for handling individual birds vary with the circumstances, although all are based on common principles. Names of gender of poultry and waterfowl are given in Table 18.1, weights in Table 18.2.

TABLE 18.1. Names of gender of domestic fowl

Bird	Male	Female	Young
Chicken	Cock, rooster	Hen	Pullet (female), cockerel (male), chick
Duck	Drake	Duck	Duckling
Goose	Gander	Goose	Gosling
Swan	Cob	Pen	Cygnet
Turkey	Tom	Hen	Poult

TABLE 18.2. Weights of poultry and waterfowl

Bird	Male (kg)	Male (lb)	Female (kg)	Female (lb)
Chickens				
Plymouth rock	4	9.5	3	7.5
Jersey black giant	6	13	5	10
White leghorn	3	6	2	4.5
Cornish	5	10	3	7.5
Turkeys				
Large strains	21	45	12	26
Medium strains	16	35	9	20
Small strains	8	17	5	11
Ducks				
Pekin	4	9	4	8
Indian runner	2	4.5	2	4
Muscovy	5	12	3	7
Geese				
Toulouse	12	26	9	20
Chinese	5	12	5	10

DANGER POTENTIAL

Chickens may peck and scratch. Roosters may develop large spurs on the legs that can seriously injure the unwary person. Roosters raised for fighting (illegal in most states) may be aggressive. Turkeys may peck, particularly at objects like rings and other jewelry, but rarely injure. Large tom

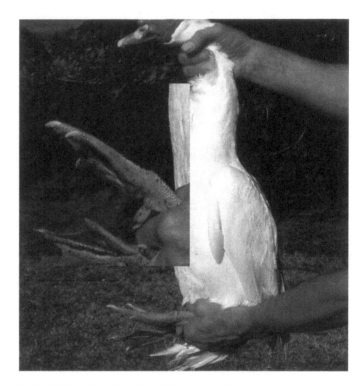

FIG. 18.1. Toenails of the Muscovy duck are adapted for perching in trees. Toenails of geese and most ducks are short and blunt.

turkeys can deliver painful wing blows and may scratch. Domestic ducks are easily handled, although some species have claws (Fig. 18.1) adapted for perching in trees and may scratch a handler. Ducks have blunt bills, so although they may peck, they rarely injure.

Geese are large. They often peck viciously with heavy, pointed bills and may also strike an intruder by rapidly flapping strong wings. A small child may be severely injured by an angry goose. I vividly recall being chased to the house by an irate gander beating me with his wings and pecking at my backside.

BEHAVIOR AND PHYSIOLOGY

Most domestic birds are docile and amenable to handling. They are gregarious and stay bunched together when approached rather than scattering. This flocking trait enables the handler to single out and capture one individual without causing it to panic or frightening the other members of the flock.

209

Waterfowl will retreat to water if harassed, so access to ponds must be prevented in order to capture them. Domestic birds rarely struggle once captured.

The trachea of a bird is composed of a series of complete cartilaginous rings that prevent collapse of the trachea. This allows a handler to grasp the neck without danger of suffocating the bird.

All birds breathe by means of a bellows-type respiratory system. (See Fig. 29.1 in Chapter 29, Wild Birds.) Be cautious when exerting pressure over the sternum.

PHYSICAL RESTRAINT
Chicken

A chicken may be grasped by the leg and wing simultaneously (Fig. 18.2). It may also be captured with a net or a hook. Once the chicken is captured, it may be held by the legs (Fig. 18.3).

A blindfolded bird will usually lie quietly. When its vision is diminished, the chicken behaves as if hypnotized. This is easily accomplished by placing a towel or cloth over the head (Fig. 18.4) or by tucking the head beneath a wing (Fig. 18.5). A torpid state may be induced by tucking the head under a wing (Fig. 18.5).

The wings of a chicken may be interlocked to temporarily prevent flight. Carefully wrap the wings around each other as illustrated in Figures 18.6 and 18.7. Do not use this technique on peafowl or large turkeys, since it may fracture the wing or dislocate the joint.

The beak of a chicken is easily opened and examined. Blood samples are obtained from the brachial vein (Fig. 18.8). Masking tape is used for positioning an anesthetized bird for surgery.

To restrain a chicken for caponization or abdominal exploration, stretch the legs backward and wrap a loop of rope or gauze around the wings, stretching the wings forward (Fig. 18.9).

Turkey

Adult turkeys are usually docile and may be approached while in a flock, especially by the usual caretaker. Slow but deliberate movements allow one to single out a bird and catch it without frightening the entire flock.

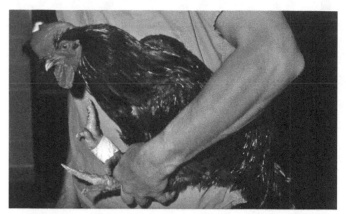

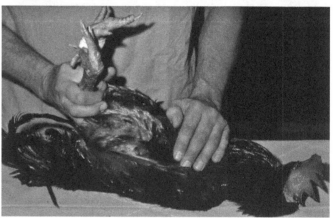

FIG. 18.3. A rooster may be carried with one hand if legs are taped together, top. A large rooster may be held on table with minimal struggling, bottom.

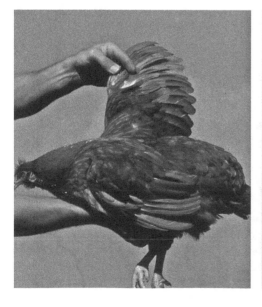

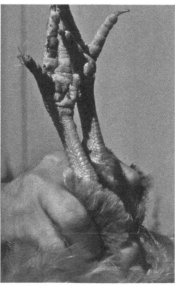

FIG. 18.2. Grasping chicken simultaneously by wing and leg.

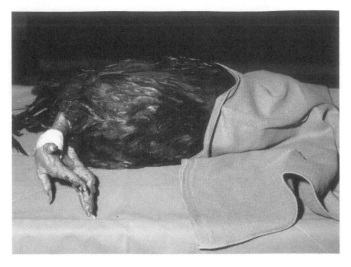

FIG. 18.4. A blindfolded chicken will lie quietly.

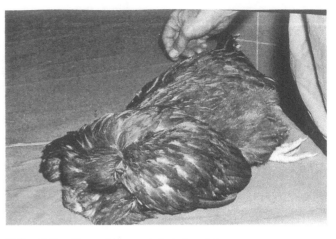

FIG. 18.5. State of hypnosis is induced by tucking head of chicken under its wing.

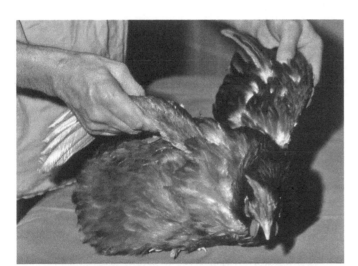

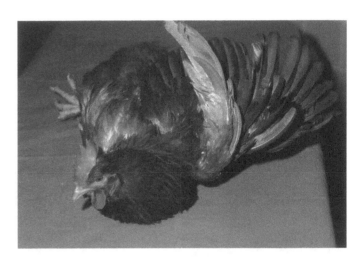

FIG. 18.7. Wings folded on a chicken.

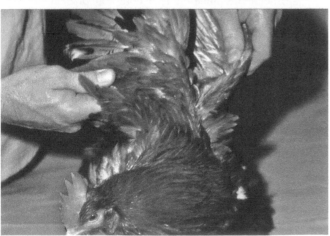

FIG. 18.6. Interfolding wings of a chicken: Grasp wings, upper. Cross wings and wrap them around one another, lower.

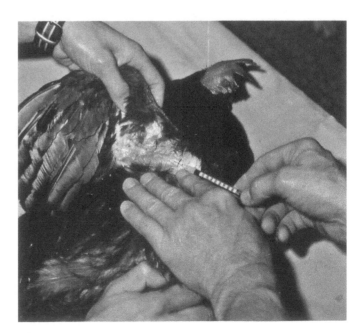

FIG. 18.8. Approach to venipuncture of brachial vein in a chicken.

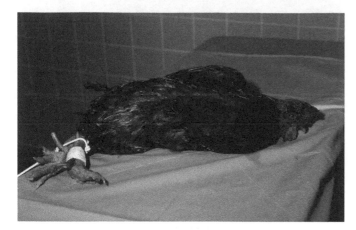

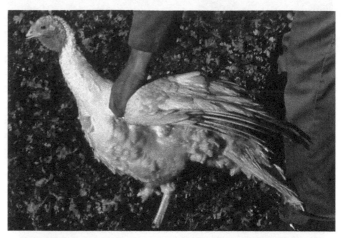

FIG. 18.9. Chicken can be stretched in lateral recumbency by securing both legs together. Another loop surrounds base of both wings.

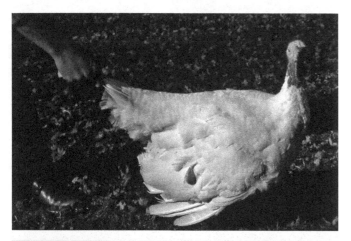

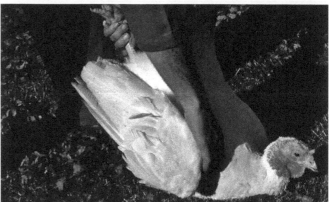

FIG. 18.11. Grasp a wing, top, and then the legs, bottom.

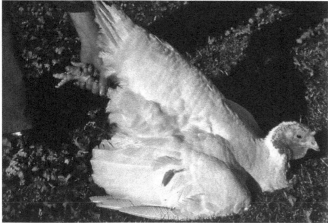

FIG. 18.10. Initial restraint of a turkey by grasping all the tail feathers, then the legs.

A large turkey may be captured as illustrated in Figures 18.10 and 18.11. A small bird may be grasped as one would a chicken. If turkeys can be herded into a small pen, the handler can approach from behind in a kneeling position (Fig. 18.12) to capture one. The heavy body of a large turkey cannot be safely suspended from the legs. Without body or wing support, the coxofemoral articulation of the hip may luxate.

Blood samples are obtained via the brachial vein. Place the bird on a table and align the humerus to face directly at the person who will withdraw the blood (Fig. 18.13). A few feathers may be plucked to expose the vein.

Artificial insemination is a common practice in commercial turkey production. Adult breeder males (toms) must be ejaculated and females (hens) inseminated. When hand-holding a hen for artificial insemination, place her body between your legs with the breast toward you (Fig. 18.14). The vent is everted for the insemination by abdominal pressure. The tom may be held in a similar manner to force ejaculation, but since toms are heavier they are usually laid on a table (Fig. 18.15), in a trough, or on a handler's lap.

To administer oral medication, hold the turkey across the lap while sitting. Hold both of the turkey's legs near its body with one hand, stretching the head and neck straight out with the other hand. An assistant then inserts a plastic tube containing the measured dose of medication through the mouth and into the crop. Hold a finger over the end of the tube to retain the fluid. When the tube is in place, remove the finger and gravity will empty the contents into the crop. The tube should be 25–27 cm (10–14 in.) long and 10 mm (3/8 in.) in diameter. Tablets can be given by pressing them into the esophagus, using the forefinger as a plunger.

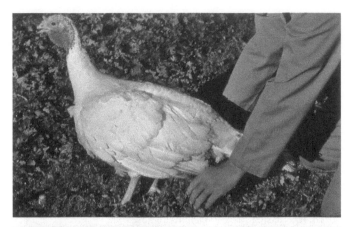

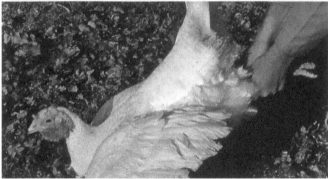

FIG. 18.12.   To capture turkey in close quarters, kneel behind bird and grasp both legs, which will cause the bird to fall to its breast.

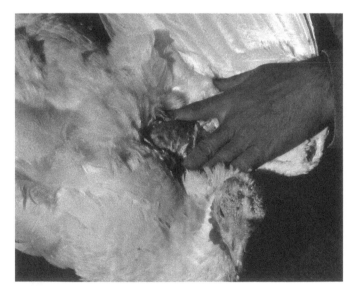

FIG. 18.13.   Turkey held in position for venipuncture of the brachial vein.

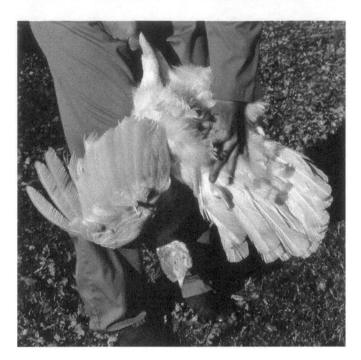

FIG. 18.14.   Hen turkey held for artificial insemination.

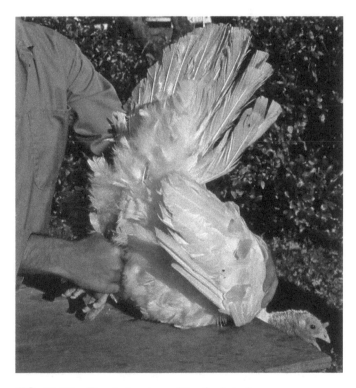

FIG. 18.15.   Tom turkey in position for inducing ejaculation.

Waterfowl[1]

Ducks and geese may be captured with nets or hooks (Figs. 18.16, 18.17). Alternatively, they may be grasped by the neck (Fig. 18.18, left; Fig. 18.19, left). If the goose is to be held for some time, or carried, grasp the wings (Fig. 18.18, right) or the legs and neck.

A large goose should be supported by the neck and wings when it is lifted (Fig. 18.18). If a heavy-bodied bird struggles, cervical injury may result. If the bird is to be carried, support the body (Figs. 18.20, 18.21); the legs may flail, but they will not injure. Keep the head of a goose restrained at all times to prevent it from reaching around to peck at your face or eyes.

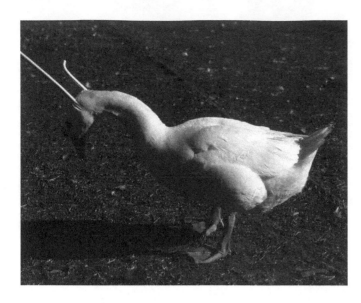

FIG. 18.16. Using hook to capture a goose.

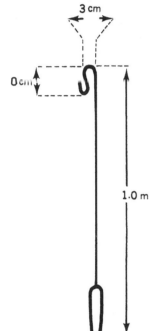

FIG. 18.17. Diagram of hook used to capture waterfowl.

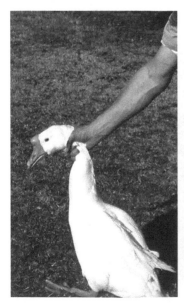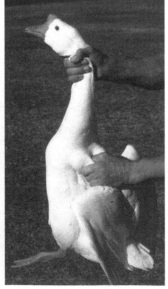

FIG. 18.18. Holding a goose by the neck.

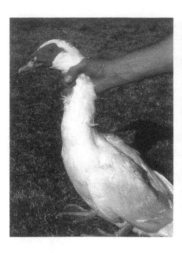
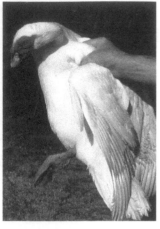

FIG. 18.19. Holding a duck by the neck, left. Lifting a duck by the wings, right.

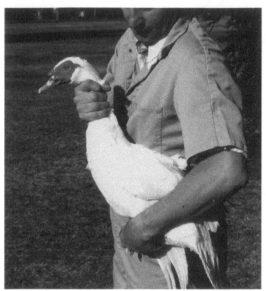

FIG. 18.20. Carrying duck by controlling head, feet, and wings.

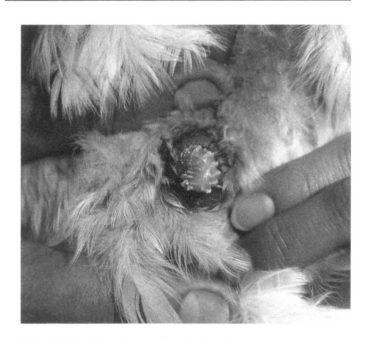

FIG. 18.22. Exposing phallus (penis) of a gander.

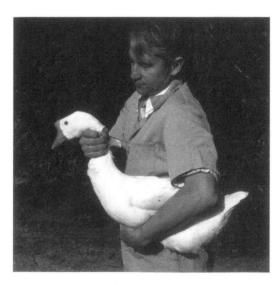

FIG. 18.21. Goose can be carried by supporting the body and controlling wings and head.

Birds frequently defecate when handled, so hold the bird in a manner that will prevent contamination of clothing.

Waterfowl may be sexed by everting the cloaca and prolapsing the phallus (penis) (Fig. 18.22).

RELEASING BIRDS

Safe release from restraint is as important as safe capture. While holding a wing and both legs, bend over and, as the bird nears the ground, release first the legs, then the wing.

TRANSPORT

Special crates have been designed for transporting poultry and waterfowl to commercial processing plants. An individual pet bird may be placed in a cardboard box or put into a burlap or cloth sack. A hole is usually cut out of a corner of the sack to allow the head of a swan, goose, or turkey to protrude. This is not necessary for chickens or ducks.

A sacked bird transported in a closed automobile trunk on a hot day is threatened with hyperthermia and endangered from carbon monoxide fumes.

CHEMICAL RESTRAINT

Restraint drugs are not used for routine handling of poultry and waterfowl.

Ketamine hydrochloride (50 mg/kg) is used as a sedative and preanesthetic medication. Anesthesia may be induced and/or maintained with isoflurane via a face mask or tracheal intubation.

REFERENCES

1. Grow, O. 1972. Modern Waterfowl Management. Chicago: American Bantam Association.
2. Leahy, J.R., and Barrow, P. 1954. Restraint of Animals, 2nd ed. Ithaca, N.Y.: Cornell Campus Store.

PART 3

Wild Animals

CHAPTER 19
Delivery Systems[1,3,4–15]

The first challenge facing anyone using chemical agents for immobilization and restraint is to administer the drug agent in a site that allows absorption. The most satisfactory technique varies from species to species and from animal to animal, according to size, distance from the operator, ability to partially confine the animal, operator skill, and effectiveness of available equipment.

ORAL

As a young practitioner, I tried oral chemical restraint for the first time in order to treat a semi-tame 40-pound juvenile chimpanzee suffering from a diseased tooth. The effective dose of phenobarbital was carefully calculated and a tablet hidden in a piece of banana. The chimpanzee readily accepted the banana and began eating it greedily. I noted that the piece containing the tablet had been taken into the mouth and gloated that I would soon have the animal in hand. As I continued to watch, the animal began chewing more carefully. In a moment the tablet appeared on her lips, and she reached up, picked the tablet out, and flipped it away in a single motion.

Numerous subsequent experiences have taught me the general futility of depending on oral medication to immobilize wild animals. Aside from the lack of acceptance of such drugs by many species, the effectiveness of oral medication is often minimal, since many chemical restraint agents are either unabsorbed or destroyed in the digestive tract. Degree of absorption may also depend on the quantity of other ingesta in the stomach.

However, sometimes oral medication is the only available choice. Some primates may be provoked to come to the side of an enclosure and scream at a strange or disliked person (usually the veterinarian), allowing medication to be squirted into the mouth. Though some of the drug may be lost, enough may be ingested to effect sedation or immobilization.

A city pond was the scene of a month-long saga involving a duck with an arrow impaled in its breast muscle. She eluded capture attempts until a recommendation was made to soak pieces of bread with a solution of amobarbital sodium (Amytal), a sleep-inducing medication (Fig. 19.1). The ducks on the pond were baited with unmedicated bread until all would readily accept the offering. Then the medicated bread was tossed to the impaled duck. Within minutes the drug took effect, and the duck was netted before her head dropped into the water.

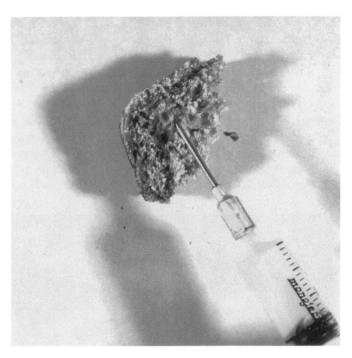

FIG. 19.1. Impregnating a piece of bread with a sedative.

Nonhuman primates are frequently conditioned to accept fruit juices and yogurt for treats and as a means of medication. Diazepam may be used as a calming drug an hour prior to anticipated immobilization. This is particularly useful in animals that normally become agitated at the prospect of immobilization.

Drugs may be placed in the food of carnivores and other species to quiet or immobilize them. However, since other delivery systems now available are more satisfactory, oral administration is generally used only for premedication.

Hand-held Syringe

Intramuscular injections may be administered quickly with a syringe held in the hand. Veterinarians accustomed to aspirating before injection, must recognize that this is not possible with wild animals. A plastic syringe will not break if knocked from the hand or if an animal kicks, strikes, or pushes it into the side of a cage. Use a large-gauge (18+) needle to deliver the liquid in the syringe quickly and use the largest syringe that will measure the quantity accurately. The plunger will have less distance to travel, and a greater

219

mechanical advantage will be obtained. Tighten the needle securely on the hub, so the pressure buildup by rapid injection will not blow the needle from the syringe.

Hand-held syringes and quick intramuscular and subcutaneous injections are commonly used for vaccinating sheep, swine, and beef cattle in chutes. Similar techniques can be used to administer drugs quickly to animals held in stalls or stanchions before they become overly excited. While standing at one side, reach across and give the injection on the opposite side of the animal's body (most animals kick out with the leg on the side pricked by the needle).

The technique follows: Grasp the syringe as indicated in Figure 19.2. Be prepared to press the plunger at the same time the needle is thrust through the skin. Many animals that have been previously injected are wary. Conceal the syringe when approaching primates or carnivores. If the animal is in a cage, wait for it to present a suitable muscular area near the side of the cage. Quickly jab the needle through the skin and at the same time make the injection. The animal will jump away, but if the thrust has been properly made, the medication will be injected before the animal can react.

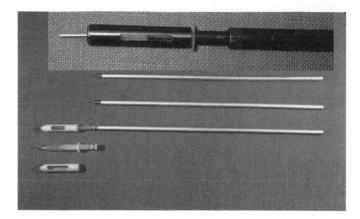

FIG. 19.3. Different types of pole or stick syringes.

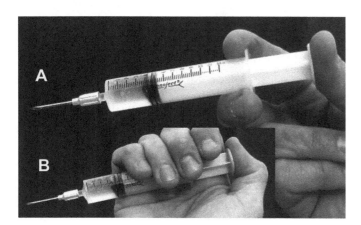

FIG. 19.2. Hand-held syringe for quick injection. **A.** proper method, **B.** Improper grasp of the syringe.

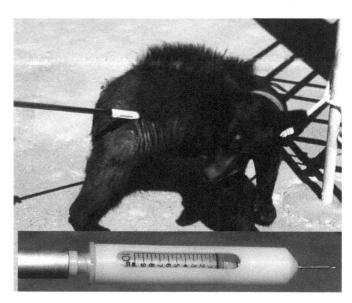

FIG. 19.4. Chemical immobilization utilizing a pole syringe.

Do not hold the syringe as illustrated in Figure 19.2B. If the animal moves, the needle may break off, or the needle may lacerate the skin or muscle. Such a hold also restricts the flexibility of the direction of thrust.

Stick Syringe (Pole Syringe)

Various homemade and commercial stick syringes act as extensions of the hand for administering drugs to dangerous animals (Figs. 19.3, 19.4). All of these syringes work on the principle of injection immediately upon insertion of the needle. A quick jab is necessary to effect administration. The operator must maintain pressure against the animal until all the solution has been injected or until the animal jumps away. If the animal jumps away before all the solution is injected, a second injection is necessary. Sharp, large-bore needles should be used for easy insertion and immediate expulsion of the drug. In many instances the animal reaches around and

bites at the syringe, damaging it. Occasionally an animal bites off the syringe and may swallow it. Hoofed animals are likely to kick out, and the quick movement may bend the needle. The needle may break off, but most devices have protecting shields around the needle to enclose and support the hub.

Blowgun[5]

Variations of the blowgun and poisoned darts have been used for both warfare and food gathering for centuries in primitive cultures (Fig. 19.5). The blowgun has now become popular with animal restrainers, since it offers certain advantages over other delivery systems.

A major advantage of the blowgun is silent projection with minimal trauma upon impact. It is adaptable for use on small animals, easily sighted, and has no mechanical parts to malfunction or that require maintenance. The only disadvantages of the blowgun are its length, short range, and the skill

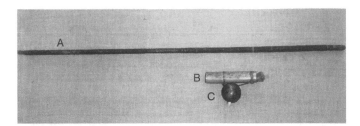

FIG. 19.5. Blowgun used by Ecuadorian Indians in the early 1900s: **A.** 2-m blowgun made by wrapping two pieces of hollowed bamboo with plant fiber yarn. **B.** Quiver to hold arrows. **C.** Hollow dried gourd. Tailpiece is made by inserting non-tipped end into a cottony plant fiber and twisting as one would make a cotton-tipped applicator stick.

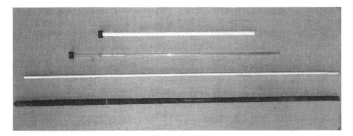

FIG. 19.6. Tubing used for blowguns: top to bottom: polyvinyl chloride plastic, Plexiglass, aluminum electrical conduit tubing, and bamboo tubing.

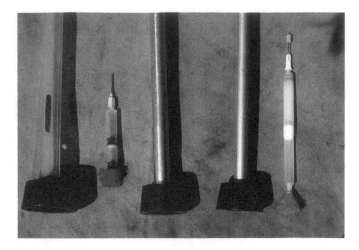

FIG. 19.7. Blowguns with mouthpieces using rubber corks. Syringes may be homemade or purchased commercially.

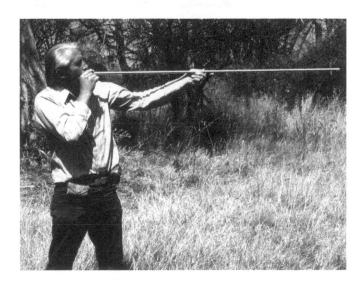

FIG. 19.8. Using a blowgun.

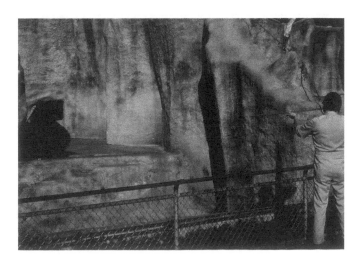

FIG. 19.9. Immobilizing a bear using a blowgun.

required of the operator. It is unwieldy in confined spaces, and the range is limited to approximately 13.7 m (15 yd). Blowguns may be purchased commercially, but aluminum, copper, stainless steel, plastic, or other types of tubing of appropriate diameter are satisfactory (Fig. 19.6). The inside of the tube must be smooth, polished if necessary, to minimize friction as the syringe is blown through it. A mouthpiece on the tube permits development of greater pressure for propulsion. The mouthpiece may be constructed from a rubber cork (Fig. 19.7).

The length of the blowgun is determined by the distance required to project the syringe, varying from 1 to 2 m (3 to 6 ft). The longer tube permits greater accuracy (Fig. 19.8). The maximum range varies with the length of the tubing and the skill of the operator, but 13.7 m (15 yd) is maximum. A blowgun may be used for chemical immobilization or medication. Figures 19.8, 19.9, and 19.10 illustrate the blowgun in use. If there is any bowing of the tube, keep the convex side of the arch lowest. Sight with both eyes open, and focus on the end of the tube.

Various commercial and home-designed syringes are used with blowguns, as shown in Figures 19.11 and 19.12.

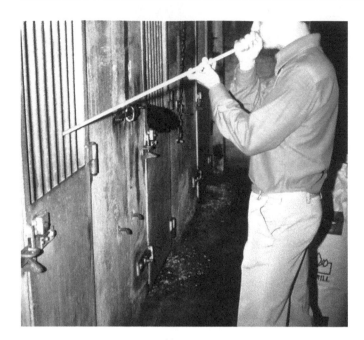

FIG. 19.10.   Immobilizing a chimpanzee using a blowgun. One must observe the movements of the animal and be prepared to project the dart at a place where the animal pauses for a moment.

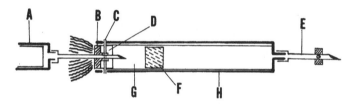

FIG. 19.11.   Haigh-designed syringe for use in blowgun: **A.** Standard syringe. **B.** Yarn stuffed into rubber plunger. **C.** Disposable needle, ends broken off. **D.** Plunger from disposable syringe. **E.** Special needle, plugged at the tip and hole bored in the side. **F.** Another syringe plunger. **G.** Chamber for injecting air or butane as ejection propellant. **H.** Disposable plastic syringe with flange removed.

Projected Syringes or Darts[6,10,15]

Equipment capable of projecting a syringe some distance and discharging the contents upon impact is essential for modern chemical restraint of wild animals. The first suitable weapons were developed by Jack Crockford and coworkers.[2] Palmer Cap-Chur equipment was the first standard equipment used in the United States, but many other systems are in use today.

There are three types of Palmer projectors (Fig. 19.13). The short-range projector (pistol) is a modified pellet gun powered by compressed carbon dioxide. The range is 13.7 m (15 yd). The long-range projector (rifle) is also powered by compressed carbon dioxide. The range is 32 m (35 yd). The extra-long-range projector is powered by percussion caps, as shown in the middle image in Figure 19.13. The strength of

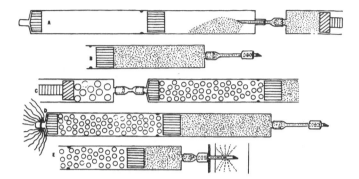

FIG. 19.12.   Diagram of a Telinject syringe. **A.** Filling the forward chamber with a drug. **B.** Drug filled and capped needle attached. **C.** Pressurizing the rear chamber with air from another syringe. **D.** Completed syringe, ready to project. **E.** Syringe strikes the skin and pushes the sleeve to expose the side port.

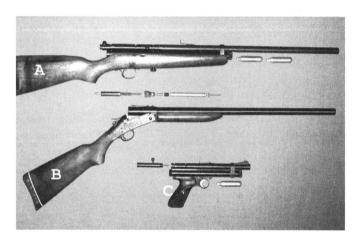

FIG. 19.13.   Palmer Cap-Chur projectors: Long range, carbon dioxide-powered, top; extra long range, powder cap-charged, middle; and short range, carbon dioxide-powered, bottom.

the caps varies according to the distance from the target. The maximum range is 73 m (80 yd).

Both the long-range rifle and the short-range pistol are loaded with the filled syringe. The breech (mechanism) is closed and the weapon cocked, sighted, and fired. When using the extra-long-range projector, the syringe is placed in the barrel with a special adaptor inserted behind it. A 0.22 blank charge is placed in the adaptor. The breech is closed and the weapon cocked, sighted, and fired. Detailed instructions on the use of the equipment are included in the instruction manual provided by the company.

The syringe itself is made up of the components illustrated in Figure 19.14. The syringe charge works on the principle illustrated in Figure 21.14B. When the syringe strikes the target, pressure against the hub of the syringe forces a small weight in back of the charge forward against a tiny spring. The sharp tip of the weight penetrates a seal, setting

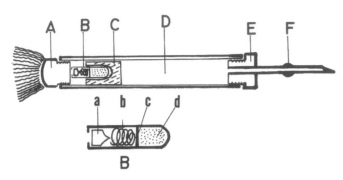

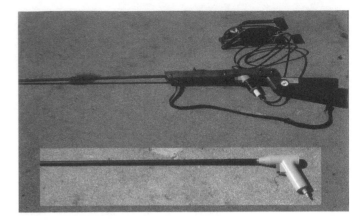

FIG. 19.14. Diagram of the mechanism of a CapChur syringe: **A.** Tailpiece. **B.** Ejection charge: (a) sharpened weight, (b) coiled spring to keep weight separated from (c) diaphragm to contain (d) charge. **C.** Plunger. **D.** Chamber for medication. **E.** Nosepiece hub. **F.** Collared needle.

FIG. 19.16. Telinject weapons utilizing compressed air power.

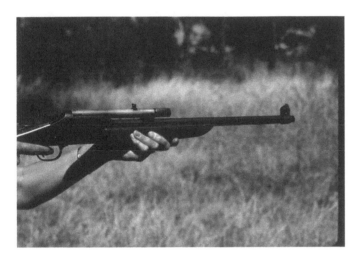

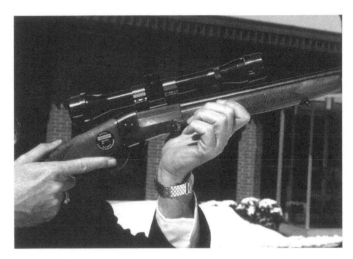

FIG. 19.15. Zulu Arms rifle (M4) with adjustable power to propel the syringe.

FIG. 19.17. Distinject rifle.

off the charge and driving the plunger forward to discharge the liquid from the syringe. If the charge is improperly placed in the neoprene plunger, the discharge will occur when the projectile is expelled from the weapon.

The Zuluarms rifle utilizes a modified over/under combination 0.22-caliber rifle and 28-gauge shotgun (Fig. 19.15). The rifle barrel is modified to serve as the power chamber (utilizing 0.22 blanks) and the shotgun barrel for the projectile. This is a well-balanced weapon that has a device for controlling the charge to the projectile chamber to allow use at distances ranging from 2 to 50 m.

Much of the immobilization within conventional zoos is accomplished by the use of systems in which compressed air or carbon dioxide cartridges provide a noiseless propelling charge. The drug is also expelled from the syringe with compressed air.

Other systems marketed in the United States include the Telinject system, as shown in Figure 19.16; the Distinject rifle, as shown in Figure 19.17; the Distinject darts, as shown

in Figure 19.18; and the Pneudart system. Another system is the PaxArms pistol manufactured in New Zealand (Fig. 19.19). Specially designed syringes spread out the impact area by allowing flanges to extrude after the dart leaves the barrel of the rifle (Fig. 19.18). Another syringe (bottom) has a collapsible rubber cup containing a dye. When the syringe strikes the animal, the dye is extruded, indicating that the animal has been injected. This is valuable when vaccinating multiple animals.

Crossbow

The crossbow has been adapted for use with various types of syringes (Fig. 19.20). Crossbows are accurate and silent. Tension may be adjusted on some models according to target distance. The disadvantages of crossbows are that they are bulky, difficult to manipulate in a restricted space, and require considerable strength to tense the bowstring.

Needles are of variable length depending on the species of animal to be immobilized (Fig. 19.21). All must have a large inside diameter so that the drug is expelled quickly.

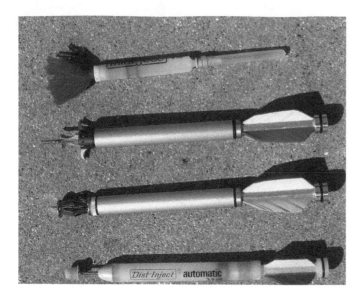

FIG. 19.18. Syringes manufactured by the Distinject company.

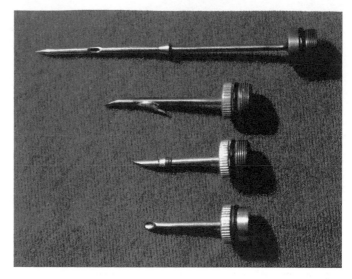

FIG. 19.21. Needles used with the Palmer CapChur system.

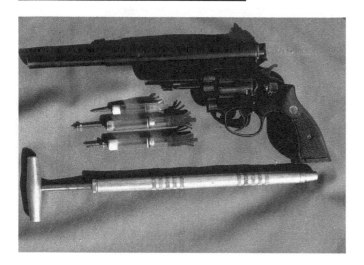

FIG. 19.19. The PaxArms pistol with syringes and a pump to charge the weapon with compressed air.

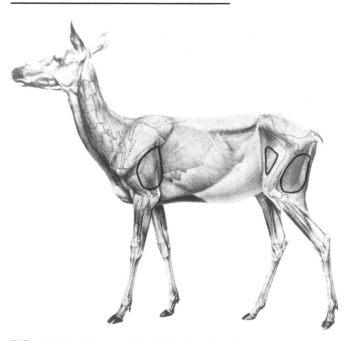

FIG. 19.22. Diagram of suitable injection sites for a deer.

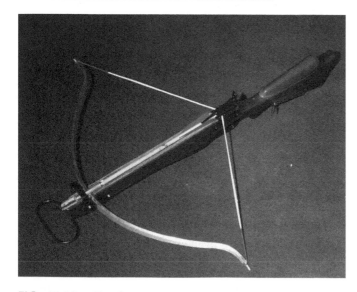

FIG. 19.20. Crossbow.

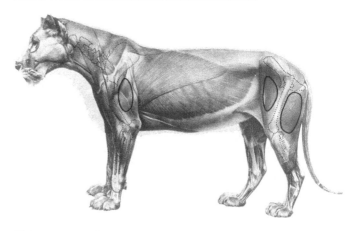

FIG. 19.23. Diagram of suitable injection sites for a carnivore.

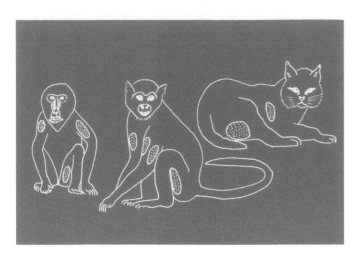

FIG. 19.24. Injection sites for primates and small carnivores.

Needles may have collars or barbs to prevent the syringe from bouncing away from the injection site before all of the drug is expelled. Barbed needles may require minor surgery for removal from the skin.

Most chemical immobilizing agents are designed for intramuscular absorption. Any large muscle mass is suitable as illustrated in Figures 19.22 to 19.24. For shooting from a helicopter, aim for the dorsal gluteal muscles or the back muscles on either side of the spinous processes of the vertebrae.

REFERENCES

1. Anderson, R.S., and Edney, A.T.B., Eds. 1991. Practical Animal Handling, 1st ed. Oxford, U.K. Pergamon Press, 198 pages, hardback.
2. Crockford, J.A., Hayes, F.A., Jenkins, J.H., and Feurt, S.W. 1958. An automatic projectile type syringe. Vet Med 53:115–19.
3. Ebedes, H. 2006. Recommendations for live game auctions. In: Kock, M.D., Meltzer, D., and Burroughs, R. Chemical and Physical Restraint—A training field manual. Greyton, South Africa, International Wildlife Veterinary Services, pp. 260–65.
4. Fowler, M.E. 1982. Delivery systems for chemical immobilization. In: Nielsen, L., Haigh, J.C., and Fowler, M.E., Eds. Chemical Immobilization of North American Wildlife, pp. 18–45. Milwaukee: Wisconsin Humane Soc.
5. Haigh, J.C., and Hopf, H.C. 1976. The blowgun in veterinary practice: Its uses and preparation. J Am Vet Med Assoc 169:881–83.
6. Harthoorn, A.M. 1970. The Flying Syringe. London: Geoffrey Bles.
7. Isaza, R. 2007. Remote drug delivery. In: West, G., Heard, D., and Caulkett, N. Zoo Animal and Wildlife Immobilization and Anesthesia. Ames, Iowa, Blackwell Publishing, pp. 61–74.
8. La Grange, M. 2006. Overview of capture methods and transport of wild animals. In: Kock, M.D., Meltzer, D., and Burroughs, R. Chemical and Physical Restraint—A training field manual. Greyton, South Africa, International Wildlife Veterinary Services, pp. 250–59.
9. Leahy, J.R., and Barrow, P. 1953. Restraint of Animals. Ithaca, New York. Cornell Campus store.
10. Lord, W. 1958. The historical development of an instrument for live capture of animals. Southeast Vet 9:147–49.
11. Rohr, F., and McKenzie, A.A. 1993. Remote injection equipment. In: McKenzie, A.A., 1993. The Capture and Care Manual. Pretoria, South African Veterinary Foundation, pp.116–30.
12. Sheldon, C.C., Sonsthagen, T., and Topel, J.A. Animal Restraint for Veterinary Professionals. 2006. St. Louis, Mosby/Elsevier, 239 pages.
13. Short, R.V., and King, J.M. 1964. The design of a crossbow and dart for immobilization of wild animals. Vet. Rec. 76:628–30.
14. Sonsthagen, T.F. 1991. Restraint of Domestic Animals. Goleta, California, American Veterinary Publications, 149 pages, paperback.
15. Young, E., Ed. 1973. The Capture and Care of Wild Animals. Capetown, South Africa: Human and Rousseau.

CHAPTER 20
Chemical Restraint

The use of drugs for restraint and immobilization has become routine for practicing wild animal veterinarians and wildlife biologists. Commonly used drugs now permit manipulative procedures that were heretofore impossible. The lives of many animals have been spared by the judicious use of drugs that minimize stress and trauma.

Although many of these agents have been widely used only during the past 50 years, restraint drugs are not new. Immobilizing agents have been used since ancient times. Primitive hunters treated the tips of arrows with poisonous extracts from plants and animals (Fig. 20.1). The art of poison-arrow hunting was practiced primarily in Africa and South America, and poisoned darts are still used by native hunters

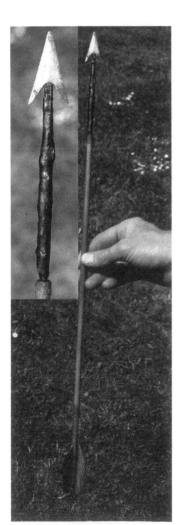

FIG. 20.1. Poisoned arrow used for hunting.

and poachers on both continents. The concentration of toxic agents in poison-dart mixtures was extremely variable, depending on the hunter's source and method of preparation. Analyses of some arrows found in Africa yielded as much as 5 g of ouabain (cardioactive glycoside) on one tip. The lethal dose for an adult human is 0.002 g.

The species of plant and animal sources of poisonous extracts were kept secret for decades. Even after the species were identified, techniques of modern chemistry were required to solve the riddles of the toxic principles.

South American hunters used plants (*Strychnos toxifera* and *Chondrodendron tomentosum*) containing curare. In some areas, hunters also collected frogs (*Dendrobates* spp.) that produced cardioactive glycosides in skin glands.

In Africa, plants (*Acocanthera* spp. and *Strophanthus* spp.) containing potent cardioactive glycosides were used. Snake venoms and other animal extracts were added to the concoctions in some instances. Small animals and birds injected with poison arrows died in as short a time as 15 minutes. Elephants sometimes survived for days.

Curare and its various derivatives were among the earliest chemical restraint agents used at the beginning of the present era.[18] Curare has many deficiencies as a restraint agent. It neither sedates nor anesthetizes, but merely paralyzes the animal. Therefore it is hazardous to use, since alarm responses, psychogenic stimulation, and other detrimental physiological neural functions continue unabated. Furthermore, the therapeutic index of curare is narrow. Respiratory arrest is common, and unless rapid assistance is provided, the animal is likely to die.

Curare is never used for chemical immobilization today, yet the techniques for drug delivery and the experience gained from working with this drug served as the foundation for modern chemical restraint practices.

This chapter is not meant to be a definitive work or a technical reference on the use of chemical agents in restraint. Books and journal articles on the development and current usage of restraint agents are available, and should be consulted.[14,24–38,47] Various computerized bibliographic services will provide references on specific animals. Articles on new drugs appear frequently. Only review or general papers and books will be used as references in this chapter. Definitions of some terms are given at the end of the chapter.

Much credit should be given to the pioneers in the development of chemical restraint agents and delivery systems.[24,27,47] Today the clinician and biologist have drugs and delivery

227

systems to fit almost any need. Some who use them do not realize the endless toil, frustration, expense, and persistence that was necessary to reach the present state of the art.

Even more important, one need not experiment or take needless risks with valuable animals by trying one drug after another. Collectively, there are persons with immobilization experience in nearly every class of vertebrates. Individuals cannot morally, ethically, or economically gain all of this experience, particularly at the expense of the lives of animals. When faced with a unique immobilization problem, help should be sought from the literature or from veterinarians at large zoos.

THE IDEAL RESTRAINT DRUG[19]

An ideal drug should have a high therapeutic index (TI) (TI = lethal dose/effective dose). A high TI allows a margin for error in estimating body weight or for individual variations in physiological response. In order to increase the TI, many chemical restraint agents are combined with other agents; combination often decreases the required dose of each agent, while increasing the effectiveness of the drugs. Therefore, the ideal restraint drug should be compatible with other useful drugs.

Because the majority of chemical restraint agents are administered intramuscularly, the ideal drug should not irritate muscle tissue. Most currently used agents meet this qualification. Some agents sting (diazepam) or cause transient local pain upon injection but cause no damage. Though a solution may not be irritating in itself, liquid injected with excessive pressure may tear muscle fibers. This may occur if charges higher than necessary are used to expel the fluid from a syringe delivered remotely. Muscle and skin may also be bruised by the impact of the syringe.

A short induction period is desirable. Movies and television programs have fostered the belief that darted animals fall immediately. With chemical restraint agents currently available, immobilization is effected 10–20 minutes following muscular injection. This time lapse allows some of the more fleet-footed animals to run for miles if unconfined. This is also a serious drawback when working with free-ranging wild animals, because after the animal is injected, it may escape into the bush and be lost to the restrainer. Furthermore, the unassisted animal may die from respiratory depression or be killed by a predator while under the influence of the drug.

The ideal drug should have an available antagonist or reversal agent, and pharmacologic investigations have indeed developed numerous reversal agents during the past 10 years. Antagonists are now available for narcotics (etorphine, carfentanil), α2 agonists (xylazine, detomidine), and benzodiazepine agents (diazepam, zolazepam).

Solution stability is important. Many restraint drugs must be used in situations where refrigeration is not available. The ideal drug should remain stable in solution for long periods.

Finally, the concentration of the ideal drug should be high enough or the effective dose be low enough to allow its use in the small-volume syringes necessary for dart injection.

That absolutely ideal drug has yet to be found. However, for individual species, one or another drug meets most of the qualifications.

INDIVIDUAL DRUG DESCRIPTION[1,5,8–11,21,27–33,39–44]

Table 20.1 lists drugs used for chemical immobilization either alone or in combination with other agents. Table 20.2 classifies tranquilizers used in animal handling. Companies supplying these agents are listed in Appendix C. Some drugs that are prohibited in the United States are available in other countries; they may not be available to practitioners in the United States at the moment because of various manufacturing, distribution, or legal problems.

Although it is possible to predict the pharmacological effect of a given drug from experimental reactions observed, it is an entirely different matter to predict the specific effects of the drug under field conditions. The physiological,

TABLE 20.1. Chemical immobilizing agents

Parent Compound	Generic Name	Trade Name	Source	How supplied
Opiates (narcotics)	Etorphine HCl	M99	Wildlife Pharmaceuticals	1 mg/ml, 10 ml
	Etorphine/acepromazine	Large Animal Immobilon[a]	Reckitt-Coleman	E-2.45, A-10 mg/ml
	Etorphine/Methotrimeprazine	Small Animal Immobilon[a]	Reckitt-Coleman	E-0.07, M-18 mg/ml
	Fentanyl citrate	Sublimaze		
	Fentanyl/droperidol	Innovar	Pitman Moore	F-0.4, D-20 mg/ml
	Carfentanil	Wildnil	Wildlife Pharmaceuticals	3 mg/ml, 10 ml
	Thiafentanil[b]	A3080	Wildlife Pharmaceuticals	
	Butorphanol tartrate	Torbugesic	Fort Dodge Laboratories	10 mg/ml, 50 ml
		Stadol	Mead Johnson	2 mg/ml, 10 ml
Cyclohexamines	Ketamine HCL	Ketaset	Bristol Laboratories	100 mg/ml, 10 ml
	Tiletamine/zolazepam[c]	Telazol	Wildlife Pharmaceuticals	100 mg/ml, 5 ml
α2 Adrenoceptor agonist	Xylazine HCl	Rompun	Wildlife Pharmaceuticals	300 mg/ml, 30 ml
	Detomidine	Dormosedan	SmithKline & Beecham	10 mg/ml, 20 ml
	Medetomidine	Domitor	Wildlife Pharmaceuticals	20 mg/ml, 5 ml

[a] Not available in the United States.
[b] Used experimentally only.
[c] Used only in combinations.

TABLE 20.2. Classification of tranquilizers used in animal handling

Parent Compound	Generic Name	Trade Name in the U.S.	Manufacturer or Distributor in the U.S.	How Supplied
Phenothiazine	Acepromazine maleate	PromAce	Aveco Co.	10 mg/ml, 50 ml
	Propionylpromazine	Combelen	Bayer	
	Perphenazine enanthate	Trilafon	Schering Corp.	5 mg/ml
	Pipothiazine palmitate[a]	Pipertii depot	May-Baker	
	Zuciopenthixol acetate[a]	Clopixol		
	Butyrophenone	Droperidol/Inapsine	Janssen	2.5 mg/ml
	Azaperone	Stresnil	Wildlife Pharmaceuticals	100 mg/ml, 20 ml
	Haloperidol lactate	Haldol	Wildlife Pharmaceuticals	5 mg/ml, 10 ml
Benzodiazepine	Diazepam	Valium	Roche Inc.	5 mg/ml, 10 ml
	Zolazepam	Telazol	Wildlife Pharmaceuticals	100 mg/ml
	Midazolam HC1	Versed	Wildlife Pharmaceuticals	1 & 5 mg/ml
Imidazole	Xylazine HC1	Rompun	Wildlife Pharmaceuticals	300 mg/ml, 30 ml
	Detomidine HC1	Dormosedan	SmithKline & Beecham	10 mg/ml, 20 ml
	Medetomidine	Domitor	Wildlife Pharmaceuticals	40 mg/ml, 3 ml

[a] Not available in the United States.

physical, and emotional condition of the animal alters the effect of any drug.

Narcotic (Opiate) Immobilizing Agents

ETORPHINE HYDROCHLORIDE (M99, IMMOBILON).[8,11,19,26,27,32,34,35,42,43] Large Animal Immobilon (etorphine plus acepromazine) is in use in Europe and Africa.

Chemistry. The formula for etorphine is tetrahydro7a-(1-hydroxy-1-methylbutyl)-6,14 endoethenooripavine hydrochloride. It is a synthetic derivative of one of the opium alkaloids (thebaine). Etorphine is a powder, readily soluble in slightly acidified water. The solution as supplied by the manufacturer is stable and may be stored at room temperature for years.

Pharmacology. Etorphine is a highly potent analgesic, with up to 10,000 times the analgesic potency of morphine hydrochloride. Etorphine produces pharmacological effects similar to those of morphine, namely, depression of the respiratory and cough centers, decreased gastrointestinal motility, and behavioral changes. Stimulation or depression of the central nervous system (CNS) varies with the species. The elephant is depressed, the eland and nyala may be stimulated to aimless walking or running, and aggressive animals usually become tractable. In addition, blood pressure is elevated, accompanied by tachycardia.

Indications. Etorphine has been tested in a wide range of species. It is particularly useful for immobilizing large ungulates such as the elephant, rhinoceros, or hippopotamus. It has been given to most species of artiodactylids with varying degrees of efficacy and safety. Etorphine is the author's preferred immobilizing agent for large bears.

Administration. Etorphine is readily absorbed from any intramuscular site. An elephant has been maintained in surgical anesthesia for as long as 4 hours by intermittent intravenous injections (1 mg every 15 minutes) or by continuous drip injection (4 mg etorphine hydrochloride in 250 ml of 0.9% sodium chloride solution, given at 1 drop per second or 1 mg every 15 minutes).[10]

The triceps muscle mass is recommended for injection of etorphine (or any immobilizing agent) in bears.[18] The likelihood of an intra-fat injection is quite high when the rear limb is used. Drug response is highly variable when the hind limb is the injection site.

Onset of anesthesia occurs 10–20 minutes after intramuscular injection. If no antagonist is administered, recovery is slow, up to 3 hours. When the antagonist is injected, the animal becomes ambulatory within 4–10 minutes.

Etorphine should not be mixed with atropine, because atropine reduces the solubility of etorphine.

Side Effects. The excitement noted in the horse and cat with the use of morphine also may be observed following administration of etorphine. This effect is dose related. Minimal doses for a species may result in excitement, tremors, and convulsions. Aimless walking or running has been observed, continuing until the animal is physically restrained (Fig. 20.2).

Inhibition of respiratory centers may directly or indirectly influence blood gases and acid-base balance. Reflex vomiting, a common disturbing side effect in morphine administration, is rare with etorphine. However, passive regurgitation is not unusual, particularly with prolonged immobilization with etorphine, probably the result of total relaxation of the cardiac sphincter of the stomach, coupled with abdominal pressure.

As with most other agents, fatal hyperthermia may occur with etorphine. An animal that has been chased or is highly excited at the time of immobilization experiences a severe buildup of body heat. Body insulation and central depression of thermoregulatory systems may inhibit heat dissipation. Smaller animals are more prone than larger species to thermal stress following the use of any chemical restraint agent.

Renarcotization. Animals immobilized with etorphine or other opiates may become renarcotized (recycling) a few hours following reversal. Renarcotization refers to the

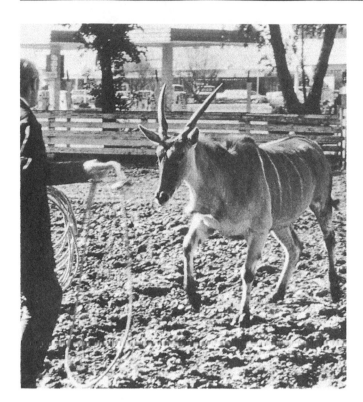

FIG. 20.2. This eland was in the aimless-walking stage of immobilization with etorphine. The animal was roped and subdued in lieu of further drugging.

resurgence of the effect of an opiate restraint agent following the administration of an antagonist (reversal agent). The causes may be numerous but generally involve the pharmacodynamics of the agonist and antagonist as follows:

1. The antagonist action subsides while there is still agonistic action.
2. The dose of the antagonist may be too low to completely counteract that of the agonist.
3. If the opiate was deposited in a site allowing slow absorption into the circulatory system (fat, subcutis), the antagonist action may cease while the agonist is still being absorbed.

Renarcotization allows the action of the opiate to continue, but only to the excitement phase, producing muscle rigidity, excessive but incoordinated muscular activity, hypertension, hyperthermia, and excessive metabolic activity leading to exhaustion and possible death. The excessive muscle activity may cause a syndrome similar to exertional myopathy with its accompanying metabolic changes that may have dire consequences to electrolytes and acid/base balance.

Etorphine is extremely dangerous to human beings. If anyone is injected accidentally, immediate medical help is essential. Etorphine, or any narcotic, should not be handled without having naloxone hydrochloride or naltrexone immediately available. In the event of an accidental injection, an initial injection of 1 mg of naloxone should be administered, followed by injections of 0.4–0.8 mg every 2–4 minutes until the victim is under hospital management. Equipment for artificial respiration should be available to deal with possible respiratory arrest.

Etorphine is readily absorbed through mucous membranes and also may be absorbed through abraded or lacerated skin. Avoid inhalation, ingestion, or contamination of the skin, particularly of the hands, which might touch the mouth. Rubber gloves should be worn when loading or washing syringes.

Antagonist. Diprenorphine (M50–50) is a specific antagonist developed for etorphine (Table 20.3). The standard dose is double the amount of etorphine injected. If diprenorphine is unavailable, naltrexone, naloxone, or nalorphine may be used.

CARFENTANIL (WILDNIL)[30–32,34,40,42,43]

Chemistry. Carfentanil is a synthetic derivative of fentanyl. Methyl 4-(1-oxopropyl) phenylaminol-1-(2 phenylethyl)-4 piperdine carboxylate-2 hydroxy-1,2,3, propanethricarbonate.

Pharmacology. Similar to etorphine, it is the most potent agent being used for immobilization in the United States. Rating fentanyl as 1 in potency, etorphine would be 15 times and carfentanil 20 times as potent.

TABLE 20.3. Antagonist/reversal agents used in animal handling

Generic Name	Trade Name	Reversal Group	Source
Diprenorphine HCl	M50–50 Revivon[a]	Opiates (etorphine)	Lemmon Corp. Reckitt & Coleman
Naloxone HCl	Narcan Narcan	Opiates	Wildlife Pharmaceuticals Abbott Laboratories
Naltrexone HCl	Trexanb	Opiates	Wildlife Pharmaceuticals
Yohimbine HCl	Antagonil Yobine	α2 agonists	Wildlife Pharmaceuticals Lloyd Laboratories
Atipamezole	Antisedan	α2 agonists	Wildlife Pharmaceuticals
Tolazoline HCl	Priscolene	α2 agonists	Wildlife Pharmaceuticals
Flumazenil	Mazicon	Benzodiazepine	(diazepam)Hoffman La Roche

[a]Not available in substance schedule. U.S.

Indications. Carfentanil became the opiate of choice when etorphine was temporarily unavailable in the United States. It is used for the immobilization of large ungulates, particularly cervids. It is usually combined with xylazine or another α2 agonist or a tranquilizer to smooth out induction and recovery.

Administration. Carfentanil may be administered via any parenteral route, preferably deep intramuscular.

Side Effects and Precautions. Side effects are similar to those produced by etorphine. There is, however, a higher prevalence of recycling or renarcotization, especially if diprenorphine or naloxone is used as a reversal agent. The use of naltrexone may prevent recycling.

Antagonists. Naltrexone is the antagonist of choice but diprenorphine, naloxone, or nalmefene may also be used. Administer 100 mg of naltrexone HCl for each mg of Carfentanil.

THIAFENTANIL (A 3080)[9,30,41-45]
Chemistry. Thiafentanil oxalate is a synthetic derivative of fentanil.

Pharmacology. Similar to etorphine, but more potent. Potency is similar to carfentanil, but has a shorter duration of action and has a greater margin of safety.

Indications. Thiofentanil oxalate is used similarly to etorphine and carfentanil. Especially useful for immobilization of giraffe, waterbuck, eland, kudu, and nyala.[33]

Administration. Thiofentanil may be administered by any parenteral route.

Side Effects and Precautions. Similar to etorphine and carfentanil but renarcotization is less common than the other opiate restraint drugs. Secondary poisoning has occurred when carcasses of deer immobilized with thiafentanil, and subsequently euthanized, were fed to captive mountain lions, *Felis concolor*.[43]

Antagonists. Naltrexone is the antagonist of choice. Reversal should occur in less than a minute.

FENTANYL CITRATE[35,40]
Chemistry. A synthetic opiate agonist, occurring as a white crystalline powder, odorless and tasteless. Soluble in alcohol, but only sparingly in water. More concentrated solutions may be prepared using DMSO.

Pharmacology. Similar to etorphine, but with 1/15 the potency of etorphine. It has less suppression of respiration but has less immobilization effect. Animals may remain standing.

Administration. Injected IM, IV for immobilization pain suppression. Fentanyl is administered transdermally via patches for pain suppression in dogs, horses, sheep, goats, and swine.

Indications. Usually used in combination with other agents and only in smaller animals such as small carnivores or herbivores. It is not suitable for zebras.[33]

Side Effects. Similar to other opiates.

Antagonists. Naltrexone (3 × the fentanyl dose or 0.04–0.07 mg/kg).

BUTORPHANOL TARTRATE (TORBUGESIC)[35]
Chemistry. Butorphanol is a synthetic opioid, derived from morphine.

Pharmacology. Butorphanol has both agonistic and antagonistic actions. As an antagonist, it may be used to reverse the effects of more potent opiates.

Indications. As a restraint agent, it is used in combination with other agents particularly if standing sedation is desired. As an agonist, it is an analgesic, and has been used in postsurgical treatment of cats and dogs. It is a controlled substance, Schedule III.

Administration. Any parenteral route.

Side Effects and Precautions. Untoward effects are minimal, but since the drug has both agonistic and antagonistic action, when used in combinations, it may have variable effects depending on the species.

Antagonists. Naltrexone is the antagonist of choice.

Cyclohexamine Derivatives
KETAMINE HYDROCHLORIDE (KETASET, KETALAR, VETALAR, KETAJECT, KETANEST)[1,3,9,12,17,40-43]
Chemistry. The formula for ketamine is 2-(o-chlorophenyl)-2-(methylamino)-cyclohexanone hydrochloride. Ketamine is a derivative of phencyclidine hydrochloride. It is a white crystalline powder, readily soluble in water.

Pharmacology. Ketamine is a nonbarbiturate dissociative anesthetic agent. The animal usually retains normal pharyngeal-laryngeal reflexes. This desirable effect minimizes inhalation of food or ingesta near the glottis. However, endotracheal intubation is difficult when ketamine is the only agent used.

Ketamine does not produce skeletal muscle relaxation; catatonia is common. Profound analgesia is rapidly produced, although analgesia of the visceral peritoneum may be less than optimal. Excessive salivation can be alleviated with atropine.

Many animals experience transitory pain upon injection of the solution. The effect on blood pressure varies from species to species. In the dog and humans, blood pressure is elevated. In the rhesus monkey, blood pressure is depressed. Nystagmus may be noted during induction.

Ketamine crosses the placenta in all species. Anesthetic effects are noted in the fetus when ketamine is used as a sedative for cesarean section or dystocia. Ketamine is not known to produce abortion when used on pregnant animals. Ketamine is detoxified in the liver, and it and its metabolites are excreted via the urine. Birds and reptiles have a renal portal system that may shunt blood (and ketamine) from the caudal regions through the kidney before reaching the systemic circulation. Thus, a dose of ketamine administered in the rear limb or caudal half of the body may not produce the desired effect in birds and reptiles.

Ketamine produces a fixed expression in the eyes. The eyelids stay open, yet the cornea usually remains moist. However, it should be routine practice to instill an ophthalmic ointment into the conjunctival sac as soon as practical following immobilization. Occasionally corneal ulceration may result from prolonged exposure. Palpebral reflexes persist. Since swallowing reflexes are usually unaffected, excessive saliva is swallowed as usual.

Induction is characterized by ataxia. The animal lies down. A characteristic licking motion is called serpentine tongue. The animal becomes insensitive to external stimulation. Lateral nystagmus appears, then disappears with increased depth of anesthesia.

Indications. Ketamine has U.S. Food and Drug Administration (FDA) clearance for use in humans, domestic cats, and nonhuman primates. However, it also has been safely and effectively used for anesthesia of numerous other species of wild animals. It is particularly effective in wild carnivores, reptiles, and birds, but is not suitable as a sole agent for most ungulates.

Administration. Ketamine is supplied as solutions of 20 mg/ml, 50 mg/ml, and 100 mg/ml concentrations. Zoo veterinarians may desiccate the solution and reconstitute it to 200 mg/ml to decrease the volume necessary for immobilizing larger species. A 200-mg/ml solution is also available commercially, from Wildlife Pharmaceuticals in Fort Collins, Colorado. Ketamine may be administered orally or parenterally. In domestic cats, the intravenous and intramuscular routes are recommended. In wild species, either intramuscular or subcutaneous routes are acceptable. Dose variation for immobilization is tremendous (2–50 mg/kg). When used as an anesthetic, intravenous re-dosage is usually required except for very short procedures. Specific doses are tabulated with each animal group.

Parenteral injections take effect within 3–5 minutes. Complete immobilization is produced within 5–10 minutes. If re-dosing seems to be necessary, do not wait for 15 minutes or the initial injection effects may have ceased. The duration of effect varies with the species and the dosage administered. The operator usually has from 15 to 30 minutes to complete a task if ketamine is not augmented with other CNS depressant drugs.

Recovery is usually smooth. An animal is usually ambulatory within 1 hour; however, recovery periods of as long as 5 hours are not rare. Some felids may show slight depression for 24 hours following anesthesia.

Side Effects and Precautions. Ketamine causes tonic clonic convulsions in a small percentage of domestic and wild felids and other carnivores.[16] Primates are less often affected. Convulsive effects can be obviated by administering diazepam (0.25–0.5 mg/kg) with the ketamine (in separate syringes). Acepromazine maleate is often used in combination with ketamine. Acepromazine decreases catatonia and provides better muscle relaxation. Theoretically, acepromazine lowers the threshold for convulsive stimulation, thus increasing the likelihood of convulsions. However, in practice, acepromazine seems to minimize the development of convulsions. Once convulsions have begun, intravenous administration of diazepam or pentobarbital sodium may be required to control seizures.

The author has observed a maniacal syndrome in a few large felid cubs when ketamine was administered as the sole immobilizing agent. Convulsive seizures gave way to wild thrashing, vocalization, and compulsive running. The cubs had to be physically restrained to prevent head trauma. The maniacal syndrome does not respond to intravenous diazepam. The cubs must be anesthetized with barbiturates or masked down with inhalant anesthesia.

Prolonged apnea is sometimes observed in large wild felids. It may be necessary to assist respiration. Endotracheal intubation is highly desirable. Salivation may be profuse, but is readily controlled with atropine.

Accidental oral ingestion or injection can produce anesthesia or immobilization in humans. Hospitalization is required. Respiration should be monitored and assistance given if necessary. Ketamine is known to produce hallucinations in humans. It is difficult to establish the occurrence of hallucinations in animals, but some primates and felids behave strangely during recovery. They may vocalize and appear to be frightened.

Ketamine may be contraindicated in animals with elevated blood pressure. Ketamine and barbiturates should not be mixed in the same syringe; they are chemically incompatible and will precipitate. Ketamine is pharmacologically compatible with other anesthetic and CNS-depressant drugs. Recovery time is prolonged when barbiturate or narcotic agents are used in addition to ketamine.

Ketamine should not be used as the sole anesthetic for reduction of fractures or luxations. Neither should it be used singly for diagnostic or surgical procedures of the pharynx, larynx, or bronchial tubes.

Hyperthermia is a side effect of ketamine anesthesia. Catatonia causes heat production. Hyperthermia is very likely to occur if seizures appear. Swine and marine mammals with heavy fat deposits cannot dissipate heat rapidly and are particularly subject to hyperthermia.

Antagonist. There is no known chemical antagonist for ketamine.

TILETAMINE HYDROCHLORIDE/ZOLAZEPAM HYDROCHLORIDE (TELAZOL, TILAZOL)[40-43]

Chemistry. Tiletamine hydrochloride is a cyclohexanone dissociative agent related to ketamine hydrochloride. The chemical formula is 2-ethylamino-2-(2-thienyl) cyclohexanone hydrochloride. It is soluble in water in up to 30% concentrations.

Zolazepam hydrochloride is a nonphenothiazine pyrazolodiazepinone tranquilizer with the formula 4-(o-fluorophenyl)-6,8-dihydro-1,3,8-trimethylpyrazolo-[3,4-e] [1,4] diazepine-7(IH)-1 monohydrochloride.

Pharmacology. The combination capitalizes on the desirable characteristics of each, while minimizing adverse side effects. Tiletamine hydrochloride used alone produces analgesia and cataleptoid anesthesia plus convulsive seizures in some animals. Combining it with zolazepam eliminates these undesirable effects.

The combination is classified as a general anesthetic. However, the eyelids usually remain open, and the corneal, palpebral, laryngeal, pharyngeal, pedal, and pinnal reflexes persist, even during deep anesthesia. As reflexes are unaffected, they cannot indicate planes of anesthesia—the classical differentiation technique. Instead, the following phases are observed: (1) induction—the time interval from injection of tiletamine-zolazepam to the onset of surgical anesthesia; (2) surgical anesthesia—the time from induction to the beginning of emergence from anesthesia; (3) emergence—the time from the end of surgical anesthesia until the animal has returned to the preanesthetic condition; (4) return of righting reflex—the animal can right itself to sternal recumbency; and (5) recovery—the time from first standing position until completely normal.

Indications. Tiletamine hydrochloride/zolazepam hydrochloride is used for chemical immobilization and surgical anesthesia in a wide variety of carnivores, artiodactylids, birds, reptiles, and amphibians.

Administration. The combination may be given orally or parenterally. The dosage is dependent on the degree of anesthesia required and the species of animal.

Onset of anesthesia occurs within 5–12 minutes after intramuscular injection. Onset following oral administration is less predictable, but effects should be observed in 15–30 minutes.

The duration of analgesia and anesthesia is directly proportional to the dose administered. The effect may last from 1 hour at low doses to as long as 5 hours with higher doses.

Side Effects and Precautions. Excessive salivation is common, but may be controlled by the administration of atropine sulfate. Rare untoward reactions include muscle rigidity, tremors, vocalization, rough recovery, vomiting, apnea, cyanosis, and tachycardia.

Of great concern is a delayed central nervous system effect, which may occur 24–48 hours following administration. The syndrome includes muscle tremors, ataxia, muscle fasciculation, weakness, anorexia, and convulsions. Sedation and nursing care are required to prevent self-trauma.

Antagonist. There is no known antagonist for tiletamine hydrochloride. Zolazepam hydrochloride may be antagonized with flumazenil.

α2, Adrenoceptor Agonists
XYLAZINE (ROMPUN) [1,34,41-43]

Chemistry. The formula is 5,6-dihydro-2-(2,7-xylidino)-4H-1,3-thiazine hydrochloride. It is a colorless crystal with a bitter taste, readily soluble in water and stable in solution.

Pharmacology. Xylazine is a nonnarcotic sedative, analgesic, and muscle relaxant. These effects are mediated by CNS depression. Animals appear to be sleeping. Stimulation during the induction stage may prevent optimum sedation, and when an animal is subsequently approached too rapidly, a seemingly sedated animal may rouse explosively, jeopardizing the safety of the operator.

Indications. Xylazine is used as a mild sedative in the horse. Higher doses effect immobilization. It is a popular immobilizing agent, used either singly or in combination with other drugs for a wide variety of species. See the animal groups for specific indications.

Administration. Xylazine may be given intravenously (IV), intramuscularly (IM), or epidurally. There is wide species variation in the optimum dosage. Immobilization occurs within 15–20 minutes after intramuscular injection. Analgesia lasts from 15 to 30 minutes, but the sleeplike state persists for 1–2 hours. Painful procedures should not be performed after 30 minutes.

Side Effects and Precautions. Occasionally muscle tremors, bradycardia, and partial A-V block occur with standard doses. Atropine should be given to dogs and cats to prevent cardiac effects. Explosive response to stimuli, particularly to auditory stimuli, may cause operator injury.

Xylazine produces an additive effect when combined with tranquilizers and barbiturates. When it is combined, dosages should be reduced and caution exercised. The analgesic effect is variable. The depth of analgesia should be ascertained before clinical diagnostic or surgical procedures are begun. A mildly sedated animal may make effective use

TABLE 20.4. Long-acting tranquilizers: source, onset, duration, dosage

Generic name	Trade name/source	Concentration of solution	Dose (mg/kg)	Onset of action	Duration of effect
Haloperidol lactate decanoate	Haldol Serenace	20 mg/ml	0.016–0.145 IM	5–10 Min.	8–18 hr
Perphenazine enanthate	Trilafon	100 mg/ml	0.058–0.19 IM	12–16 hr	7 d
Pipothiazine palmitate	Piportil	50 mg/ml in sesame oil		48–72 hr	21–28 d
Zuclopenthixol acetate	Clopixol		0.128 IM only	1 hr	3–4 d

of defensive mechanisms if pain is inflicted. Analgesia of the distal extremities of the horse is variable.

Xylazine has not been cleared for use in food-producing animals.

Antagonists. Yohimbine, tolazoline, and idozoxan are all used to reverse the action of xylazine.

DETOMIDINE HYDROCHLORIDE (DOMORSEDAN)[41–43]
Chemistry. An imidazoline derivative $\alpha2$ adrenergic agonist.

Pharmacology. Similar to that of xylazine but is 10 times more potent. It produces a dose-dependant sedative and analgesic effect.

Indications. Has been used for sedation in dogs, cats, horses, cattle, and numerous species of wild animals.

Administration. Any parenteral route.

Side Effects and Precautions. Similar to xylazine. There may be a transient rise in blood pressure, which may be followed by bradycardia.

Antagonist. Atipamezole.

MEDETOMIDINE HCL (DOMITOR).[28,41–43]
This is a superb immobilizing agent especially when used in combination with other agents.

Chemistry. The formula for medetomidine is 4-[-1(2,3-dimethyiphenyl)ethyl]-1H-imidazole hydrochloride.

Pharmacology. Medetomidine is an $\alpha2$ adrenoceptor agonist producing sedation, analgesia, relief of anxiety, bradycardia, hypotension, and hypothermia. Detoxification takes place in the liver, with metabolites excreted in the urine. It is the newest and most potent in the line of $\alpha2$ adrenoceptor agonists, with action more specifically on receptors associated with sedation and analgesia.

Indications. Medetomidine is rarely used as the sole immobilizing agent. Commonly it is combined with ketamine. It has a high therapeutic index and is appropriate for use in a broad range of animal species.

Administration. Medetomidine may be administered intravenously or intramuscularly. Induction time to sedation may be 2–5 minutes with maximum effect within 15 minutes of an intramuscular injection.

Side Effects and Precautions. Medetomidine is one of the safest immobilizing agents being used. Ruminants, carnivores, and primates have tolerated 5–10 times overdosages. Bradycardia is an inherent mode of action unless it is combined with ketamine. Regurgitation has occurred in a small number of ruminants. Abortion has not been produced.

Antagonist. Atipamezole is the antagonist of choice.

Muscle Relaxant/Paralyzing Agents
Muscle-paralyzing drugs were the first immobilizing agents used by native hunters. In the modern era, they were also the first agents to be employed for capturing animals. These drugs have great potential for abuse because no analgesia or anesthesia is associated with their use. Nonetheless, there are bona fide indications for these effects, especially when combined with general anesthesia. Table 20.4 lists drugs that are currently available and being used for immobilization or muscle relaxation during anesthesia.

SUCCINYLCHOLINE CHLORIDE/SUXEMETHONIUM (SUCOSTRIN, ANECTINE, QUELICIN, SCOLINE).[1,3,7,38,39–43]
Succinylcholine is historically significant and still has a limited but specific use in chemical immobilization.

Chemistry. Succinylcholine chloride is the dicholine chloride ester of succinic acid. It is a white, odorless powder; sensitive to light; and readily soluble in water. Unrefrigerated, succinyicholine chloride in solution has a short shelf life. It is easily hydrolyzed in an alkaline solution; therefore it is chemically incompatible with barbiturates if mixed in the same syringe. Other similar drugs (suxamethonium, decamethonium) have been used in North America and other countries.

Pharmacology. Succinylcholine acts by depolarizing the motor endplate and disrupting impulse transmission to the skeletal muscles. There is no analgesia or anesthesia. The animal retains consciousness and may be affected by auditory, visual, and psychological stimulation. For any painful procedure, the use of succinylcholine unaccompanied by suitable anesthesia is barbaric.

The animal may exhibit all the signs of alarm except those related to skeletal muscle response. Thus tachycardia and elevated blood pressure are potential hazards of use.

Succinylcholine and related drugs are detoxified by plasma cholinesterase or pseudocholinesterase. Animals vary tremendously in the levels of this enzyme present in the plasma. This may account for the wide variation in effective dosage and persistence of action of the drug in various species. Ruminants have a low pseudocholinesterase level, and thus experience prolonged succinylcholine action. The pattern of muscle paralysis proceeds from the head to the neck, shoulders, limbs, abdomen, thorax (respiratory), and finally to the diaphragm. Artificial respiration equipment must always be available when working with this drug.

The first visible reaction to the drug is muscle fasciculation, described as very painful by human volunteers. The plasma potassium level rises, which may have marked action on cardiac muscle.[12]

Indications. Succinylcholine is useful in providing additional muscle relaxation in the anesthetized surgical patient. Anesthesia must be carefully monitored lest succinylcholine mask pain reflexes and the surgery become inhumane. Succinylcholine is used to immobilize crocodilians and chelonians (tortoises, turtles). Succinylcholine chloride was once used in equine practice to immobilize stallions for castration.

The availability of tranquilizing agents has reduced the need for, and the use of, this drug in equine practice. At one time, succinylcholine was the only immobilizing agent approved by the Bureau of Land Management (United States Department of Agriculture) for handling feral horses on western ranges. A dose of 0.65 mg/kg administered intramuscularly produced immobilization in approximately 2 minutes, and the effect lasted for 6–24 minutes, allowing collecting of blood samples and aging via the teeth.

Some fatalities have occurred with its use in the horse, especially when organic phosphate anthelmintics were administered within the previous 30 days. The author once administered the feral horse dose to a Percheron stallion that was slated for castration but was totally unmanageable. Immobilization proceeded as expected and the horse became apneic. An endotracheal tube was placed and artificial respiration begun, but the horse failed to respond and died. No lesions were found at necropsy.

Succinylcholine is the most rapidly acting immobilizing agent available. Succinylcholine and similar agents have been used extensively in wild animal immobilization in the past, but newer, nonparalyzing agents have supplanted them. Succinylcholine has a marked variation in dosage and requires extensive experience for safe, effective use. Solutions are unstable and quickly lose potency, further complicating determination of the proper dosage. Nevertheless, this agent is still useful for rapid immobilization.

Administration. The dosage range is tremendous and is listed in appropriate animal groups. The chemical, supplied as a powder in a stoppered vial, is reconstituted as used. The solution must be kept cool, preferably refrigerated, and free from light exposure.

Intravenous administration results in immobilization within 1–2 minutes. Intramuscular injections require 3–10 minutes. The duration of immobilization is variable, depending on the concentration of plasma cholinesterases. In the horse, the effect lasts for 3–5 minutes. A calf remained in flaccid paralysis for 45 minutes from a single injection of succinylchloline chloride. The calf required artificial respiration throughout this period.

Recovery is rapid and complete. Although there is no CNS effect, animals are less aggressive for a few minutes after recovery. Animals appear to be bewildered by the whole experience. Psychological stress is associated with being unable to fight or flee—the normal alarm response.

Side Effects and Precautions. Cessation of respiration is a natural result of succinylcholine chloride immobilization. Procedures should not be attempted without resuscitation equipment available. Elevated blood pressure with ruptured aneurysms (weakened arteries) has occurred in the horse.

Prolonged effects, resulting from cholinesterase inhibitors in the plasma, are a sequel to immobilization induced shortly after administering organic phosphate anthelmintics.

This drug should never be used without thorough knowledge of the correct dosage for the species to be worked on. Equipment to assist with respiration should always be immediately available.

Antagonist. There is no specific antagonist.

GALLAMINE (FLAXEDIL)[41–43]
Chemistry. Gallamine is a complex nitrogen-containing compound with one benzene ring.

Pharmacology. A non-depolarizing neuromuscular blocking agent that competes with acetylcholine for available cholinergic receptors at the postsynaptic membrane. It is in the same class with d-tubocurarine. Gallamine causes loss of muscle tone, followed by paralysis.[35] It is important to recognize that gallamine does not diminish sensory perception and should not be used without analgesia when painful procedures are performed.

Indications. Gallamine is limited to use in immobilizing crocodilians.

Administration. By intramuscular injection at the base of the tail.

Side Effects and Precautions. The muscles of respiration are paralyzed thus assisted respiration may be required.

Fortunately crocodilians normally are capable of breath holding for many minutes.

Antagonist. Neostigmine.

Reversal Agents (Antagonists)

The safety of chemical immobilizing agents has been greatly enhanced by the development of suitable reversal agents for most of the currently used drugs. Table 20.3 lists a number of the reversal agents currently available or undergoing field trials.

Diprenorphine HCL

Chemistry. The formula for diprenorphine is N-(cyclopropylmethyl)6,7,8,14-tetrahydro-7-a-(1-hydroxy-1-methylethyl)-6,14-endoethanonororipavine hydrochloride.

Pharmacology. Diprenorphine is a narcotic antagonist, used to reverse the effects of etorphine. It also has agonistic action if administered solely or if an overdose is administered to counteract etorphine.

Indications. Diprenorphine was developed as a specific antagonist for etorphine. It will also reverse other narcotics and may be used in an emergency for humans accidentally injected with etorphine. It must be used carefully because it also has agonistic effects.

Administration. Diprenorphine is injected intravenously if possible, otherwise intramuscularly. The recommended dose is double the injected dose of etorphine. When injected intravenously, reversal usually occurs within 1–4 minutes. Intramuscular injection requires 15–25 minutes for reversal effects.

Side Effects. No adverse effects should be noted unless an overdose is administered.

Antagonist. Naloxone is an antagonist for diprenorphine.

NALTREXONE HCL

Chemistry. A synthetic opiate antagonist. Occurs as white crystals and has a bitter taste. Soluble in water at 100 mg/ml.

Pharmacology. It competitively binds to opiate receptors in the CNS, thus preventing both exogenous and endogenous opiates from acting. It is particularly effective in preventing renarcotization when using carfentanil.

Indications. It is one of the more effective opiate antagonists. It is now considered the drug of choice for treatment of accidental injection of opiates in humans.

Administration. It may be administered IM, IV, or IP.

Side Effects and Precautions. At usual doses it is relatively free of adverse effects.

NALOXENE HYDROCHLORIDE (NARCAN)[16,19,23]

Chemistry. The formula for naloxone is N-allylnoroxymorphone hydrochloride, a synthetic congener of oxymorphone.

Pharmacology. Naloxone is a true narcotic antagonist, with none of the agonistic effects that some other narcotic antagonists may produce.

Indications. Naloxone is used solely as an antagonist to narcotic immobilizing agents.

Administration. Intravenous, intramuscular, and subcutaneous routes for injection are used. Induction time for naloxone is within 2–3 minutes when injected intramuscularly. The dose of naloxone is 0.006 mg/kg. For a human accidentally injected with etorphine or carfentanil, an initial injection of 1 mg of naloxone should be administered intravenously, followed by injections of 0.4–0.8 mg every 2–4 minutes until the victim is under hospital management.

Antagonist. None.

TOLAZOLINE HCL (TOLAZINE)

Chemistry. Is structurally related to phentolamine and occurs as white to off-white crystalline powder. It is freely soluble in water and alcohol.

Pharmacology. Tolazoline is a competitive α2 and α2 adrenergic blocking agent. It also relaxes vascular smooth muscle producing a peripheral vasodilatation.

Indications. In restraint it is used to antagonize α2 adrenergic agonists (xylazine, medetomidine, detomidine).

Administration. IV or IM.

Side Effect and Precautions. Transient tachycardia, gastrointestinal hypermotility.

Antagonist. None.

YOHIMBINE (ANTAGONIL)

Chemistry. Yohimbine is a 17-Hydroxyl-20-yohimban-16 carboxylic acid methyl ester.

Pharmacology. Yohimbine was resurrected from the discarded drug locker when it was found to have α adrenoceptor antagonist activity and became the first drug to be utilized for reversing the effects of xylazine. It is relatively nonselective in its action and is not effective in all species.

Indications. Yohimbine has been given to numerous species to reverse the respiratory depression effects of xylazine and ultimately to assist in complete recovery of the animal from immobilization. The variable response of individual species will be addressed in animal group discussions.

Administration. Yohimbine may be administered intramuscularly, but a more immediate reaction occurs with intravenous injection.

Side Effects and Precautions. There are few side effects. The major weakness of yohimbine is failure of effect in some species.

Antagonist. None.

ATIPAMEZOLE[28,34,35,40,42,43]

Chemistry. Chemically, atipamezole is 4-(2-ethyl-2,3-dihydro-1H-inden-2-Yl)-1H-imidazole hydrochloride.

Pharmacology. Atipamezole competitively inhibits $\alpha 2$ adrenergic receptors and is thusly a reversal agent for $\alpha 2$ adrenergic agonists such as medetomidine, detomidine, and xylazine.

Administration. It should be administered intravenously for optimal response, but may be given intramuscularly in doses 4–5 times the dose of medetomidine.

Side Effects and Precautions. There is no contraindication for this drug, but it is not recommended that atipamezole be used in pregnant or lactating animals.

FLUMAZENIL

Chemistry. It is a benzodiazepine antagonist, a derivative of 1,4-imidazobenzodiazepine.

Pharmacology. Flumazenil is a competitive blocker of benzodiazepines at the their receptor site in the CNS.

Indications. In restraint it is used as an antagonist for benzodiazepines (diazepam, midazolam).

Administration. IM or IV.

Side Effects or Precautions. Slight pain at the site of injection. Rarely produces seizures when overdosed.

NEOSTIGMINE BROMIDE AND N. METHYLSULFATE[42,43]

Chemistry. It is a synthetic quaternary ammonium parasympathomimetic agent. It occurs as a white crystalline powder that is odorless but has a bitter taste. They are soluble in both aqueous and alcoholic solutions.

Pharmacology. Neostigmine competes with acetylcholine for acetycholine esterase. It produces the same actions as other parasympathomimetic agents.

Indications. Its only use in restraint is as a reversal agent for gallamine, which is used as an immobilizing agent in crocodilians.

Administration. IM.

Side Effects and Precautions. An overdose may cause all the effects of parasympathomimetic stimulation (diarrhea, excessive salivation, lacrimation, bronchospasm, hypotension, and muscle cramps). It should not be used to reverse succinylcholine immobilization.

Antagonist. Atropine sulfate.

Tranquilizers[1]

Tranquilizers are often used to calm aggressive domestic animals. (See Table 20.2.) Tranquilizers are frequently used in combination with immobilizing drugs to counter undesirable pharmacologic effects of the primary drug. A new and important use of long-acting tranquilizers is to calm animals during stressful periods. Many classes and brands of these agents are available. The pharmacology and clinical use of tranquilizers are important, but a complete listing is outside the purview of this book, however, a few formulations will be discussed. The reader is referred to textbooks on anesthesia and pharmacology for detailed discussions of tranquilizers.[1,15,40,41]

ACEPROMAZINE MALEATE (ACETYLPROMAZINE MALEATE)

Chemistry. The formula for acepromazine maleate is 10-[3-(dimethylamino) propyl]phenothiazin-2-Yl-methyl keton maleate. It is an acetyl derivative of promazine; a yellow crystalline powder.

Pharmacology. Acepromazine maleate is a potent tranquilizing agent that depresses the CNS, producing muscular relaxation and reducing spontaneous activity. It exhibits antiemetic, hypotensive, and hypothermic properties.

Indications. Acepromazine maleate is rarely used singly for immobilization purposes; rather it is usually used in combination with etorphine or ketamine. Its muscle-relaxing characteristic is of particular value when used with ketamine. Acepromazine maleate is used extensively in domestic dogs, cats, and horses as an antiemetic, to inhibit pruritus, and to control intractable animals for examination and minor surgical procedures.

Administration. This agent may be injected intravenously, intramuscularly, or subcutaneously. A tablet form is available for oral administration, but the effects of oral administration are somewhat unpredictable. Dosage varies with species. The parent compound, promazine, is available in a granulated form for inclusion in the diet and is more suitable than acepromazine maleate for this route of administration.

Acepromazine maleate is commonly used as a preanesthetic agent. Since it potentiates the action of barbiturates, dosages of both the barbiturate and acepromazine maleate should be decreased.

When given intravenously, effects are noted within 1–3 minutes. Intramuscularly, full effect requires 15–25 minutes. Oral effects appear within 30–60 minutes. The general dosage for domestic animals is (1) dog: 0.5–1.0 mg/kg; (2) cat: 1.0–2.0 mg/kg; (3) horse: 0.04–0.08 mg/kg.

Side Effects and Precautions. Caution should be exercised when acepromazine is combined with other hypotensive agents. Occasionally, instead of producing CNS depression, it acts as a stimulant and hyperexcitability ensues.[17]

Acepromazine should not be used to control convulsions caused by organic phosphate insecticide poisoning.

Antagonist. There is no known antagonist.

AZAPERONE (STRESNIL)[40]
Chemistry. Azaperone is a butyrophenone neuroleptic, occurring as a white to yellowish-white macrocrystalline powder.

Pharmacology. Produces sedation and tranquilization. It also has antiemetic action.

Indications. Its greatest use is in combination with other chemical restraint agents.

Administration. Should only be administered IM.

Side Effects and Precautions. May see transient salivation and shivering in pigs. It has minimal analgesic action.

DIAZEPAM (VALIUM, TRANIMAL, TRANIMUL)
Chemistry. The formula for diazepam is 7-chloro-1,3 dihydro-1-methyl-5-phenyl-2H-1,4-benzodiazepin-2-one. It is a colorless crystalline compound and has limited stability in solution.

Pharmacology. Diazepam acts on the thalamus and hypothalamus, inducing calm behavior. Unlike some other tranquilizers, it has no peripheral autonomic blocking action. Transient ataxia may develop with higher doses as muscle relaxation progresses. Spinal reflexes are blocked. Diazepam is an effective anticonvulsant.

Indications. Diazepam may be given orally, intravenously, or intramuscularly. Oral administration is not recommended for immobilization but may be used to calm an animal prior to immobilization. The dosage varies from 0.05 to 3.5 mg/kg, depending on the species and the degree of excitement at the time of injection. Onset is within 1–2 minutes when given intravenously. If given intramuscularly effects appear in 15–30 minutes, depending on the dose. Diazepam is metabolized slowly in the normal liver. Clinical effects usually disappear within 60–90 minutes. Diazepam has anticonvulsive action, thus is indicated for controlling ketamine-induced seizures.

Side Effects and Precautions. Venous thrombosis and phlebitis at the injection site are complications of use. Diazepam is chemically incompatible with most other immobilizing agents, and should not be mixed with them in the same syringe nor in intravenous solutions. Some pain is associated with intramuscular injections, and a transient inflammatory reaction may develop at the site. Diazepam is contraindicated in patients suspected of having glaucoma.

Antagonist. Flumazenil (Mazicon) is a new specific antagonist to benzodiazepine tranquilizers.

MIDAZOLAM HCL (VERSED)
Chemistry. The formula for midazolam is 8-chloro-6-(2-fluoropehenyl)-1-methyl-4H-imidazo [1,5-a]benzodiazepine hydrochloride. It is a white to light yellow crystalline compound that is soluble in water.

Pharmacology. Midazolam is a short-acting benzodiazepine CNS depressant, similar to diazepam, but more potent.

Indications. Same as for diazepam.

Administration. Any parenteral route. Midazolam is a schedule IV drug in the Controlled substance Act of 1970.

Side effects and precautions. Prolonged sedation, incoordination, nausea, vomition and coughing may be seen.

Antagonists. Flumazenil (Mazicon)

PERPHENAZINE ENANTHATE (TRILAFON)[8,11,16,40–43]
Pharmacology. Perphenazine was first marketed as a tranquilizer for cattle 35 years ago. Unfortunately, it was also given to horses, in which it produced a nonreversible paralysis of the retractor penis muscle in stallions. It was subsequently withdrawn from the veterinary market in the United States, but has recently been restored.

Indications. Investigations in South Africa indicate it has a marked calming effect on hoofed stock lasting for up to 72 hours.

Administration. The intramuscular route is most commonly used in animals.

Side Effects and Precautions. Perphenazine should not be used in equids.

Antagonist. None.

HALOPERIDOL (HALDOL, SERENACE)[23]

Pharmacology. Haloperidol is a butyrophenone derivative with actions similar to those of azaperone, but it is more potent and the effects last longer (8 to 18 hours).

Indications. It is used in human medicine as an antipsychotic. In wild animals it is used to quiet highly excitable or aggressive animals for transport episodes of short duration. It may be administered simultaneously with another neuroleptic such as perphenazine that has a slower induction (1–3 days), but has a duration of action lasting for 2–3 weeks. It should not be mixed with opiates as they are chemically incompatible.

Administration. Haloperidol may be administered IM or orally in the lactate form. It is also marketed as a decanoate salt, but this may cause severe anorexia in some species (elephants).

Side Effects. Animals should be monitored for several hours following administration of haloperidol and other long-acting neuroleptics because the drugs may have an effect on the extra-pyramidal system, causing restlessness, anxiety, disorientation, repetitive muscle spasms and postures of the head, neck, and face, muscle rigidity, opisthotonus, tremors, a shuffling gait, and recumbency. These signs may be observed in 1–4 hours following administration.

Reversal Agent. There is no specific reversal agent for this drug. However, the extrapyramidal effects may be treated with diphenyl hydramine (Benadryl, Baxter Health Care, Deerfield, IL, 60015), which is a commonly used antihistamine but also has an anticholinergic action to relax muscle tension. The dose for an adult rhinoceros is 500 mg total dose, IV.[46]

Support Drugs

Table 20.5 lists emergency and support drugs used in animal immobilization.

ATROPINE SULFATE

Chemistry. Atropine sulfate is a white crystalline powder, stable in aqueous solution.

Pharmacology. Atropine is a parasympatholytic drug with action equivalent to blockage of the parasympathetic autonomic nervous system. It decreases salivation, sweating, gut motility, bladder tone, gastric secretions, and respiratory secretions. Vagal blockage produces tachycardia. Mydriasis occurs.

Indications. Atropine diminishes excessive secretions induced by ketamine and phencyclidine. It is also commonly used as a preanesthetic medication to prevent reflex vagal stimulation of the heart (cholinergic bradycardia) during induction.

Administration. Atropine may be administered orally or parenterally at dosages of 0.04 mg/kg. Effects may be seen within 1–15 minutes, depending on the route of administration.

Side Effects and Precautions. Animals that dissipate excess heat and moisture by sweating may develop hyperthermia because of inhibition of the sweat glands. Dilated pupils should be protected from direct sunlight to prevent retinal damage. Atropine is contraindicated for patients with glaucoma.

Antagonists. Parasympathomimetic drugs (pilocarpine, physostigmine) may aid in counteracting the effects of atropine, but atropine is difficult to reverse.

Hyaluronidase (spreading factor). Hyaluronidase is an enzyme that hydrolyzes hyaluronic acid, a viscous polysaccharide found in intercellular spaces. At one time hyaluronidase was used extensively to hasten the absorption of fluids administered subcutaneously. When mixed in the solution (150 units/ml) with an immobilizing agent, induction time may be reduced by 50%.[34]

DOXOPRAM HCL (DOPRAM). Doxopram is a respiratory and cardiac stimulant that may be indicated when an immobilized animal experiences respiratory depression. It is not a reversal agent or antagonist to any drug. A dose of 1 mg/kg should be administered intravenously. The author observed a field immobilization of an African lion with

TABLE 20.5. Emergency and support drugs used in animal immobilization

Drug Generic name	Drug Trade name	Concentration	Indication	Dose (mg/kg)
Atropine sulfate	Atropine generic	2 mg/ml	Bradycardia, antidote for organophosphate poisoning	0.02–0.04 IV, IM, SQ
Epinephrine HCl	Adrenaline, Epinephrine, generic	1 : 1000 (1 mg/ml)	Cardiac arrest, anaphylaxis	Equine. 0.1, IV, IM
Doxapram HCl	Doxopram	20 mg/ml	Respiratory depression	Equine. 0.5–1.0 IV at 5-minute intervals
Diazepam HCl	Valium	5 mg/ml	Convulsions, catatonia	0.1–0.2, IV
Lidocaine HCl	Xylocaine lidocaine generic	20 mg/ml	Ventricular arrhythmia	0.25–0.5 IV, q 15 m. as needed
Sodium bicarbonate	Na bicarbonate, generic	1 mEq/ml	Metabolic acidosis	0.5–1.0 mEq/kg, slowly, IV
Calcium gluconate or Ca borogluconate	Ca gluconate, generic	23%, 8 mEq/ml, Ca 10%, 0.43 mEq/ml	Hypocalcemia	0.7 mEq/kg, slowly IV
Hyaluronidase	Wydase	150 NF units/ml	Enhance absorption of agents (Hoare 99, Morton 91)	

xylazine, when the cat suffered a cardiac arrest. The biologist conducting the immobilization administered doxopram intramuscularly, but because circulation had ceased, it was ineffective. Intracardiac injection of doxopram plus cardiac massage aided in the cat's recovery.

MISCELLANEOUS CONSIDERATIONS

Combinations of immobilizing agents are frequently used in zoo practice. None have been cleared by the FDA. There is, however, a decided advantage in using combinations that allow dosage reduction. Skill and experience are prerequisites to successful combination of immobilizing agents. Few clear-cut guidelines are available.

Curare (d-tubocurarine) and nicotine alkaloid are drugs that were used in the early development of chemical restraint. Both drugs have been supplanted with safer and more effective drugs. Animal control officers face a dilemma since nicotine alkaloid is the only drug available for lay use without veterinary supervision, yet the therapeutic index is low. Wide experience with this drug in a species such as the dog allows the development of sufficient skill to keep mortality rates low. When attempts are made to use nicotine alkaloid in wild species or in domestic species other than the dog, mortality rates rise to unacceptable levels.

Despite the tremendous historical importance of these drugs in the developmental stages of chemical restraint, neither curare nor nicotine can be recommended as suitable immobilizing agents.

Immobilizing Free-ranging Wild Mammals[5,32–35,41–43]

The immobilization of free-ranging wild animals may be unlike dealing with the same species in a captive or controlled situation. Before any actual procedure is carried out, the following factors should be considered:

1. Visual evaluation of the physical conditions
2. Terrain to be dealt with
3. Degree of excitement to be expected
4. Estimate of the age, weight, and sex of the animal(s)
5. Potential hazards or obstacles that may be encountered
6. Potential pre-existing diseases that may be present
7. Social interactions with other animals
   a. Hierarchical considerations
   b. Potential predators
   c. Ability to return the animal to its social group

The art of successful immobilization of free-ranging wild mammals requires a detailed knowledge of the behavior and biology of the species to be immobilized plus considerable experience in the use of immobilizing agents and the equipment for the administration of the agent.

Space does not permit a detailed treatise on the myriad species that may require immobilization. The reader is referred to monographs on the subject; for African animals (McKenzie[34], Kock[32]), for South American Animals[15] (Fowler[19]), for North America[33,42,43] (Fowler[21]).

Generally, free-ranging species require higher dosages of chemical restraint agents than their captive counterparts. Accurate weight determination is impossible in the field until the animal is in hand. Rather, the immobilizer must know the weight range of the species and sex they are working with. A total dose of the agent to be used is selected rather than a mg/kg dose. Drugs should be selected that have a wide margin of safety and preferably have an effective reversal agent that is available. Drugs that have a rapid induction time are preferred. Hyaluronidase is frequently added to the mixture of drugs to speed induction.

Special circumstances must be foreseen such as a hippopotamus retreating to water, if available, following injection. Likewise a polar bear in the Arctic may exhibit the same response. **THE RESTRAINER MUST KNOW THE NORMAL ANIMAL.**

Rarely is a single drug used for free-ranging immobilization. Drug combinations allow lower dosages of individual agents and also counteract undesirable pharmacologic effects of individual agents.

Pet/trained Wild Animals

It is unwise to administer tranquilizers to wild animal pets or trained wild animals. Whereas the animal may respond appropriately to the trainer or owner, when tranquilized, the animal's inhibitions may disappear and wild behaviors become manifest. If physical restraint facilities (squeeze cages, nets, snares) are not available, full immobilization should be used.

Owners, handlers, and trainers frequently feel that they have complete control of their animal, but the presence of a stranger (veterinarian) may not be tolerated. The author had a trained circus chimpanzee presented for suspected kidney failure. The owner/trainer was told that a blood sample was needed. "No problem," the owner said. "I'll draw the blood." The chimpanzee allowed the owner to attempt to draw blood, but he couldn't locate the vein.

I had the owner sit down with the chimpanzee at his side and me on his other side. He pulled the arm over his lap so that I could reach it. I drew the blood sample, but about that time the chimpanzee realized that there were too many hands on his arm. He made a lunge for me, but fortunately he was leashed and unable to complete his attack. The owner was allowed to stick needles in the chimpanzee's arm but a stranger was unacceptable.

ACCIDENTAL EXPOSURE OF HUMANS TO RESTRAINT AGENTS. All restraint agents may be hazardous or even lethal to people if accidentally injected into, or in some cases, sprayed onto mucous membranes or the conjunctiva. To prevent accidental exposure of restraint agents to humans, see Table 20.6. The narcotics are especially dangerous. Note that etorphine is not absorbed through the intact skin, but is

TABLE 20.6. Prevention of accidental human exposure

1. Prepare for the procedure.
2. Anticipate challenges.
3. All personnel should be trained in basic first aid.
4. Have all personnel assigned to specific tasks.
5. Have all personnel trained in their specific task.
6. No procedure involving narcotics should be conducted without a minimum of two persons capable of dealing with accidental human exposure (including human intravenous capability, and cardiopulmonary resuscitation training).
7. Never eat, drink, smoke, or rub your eyes when working with restraint agents.
8. Wear latex gloves and protective glasses when loading syringes and darts.
9. Always have human antidotes readily available when handling darts.
10. Do not push air into vials of powerful drugs.
11. Don't put loaded syringes or darts in a pocket or in mouth.
12. Assume that all weapons are loaded until determined to be otherwise.
13. Label all darts, syringes, and containers with drug and date.
14. Dispose of animals that die during an immobilization procedure to preclude other animals from ingesting it.

absorbed through mucous membranes and abraded or lacerated skin. Wash off any spilled drug as soon as possible. The antidote of choice for narcotic poisoning in people is naltrexone.[13,32,36]

The symptoms of narcotic poisoning in humans are dizziness and incoordination, nausea and vomiting, pinpoint pupils, slow and shallow breathing, bluish tinge to the skin, drop in blood pressure, loss of consciousness, heart failure, terminal dilatation of pupils, and death.[37]

A first aid kit should always be available during field immobilization procedures (Table 20.7). It may not always be possible to carry a large first aid kit when stalking an animal, but an emergency kit should be carried, including one vial of naltrexone (50 mg/ml), two clean 2-ml plastic syringes, two 21-gauge (0.8 mm) needles, a rubber tourniquet, and a clamp.[36]

TABLE 20.7. Suggested first aid kit for field immobilization[36]

Supplies
Saline solution, 2 liters
IV sets (2)
Needles, 21-gauge (0.8-mm) and 18-gauge (1.2-mm)
Plastic syringes, 2.5 to 10 ml
Elastoplast with scissors
Tourniquet and clamp
Stethoscope
Face mask and breath bag
Instructions for dosages of drugs

Drugs
One Vial of naltrexone, 50 mg/ml
250 mg hydrocortisone
40 mg diazepam
5 mg atropine
20 mg epinephrine
10 mg neostigmine
Water, sufficient to wash drugs from exposed skin and mucous membranes
Saline solution, 2 liters

An example of why an emergency kit should be carried follows. The author was involved in a helicopter immobilization of a North American bull elk. The animal was darted with etorphine. The animal was placed in a sling to be transported back to a staging area. The helicopter could not carry the elk

and the two veterinarians who were the restrainers at the same time, so they stayed on the ground to be picked up later.

The dart that was used was kept by a colleague and he absent-mindedly opened it while waiting. Not all of the drug had been discharged, and it spilled onto his hands. Neither of us had the antidote, nor did we have any way of communicating our predicament to the base. Neither was water available. He had some abrasions on his hands, but the only thing we could do was to rub sand on the hands to remove the drug. We reviewed the procedure for CPR, but fortunately it was unnecessary.

EUTHANASIA

It is always emotionally traumatic to all concerned when it becomes necessary to end the life of any animal. Those responsible for carrying out euthanasia must appreciate the associated emotions and act appropriately. It should always be performed humanely with minimal pain and distress. An appropriate euthanizing procedure should result in a rapid loss of consciousness followed by cardiac and respiratory arrest.[4]

Euthanasia should be performed in accordance with applicable national, state, and local laws including acquisition, storage and use of drugs, occupational safety, and disposal of euthanized animals. Death must be verified by vital signs, such as heartbeat or other parameters according to the species being euthanized. For instance, lack of breathing (apnea) is not a suitable parameter for determining death in reptiles or marine mammals because apnea is a normal physiologic state for them.

When owners or others who have been closely associated with an animal choose to be present at the euthanasia, every effort should be made to explain in detail how the procedure will be carried out and what reactions may be expected in the animal. In a public setting, such as at a zoo or race track, when dealing with a stranded marine mammal or an injured wild animal, consider the feelings and potential responses of the public and take steps to minimize adverse reactions.

Federal and state agricultural employees may be involved in mass euthanasia of poultry and livestock in the face of a foreign animal disease outbreak, natural disaster, or act of bioterrorism. Nonetheless, humane euthanasia should be performed.

The basic mode of action of euthanizing agents fit into one of the three following mechanisms:

1. Those that produce hypoxia or anoxia (do not use muscle relaxants, strychnine, nicotine, or magnesium salts).
2. Direct depression of neuronal function (anesthetic agents, T61, carbon monoxide).
3. Destruction of brain activity (gunshot, stunning, electricity).

Many different methods have been used depending on circumstances and species.

Inhalant Agents

Inhalants are used directly to euthanize animals when administered in high concentrations. Any of the inhalant anesthetic agents used in veterinary medicine are suitable. Inhalants may also be used to anesthetize an animal preparatory to administering another lethal substance (such as saturated potassium chloride [KCl] solution).

Injectable Agents

Barbiturates are the drugs of choice for euthanizing dogs, cats, other small animals and horses. Barbiturates have the advantage of being less expensive than many other agents, rapid acting, and causing minimal discomfort to the animal. The disadvantages are that these drugs must be administered intravenously or intraperitoneally, and are not readily available except to veterinarians. The cost of barbiturates may be prohibitive for an animal the size of an elephant or giraffe. Table 20.8 lists comparative costs of restraint agents available in the U.S. as of November 2007.

In a day when immobilizing agents are available in all but the most remote locations on the globe, the humane method of euthanasia for elephants or other megavertebrates is to first immobilize with an agent that renders the elephant totally unconscious (etorphine, carfentanil, xylazine, detomidine). A catheter should be placed in an accessible vein quickly, following recumbency. Incise down to the vein if blood pressure drops or there is a problem with inserting the catheter through the skin. Then a saturated solution of KCl is injected intravenously. In a few seconds the heart will stop and death is instantaneous.

Powdered KCl is readily available from chemical companies or a pharmacy without a prescription. It need not be medical grade, and sterility is not necessary. A saturated solution is prepared by adding 180 g of KCl to 600 ml of hot water, which provides 0.3 g/ml of solution. The dose required to stop the heart is 44 mg/kg (20 mg/lb). For instance, a 3,000-kg elephant would require 440 ml of the 0.3 g/ml saturated solution. In practice, the solution is administered in excess, so it would be appropriate to make a double quantity of KCl solution to account for possible spillage. This method of euthanasia is humane, suitable for any large domestic or wild animal, and is in compliance with the American Veterinary Medical Association's (AVMA) Guidelines for Euthanasia.[4] The animal must be anesthetized and fully unconscious before injecting the KCl solution.

Physical Methods

Although several physical methods are mentioned in the AVMA Guidelines for Euthanasia, those that I would recommend include gunshot, stunning by a blow to the head, and cervical dislocation. All of the physical methods require a person who is well trained in carrying out the procedure and has knowledge of the anatomy of the head region and brain location. These procedures are more appropriate for infants or juvenile animals, or species with fragile head bones. The appropriate site on the skull for most ruminants and equids is illustrated in Figure 20.3.

An unpleasant experience illustrates the need for training. While traveling the Canadian transcontinental highway, I came upon man cradling a moose calf that had been struck by an automobile. The calf had three broken legs and possibly other injuries that warranted euthanasia. I had a single bitted axe in my vehicle so I said I could euthanize the calf with a blow to the head. The person said, "No, we must wait for the police." When the officer arrived, I explained to why the animal should be euthanized and he agreed. He told everybody to step back and instead of going up to the calf and placing a bullet in the proper place on the skull, he stepped back three or four meters and began shooting. He emptied his service revolver on the calf before it died.

TABLE 20.8. Comparative cost of chemical restraint agents that are available in the United States, Nov. 2007. Prices subject to change without notice

Agent, generic/trade	How supplied	Retail cost per container	Retail cost per milligram
Etorphine	10.0 ml, 10.0 mg/ml	$400.00	$4.00
Carfentanil	10.0 ml, 3.0 mg/ml	$500.00	$16.67
Thiafentanil	Experimental	Experimental	Experimental
Butorphanol	6.0 ml, 50.0 mg/ml	$350.00	$1.16
Ketamine	30.0 ml, 200 mg/ml	$140.00	$0.02
Tiletamine/zolazepam	5.0 ml, 100 mg/ml	$45.00	$0.09
Xylazine	30.0 ml, 300.0 mg/ml	$1250.00	$0.05
Detomidine	20.0 ml, 10.0 mg/ml	$229.10	$1.16
Medetomidine	5.0 ml, 20.0 mg/ml	$400.00	$4.00
Acepromazine	50.0 ml, 10.0 mg/ml	$8.59	$0.02
Azaperone	20.0 ml, 100.0 mg/ml	$20.00	$0.01
Haloperidol	10.0 ml, 10.0 mg/ml	$67.00	$0.33
Diazepam	10.0 ml, 20.0 mg/ml	$14.40	$0.06
Midazolam	10.0 ml, 50.0 mg/ml	$300.00	$0.60
Naltrexone	10.0 ml, 50.00 mg/ml	$100.00	$0.20
Naloxone	1.0 ml, 1.0 mg/ml	$18.00	$18.00
Yohimbine	30.0 ml, 10.0 mg/ml	$150.00	$0.50
Atipamezole	10.0 ml, 5 mg/ml	$133.00	$2.60
Tolazoline	30.0 ml, 200 mg/ml	$40.00	$0.01
Flumazenil	10.0 ml, 0.1 mg/ml	$100.92	$10.09

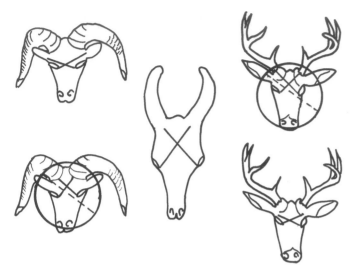

FIG. 20.3. Sites for a gunshot or blow to the head for euthanasia in ungulates. From the base of the ear to the medial canthus of the eye.

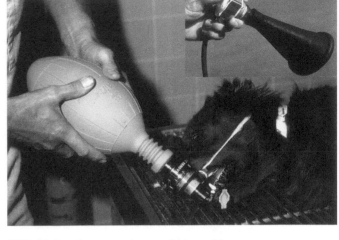

FIG. 20.4. A pressure bag used to provide positive pressure respiration in an apneic animal. Bird unit demand valve for assisted respiration, inset.

For more information about euthanasia, consult the AVMA Guidelines for Euthanasia.[4]

ASSISTED RESPIRATION

It may become necessary to assist in pulmonary exchange of an immobilized animal. Apnea (not breathing) may occur at any time, but particularly during induction. One person on the immobilizing team should be assigned to carefully monitor respiration. If the animal stops breathing, the observer should hold his/her own breath. When the observer can no longer hold his/her breath, assisted respiration must be begun.

First, slap the chest of a mammal to stimulate breathing. If that is unsuccessful, initiate artificial respiration. In small mammals squeeze the chest from side to side. For ungulates avoid pressure on the caudal rib cage, because this may put pressure on the stomach and encourage regurgitation. Instead, place the animal on its right side. Stand at the back near the withers, and reach over and grab the last rib of the ribcage and lift. Next release the hold and press on the chest just behind the shoulder. Repeat the process 10–20 times per minute. Lifting the rib cage expands the chest and causes air to rush into the lungs. Pressing on the chest behind the shoulder expels the air without putting pressure on the stomach.

For birds, place the bird on its back and gently press on the sternum (keel). Then release the press. This is the normal breathing pattern of a bird. Repeat 30 or 40 times per minute, depending on the size of the bird.

Continued apnea requires tracheal intubation with an endotracheal tube, and pressure to inflate the lungs (Fig. 20.4).

Someone on the immobilizing team should be able to place an endotracheal tube rapidly and accurately. This requires knowledge of the pharyngeal anatomy of the species

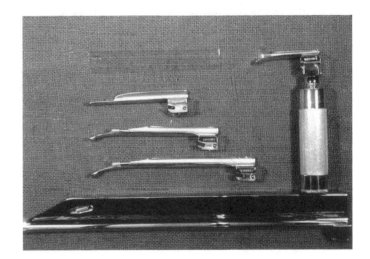

FIG. 20.5. Laryngoscopes for small and large animals.

being immobilized. If the tracheal opening can be visualized, a laryngoscope of an appropriate size (Fig. 20.5) may be inserted through the mouth and the endotracheal tube inserted.

In some species, notably the llama or alpaca, the soft palate is elongated and may be hooked beneath the epiglottal cartilage (Fig. 20.6). This obstructs the opening into the trachea so the soft palate must be lifted dorsally with the blade of the laryngoscope for insertion.

To place the endotracheal tube in llamas, alpacas, and other species with limited space in the pharynx, insert a small catheter into the trachea and thread an endotracheal tube over it. The procedure is as follows: Take two stiff polypropylene catheters (8–19 French, 50-cm long) and couple them end to

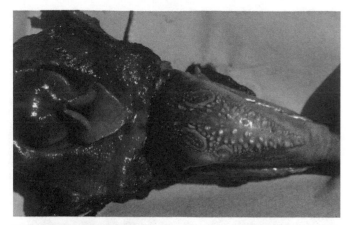

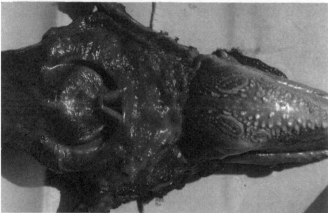

FIG. 20.6.   Positions of the soft palate in a llama, top. Beneath the epiglottal cartilage, bottom, above the epiglottal cartilage.

end with tape. Insert a long-bladed (45 cm; 18 in.) laryngoscope through the mouth to the base of the tongue and depress the tongue. Avoid touching the epiglottal cartilage as this may cause reflex regurgitation.

If the opening to the trachea is not visible, lift the soft palate dorsally and expose the opening. Then insert the catheter into the trachea. The laryngoscope may be removed and the appropriately sized endotracheal tube threaded over the catheter and into the trachea.

This technique is applicable for species as small as a mouse or as large as an elephant. In the mouse, an otoscope cone may be used as the speculum. In the elephant, the mouth is held open with ropes, and an equine foal stomach tube is carried into the pharynx manually and pushed into the trachea. The largest equine endotracheal tube is then threaded over the stomach tube. An endotracheal tube may also be placed manually in large adult carnivores (bears, tigers, lions).

A check should be made for air movement through the endotracheal tube before the catheter is removed. The cuff should be inflated and the tube tied or taped to the lower jaw. All species must be anesthetized before attempting any of these procedures.

LEGAL ASPECTS OF USING IMMOBILIZING DRUGS IN THE UNITED STATES[2]

Few of the available immobilizing agents have been given FDA clearance for use in other than specific domestic species, wild animals, or humans. Drug companies are unable or unwilling to justify the expense of carrying out the extensive testing necessary to license a drug for use on wild animals. However, immobilizing agents must be used by the zoo veterinarian if proper health care is to be given.

Immobilizing drugs are potent and dangerous. None can be purchased or used without prescription on the order of a licensed veterinarian. Additionally, some are classified as controlled drugs by the Drug Enforcement Administration (DEA) of the U.S. federal government. (See Tables 4.1, 4.2.) Drugs classified as controlled substances are controlled by both federal and state law. Use of controlled substances requires a special federal registration (BND number).

The federal law is encompassed in the Controlled Substances Act of 1970, which is administered by the DEA branch of the Department of Justice. The federal law serves as a model for state law, but states may enact more stringent regulations. In any case, the stricter law always prevails.

The Controlled Substances Act of 1970 places dangerous drugs in categories known as schedules and specifies regulations for their possession, use, and dispensing. The list is amended periodically, especially when it becomes apparent that substance abuse is occurring.

Schedule I drugs (heroin, LSD, and marijuana) have no accepted medical use in the United States and are outlawed. Schedule II drugs are potent narcotics and short-acting barbiturates. This group also includes the amphetamines. Six restraint drugs fall into this schedule (etorphine, fentanyl, fentanyl/droperidol, diprenorphine, carfentanil, thiofentanil). Etorphine, carfentanil, and diprenorphine are in a special category within Schedule II. These drugs have been removed from Schedule I and placed in Schedule II to allow clinical usage, but security must be consistent with Schedule I regulations.

Etorphine, carfentanil, thiofentanil, and diprenorphine can be purchased only by those having a valid DEA registration. Furthermore, such persons must comply with the following guidelines and be specifically investigated and approved by the DEA.

1. Federal law restricts this drug to use by or on the order of a licensed veterinarian.
2. Distribution of the product will be limited to veterinarians engaged in zoo and exotic animal practice, wildlife management programs, and research. Nonveterinarians who desire to work with the aforementioned drugs are required to obtain the substance through a licensed and approved veterinarian, along with the official DEA 222C Narcotics Order form. On the order form, the veterinarian must name the

individual for whose use the substance is being obtained.

3. All registrants desiring to handle etorphine, carfentanil, or diprenorphine are required to use a safe or steel cabinet equivalent to a U.S. Government Class 5 security container. This container is rated at 10 work minutes against forced entry, 30 work minutes against surreptitious entry, and 20 work hours against radiological techniques. In lieu of a U.S. Government Class 5 safe or steel cabinet, a bank safety deposit box is acceptable for storage of the drug.

4. All authorized registrants handling etorphine, carfentanil, or diprenorphine are required to maintain complete and accurate records to ensure full accountability for the substance. These records must include specific quantities administered and any amount lost when a target is missed. It is important that the records be complete so that at any time the registrant can fully account for the total amount of the product received.

Schedule III drugs are less dangerous narcotics and ultra short-acting barbiturates, including methohexitol. Schedule IV drugs are dangerous, but are less subject to potential abuse. Diazepam and ketamine are in this schedule.

Controlled Substances Act Summary

By law, anyone who deals with controlled substances in any way is required to register with the DEA, that is, practitioners, wholesalers, researchers, manufacturers, and importers. The only person who can legally possess these substances without such registration is the ultimate consumer who possesses a legitimate prescription.

Veterinarians who wish to become registered must (1) be licensed to practice by the state, (2) be free of felony convictions for drug-related offenses, (3) have separate registration for each address where practice is conducted, (4) pay a fee, (5) apply for registration on application form BND-224 (available from the Registration Branch, Drug Enforcement Administration, P.O. Box 28083, Central Station, Washington D.C. 20005), and (6) specify which schedules of drugs one wishes to use. Chemical restraint drugs are included in Schedules II, III, and IV.

All records and inventories must be kept for 2 years. An inventory must be made biannually. Records of receipt of all drugs in Schedule II must be kept separate from all other business records and the actual date of receipt recorded. Records of receipt of drugs in Schedules III and IV must be kept in an "easily retrievable manner." All drugs in Schedule II must be ordered on an official BND-222 order form, and this must be signed by the registrant. Any practitioners who have controlled substances in their possession must store them in a safe or a substantially constructed, locked cabinet. Any theft of controlled substances must be reported to a regional office of the DEA at the time the theft is realized. Local police must also be notified.

All laws controlling drugs are subject to change. Contact regional offices of the DEA for current regulations.

DEFINITION OF TERMS

Analgesia: Absence of pain.

Analgesic: A drug abolishing pain without producing unconsciousness or sleep.

Anesthesia: Without sensation or loss of sensation, with an accompanying reversible depression of nervous tissue, either locally or generally.

Antagonist: An agent that counteracts or blocks the action of another agent.

Antidote: A remedy that neutralizes or counteracts the effects of a poison.

Ataractic: An agent capable of producing ataraxia (tranquilizers fit this classification).

Ataraxia: Impassiveness or calmness; perfect peace or calmness of mind; detached serenity without depression of mental faculties or clouding of consciousness.

Catalepsy: A condition characterized by waxy rigidity of muscles. The extremities tend to remain in any position in which they are placed.

Cataleptic: A drug inducing catalepsy (phencyclidine analogs are cataleptics), or a person or animal in a state of catalepsy.

Hypnosis: A condition resembling deep sleep, resulting from moderate depression of the central nervous system.

Narcosis: Has a variable meaning but is generally similar to analgesia, accompanied by deep sleep.

Narcotic: An agent that produces narcosis, but usually applied to agents having actions similar to morphine (opiates).

Neuroleptic (Neuro + Lepsis: a taking hold): A drug or agent that produces signs resembling those of disorders of the nervous system (tranquilizers fit into this category).

Neuroleptoanalgesia: A state produced by the combination of a neuroleptic and an analgesic (Innovar-Vet is an example of a drug that induces neuroleptoanalgesia).

Reversal agent: A drug that reverses the action of another drug.

Sedation: A mild degree of central nervous system depression, in which an animal is awake but calm, free of nervousness, and incapable of fully responding to external stimulation.

CONCLUSIONS

It is not appropriate nor possible to cover all aspects of standing sedation or immobilization for short-term procedures of a given species in this text. It is not the intent of this book to discuss detailed anesthesia. Suffice it to say that the chemical restraint agents and combinations thereof mentioned in the species chapters represent those used by the author or the experience of others with detailed knowledge of the species.

Other protocols have been used and no claim is made for including all possible drugs and combinations. For more detailed information, particularly for anesthesia, consult the references, particularly West[42] and Tranquilli.[41]

Selection of a drug regimen should depend on the physical condition of the animal, the experience of the restrainer, the type of assistance available, the equipment available, and the cost of the drug. Most crucial to successful immobilization is the ability to monitor the patient until it returns to normal activity.

The drugs mentioned are routinely used, but may be under stringent regulations as to who and how they may be used. Contact a local zoo veterinarian if questions arise.

REFERENCES

1. Adams, H.R. 2001. Veterinary Pharmacology and Thereapeutics, 8th Ed. Ames, Iowa State University Press.
2. Anonymous. 1975. U.S. drug enforcement agency guidelines for handling and using M99 and M50–50. (Mimeo) U.S. Dept. of Justice.
3. Anonymous. 1993. Compendium of Veterinary Products, 2nd ed. Port Huron, Michigan: North American Compendiums.
4. Anonymous. 2007. AVMA Guidelines for Euthanasia. Schaumberg, Illinois, American Veterinary Medical Association.
5. Allen, J.L., Janssen, D.L., Oosterhuis, J.E., and Stanley, T.H. Immobilization of captive nondomestic hoofstock with carfentanil. Proc Annu Meet Am Assoc Zoo Vet Calgary, Canada, p. 343.
6. Atkinson, M., Kock, M.D., and Meltzer, D. 2006. Principles of chemical and Physical restraint of wild animals. In: Kock, M.D., Meltzer, D. and Burroughs, R. Chemical and Physical Restraint—A training field manual. Greyton, South Africa, International Wildlife Veterinary Services, pp. 96–115.
7. Berger, J., Kock, M., Cunningham, C., and Dodson, N. 1983. Chemical restraint of wild horses: Effects on reproduction and social structure. J Wildl Dis 19(3):265–68.
8. Blumer, E.S. 1991. A review of the use of selected neuroleptic drugs in the management of non-domestic hoofstock. Proc Am Assoc Zoo Vet, pp. 326–32.
9. Burroughs, R., Morkel, P., Kock, M.D., Hofmeyr, M., and Heltzer, D. 2006. Chemical immobilization—Individual species requirements. In: Kock, M.D., Meltzer, D. and Burroughs, R. Chemical and Physical Restraint—A training field manual. Greyton, South Africa, International Wildlife Veterinary Services, pp. 116–211.
10. Bush, M., Citino, S.B., and Tell, L. 1990. Telazol and telazol/rompun anesthesia in nondomestic cervids and bovids. Proc An Meet Am Assoc Zoo Vet South Padre Island, Texas, pp. 251–52.
11. Buss, P., and Morton, D. 2006. Basic pharmacology. In: Kock, M.D., Meltzer, D. and Burroughs, R., Eds. Chemical and Physical Restraint—A training field manual. Greyton, South Africa, International Wildlife Veterinary Services, pp. 8–16.
12. Carpenter, R.E., and Brunson, D.B. 2007. Exotic and zoo animal species. In: Tranquilli, W.J., Thurman, J.C. and Grimm, K.A., Eds. 2007. Lumb and Jones' Veterinary Anesthesia and Analgesia, 4th Ed. Ames, Iowa, Wiley-Blackwell Publishing, pp. 785–806.
13. Caulkett, N., and Shury, T. 2007. Human safety during wildlife capture. In: West, G., Heard, D. and Caulkett, N., Eds. Zoo Animal and Wildlife Chemical Immobilization and Anesthesia. Ames, Iowa, Blackwell Publishing, pp. 123–30.
14. Crockford, J.A., Hayes, F.A., Jenkins, J.H., and Feurt, S.W. 1958. An automatic projectile type syringe. Vet Med 53:115–19.
15. Cubas, Z.S., Silva, J.C.R., and Catão-Dias, J.L. 2007. (Treatis on Wild Animal Veterinary Medicine) Tratado de Animais Selvagens Medicina Veterinária. São Paulo, Brazil, Editora Roca LtdA. (in Portuguese)
16. Ebedes, H., Ed. 1992. The use of tranquilizers in wildlife. Dept. Agricultural Development, Director of Agricultural Information. Pretoria, Republic of South Africa.
17. Fazekas, J.F., Shea, J.G., Ehrmantraut, W.R., and Alman, R.W. 1957. Convulsant action of phenothiazine derivatives. J Am Med Assoc 165:1241–45.
18. Fowler, M.E., and Hart, R. 1973. Castration of an Asian elephant using etorphine anesthesia. J Am Vet Med Assoc 163:539–43.
19. Fowler, M.E. 1995. Chemical restraint. In: Fowler, M.E. Restraint and Handling of Wild and Domestic Animals, 2nd Ed. Ames, Iowa State University Press, pp. 36–56.
20. Fowler, M.E. 1981. Problems with immobilizing and anesthetizing elephants. Proc Am Assoc Zoo Vet Seattle, Washington, pp. 87–91.
21. Fowler, M.E. 1998. Medicine and Surgery of South American Camelids, 2nd Ed. Ames, Iowa State University Press, pp. 98–100.
22. Fowler, M.E., and Cubas, Z.S. 2001. Biology, Medicine and Surgery of South American Wild Animals. Ames, Iowa State University Press.
23. Fowler, M.E., and Mikota, S.K., Eds. 2006. The Biology, Medicine and Surgery of Elephants, Ames, Iowa, Blackwell Publishing, p. 114.
24. Haarthoorn, A.M. 1965. Application of pharmacological and physiological principles in restraint of wild animals. Wildl Monog 14, p. 74.
25. Haarthoorn, A.M. 1966. Restraint of undomesticated animals. J. Am. Vet. Med. Assoc. 14(9):875–80.
26. Harthoorn, A.M. 1970. The Flying Syringe. London: Geoffrey Bles.
27. Haarthoorn, A.M. 1976. The Chemical Capture of Animals. London: Bailliere, Tindall.
28. Haigh, J.C. 1982. Mammalian immobilizing drugs: Their pharmacology and effects. In: L. Nielsen, J.C. Haigh and M.E. Fowler, Eds. Chemical Immobilization of North American Wildlife, pp. 46–62. Milwaukee, Wisconsin Humane Soc.
29. Jalanka, H.H. 1993. New alpha, adrenoceptor agonists and antagonists. In: M.E. Fowler, Ed. Zoo and Wild Animal Medicine, Current Therapy 3, pp. 477–80. Philadelphia, W.B. Saunders.
30. Janssen, D.L., Raath, J.P., deVos, V., Swan, G.E., et al. 1991. Field studies with the narcotic immobilizing agent A3080. Proc. Annu Meet Am Assoc Zoo Vet Calgary, Canada, pp. 340–41.
31. Kock, R.A., Morkel, P., and Kock, M.D. 1993. Current immobilization procedures used in elephants. In: Fowler, M.E., Ed. Zoo and Wild Animal Medicine Current Therapy Vol. 3. W.B. Saunders Company, Philadelphia, PA, USA, pp. 436–41.
32. Kock, M.D., Meltzer, D., and Burroughs, R. 2006. Chemical and Physical Restraint of Wild Animals. Greyton, South Africa, Zimbabwe Veterinary Association Wildlife Group and International Wildlife Veterinary Services.
33. Kreeger, T.J., Arnemo, J.M., and Raath, J.P. 2002. Handbook of wildlife chemical immobilization, International edition. Wildlife Pharmaceuticals Inc., Fort Collins, Colorado, U.S.A., 412 pages.
34. McKenzie, A.A., Ed. 1993. The capture and care manual: capture, care, accommodation and transportation of wild African animals. Pretoria, Wildlife Division Support Services, South African Veterinary Foundation, Pretoria, 729 pages.

35. Metzler, D. 2006. Applied pharmacology. In: Kock, M.D., Meltzer, D. and Burroughs, R., Eds. Chemical and Physical Restraint—A training field manual. Greyton, South Africa, International Wildlife Veterinary Services, pp. 43–67.

36. Morkel, P., Kock, M., and McTaggart, J. 2006. Safety and first aid in the field. In: Kock, M.D., Meltzer, D. and Burroughs, R. Chemical and Physical Restraint—A training field manual. Greyton, South Africa, International Wildlife Veterinary Services, 77–95.

37. Parker, J.B.R., and Haigh, J.C. 1982. Human exposure to immobilizing agents. In: Nielsen, L., Haigh, J.C. and Fowler, M.E., eds. Chemical Immobilization of North American Wildlife, Milwaukee, Wisconsin Humane Soc. pp. 119–36.

38. Pistey, W.R., and Wright, J.F. 1961. The immobilization of captive wild animals with succinylcholine. Can J Comp Med 25:59–68.

39. Pitts, N.I., and Mitchell, G. 2002. Pharmacokinetics and effects of succinylcholine in African elephant (*Loxodonta africana*) and impala (*Aepyceros melampus*). Eur J Pharm Sci 15(3):251–60.

40. Plumb, D.C. 2005. Veterinary Drug Handbook. 5th Ed. Ames, Iowa, Blackwell Publishing.

41. Swan, G.E. 1993. Drugs used for the immobilization, capture, and translocation of wildlife. In: McKenzie, A.A., Ed. The Capture and Care Manual. Pretoria Wildlife Division Support Services, South African Veterinary Foundation, pp. 2–64.

42. Tranquilli, W.J., Thurman, J.C., and Grimm, K.A., Eds. 2007. Lumb and Jones' Veterinary Anesthesia and Analgesia, 4th Ed. Ames, Iowa, Wiley-Blackwell Publishing.

43. West, G., Heard, D., and Caulkett, N., Eds. 2007. Zoo Animal and Wildlife Chemical Immobilization and Anesthesia. Ames, Iowa, Blackwell Publishing.

44. Wolfe, L.L., Lance, W.R., and Miller, M.W. 2004. Immobilization of mule deer with thiafentanil (A3080) plus xylazine. J Wildlife Dis 40(2):282–7.

45. Wolfe, L.L., and Miller, M.W. 2005. Suspected secondary thiafentanil intoxication in a captive mountain lion *Puma concolor*. J Wildlife Dis 41(4):829–33.

46. Woodbury, M. 2007. Euthanasia. In: West, G., Heard, D. and Caulkett, N., Eds. Zoo Animal and Wildlife Chemical Immobilization and Anesthesia. Ames, Iowa, Blackwell Publishing, pp. 37–42.

47. Young, E., Ed. 1973. The Capture and Care of Wild Animals. Capetown, South Africa: Human and Rousseau.

48. Zuba, J., and Oosterhuis, J.E. 2007. Treatment options for adverse reactions to haloperidal and other neuroleptic drugs in non-domestic hoofstock. Annual Proceedings Am Assoc Zoo Vets 2007, Knoxville, Tenn, pp. 53–7.

CHAPTER 21

Monotremes and Marsupials

CLASSIFICATION (NUMBERS IN PARENTHESIS DENOTE NUMBER OF KNOWN SPECIES)

Order Monotremata
  Family Tachyglossidae: echidna (5)
  Family Ornithorhynchidae: platypus (1)
Order Marsupialia
  Family Didelphidae: New World opossum (65)
  Family Dasyuridae: marsupial mouse, Tasmanian devil, numbat (49)
  Family Notocryctidae: marsupial mole (2)
  Family Peramelidae: bandicoot (20)
  Family Caenolestidae: rat opossum (7)
  Family Phalangeridae: phalanger, koala (48)
  Family Phascolomidae: wombat (2)
  Family Macropodidae: wallaby, wallaroo, kangaroo (55)

Adult males are referred to as males, bucks, or boomers; adult females as females, does, or flyers. The infant kangaroo is called a joey; the infant koala a cub.

Some weights of monotremes and marsupials are listed in Table 21.1.

TABLE 21.1. Some weights of monotremes and marsupials

Animal	Kilograms	Pounds
Echidna	2.5–6	6–13
Platypus	0.5–2	1.4
Tasmanian devil		
Male	6.35–9.07	14–20
Female	4.53–5.44	10–12
Bandicoot	0.55	1
Koala	5–15	9–33
Common wombat	15–35	33–35
Red-necked wallaby	4–24	14–24
Red kangaroo	23–70	51–154
Grey kangaroo	23–70	51–154

MONOTREMES

Monotremes are primitive egg-laying mammals, represented by the platypus (restricted to the Australian continent) and the echidna (five species distributed throughout Australia, Tasmania, and New Guinea).

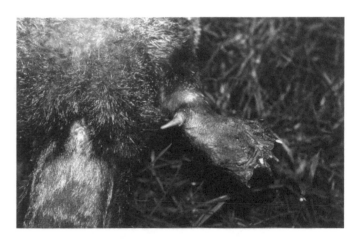

FIG. 21.1. Venom spur on the medial aspect of the tarsus of a male platypus.

Danger Potential

Venom of the male platypus is delivered through a hollow curved spur (Fig. 21.1) on the medial aspect of the tarsal (hock) joint of the hind leg. The spur is normally carried against the leg. When the animal becomes agitated, the spur erects. The platypus kicks with a jabbing motion, usually with both hind legs.

The venom gland is located on the medial aspect of the thigh and is emptied by a duct into a small reservoir situated below the spur. A second duct connects the reservoir to the spur.

The hind legs of the platypus are short. It is safe to pick up the animal by the tail while supporting the body with the other hand. The platypus is not particularly aggressive, but persons have been envenomated as a result of careless handling. Human envenomation is not likely to be lethal. Signs reported are immediate intense pain, swelling at the wound, numbness around the wound, and a feeling of faintness.

The echidna possesses a diminutive spur and crural venom gland, but there are no reports of human envenomation by these animals. Echidnas cannot bite. Their diet consists primarily of small insects and other invertebrate species. The elongated snout is designed to probe in the soil or beneath objects, searching for prey.

249

Spines of the echidna are not barbed like those of the porcupine but are sharp enough to injure the ungloved hand. The echidna is an efficient burrower with strong claws, which can injure a handler by raking if care is not taken.

Physical Restraint

The platypus is fragile and easily upset, but it may be netted from the aquatic environment and picked up gently by grasping the tail base firmly from above. To prevent the animal from reaching clothes or surrounding objects, grasp a hind foot and extend the limb to determine the presence of the spur. The platypus responds adversely to excessive handling.

Echidnas are best picked up from a hard surface. Grasp a hind leg by first touching the animal on the forehead, which causes an immediate reflex to extend a hind leg rearward. The response may be repeated if the leg is not grasped on the first try. The other hand may then be inserted beneath the abdomen to support the body.

Alarmed echidnas either dig themselves into the ground, if the soil is soft enough, or roll into a tight ball with all the spines projecting outward (Fig. 21.2). If the animal cannot be induced to relax, it must be chemically immobilized for examination. An echidna buried in soil may be carefully removed with a shovel or induced to come to the surface by filling the hole with water.

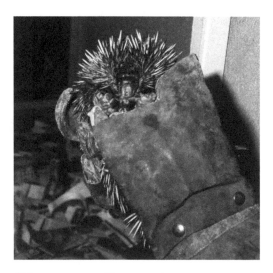

FIG. 21.2. Handling an echidna.

MARSUPIALS

There are 248 species of marsupials. Size variation is extreme, ranging from 25 g to 70 kg.

Danger Potential

Scratching with strong claws is the primary mode of defense for most marsupials. The large macropods can injure severely by kicking with the hind legs as well as by clawing with both forefeet and hind feet. Some large species, such as the eastern gray kangaroo and the red kangaroo, sit back on their hind limbs and tails to kick and claw. The power of the kick can knock a human down, and the claws may disembowel an adversary. If an aggressive kangaroo attacks an unprotected person, striking the animal in the neck with a fist may drive it off. Hitting the body is ineffective.

All marsupials are capable of biting. A number of species are carnivorous, with strong jaw muscles and sharp teeth. Herbivores are somewhat less inclined to bite than carnivores, and since their teeth are not adapted for tearing, they inflict less severe damage.

Anatomy and Behavior

Marsupials exhibit diverse morphologic and physiologic characteristics. The marsupials of the Australian continent and contiguous islands evolved in the absence of other mammalian species. Various species developed adaptations that allow them to exploit different habitats. Some marsupials are rodent-like in all their behavioral repertoire; others have become carnivorous, serving in the role of predator; still others are herbivorous, existing on sparse grass and herbaceous material much as do the large grazers in the order Artiodactyla. Marsupials are characterized by a unique reproductive biology that provides for the final development of the fetus in a specialized pouch called a marsupium. The structure and location of the pouch vary from species to species. In all cases this may present special problems during restraint, because the presence of a fetus in the pouch is not easily recognized.

Upon arrival in the pouch, the fetus attaches firmly to one of the nipples, establishing a semi-permanent bond. Rough handling may cause the fetus to pull away from the nipple and even be extruded from the pouch. If the fetus cannot be immediately reattached, it will die. The female will not replace the expelled fetus on her own, and it may not be possible for the very young infant to reestablish a connection if jostled loose. More mature infants, if not killed outright, may be traumatized.

Physical Restraint[12,13]

The only North American marsupial is the Virginia opossum.[4,6] This medium-sized omnivorous marsupial has a formidable array of 50 small sharp teeth.[6] A cornered opossum is dangerous, but it may be handled and captured quite easily with a net. If suspended from the tail, the opossum may climb up its own tail and bite a handler; if the animal's feet are on a firm surface, it will pull away from pressure on the tail.[6] An opossum may be held by placing a gloved hand on either side of the head and neck.

An opossum in a restricted enclosure may be snared (Fig. 21.3). Once the snare is around the neck, grasp the tail and hold it alongside the handle of the snare to help control the animal.

Free-ranging opossum frequently prey on birds and their eggs, making them unwelcome inhabitants of zoo grounds.

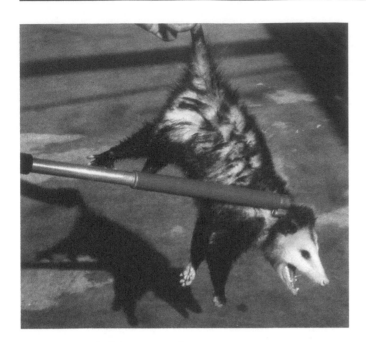

FIG. 21.3. Virginia opossum in a snare.

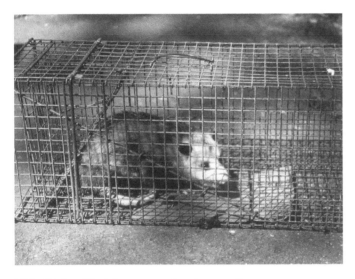

FIG. 21.4. Virginia opossum in a humane live trap.

Baited live traps are frequently used to capture them for relocation (Fig. 21.4).

Small rodent-like species such as quolls, kowaris, and antechinus are handled in much the same manner as wild rats.[13] Gloves, towels, tubes, and other special devices may be purchased or improvised for handling these small marsupials. (See Chapter 18.)

Small- to medium-sized marsupials such as Australian possums are easily handled by quickly grasping the tail and lifting the rear legs off the ground. If the animal is allowed to grasp with the forelegs, it will pull forward and it may then be grasped around the neck for more restrictive handling.

Keep tension on the tail or the animal can reach up and scratch the hand holding the neck. A possum is capable of climbing its own tail.[2]

The Tasmanian devil is reputed to be a ferocious carnivore. The reputation is only partially deserved, since this animal may be handled and moved with some ease. When threatened, the Tasmanian devil opens its mouth wide, exposing an array of carnivorous teeth to frighten off the attacker. A household broom or long-handled scrub brush may be used to ward off the mouth attack while maneuvering the animal into a position that enables a handler to grasp the tail and lift the animal off the ground. If suspended, the Tasmanian devil cannot turn on itself and climb the tail to bite the handler. The animal may be further restricted by placing a hand at the back of the head.

The Tasmanian devil is easily netted, but it is difficult to encircle the very short neck with a hand to extract it from the net. In a confined space it is more efficient and effective to place a snare over its head (Fig. 21.5) and stretch its hind legs (Fig. 21.6). One can then manipulate, examine, or collect blood samples from the Tasmanian devil as desired.

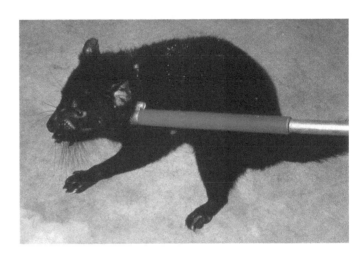

FIG. 21.5. A snare may be used on a Tasmanian devil.

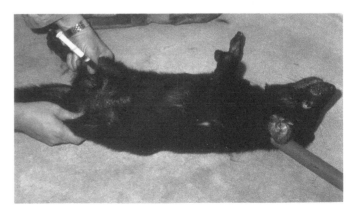

FIG. 21.6. Tasmanian devil being bled from the femoral vein.

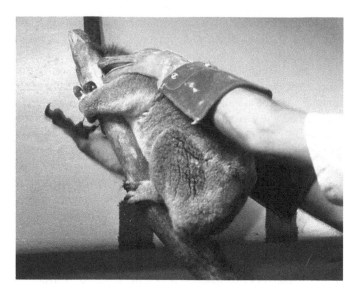

FIG. 21.7.   Approaching a perched koala, using gloves.

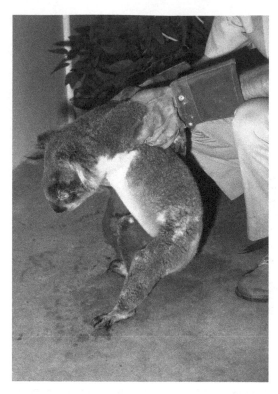

FIG. 21.8.   Holding forelimbs of a koala behind the back.

Phalangers are small to medium-sized animals.[11] Many are arboreal and thus have sharp grasping claws. Nets and snares are suitable restraint tools. Some phalangers may be grasped with gloved hands. Bush-tailed phalangers may be grasped bare-handed around the back of the neck with one hand while grasping the rump or base of the tail with the other.[11]

The koala, though rather phlegmatic, is capable of biting and scratching. Gloves may protect from bites and scratches. It likes to cling to soft furry objects and may tear clothing if the handler is wearing a sweater.

Field researchers use one of two methods to capture koalas in the wild. A canvas sack attached to a long pole is placed above the koala to cause it to retreat down the trunk, or a snare on the end of a long pole is used to grasp the neck and pull the koala from the branch. Once in hand, the koala is placed in a burlap or canvas sack.

Captive koalas generally adapt to human handling, but a few are cantankerous and should be approached with gloves (Fig. 21.7). The arms are held behind the back (Fig. 21.8). A docile koala may be picked from a branch by an experienced handler without gloves. The koala is approached from behind, the arms grasped and pulled free of the branch and away from the body. The animal is then lifted by the arms and immediately placed in the handler's cocked arm to provide it comfort and security (Fig. 21.9). Training for this type of restraint should begin with juveniles. If an extended period of restraint is required, the animal may be placed in a canvas sack or finely meshed net.

A koala should not be grasped around the middle. Young koalas may be held like rabbits by grasping the forelimbs and hind limbs on each side with one hand and fixing the head with the thumbs.

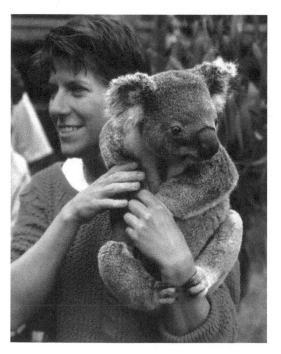

FIG. 21.9.   Allowing a koala to perch on a cocked arm.

Wombats are heavy-bodied burrowing marsupials.[19] Although they are not overly aggressive, they possess strong limbs with claws designed for digging and burrowing. Captive wombats have been known to charge, bite, and grasp handlers.

The claws can inflict serious injury on another animal or a careless restrainer.

A tapering canvas bag with laced-up inspection ports is a useful device for handling wombats.[19] If the bag is placed over the head of the wombat, it will climb inside until it is firmly wedged.

Nets and squeeze cages are effective for moving wombats from one place to another or for restricting them for medication or examination. To pick up a wombat and put it into a crate, approach it from above and behind. Grasp the animal around the body just behind the front limbs and hold it against the chest. The wombat is not generally inclined to bite, but it may. If held in this position, the short neck and decreased mobility of the head prevent it from doing so.

All of the macropods are efficient jumpers. The hind limbs are highly developed, capable of carrying the animal through the air for great distances. The hind limbs are also used as weapons.[2,5,8]

A sheet of burlap or opaque plastic is an effective tool for herding a mob (group) of macropods from one enclosure into another. Wallabies may be moved from one place to another by letting them crawl or hop along while directing them by the tail (Fig. 21.10).

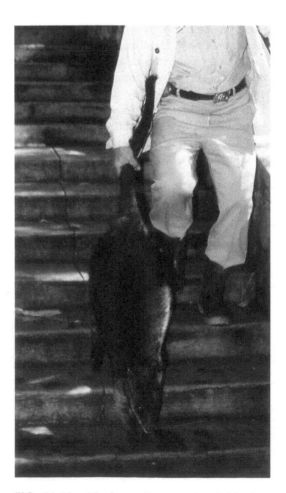

FIG. 21.10. Moving wallaroos and wallabies by directing them with an elevated tail.

Before capturing macropods, it is desirable to confine them in an enclosed solid-walled structure.[10] Capturing macropods from an enclosure surrounded by wire netting or cyclone fencing is hazardous; the animals may not recognize such a fence as a barrier and, in their excitement and fright, may jump against the fence, causing serious injury to themselves or to immature young in the pouches of females.

Nets are useful for the initial capture of wallabies or other small species. A net with a very fine mesh should be used to avoid entangling the claws. The macropod's agility and ability to jump may tax the skills of a person attempting to net it; once the animal is caught, the tail may be grasped and the animal removed from the net. After the tail is grasped, the limbs may be grabbed and the animal stretched (Fig. 21.11).

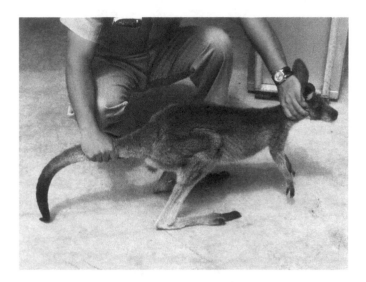

FIG. 21.11. Restraining a small kangaroo.

Small macropods may traumatize their spines if they are allowed to kick out with the hind legs while being captured or held by the tail. Agile wallabies in particular have suffered from posterior paralysis as a result of such injury. Large macropods may be held by the tail but should be turned to the side (Figs. 21.12, 21.13).

Three experienced handlers can enter a group of large macropods to capture them by hand. Two, acting as a team, simultaneously grasp a selected animal by the tail, while the third person surrounds the animal's body with his arms or grasps and stretches the hind legs. A kangaroo may constantly turn to face and defy restrainers, preventing them from getting behind it to grasp the tail. A great degree of self-confidence is required for one person to close in and parry with such an animal, distracting its attention to allow the team to grasp the tail from behind.

A forked stick (see Fig. 29.22) similar to that used to push away an ostrich may be used to push a large male off balance until another person can grab the tail.[2] Once it is captured, a large kangaroo can be kept off balance by bringing

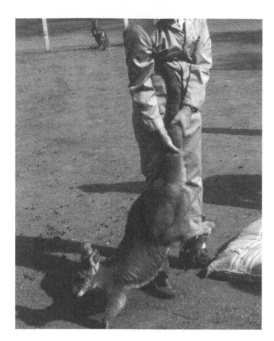

FIG. 21.12. Macropod is handled by lifting its hind feet off the ground, directing the hind legs away from the handler.

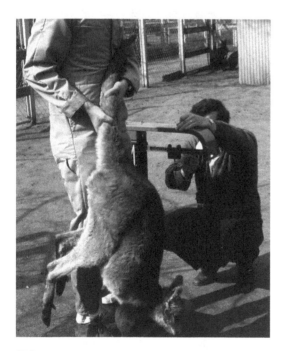

FIG. 21.13. Weighing a macropod.

the tail forward between the hind legs and taping it to the body. This technique is valuable if repeated handling is necessary within a few hours.

A large aggressive kangaroo may be safely caught by two people approaching the animal with a large burlap or light canvas sheet, which is quickly wrapped around the animal; it is then tipped off balance and placed in a large sack.[2]

The length of time that anyone can hold a large macropod off the ground is limited. If prolonged examination or manipulation is required, the animal must be subdued and held recumbent on the ground. If at all possible, the animal should be placed on a padded surface such as an old mattress, to prevent trauma during restraint (Fig. 21.14). The tail can

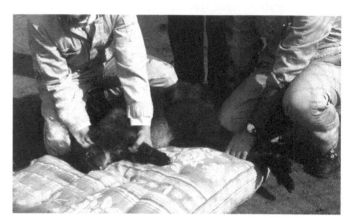

FIG. 21.14. Holding a kangaroo on a mattress.

be held by one person while another grasps the hind legs and a third person holds the front legs and restricts mobility of the head. A burlap bag may be placed over the head and forequarters to assist the person holding the head.[2]

A macropod that cannot be approached to grasp its tail may be squeezed into a corner with the use of solid shields, canvas, or a mattress. A mattress may be used to press the animal against the wall and hold it for grasping (Fig. 21.15). A mattress is also desirable when a large animal must be chemically immobilized. During the induction state of immobilization, the animal may become hyperactive; unless

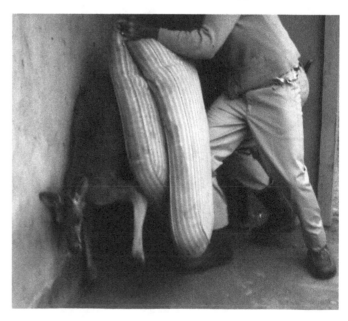

FIG. 21.15. Pressing a kangaroo against a wall with a mattress.

activity is restricted, it may jump against walls and fences. When this type of activity develops, a mattress may be placed over the animal to hold it until it succumbs to the drug.

When a joey is mature enough to leave and return to the pouch, it may be handled and examined independently. To remove the joey from the pouch, grasp the youngster by the tail and give it a quick jerk. Orphaned joeys are frequently kept in an artificial pouch made from a towel (Fig. 21.16).

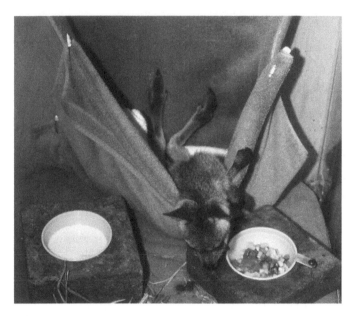

FIG. 21.16. Artificial pouch for a joey.

Blood Collection

Blood may be collected from the platypus bill. The animal is placed in a cloth bag (pillow case) with a corner cut out for the bill to protrude. The bill should be supported on a foam pad. A 23- to 26-gauge needle and a 2-ml syringe are recommended. The needle should be inserted through the rostral or rostrolateral margin of the upper bill, then gradually withdrawn while maintaining negative pressure on the syringe. If unsuccessful, another site, a centimeter away, may be tried.[20,21]

Echidnas should be immobilized to allow easy access to the superficial veins on the forelimb or on the chest.[20,21] The femoral vein is accessible in all mammals if restraint is optimal.

Blood may be collected from the femoral vein of small marsupials, or a toenail may be clipped. Venipuncture in possums and macropods may be accomplished via the recurrent tarsal vein or the lateral tail vein. The lateral tail vein is easily accessed in macropods if the animal is in a sack and the tail can be extracted through a small hole.[2]

The koala has superficial veins on the forelimb that may be accessed for blood collection.

Venipuncture in macropods may be carried out by a number of methods. Restraining the animal in lateral recumbency and stretching the head slightly exposes the jugular vein on the ventrolateral surface of the neck. In large animals the saphenous vein may be raised on the medial aspect of the tibia by applying pressure around the stifle. The femoral vein is accessible in all species, immediately posterior to and medial to the femur. Kangaroos have a medial tail vein that may be used to obtain blood samples, but it should not be used to administer intravenous medication.

Transport

Platypuses may be transported in cloth bags for short distances, but for longer trips, small smooth-sided boxes are desirable.[20,21] Echidnas may also be transported in small boxes or in plastic garbage cans with the lid securely fastened. In both cases it is essential to maintain ambient temperatures below 25°C throughout the trip and provide adequate ventilation in the box.

Marsupials may be transported in crates such as for other mammals of comparable size.[1] Crates with wire ends are hazardous for shipping or holding macropods. If they become frightened or excited, they will jump against the wire in an attempt to escape. Macropods are subject to capture myopathy.[14]

Chemical Restraint[3,4,7–10,15–18]

Table 21.2 lists restraint agents and the dosage for various groups of monotremes and marsupials. Ketamine or combinations of ketamine and xylazine are used most frequently, but tiletamine/zolazepam is often used.[3,4]

Etorphine hydrochloride and acepromazine maleate were used in another study to capture red kangaroos.[22] The dosages were 0.04 mg/kg etorphine and 0.16 mg/kg acepromazine.

TABLE 21.2. Selected chemical restraint agents used for immobilizing marsupial[7,8,9,10,16]

Agent	Dose (mg/kg), IM	Comments
Isoflurane	5% induction, 2.5% maintenance	Use a face mask
Ketamine/xylazine	10.0/4.0	Macropods
	5.0/5.0	Koalas
Ketamine/medetomidine	2.0–3.0/0.05–0.1	
Tiletamine/zolazepam	2.0–8.0	Wombats
(Telazol)	10.0–20.0	Possums*
	4.0–10.0	Koalas
	5.0–7.0	Echidna
Telazol/xylazine	5.0/0.5	general

*High doses used on free-ranging possums.

The animals were not immobilized but were sedated and able to be handled.

Ketamine has been shown to be a safe agent in red kangaroos (15 mg/kg) and wallaroos (19 mg/kg).[3] My own experience verifies that ketamine (10–15 mg/kg) is satisfactory for handling wallaroos.

Effective anesthetic-immobilizing agents in the Virginia opossum include ketamine hydrochloride (20–25 mg/kg) and fentanyl-droperidol (0.4 mg/kg and 20 mg/kg, respectively).[4] General anesthesia is usually accomplished by masking the animal down with isoflurane or similar newer inhalation agents (Fig. 21.17).

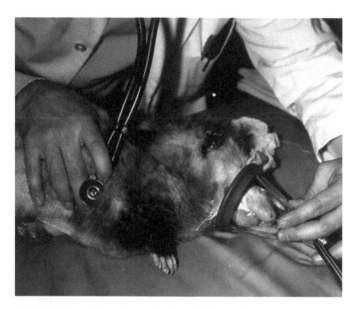

FIG. 21.17.   Inhalant anesthesia administered with a mask.

REFERENCES

1. Anonymous. 2007. Live Animal Regulations, 34th ed. Montreal: International Air Transport Association.
2. Calaby, J.H., and Poole, W.E. 1971. Keeping kangaroos in captivity; marsupials in captivity. Int Zoo Yearb 2:5–12.
3. Denny, M.J.S. 1973. The use of ketamine HCl as a safe, short duration anesthetic in kangaroos. Br Vet J 129:362–65.
4. Feldman, D.B., and Self, J.L. 1971. Sedation and anesthesia of the Virginia opossum, Dideiphis virginiana. Lab Anim Sci 21:717–20.
5. Firth, J.H., and Calaby, J.H. 1969. Kangaroos. Melbourne, Australia: Cheshire.
6. Fritz, H.I. 1971. Maintenance of the common opossum in captivity; marsupials in captivity. Int Zoo Yearb 2:32–33.
7. Holz, P. 1992. Immobilization of marsupials with tiletamine and zolazepam. J. Zoo Wildl Med 23:426–28.
8. Holz, P. 2003. Marsupalia. In: Fowler, M.E., and Miller, R.E., Eds. 2003. Zoo and Wild Animal Medicine. 5th Ed. St. Louis, Saunders/Elsevier. pp. 290–92.
9. Holz, P. 2007. Monotremes. In: West, G., Heard, D., and Caulkett, N. 2007. Zoo Animal and Wildlife Immobilization and Anesthesia. Ames, Iowa, Blackwell Publishing, pp. 337–40.
10. Holz, P. 2007. Marsupials. In: West, G., Heard, D., and Caulkett, T. 2007. Zoo Animal and Wildlife Immobilization and Anesthesia. Ames, Iowa, Blackwell Publishing, pp. 341–46.
11. Hope, R.M. 1971. The maintenance of the brush-tailed opossum in captivity; marsupials in captivity. Int Zoo Yearb 2:24–25.
12. Keep, J.M., and Fox, A.M. 1971. The capture, restraint and translocation of kangaroos in the wild. Aust Vet J 47:141–44.
13. Lyne, A.G. 1971. Bandicoots in captivity; marsupials in captivity. Int Zoo Yearb 2:41–43.
14. Munday, B.L. 1972. Myonecrosis in free-living and recently captured macropods. J Wildl Dis 8:191–92.
15. Richardson, K.C., and Cullen, L.K. 1981. Anesthesia of small kangaroos. J Am Vet Med Assoc 179:1162–65.
16. Shima, A.L. 1999. Sedation and anesthesia in marsupials. In: Fowler, M.E., and Miller, R.E., Eds. Zoo and Wild Animal Medicine—Current Vet. Therapy. 4th Ed. Philadelphia, WB Saunders. pp. 333–36.
17. Watson, C.R.R., and Way, J.S. 1971. Anesthetics for kangaroos; marsupials in captivity. Int Zoo Yearb 2:12–13.
18. Watson, C.R.R., and Way, J.S. 1972. The unusual tolerance of marsupials to barbiturate anesthetics. Int Zoo Yearb 12:208–211.
19. Wells, R.T. 1971. Maintenance of the hairy-nosed wombat in captivity; marsupials in captivity. Int Zoo Yearb 2:30–31.
20. Whittington, R.J. 1988. The monotremes in health and disease. In: The John Keep Refresher Course for Veterinarians, Proceeding 104, pp. 727–87, Sydney, Aust., Post Graduate Committee in Veterinary Science.
21. Whittingham, R.J. 1993. Diseases of monotremes. In: M.E. Fowler, Ed. Zoo and Wild Animal Medicine 3rd ed., pp. 269–76. Philadelphia: W.B. Saunders.
22. Wilson, G.R. 1974. The restraint of red kangaroos using etorphine-acepromazine and etorphine-methotnimeprazine mixtures. Aust Vet J 50:454–58.

C H A P T E R   2 2
Small Mammals

CLASSIFICATION (NUMBERS IN PARENTHESES DENOTE NUMBER OF KNOWN SPECIES)

Order Insectivora

    Superfamily Tenrecoidea: solenodon, tenrec, other shrews (29)

    Superfamily Chrysochioroidea: golden mole (15)

    Superfamily Erinaceoidea: hedgehog (19)

    Superfamily Macroscelidoidea: elephant shrew (21)

    Superfamily Soricoidea: shrew, mole (284)

Order Dermoptera

    Family Cynocephalidae: flying lemur (2)

Order Chiroptera: bats

    Family Megachiroptera: fruit bat (150)

    Family Microchiroptera: insectivorous bat (831)

Order Edentata

    Family Myremecophagidae: anteater (4)

    Family Bradypodidae: sloth (7)

    Family Dasypodidae: armadillo (21)

Order Pholidota

    Family Manidae: pangolin (7)

Order Lagomorpha

    Family Ochontonidae: pika (14)

    Family Leporidae: rabbit, hare (52)

Order Rodentia

    Suborder Sciuromorpha: squirrel, marmot, chipmunk, gopher, beaver, kangaroo rat, springhaas (366)

    Suborder Myomorpha: rat, mouse, hamster, lemming, mole (1,183)

    Suborder Hystricomorpha: porcupine, cavy, capybara, chinchilla, agouti, guinea pig (180)

Order Tubulidentata

    Family Orycteropodidae: aardvark (1)

Order Hyracoidea

    Family Procaviidae: hyrax (6)

Most small mammal adults are referred to as male and female. The young and newborn are called infants, offspring, youngsters, or juveniles.

A few introductory remarks will indicate some techniques common to many species. Specialized problems or procedures will be described for taxonomic groups.

Biting, scratching, and clawing are common defensive and offensive actions by small mammals.

Many species may be handled with gloves. Nets and snares are useful, the type varying with the size and behavior of the animal. All the insectivores have tiny sharp teeth. If agitated, they may bite at hard objects and injure their teeth.

INSECTIVORA[1,2,7,11,15,17]

Tenrecs,[11] shrews,[17] and hedgehogs[9,11,15] are primitive insectivorous mammals. Shrews are tiny rodent-like creatures with an extremely high metabolic rate.[2,17] They cannot tolerate extensive manipulation because they may overheat and become hypoglycemic in a short time. Shrews are handled with techniques similar to those used for rodents (e.g., plastic tubes or other similar devices). These techniques minimize direct handling, which distresses this species. Light gloves protect the hands if it is necessary to grasp the animal.

The following species of shrews and solenodons are known to be venomous:[7] American short-tailed shrew, *Blarma brevicauda*; European water shrew, *Neomys fodiens*; masked shrew, *Sorex cinereus*; Haitian solenodon, *Solenodon pardoxus*; and elephant shrew, *Macroscelides* spp. Probably other species are also venomous, at least to their prey species.[7] The venom apparatus in shrews and solenodons consists of modified submaxillary salivary glands. The ducts of these glands open near the incisor teeth, which may be grooved or channeled to assist in the deposition of venom. Envenomation of a human being is usually of little consequence, but precautions should be taken.

Hedgehogs hibernate for 4–5 months of the year and may appear to be ill as a result of their inactivity.[11,15] The weight of an adult hedgehog varies from 800 to 1,700 g.[15]

Tenrecs and hedgehogs have teeth and may bite. Many individuals kept in captivity for a long period become docile and may be handled gently with the bare hand. However, if it becomes necessary to severely restrict movement, it is advisable to wear a glove (Fig. 22.1).

Modified hairs of hedgehogs and tenrecs are spiny. The spines or quills are not cast and are neither sharpened nor barbed like the quills of New World porcupines. Hedgehogs characteristically make a sudden jerking motion when touched, to make the intruder cognizant of their prickly nature.

Tenrecs and hedgehogs protect themselves by rolling up into a tight ball, exposing only quills. This is accomplished by a unique superficial muscle layer. These animals cannot be placed into a squeeze cage because as soon as they sense strange surroundings or pressure, they immediately roll into a ball. Nothing but spines is exposed for examination. Exerting more pressure crushes the animal. These animals can be

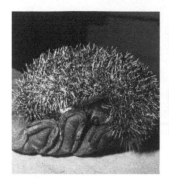
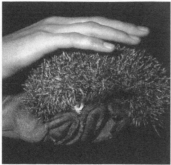

FIG. 22.1. The quills of a hedgehog are not barbed nor extremely sharp. Nonetheless, gloves are usually recommended for handling them.

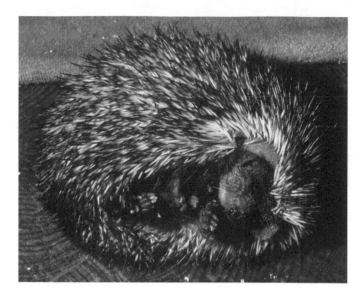

FIG. 22.2. A hedgehog sedated with ketamine.

examined only if they are completely relaxed. Otherwise they must be chemically immobilized.

Chemical Immobilization

The chemical restraint agents and combinations mentioned in this chapter represent those used by the author or experienced veterinarians with detailed knowledge of the species. Other protocols have been used and no claim is made for including all possible drugs and combinations. For more detailed information, particularly for anesthesia, consult the references.

The safest and most effective immobilization of shrews and hedgehogs is with 5.0% isoflurane in oxygen. The viewing cage may be placed in an anesthetic chamber or inside a plastic bag. When relaxation occurs, reduce the flow to 2.5% and place a mask over the face to maintain anesthesia for the required time. Work with the shrew on a heating pad, for isoflurane enhances blood flow to the skin and rapid body cooling.[17] Alternatively, ketamine alone (10–20 mg/kg) or in combination with xylazine (1.0 mg/kg) may be administered intramuscularly, providing sedation for 20–30 minutes. Table 22.1 lists other restraint agents and dosages.

Intramuscular injection into the superficial muscle can be made between the spines of a hedgehog (Fig. 22.2). Drugs should not be injected into the neck region, for this is the site of accumulation of brown fat.

The sex of a tenrec or hedgehog may be determined by placing the animal in a box with a transparent bottom (plastic or glass). Once the animal has relaxed, the box can be lifted and the external genitalia viewed from below.[10]

DERMOPTERA—FLYING LEMURS[2]

Gloves and nets are used to handle these animals.

CHIROPTERA—BATS[6,12,20–22,27]
Danger Potential

All species of bats bite. It is necessary to control the head at all times. Vampire bats and some species of insectivorous bats are known to carry rabies virus. Bites from infected animals may prove lethal. Although fruit bats have not been reported to harbor the rabies virus, they have been implicated as carriers for lyssaviruses in Southeast Asia.

ANATOMY AND BEHAVIOR

Bats are the only mammals capable of sustained flight. The delicate bones of the forelimb support an elastic wing membrane called a patagium. Some species possess a highly refined echolocation sense, which makes capture with nets extremely difficult. Most bats are nocturnal, thus bright lights

TABLE 22.1. Selected chemical restraint agents for insectivores and flying lemurs[2]

Agent	Sedative dose (mg/kg), IM	Immobilizing dose (mg/kg), IM
Isoflurane		5% induction, 2.5% maintenance, mask, Preferred (13)
Diazepam	0.5–2.0	(11)
Ketamine	5.0–20.0	
Tiletamine/zolazepam		1.0–5.0
Xylazine		0.5–1.0
Ketamine/xylazine		5.0/0.5
Ketamine/medetomidine		2.0/0.2
Ketamine/midazolam		20.0/1.0–2.0, IM (11)

are useful to confuse bats while they are being grasped. Bats possess unique physiological adaptations that make them desirable for biomedical research. Some bats are hibernators, others become torpid or hypothermic daily. This heterothermic adaptation is unique among mammals and is utilized to conduct studies of infectious agents.

Physical Restraint of Fruit Bats[6,12]

If the bat is in a cage that does not permit flight, it may be grasped with gloved hands. A towel or laboratory coat may be thrown over the bat to restrict its activity before grasping it. In flight enclosures a bright light may be shone on a perched animal and the animal grasped while it is dazed by the intense light. Nets may be used, but the hoop must be large enough to capture the bat without traumatizing the wings. The net should be made of a closely woven fabric; otherwise the claws will become hopelessly entangled.

Physical Restraint of Insectivorous Bats

Experienced handlers grasp most species at the nape of the neck with bare or gloved hands (Fig. 22.3).

The novice should wear a leather glove. Bats move rapidly, even when crawling, and may crawl past the handler's gloved hand to bite an exposed wrist or arm. A leather jacket and gauntleted gloves may obviate this action. Small bats may be grasped by the nape of the neck with a long thumb forcep to transfer a bat from one cage to another (Fig. 22.4). This technique may also be used to capture a bat, enabling the handler to grasp the animal as it struggles to free itself from the forceps.

A towel or cloth may be dropped over insectivorous as well as frugivorous bats. Nets are also suitable capture equipment.

Mist nets and other elaborate devices have been designed for capturing free-ranging bats.[6]

Physical Restraint of Vampire Bats

Vampire bats are less fragile and liable to injury than insectivorous bats. Extreme caution must be used when handling vampire bats because they may transmit rabies. Nets,

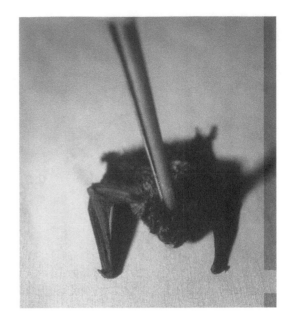

FIG. 22.4.   Handling a small bat with a long thumb forcep.

forceps, and/or thick gloves offer some protection when handling these animals. Vampire bats can run and jump even when so engorged with food they are unable to fly.

Blood Collection

Venipuncture to collect a blood sample from a bat is made possible by stretching the wing and locating the vein on the anterior edge between the carpus and shoulder (Fig. 22.5).

Transport

Bats may be carried in light cloth sacks or cardboard boxes. They will not gnaw or chew their way out.[22]

Chemical Restraint[6,12]

Tranquilization and immobilization are seldom imposed on bats. Ketamine hydrochloride (5–15 mg/kg) has been used.

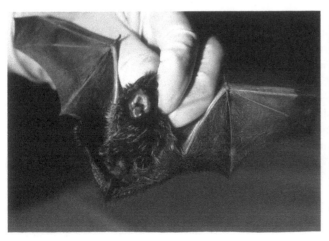

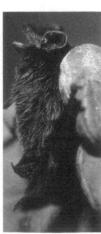

FIG. 22.3.   Grasping a small bat with rubber-gloved thumb and forefinger, left. Grasping with a leather glove, right.

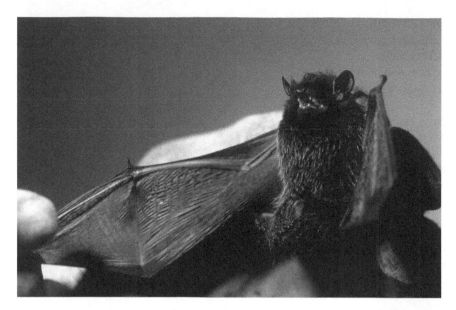

FIG. 22.5.   Handling a bat with rubber gloves exposing the vein on the leading edge of the wing.

TABLE 22.2.   Selected chemical restraint agents for bats[12]

Agent	Dose (mg/kg), IM
Isoflurane	5% induction, 2.5% maintenance, face mask
Ketamine	15.0–40.0
Ketamine/xylazine	10.0/2.0
Tiletamine/zolazopam	40.0, orally

Salivation and catatonia may be pronounced. Diazepam alleviates catatonia. See Table 22.2 for other chemical restraint agents.

Isoflurane is the anesthetic agent of choice in a chamber using a calibrated vaporizer.

EDENTATA—ANTEATERS, SLOTHS, ARMADILLOS[1,8–10,19,20,25]

Anteaters eat termites and ants. Some, such as the tamandua, are arboreal; others are strictly terrestrial.[8,9]

The tamandua is a diminutive anteater with claws on the forefeet for opening termite nests and a prehensile tail (Figs. 22.6, 22.7). The claws are not so enlarged nor used in so aggressive a manner as the claws of the giant anteater. When a tamandua is frightened or threatened, it stands up with outspread arms. The enemy is grasped by the strong claws and held away from the body. The tamandua is handled by firmly holding the back of the head and tail simultaneously, preventing the animal from twisting around to grasp an arm with the front claws. Any manipulation of the ventral aspect of the animal requires grasping the front feet, preferably with a gloved hand. The tamandua is not aggressive, and minor procedures can be carried out with no physical restriction whatsoever. Intramuscular injections may be given by a quick jab. Examination may usually be conducted at close quarters without significant danger.

The giant anteater weighs up to 90 kg (200 lb) and is well known for its unpredictable and frequently aggressive

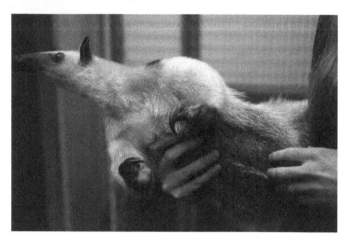

FIG. 22.6.   The tamandua has strong claws but is not as aggressive as the giant anteater.

actions. It has no teeth and is unable to bite, but it possesses extremely long, strong recurved claws on the forefeet that are especially designed for tearing open termite mounds (Fig. 22.8). If threatened, it grasps and pulls an enemy into its body. A person caught in such an embrace could not escape unaided. The dulled claws of an anteater were once driven into the bone of my wrist, so I can attest to the speed and strength of its forefeet. More than one zookeeper has been chased from an enclosure by a giant anteater.

A giant anteater may be restricted by directing it into a narrow screened enclosure or box by means of a plywood shield and held in the box by bars placed in the opening. Such a box is suitable for sexing a giant anteater but does not allow sufficient exposure to conduct a general physical examination. A squeeze cage for the giant anteater is illustrated in Figures 22.9 and 22.10.

If blood samples or comprehensive examination are required, the animal may be stretched by placing a snare on each foot. This is not difficult to do, since these animals are

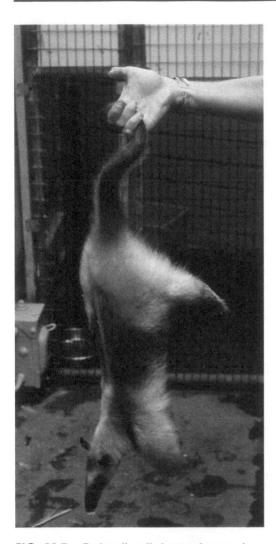

FIG. 22.7. Prehensile-tailed tamandua may be moved via the tail.

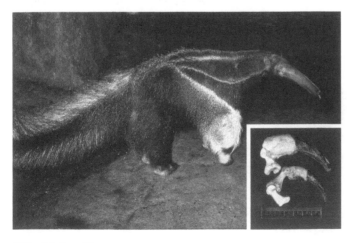

FIG. 22.8. Giant anteater.

somewhat slow moving. A handler can let the animal step into the loop of a snare with each foot. Nets are unsatisfactory for capturing a giant anteater; it is likely to tear the net to shreds with the forefeet.

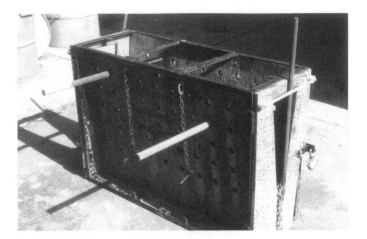

FIG. 22.9. A squeeze cage designed for the giant anteater.

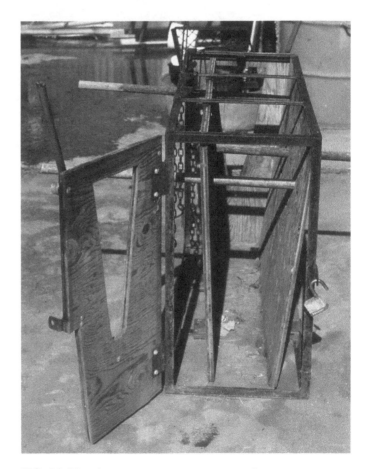

FIG. 22.10. An anteater squeeze cage opened to see the movable sides.

The sloth appears to be slow and docile.[10,20] On the ground it is clumsy or even helpless. The natural response of a threatened sloth is to curl up into a tight ball. When angered, however, it can move very quickly and slash accurately with the front claws. It also has a tendency to grasp an opponent and draw it close enough to bite.

The sloth's claws are highly adapted for grasping branches of trees. It is extremely difficult to detach a sloth that is clinging to a branch or post in an enclosure. If the sloth may be enticed to move onto a detachable pole, it can be carried on the pole to an area where the floor is smooth. Then a snare or catch strap may be attached to each of the limbs and the animal spread-eagled on the floor. If the animal is to be held with the hands, the handler is advised to wear gloves to avoid being pinched by the curved claws. The sloth may be sedated with ketamine (5–15 mg/kg) administered by a pole syringe or anesthetized in an anesthetic chamber with isoflurane (Fig. 22.11).[10,20]

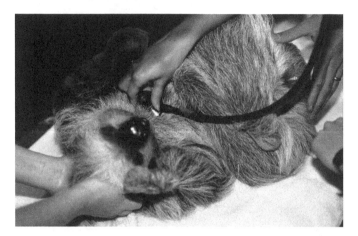

FIG. 22.11. A sloth being examined under ketamine sedation.

Twenty-one species of armadillos, varying in size from 4 to 60 kg, are found in North and South America.[1] Armadillos are insectivorous or omnivorous. They have short necks and heavy, sharpened claws adapted for burrowing. The dorsal surface of the armadillo is covered by a segmented armored membrane.

The armadillo has molar teeth but no incisors and seldom bites.[1] Its tail is useful for restraint practices since it can be grasped and held to prevent the animal from curling up into a tight ball.

Armadillos have poor eyesight and are primarily nocturnal. They are accustomed to a tropical habitat and are susceptible to cold stress. Strict confinement in small squeeze cages may be detrimental to these animals since they will continually scratch and claw at the enclosure in attempts to escape.

The three-banded armadillo rolls into a tight, completely enclosed ball when frightened (Fig. 22.12). Complete examination of this animal is impossible without the aid of chemical immobilizers or the use of strong physical force to unwind the ball. The nine-banded armadillo and the giant armadillo are incapable of rolling into a complete ball and may be unrolled by grasping the plates near the midsection (Figs. 22.13, 22.14). Free ranging nine-banded armadillos may move quite rapidly and are capable of jumping as high as 0.5 m. The armadillo has developed the ability to stop breathing for 5–10 minutes. Breath-holding is probably utilized during periods of intensive burrowing when the nostrils are buried in the earth.[1] This breath-holding technique enables the

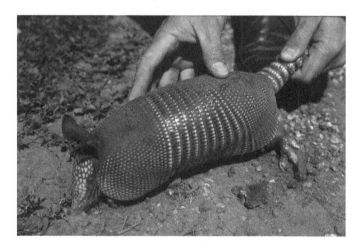

FIG. 22.13. Grasping a nine-banded armadillo by the tail.

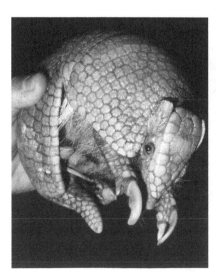

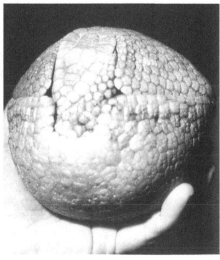

FIG. 22.12. Three-banded armadillo rolls up into a tight ball, difficult to open without sedation or injury to animal.

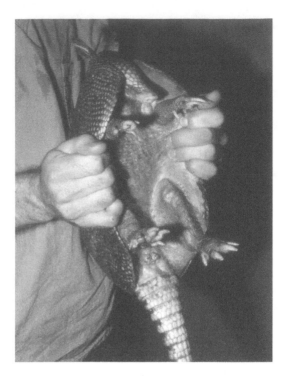

FIG. 22.14. Grasping nine-banded armadillo near its midsection.

animal to enter complete torpidity, characterized by no apparent respiration, when it is disturbed. This phenomenon must be understood by the animal restrainer, since restraint may trigger the breath-holding reflex and subsequent torpidity, giving the impression that the animal has died. Cardiac function remains, and the animal will probably begin to breathe again within a few minutes. Obviously this phenomenon must be differentiated from unconsciousness resulting from other conditions. If injured during restraint, an armadillo should be separated from others; cannibalism of injured or disabled individuals is common within captive groups.

Chemical Restraint[1,8–10,19,20,25]

Edentates may be immobilized with isoflurane in an anesthetic chamber, but armadillos and sloths are capable of holding their breath for a considerable time. See Table 22.3 for other agents.

TABLE 22.3. Selected chemical restraint agents for immobilizing edentates[8,9,25]

Agent	Dose (mg/kg), IM
Isoflurane	5% induction, 2.5% maintenance, face mask
Ketamine	10.0–20.0
Ketamine/xylazine	5.0–10.0/1.0
Ketamine/medetomidine	1.0–2.0/0.03–0.04
Ketamine/midozolam	5.0–10.0/0.2
Tiletamine/zolazepam	2.5–5.0

PHOLIDOTA PANGOLINS[16,24]

Pangolins are insectivores without teeth. Their natural diet consists of termites and ants. Heavy claws of the forefeet

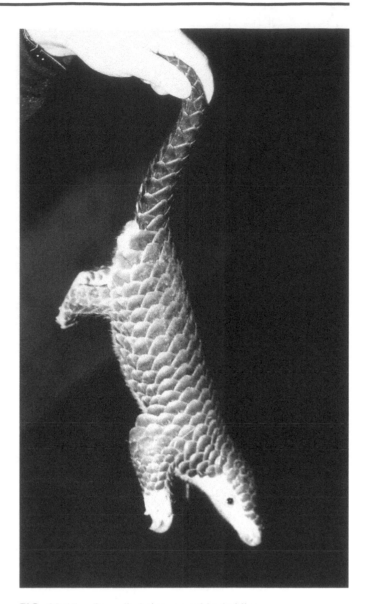

FIG. 22.15. Pangolin being moved by holding tail.

are used for digging. All pangolins are nocturnal, and most species are arboreal. The pangolins occupy the ecological niche in Africa and Asia filled by the anteaters in the New World.

The scales of pangolins are razor sharp. A pangolin may be picked up by its tail, but often when touched, the animal curls up into a ball. (Figs. 22.15, 22.16). Wear a light glove when physical handling is advised. Induce the curling response; then gently uncurl the animal, taking care to avoid the claws. Pangolins are likely to spray urine in defense.

Some individuals accustomed to people will permit touching and examination without rolling into a ball. Assumption of the defensive posture, however, is the usual response to being touched.

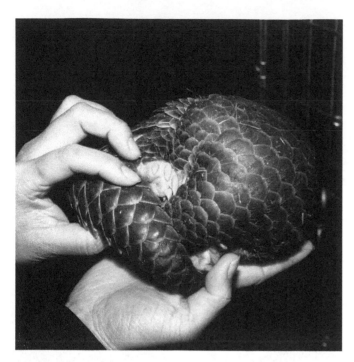

FIG. 22.16.   Pangolin tucked into a ball.

Ketamine hydrochloride (5.0–15.0 mg/kg) or tiletamine-zolazepam (2.0–10.0 mg/kg) are suitable immobilizing agents.

LAGOMORPHA—RABBITS, HARES, PIKAS[14]

Rabbits and hares are not aggressive animals and are unlikely to bite, but they do have long, sharp incisor teeth and if annoyed sufficiently may bite. However, the prime danger to the handler is from scratching. A mature hare may lash out and scratch viciously with its powerful hind feet.

Rabbits are prone to injure themselves by bolting against walls and fences with sufficient force to contuse the brain or fracture the cervical vertebrae. A physically restrained hare may self-inflict back injuries, including fractures or dislocations, by simply flexing the loin muscles.

Manual restraint of the smaller rabbits and hares is simple. Gauntleted light gloves will prevent scratches. Techniques used for restraining domestic rabbits have some applicability, but caution must be used because a wild animal will probably resist vigorously and may injure itself. It is important to support the body when applying restraint techniques. Never suspend a rabbit or hare from its ears.

Isoflurane administered in an anesthetic chamber is the agent of choice for immobilizing rabbits.[14]

RODENTIA

Rodentia, which includes over 1,500 species, is the largest order of mammals. Rodents vary in size from a mouse weighing 10–15 g to a capybara weighing 75 kg.

Danger Potential

All rodents have incisor teeth specialized for chewing and gnawing. Large species such as capybaras, beavers, and porcupines may cause serious injury by biting.

Many species of rodents are burrowers, with sharpened claws that may scratch the handler. Specialized defense mechanisms will be described in discussions of individual species.

Physiology and Behavior

Rodents are usually small, with high metabolic activity. They frequently struggle violently during restraint, and the tendency to exert excessive pressure with gloved hands or nets, which can interfere with respiration, should be resisted. Perhaps the most important fact to remember is that rodents possess no specialized thermoregulatory mechanisms. Thermal regulation is achieved by behavioral activity; they seek a source of heat when cold or retreat from a hot environment. Excitation and extreme activity during restraint procedures predisposes them to hyperthermia inasmuch as they are unable to dissipate excess heat. The predisposition is intensified if the rodent is one of the many species with heavy fur pelts.

Physical Restraint[3,4,13,18,23,26,28]

A person experienced in dealing with laboratory rodents should be cautioned that wild rodents cannot be handled with the same casualness permitted by laboratory animals. Gloves that provide protection from the bite of a laboratory species may be totally ineffective with a wild squirrel or a marmot. Wild rats, mice, and lemmings are generally handled with gloves (Fig. 22.17); however, the less they are subjected to handling, the better. When adapted to laboratory care, they may be handled bare-handed (Fig. 22.18). Squirrels should not be captured or held by their tails. The skin over the tail is friable and may strip off the tail.[10]

Most rodent species may be netted, but the claws often become entangled in nets. A fine mesh that minimizes entanglement is best for capturing rodents. Small rodents are easily traumatized if struck by the hoop of a net. As with other species, the animal should be grasped securely around the head and neck through the net, and the net carefully worked off.

A large capybara (Fig. 22.19) may be netted and physically restrained, as depicted in Figure 22.20.[28] Heavy-bodied marmots and woodchucks are difficult to remove from a net. A more effective method for handling these animals is a specialized squeeze cage (Fig. 22.21) that is adjustable for various sizes of animals. Plastic tubes are useful for transporting smaller rodents as well as for conducting examinations, taking radiographs, or administering anesthesia.

Snares are rarely used to capture rodents. Most have short necks, precluding safe use of a snare. A snare may easily tear the skin of an African crested porcupine. Specialized squeeze cages or boxes have been developed by those who work with captive rodent species in laboratories. The designs

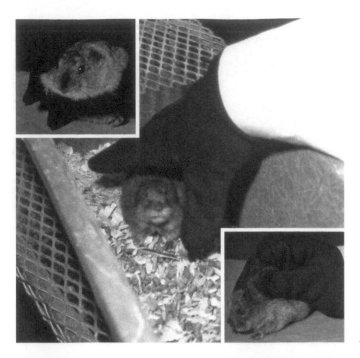

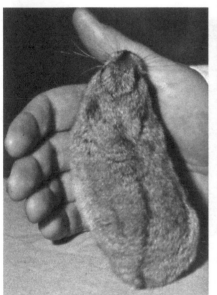

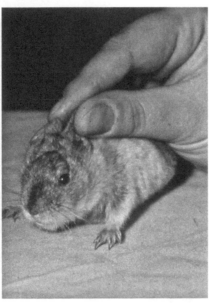

FIG. 22.17. Gloves should be worn when handling aggressive rodents or those of unknown behavior.

FIG. 22.18. Small docile rodents like this laboratory-reared lemming may be handled bare-handed.

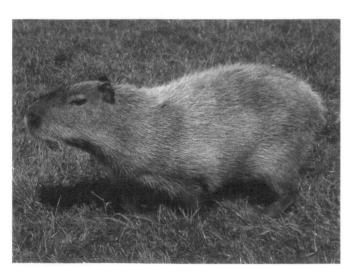

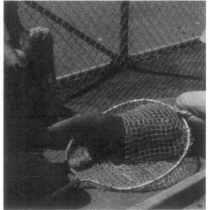

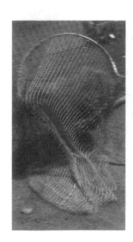

FIG. 22.19. Capybara.

FIG. 22.20. Manual restraint of a netted capybara.

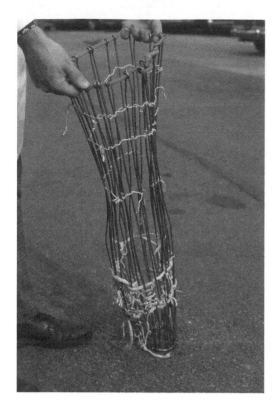

FIG. 22.21.   Special squeeze device for a woodchuck—designed by the Penrose Research Foundation, Philadelphia.

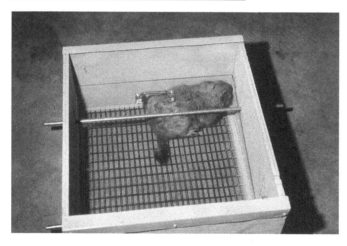

FIG. 22.22.   Prairie dog in a hand-made squeeze cage.

of squeeze cages are myriad and are usually the result of personal observation of the behavior and anatomical structure of a particular species. The device illustrated in Figures 22.22 to 22.25 is adaptable for a number of small mammalian and reptilian species. It consists of a wooden frame with a plasticized wire bottom and a Plexiglas shield used to press the animal. Plexiglas permits visual communication with the animal, so excessive pressure is not applied. Rods keep the plastic shield in place once the animal is squeezed. Prairie dogs may also be grasped with gloved hands (Fig. 22.26).[3]

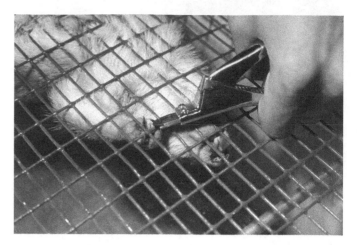

FIG. 22.23.   Clipping a toenail.

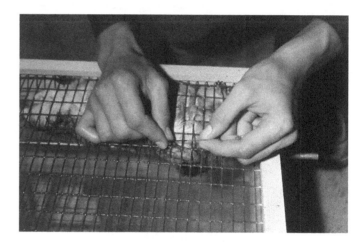

FIG. 22.24.   Collecting blood from the toenail of a prairie dog.

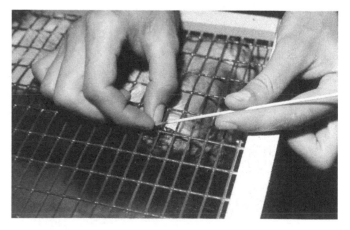

FIG. 22.25.   Cauterizing the clipped toenail with a silver nitrate stick.

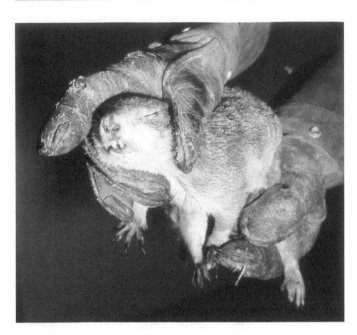

FIG. 22.26. Hand holding a prairie dog using gloves.

The box is inverted to expose the abdomen. If exposure of the dorsal surface is needed, the box is inverted and the squeeze is released slightly, allowing the animal to flip over. The squeeze is then reapplied, pressing the dorsal surface against the wire screen.

Do not lift a beaver by the tail.[26] Beavers are heavy bodied, and the weight may cause spinal injuries. Restrain the beaver with a snare or preferably a catch strap around the neck. The animal may be lifted and held by a firm grip at the base of the tail as well for additional restraint.

Grasp the muskrat by the tail and pull the animal backward as it struggles to escape, placing the other lightly gloved hand over the back to press the animal to the surface (Figs. 22.27, 22.28). To pick up the animal, surround the neck with thumb and forefinger, maintaining the pull on the tail and keeping the legs stretched to the front.

A chinchilla in a cage may exhibit defensive or even aggressive behavior when approached by a stranger. I had a personal pet, which, when first acquired, would stand on its hind legs in the back of the cage and urinate on the hands of anyone who attempted to catch it. This individual would also use its forepaws to box with our pet cat through the bars of the cage.

The fur of the chinchilla is extremely delicate. Individual fibers can be pulled from the hide at a touch. Picking up the chinchilla by the body will result in the loss of some of the fur. The proper method of picking up a chinchilla is by grasping the animal at the base of the tail (Fig. 22.29). If you are unfamiliar with the animal, wear a light leather glove. Once the chinchilla is grasped, it may be held on the hand, maintaining the grip on the tail (Fig. 22.30).

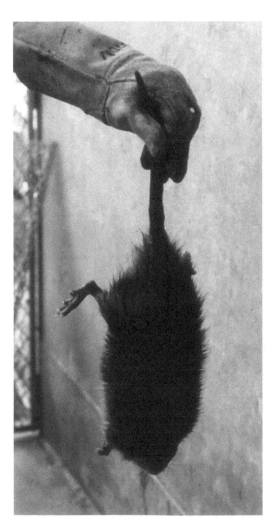

FIG. 22.27. Muskrat may be lifted by the tail or pinned, using the tail and gloved hand.

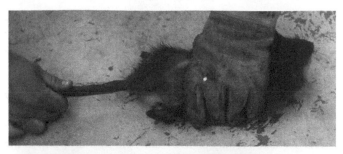

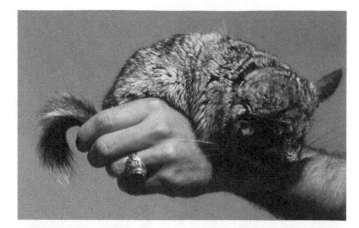

FIG. 22.28.   Once a muskrat is pinned, it may be manipulated into other positions.

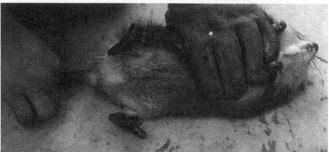

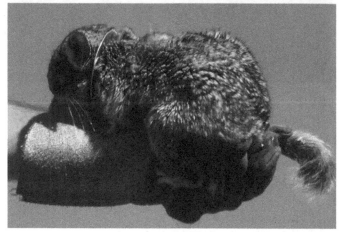

FIG. 22.30.   Holding a chinchilla bare-handed, top, with gloved hand, bottom.

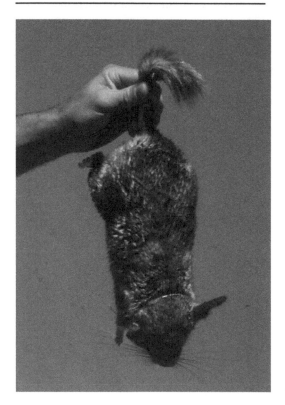

FIG. 22.29.   Initial capture should always be via the tail.

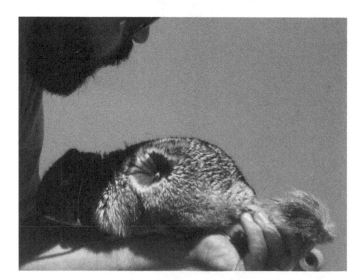

FIG. 22.31.   Fur may be examined by gently blowing to separate fibers.

If the coat or skin requires examination, blow on the fur to separate individual fibers and look at the skin (Fig. 22.31). By simply blowing in different locations, the whole body surface can be adequately examined.

If further manipulation or more restrictive restraint is necessary, grasp the animal by the ears as illustrated in Figure

22.32. If a chinchilla must be securely held, wrap it in a towel to avoid damaging the fur. Chinchillas are commonly plagued with dental problems. Dental specula are illustrated in Figure 22.33.

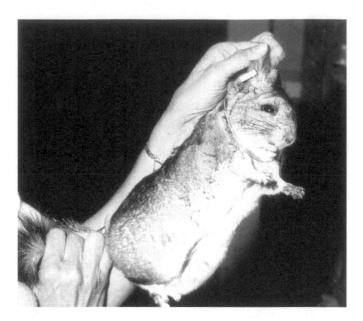

FIG. 22.32. Holding a chinchilla by the ears and tail.

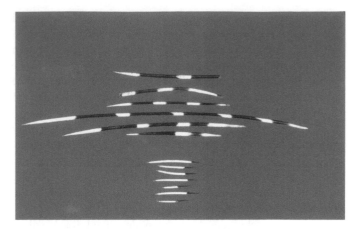

FIG. 22.34. Quills of an African porcupine, top. Barbed quills of an American porcupine, bottom.

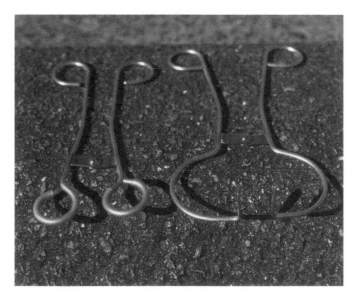

FIG. 22.33. Chinchilla dental specula: Forceps on left is placed behind incisor teeth to open the mouth. Forceps on right is inserted into the cheek pouch to pull out cheek for better visualization of the teeth.

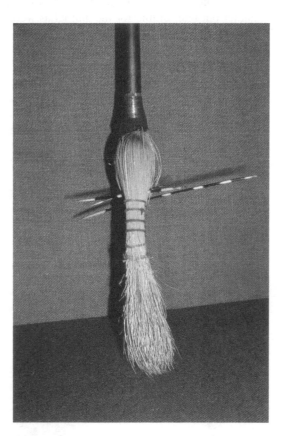

FIG. 22.35. Quills of an African porcupine driven through a broom.

Porcupines have evolved quills to use as a protective mechanism against enemies.[23] Old World crested porcupines have large smooth quills 30–45 cm (1–1.5 ft) long (Fig. 22.34). When frightened, they erect the quills and run backward, driving the long solid quills through the boots or legs of anyone approaching. The sudden rush can force the quills through a heavy leather boot or a broom (Fig. 22.35). The only adequate protection against such quills is a piece of heavy plywood or metal. An excited crested porcupine warns of impending attack by impatiently rattling the hollow tail quills.

Old World porcupines may be transferred quite easily; they are nocturnal and will readily enter a dark box in the cage. Close examination is possible if the box is constructed as a wire inner enclosure with removable covers.

Quills of the North American porcupine are much shorter than those of the crested porcupine. The quills are hazardous, both to the restrainer and to the animal itself. The porcupine is not capable of projecting the quills, but if it flips the tail and touches the handler, quills will impale the tissue. Furthermore, the quills have microscopic reverse barbs that catch in the flesh and cause the quills to migrate through the tissue unless they are quickly removed. Porcupine quills can be driven through heavy canvas and leather gloves, so neither of these provides adequate protection.

If two or more porcupines are in an enclosure, they should be separated before attempting to capture one; otherwise the excitement may cause one porcupine to bump into another, resulting in discharge of the quills by one or both and subsequent injury to the porcupines. Quills scattered on the floor can penetrate the feet of the porcupines.

Various techniques have been described for handling porcupines, most of them apparently by persons who have never handled one. Some have recommended throwing a canvas over the porcupine. Such a technique is not only dangerous to the handler but undesirable for the animal as well. All the quills that touch the canvas will be pulled from its body, causing dermal hemorrhage.

A technique successfully practiced by experienced persons is to approach the porcupine from the rear after it has headed toward a corner. Usually the porcupine drags its tail on the ground, but when the animal is disturbed, the tail is flipped upward. Anything that comes in contact with that tail will receive an injection of quills. To guard against this, keep the hand on the ground at the same level as the tail and gently reach up to grasp some of the under hairs and quills and pull backward (Fig. 22.36). The animal will attempt to flip its tail upward as soon as it feels the touch, so maintain sufficient

tension to keep the tail from pulling away. A wooden stick may be used to hold the tail down. It may be necessary to regrasp the tail with the other hand in order to achieve a firmer hold. As long as the tail is grasped firmly, it cannot be flipped to discharge quills. Maintain pressure on the tail and gently lift the animal off its feet by sliding the other hand beneath the tail and up under its body (Fig. 22.37). The ventral surface is free of quills.

A squeeze cage with smooth inner walls may also be used to restrict a porcupine's movement. The quills should be pressed in the right direction to lie smoothly against the body.

Manual restraint of a North American porcupine has been carried out with multiple snares—one snare around the base of the tail and others on each foot to stretch the animal. It may be placed in dorsal recumbency, exposing the ventral surface for various procedures such as obtaining blood samples or tuberculin testing (Fig. 22.38).

The Brazilian tree porcupine has quills that are neither sharp nor barbed. The quills are more like those of hedgehogs or tenrecs. These animals may be handled quite easily with leather gloves.

Chemical Restraint[13]

See Table 22.4. for chemical restraint agents used in rodents. Caution is advised when chemically immobilizing the African crested porcupine. I administered ketamine to two animals with a pole syringe while standing behind a shield. When the animals became immobile, large (12-cm) lacerations were observed at the two injection sites. The response

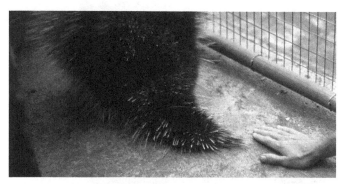

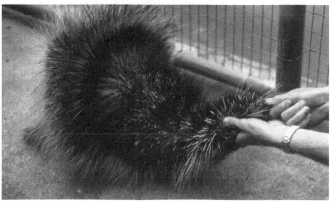

FIG. 22.36.   Initial step in capturing a North American porcupine: Keep the hand low and grasp hairs at tip of tail. Work the other hand carefully up the underside of tail until a firm grasp is possible.

TABLE 22.4.   Chemical restraint agents for rodents[13]

Agent	Dosage (mg/kg)	Comments and References
Isoflurane		5.0% induction, 2.5% maintenance
Tiletamine/zolazepam	50.0–80.0, general, IP	
	20.0–40.0 Guinea pig, IP	
	4.0–6.0 Beaver, porcupine, capybara, IM	
Ketamine/midazolam	40.0–50.0/3.0–5.0 guinea pig	
Ketamine/medetomidine	3.0–4.0/0.03–0.04 Beaver, porcupine, capybara, IM	
Ketamine/xylazine	50.0–150.0	
	20.0–40.0/3.0–5.0	
	Guinea pig, IV	
	5.0–10.0/1.0–2.0	
	Beaver, porcupine, capybara, IM	

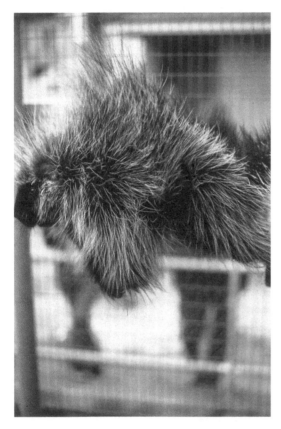

FIG. 22.37.   Final step in porcupine restraint: Insert a hand between hind legs underneath the abdomen to support the body.

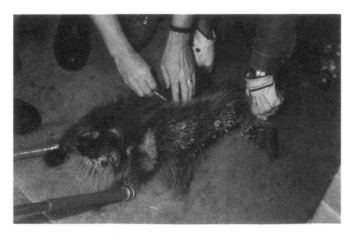

FIG. 22.38.   Capturing a North American porcupine with snares.

of the porcupines upon feeling the injection was to contract the heavy subcutaneous muscle to rattle the quills. Apparently, the large-bore needle acted as if it were a cheese or cake cutter, and lacerated the skin and muscle. Subsequently, blow darts were used without such damage.

TUBULIDENTATA[16,24]

The aardvark is a medium-sized animal especially adapted for digging and burrowing. It has heavy claws, a thick body, and a short neck, making restraint rather difficult. When the animal's activity is restricted, it begins twisting and turning, expending great bursts of energy. The aardvark will begin to thrash wildly if snared; unless the restrainer is extremely careful, the animal will strangulate.

The aardvark has incisor teeth, but its mouth cannot open widely enough to be of any real danger.

The cone-shaped canvas bag described for restraining the wombat (see Chapter 17) is useful for controlling an aardvark. See Table 22.5 for chemical restraint agents used in aardvarks.

TABLE 22.5.   Chemical agents for the aardvark[24]

Agent	Dose (mg/kg), IM	Reversal
Tiletamine/zolazepam	4.0–5.0	Flumazenil 0.1 mg/kg
Ketamine/medetomidine	1.0–3.0/0.025–0.06	Atipamezole 0.15–0.4 mg/kg
Ketamine/midazolam	15.0–20.0/0.28–0.68	
Ketamine/diazepam	11.0/0.26	

HYRACOIDEA[5]

Hyraxes present no any major restraint problems, but they are highly susceptible to stress and should be handled as little as possible.[5] Strangers inside a cage may unnecessarily alarm the animals. It is desirable for a hyrax to be captured by the usual keeper.

Hyraxes may be gently directed into boxes or transfer cages without becoming alarmed.[5] A net is satisfactory for capturing them from an enclosure. They may be removed from the net and manipulated using gloves, or they may be handled bare-handed because they are not likely to scratch (Figs. 22.39, 22.40).

See Table 22.6 for chemical restraint agents used in hyraxes.

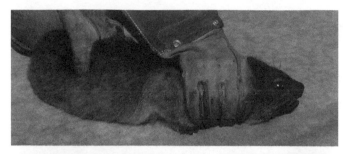

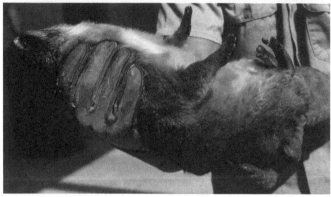

FIG. 22.39.   Hyrax handled with gloves.

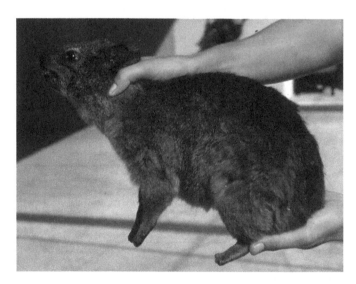

FIG. 22.40.   The hyrax is not likely to scratch, thus it may be safely held bare-handed after capture.

TABLE 22.6.   Chemical restraint agents for immobilization of hyraxes[5]

Agent	Dose (mg/kg), IM
Isoflurane	5.9% induction, 2.0% maintenance. Use a mask.
Tiletamine/zolazepam	5.0–10.0
Ketamine	10.0
Ketamine/diazepam	5.0–20.0/1.0–3.0
Ketamine/xylazine	5.0–10.0/3.0–5.0
Ketamine/medetomidine	5.0/0.35

REFERENCES

1. Anderson, J.M., and Benirschke, K. 1966. The armadillo, *Dasypus novemcinctus*, in experimental biology. Lab Anim Care 16:202–16.
2. Barbiers, R. 2003. Insectivora and Dermoptera. In: Fowler, M.E., and Miller, R.E., Eds. Zoo and Wild Animal Medicine. 5th Ed. St. Louis, Saunders/Elsevier. pp. 304–20.
3. Carpenter, J.W., and Martin, R.P. 1969. Capturing prairie dogs for transplanting. J Wildl Manage 33:1024.
4. Caudill, C.J., and Gaddis, S.E. 1973. A safe efficient handling device for wild rodents. Lab Anim Sci 23:685–86.
5. Collins, D. 2003. Hyracoidea (Hyraxes). In: Fowler, M.E., and Miller, R.E., Eds. Zoo and Wild Animal Medicine. 5th Ed. St. Louis, Saunders/Elsevier. pp. 550–52.
6. Constantine, D.G. 1958. An automatic bat-collecting device. J Wildl Manage 22:17–22.
7. Fowler, M.E. 1993. Veterinary Zootoxicology, Boca Raton, Fla.: CRC Press, pp. 230–32.
8. Gillespie, D.S. 1993. Diseases of edentata. In: Fowler, M.E., Ed. Zoo and Wild Animal Medicine, 3rd ed., Philadelphia, W.B. Saunders, pp. 304–09.
9. Gillespie, D.S. 2003. Xenarthra (edentata). In: Fowler, M.E., and Miller, R.E., Eds. Zoo and Wild Animal Medicine. 5th Ed. St. Louis, Saunders/Elsevier. pp. 399–400.
10. Hanley, C. S., Siudak-Campfield, J., Paul-Murphy, J., Vaughan, C., Ramirez, O., and Sladky, K.K. 2006. Immobilization of free-ranging Hoffmann's two-toed sloths *Choloepus hoffmanni* and brown-throated three-toed sloths *Bradypus variegatus* using medetomidine-Ketamine: A comparison of physiologic parameters. 2006 Proceedings Am Assoc Zoo Vets, pp. 224–25.
11. Heard, D.J. 2007. Insectivores (hedgehogs, moles, tenrecs). In: West, G., Heard, D., and Caulkett, N. Zoo Animal and Wildlife immobilization and Anesthesia. Ames, Iowa, Blackwell Publishing, pp. 507–22.
12. Heard, D.J. 2007. Chiropterans (bats). In: West, G., Heard, D., and Caulkett, N. Zoo Animal and Wildlife immobilization and Anesthesia. Ames, Iowa, Blackwell Publishing, pp. 359–66.
13. Heard, D.J. 2007. Rodents. In: West, G., Heard, D., and Caulkett, N., Eds. Zoo Animal and Wildlife Chemical Immobilization and Anesthesia. Ames, Iowa, Blackwell Publishing, pp. 655–62.
14. Heard, D.J. 2007. Lagomorphs. In: West, G., Heard, D., and Caulkett, N., Eds. Zoo Animal and Wildlife Chemical Immobilization and Anesthesia. Ames, Iowa, Blackwell Publishing, pp. 647–54.
15. Isenbuegel, E., and Baumgartner, R.A. 1993. Diseases of the hedgehog. In: Fowler, M.E., Ed. Zoo and Wild Animal Medicine, 3rd ed., Philadelphia: W.B. Saunders, pp. 294–301.
16. Langan, J.N. 2007. Tubulidentata and Pholidota. In: West, G., Heard, D., and Caulkett, N. Zoo Animal and Wildlife immobilization and Anesthesia. Ames, Iowa, Blackwell Publishing, pp. 355–58.
17. Meehan, T.P. 1993. Medical problems of shrews. In: Fowler, M.E., Ed. Zoo and Wild Animal Medicine 3rd ed., Philadelphia, W.B. Saunders, pp. 302–03.
18. Melchior, H.R., and Iwen, F.A. 1965. Trapping, restraining, and marking arctic ground squirrels for behavioral observations. J Wildl Manage 29:671–78.
19. Merritt, D.A., Jr. 1972. Edentate immobilization at Lincoln Park Zoo, Chicago. Int Zoo Yearb 12:218–20.
20. Merritt, D.A. 1974. A further note on the immobilization of sloths. Int Zoo Yearb 14:160–61.

21. Orr, R.T. 1958. Keeping bats in captivity. J Mammal 39:339–44.
22. Pye, J.D. 1967. Bats. In: The UFAW Handbook on the Care and Management of Laboratory Animals, 3rd ed., London, E & S Livingstone, pp. 491–501.
23. Shadle, A.R. 1950. Feeding, care and handling of captive porcupines (Erethizon). J Mammal 31:411–16.
24. Stetter, M.D. 2003. Tubulidentata (aardvark). In: Fowler, M.E., and Miller, R.E., Eds. Zoo and Wild Animal Medicine. 5th Ed. St. Louis, Saunders/Elsevier. p. 539.
25. West, G., Carter, T., and Shaw, J. 2007. Edentates (Xenarthra). In: West, G., Heard, D., and Caulkett, N. Zoo Animal and Wildlife immobilization and Anesthesia. Ames, Iowa, Blackwell Publishing, pp. 349–54.
26. Whitelow, C.J., and Pengelley, E.T. 1954. A method for handling live beaver. J Wildl Manage 18:533–34.
27. Wimsatt, W.A. 1970. Biology of Bats, vols. 1, 2. New York, Academic Press.
28. Zara, J. 1973. Breeding and husbandry of the capybara at Evansville Zoo. Int Zoo Yearb 13:137–39.

CHAPTER 23

Carnivores

CLASSIFICATION (NUMBERS IN PARENTHESES DENOTE NUMBER OF KNOWN SPECIES)[35]

Order Carnivora

    Family Canidae: dog, fox, wolf (37)

    Family Ursidae: bear (7), giant panda (1)

    Family Aluridae: lesser panda (1)

    Family Procyonidae: raccoon, kinkajou (17)

    Family Mustelidae: skunk, otter, weasel (68)

    Family Viverridae: civet, mongoose (82)

    Family Hyaenidae: hyena (4)

    Family Felidae: cat (36)

TABLE 23.1. Names of gender for carnivores

Animal	Male	Female	Newborn or Young
Dog	Dog	Bitch	Pup, puppy
Fox	Reynard	Vixen	Kit, cub, pup
Wolf	Lobo	Female	Pup
Bear	Boar	Sow	Cub
Raccoon	Boar	Sow	Cub
Hyena	Male	Female	Pup
Skunk	Male	Female	Pup, kit
Otter	Male	Female	Pup
Ocelot, bobcat, mountain lion	Tom, male	Queen, female	Kitten
Tiger and other large cats	Male	Female	Cub, kitten
Cheetah	Male	Female	Kitten

TABLE 23.2. Weights of carnivores

Animal	Kilograms	Pounds
Wolf	27–80	60–176
Gray fox	2.5–7	6–15
Coyote	9–12.7	20–28
American black bear	90–150	200–330
Grizzly bear	225–325	495–715
Polar bear	300–720	660–1,580
Sun bear	27–65	59–143
North American raccoon	15–22	33–48
Coatimundi	3–11.3	7–25
Cacomistle	0.87–1.1	2–3.0
Kinkajou	1.4–2.7	3–6
River otter	4.5–15	10–33
Sea otter	16–37	35–81
Striped skunk	0.75–2.5	2–6
Wolverine	14–27.5	30–60
Mongoose	0.34–4.5	0.75–10
Aardwolf	8	18
Spotted hyena	0–80	132–175
Cheetah	40–50	88–110
African lion	181–227	400–500
Tiger	225–340	500–750

Although most members of the order Carnivora are carnivorous, some species are omnivorous and/or insectivorous. The order has worldwide distribution. Carnivores are popular zoo exhibits. Names of gender are listed in Table 23.1. Weights are listed in Table 23.2.

Carnivores should not be handled immediately after they have ingested a meal. Regurgitation is a common reaction to fright or other emotional upsets and may result in aspiration pneumonia. Small carnivores may be shifted to or from swinging door cages using the technique described in Chapter 2.

DANGER POTENTIAL[6,10,22,33,39,40,44]

Teeth specialized for grasping and tearing prey are characteristic of all carnivores. The enlarged canine teeth are formidable weapons used for offense and defense as well as for food gathering.

The jaw muscles are well developed and tremendously strong. A hyena is capable of crushing the tibia of prey species with one snap. On one occasion I inserted a heavy stainless steel dental speculum, designed for a large cow, into the mouth of an immobilized bear. The bear suffered a convulsive seizure, bit down on the speculum, and completely collapsed it.

Wolves have extraordinarily powerful jaws. I have seen a medium-sized wolf collapse the bars of a cage especially designed to house rabid domestic dogs. Wolves can demolish a heavy stainless steel feeding bowl within a few moments.

The paws of most members of this order are fitted with claws that can rip and tear. All felids have dangerous claws. The larger carnivores are fully capable of killing a person who is careless when approaching or handling them.

In zoos large carnivores are customarily exhibited in an outdoor enclosure, with a bedroom as part of the exhibit area. A work area is usually constructed contiguous to the enclosure. When entering the work area, it is important for a handler to know exactly where the animal is in the enclosure and which doors are open or closed. Some tragic mistakes have been made by individuals who entered a work area under the assumption that the animal was barred from access to that area, only to find themselves confronted with a large cat or a bear.

Unless one has had extensive experience with members of this order, it is difficult to appreciate the speed and agility of these animals. Such speed and agility should be understandable, inasmuch as they must gather food by pouncing upon and grasping their prey, but many people fail to realize that most species can lash out with the claws much faster than a person can jump away. In addition, these animals have a mobile head that can reach forward or to the side quickly to bite.

It may be necessary to partially open the door to a carnivore cage to retrieve an object or to provide exposure for darting an animal. Be cautious! The animal may paw the door open wider and escape or attack. Keep a swinging door from opening too far by chaining it with a loose chain. Insert a rod through the netting or bars of a guillotine door so the door can be lifted only a specified distance.

Many carnivores have anal glands, which may be simply a cutaneous invagination with multiple ducts opening on the surface or a discrete glandular vesicle with a single duct to the surface. The secretions are exuded to define territorial limits by scent marking. Skunks and related mustelids eject the unpleasant secretion defensively.

CANIDAE—DOG, FOX, WOLF[3,4,13,14,18,19,29–32]

Various wild members of this family have been raised and trained by people, and many owners sincerely believe such an animal is as safe to handle as the domestic dog. This is far from the truth! Strangers who must handle such animals must assume they are wild and may suddenly revert to innate defensive behavior. Tamed wild canids are capable of inflicting serious injury.[14]

A pet wolf brought to me for examination was docile as long as the owner was present. The animal required hospitalization. As soon as the client left, the wolf became vicious and could be given medication only when restrained with snares and a squeeze cage.

Semi-domesticated foxes raised for fur are handled as shown in Figure 23.1. Special tongs and snares are also used as needed. Zoo animals or captured free-ranging species should be handled carefully with nets (Fig. 23.2), snares, or squeeze cages.

Gloves may be worn while grasping smaller species after initial capture with a net or snare (Fig. 23.3). All carnivores can bite through heavy leather gloves, which are worn primarily to guard against scratching (Fig. 23.4).

A muzzle made of a small rope or gauze bandage will prevent a wild canid from biting. It may be wise to apply a muzzle as soon as the animal has partially recovered from chemical immobilization. However, caution must be exercised lest the animal overheat as a result of the inability to pant, the normal thermoregulatory mechanism for canids. Larger members of this family should be handled only with special squeeze cages or by chemical restraint.

Blood may be collected as in a dog from the cephalic vein on the forearm, as shown in Figure 23.5, or from the saphenous vein on the medial aspect of the tibia, as shown in Figure 23.6.

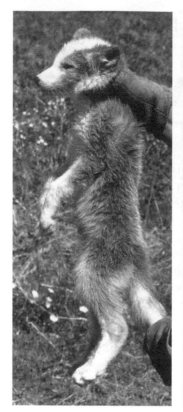
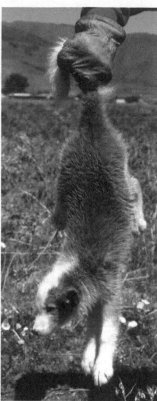

FIG. 23.1. A ranch-raised fox may be grasped by the tail and gently swung to keep it off balance until the back of the head is grasped.

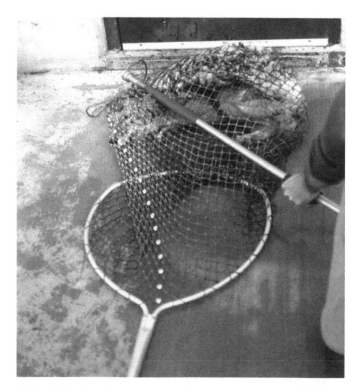

FIG. 23.2. Small canids are easily netted.

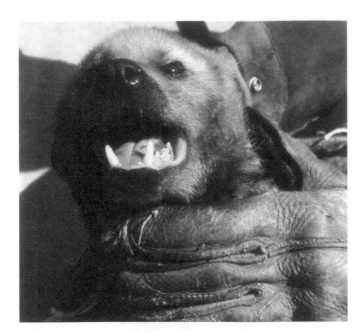

FIG. 23.3. A wild canid held tightly with gloved hands for examination and treatment.

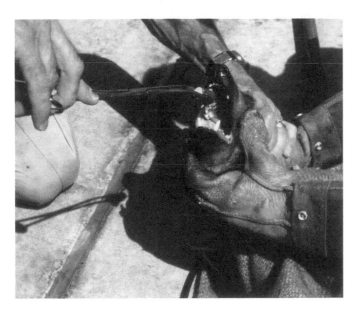

FIG. 23.4. A bush dog being hand held to administer a capsule.

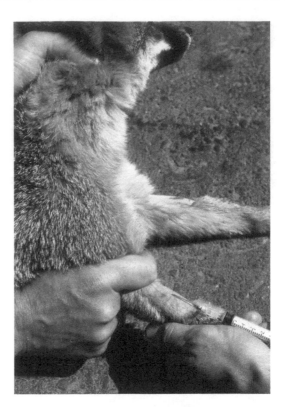

FIG. 23.5. Venipuncture of the cephalic vein.

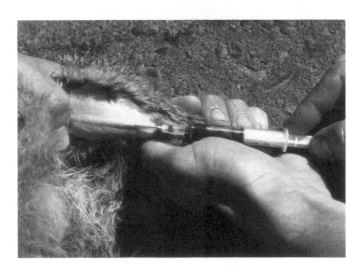

FIG. 23.6. Venipuncture from the saphenous vein.

URSIDAE—BEARS[7,16,17,20,35–37,43]

Bears have tremendous strength. Mature bears are capable of bending bars and tearing off screens with their heavily clawed forepaws. Although bear claws are not sharpened and re-curved like those of the large cats, the power of their paws and limbs makes bears dangerous to handle. Large bears such as grizzly or polar bears are capable of killing with a single swat of the paw (Fig. 23.7).

Immature bears may be hand held or controlled by nets or snares (Fig. 23.8). Mature bears should be handled only by the use of special squeeze cages[5] or by chemical restraint[16] (Figs. 23.9, 23.10). Squeeze cages used for bears must be especially strong; cages designed for large cats are usually not adequate. The use of chemical immobilization has minimized the need for such devices.

A large bear is usually transported in a heavy crate. The crate must be especially constructed of strong materials to prevent the bear from tearing it apart and escaping. Many bear crates are lined with galvanized sheeting, welded at the seams

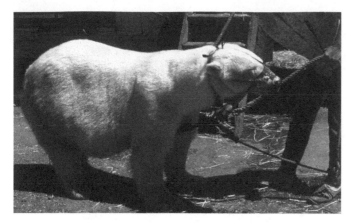

FIG. 23.7. Although muzzled, this polar bear could still kill a person with a blow from a paw.

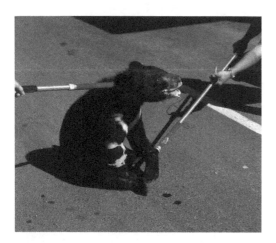

FIG. 23.8. Small bear restrained with snares.

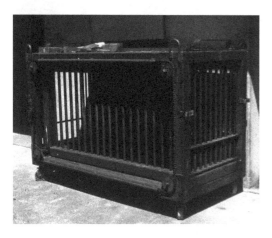

FIG. 23.9. Squeeze cages for large bears must be heavily constructed.

to prevent the animal from ripping it off by prying a claw beneath a seam.

To load a bear, the crate must be firmly secured to the cage opening with chains or ropes (Fig. 23.11). Otherwise the bear may run full tilt into the crate and, by the force of its

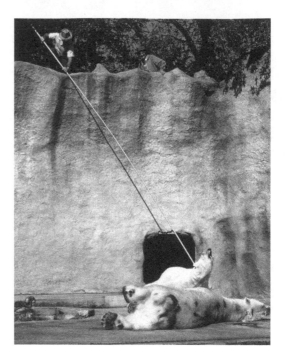

FIG. 23.10. Immobilized polar bear. (Check the stage of immobilization before entering an enclosure with this dangerous animal.)

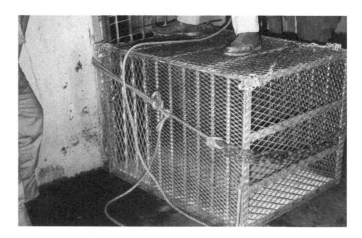

FIG. 23.11. Bear crate chained to the door.

body crashing against the opposite end, push the cage away from the opening and escape. A high-pressure water system is useful for directing a bear into a crate. It may be necessary to chemically immobilize a large bear before it can be placed into the crate.

Orphan cubs must be bottle fed from the proper position (Fig. 23.12). If the animal is placed on its back, the milk may be inhaled into the lungs, causing aspiration pneumonia.

Blood is obtained from the tongue vein, as shown in Figures 23.13 and 23.14; the saphenous vein, as shown in Figure 23.15; or the femoral vein.

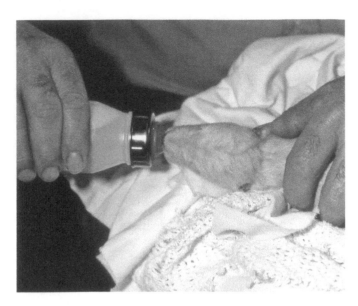

FIG. 23.12. Polar bear cub in proper nursing position.

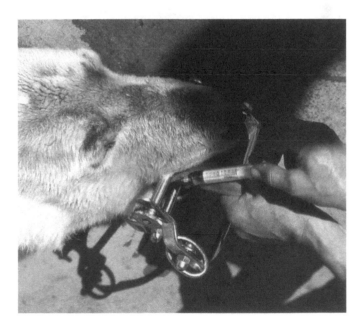

FIG. 23.13. Collecting blood from the tongue vein of an anesthetized polar bear.

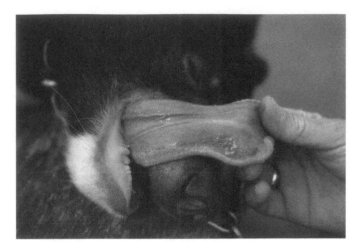

FIG. 23.14. Ventral tongue vein in a bear.

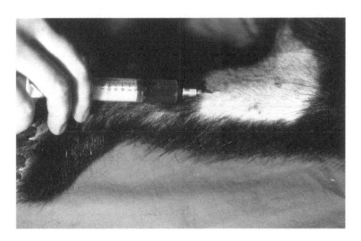

FIG. 23.15. Collecting blood from the saphenous vein of a bear.

TABLE 23.3. Selected chemical restraint agents for immobilization of canids[3,26,28]

Agent	Dose (mg/kg), IM	Comment
Tiletamine/zolazepam	10.0	General dose for all canids
Ketamine/xylazine	6.6–10.0/1.25–2.0	
Ketamine/medetomidine	2.5/0.08	
Ketamine/acepromazine	20.0/0.1	General dose for all canids

Table 23.4. Chemical restraint agents for immobilization of bears[6,16,17,22,33,41]

Agent	Dose (mg/kg), IM
Tiletamine/zolazepam	5.0–9.0
Ketamine/xylazine	5.0–10.0/2/0–11.0
Ketamine/medetomidine	3.0–4.0/0.012–0.15
Etorphine	0.02–0/06

Chemical Restraint and Anesthesia

Many chemical agents have been used successfully to immobilize bears. (See Tables 23.3 to 23.9.) Anesthesia is handled in the same manner as for dogs. General anesthesia is optimally performed by endotracheal intubation and inhalation anesthesia (Fig. 23.16). An endotracheal tube may be carried into the pharyngeal cavity by hand, with the mouth held open using a sturdy oral speculum such as the Hauptner cattle speculum after deep immobilization (Fig. 23.17).

TABLE 23.5. Selected chemical restraint agents for immobilizing giant pandas

Agent	Dose (mg/kg), IM
Ketamine	2.4–6.0
Ketamine/xylazine	3.9–5.0/0.39–0.7
Ketamine/diazepam	6.0–7.0/0.2
Tiletamine/zolazepam	5.8 ± 1.3

TABLE 23.6. Chemical restraint agents to immobilized procyonids and viverrids[9,15]

Agent	Dose (mg/kg), IM
Ketamine	10.0–30.0
Ketamine/diazepam	10.0/0.5
Ketamine/xylazine	10.0/1.0–2.0
Ketamine/xylazine	2.5–5.0/0.025–0/05
Tiletamine/zolazepam	3.0–5.0

TABLE 23.7. Chemical restraint agents for immobilization of mustelids[19,39,40,41]

Agent	Dose (mg/kg), IM
Ketamine/diazepam	10.0–12.0/0.3–0.6
Ketamine/midazolam	6.0–15.0/0.1–0.5
Ketamine/xylazine	10.0/1/0–2.0
Ketamine/medetomidine	2.5–10.0/0.025–0.1
Tiletamine/zolazepam	2.2–4.4

TABLE 23.8. Chemical restraint agents for immobilization of hyenas

Agent	Dose (mg/kg), IM
Tiletamine/zolazepam	4.0–6.0
Ketamine/xylazine	8.0–10.0/0.5–1.0
Etorphine/xylazine	0.05/0.63

TABLE 23.9. Selected chemical restraint agents for immobilization of felids[18,23,31,36,38,43]

Agent	Dose (mg/kg), IM	Comment
Ketamine/xylazine	4.0–6.0/0.5–1.0	
Ketamine/medetomidine	2.5/0.07	
Tiletamine/zolazepam	2.0–10.0	Higher doses in cheetahs may cause apnea for 15–60 minutes; Respiratory assistance may be needed
Azaperone	0.5–0.1	Sedative dose
Medetomidine	0.05–0.1	Sedative in cheetahs[34]

PROCYONIDAE—RACCOON, KINKAJOU, COATIMUNDI[8,9,15,27]

Members of this family are small to medium sized. Do not underestimate the danger of being bitten by a procyonid. Even hand-raised individuals may revert to wild behavior and inflict serious injury. I am aware of one North American raccoon that disfigured its owner's face for life in an unprovoked attack. Though raised from infancy, the raccoon laid open the lady's cheek as she held it lovingly in her arms.

Most procyonids are easily handled with nets or squeeze cages. Snares may also be used; however, most procyonids have highly prehensile forepaws and are capable of grabbing the loop of the snare and pushing it away or of pulling it off the head. An Elizabethan collar is used to prevent self-mutilation while wounds heal or during postsurgical care (Fig. 23.18).

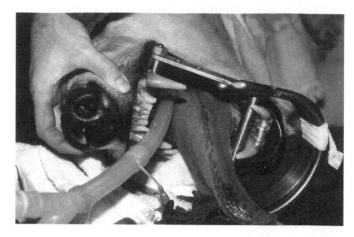

FIG. 23.16. Endotracheal intubation in a polar bear.

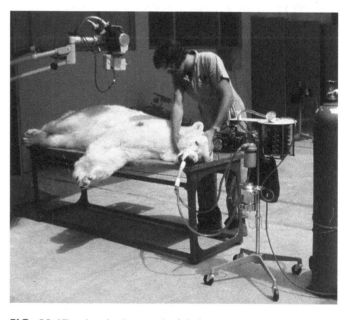

FIG. 23.17. A polar bear under inhalant anesthesia.

MUSTELIDAE—SKUNK, WEASEL, OTTER[1,12,21,27,40–42]

Mustelids are small to medium-sized carnivores that are dangerous to handle. They have needle-sharp teeth and are agile and aggressive.

All members of this family may be handled with nets, snares, or squeeze cages. Chemical immobilization is also effective. Pets may be manually handled with caution (Fig. 23.19).

Skunks bite readily.[18] Since they are one of the major reservoirs of rabies, they should be handled with great care.[1,24] Skunks defend themselves primarily by spraying the secretions of the anal sacs at enemies.[13] This sticky, irritating liquid

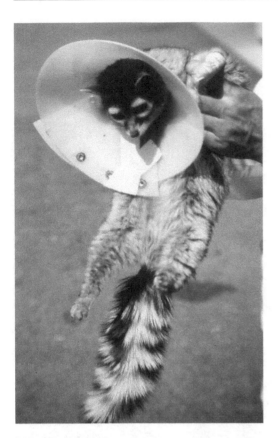

FIG. 23.18. Elizabethan collar on a cacomistle.

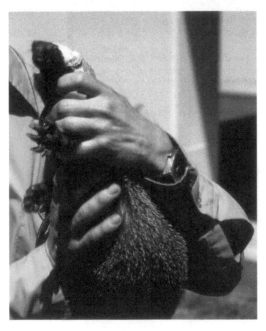

FIG. 23.19. Pet grison—handheld by owner. (Generally unsafe, since the owner rarely is qualified to maintain a proper grip.)

can be projected accurately for a distance of up to 4 m (13 ft) and under favorable weather conditions can be smelled as far as 2 km (1 mile) away. The defensive position assumed by a threatened skunk is with hindquarters facing the enemy, feet planted firmly on the ground, and tail straight up in the air. It usually stamps with the front feet in warning before spraying. The spotted skunk lifts the hindquarters off the ground to spray. The musk sac is surrounded by heavy muscle layers. The spraying action is similar to that resulting from compression of a bulb syringe. Some believe that a skunk lifted up by the tail cannot spray. Not true! It can! Immature skunks 8–10 weeks of age are not likely to spray though capable of doing so. Capture intact skunks with a net[24] from behind a shield of plate glass or plastic, or wear goggles and protective rain gear.

The only safe way to handle an intact mature skunk is to sedate or anesthetize it. If the skunk is presented in a box, enclose the box in a plastic bag and insert a wad of cotton soaked with isoflurane. Watch carefully for signs of anesthesia and remove the skunk from the box only after it is sedated.

Ketamine hydrochloride (5.0–15.0 mg/kg) is an effective intramuscular anesthetic. Infant skunks may be wrapped in a towel for intramuscular injection. Mature skunks must be sedated first with a volatile anesthetic.

Clinical signs exhibited by those sprayed with skunk musk include skin burns, temporary blindness, nausea, convulsions, and loss of consciousness. If sprayed, wash spray from the eyes with copious amounts of water. Lacrimal secretions will also clear the eyes of the material within 15 minutes. Rinse the secretion from skin surfaces as well.

The pungent, acrid skunk musk is composed of many compounds, but the principal one is normal butyl mercaptan (butanethiol). The mercaptan can be made soluble, harmless, and odorless by applying strong oxidizing agents such as the alkaline sodium or potassium salts of halogens. Sodium hypochlorite (household bleach) is the most readily available, in a concentration of 5.25% chlorine. Dilute to approximately 500–1,000 ppm of available chlorine before applying. The chlorine oxidizes the mercaptan, breaking sulfur free from the carbon chain to form sulfate or sulfone compounds that are odorless. These compounds are water-soluble and can be removed by repeated washings with copious quantities of water. Delicate fabrics and colored clothing may be damaged by this bleaching action. Commercial deodorizers are available.

If the hair of an animal has been sprayed, a superficial clip may remove the bulk of the contamination. Close-clip the hair if necessary and rinse with a dilute bleach solution followed by repeated shampooing.

When a person's hair has been sprayed, the problem is compounded. A strong bleach solution will damage the hair, and one usually does not wish to close-clip the hair. Some have recommended repeated washing in tomato juice; thorough shampooing and rinsing, accompanied by application of a mild bleach solution, may prove to be the most practical method for removing skunk odor.

Skunks kept in captivity are usually descented by surgical removal of the anal glands. Descented skunks may be handled like any other mustelid.

Some mink are semi-domesticated for the production of fur. Although mink are small, they have relatively large canines, capable of inflicting severe lacerations.

Snares may be used to move mink, although special transfer cages are probably more satisfactory. The experienced handler can remove mink from a cage as illustrated in Figures 23.20 to 23.23. Using a gloved hand, the handler grasps the mink by the tail and quickly pulls it from the cage. As it attempts to climb back into the cage, the handler's other hand grasps the animal behind the neck with the thumb and finger around the head. This sequence must be carried out quickly, because the animal is fully capable of biting the hand through the glove. Special restraint tubes have been utilized when repeated handling is required.

Mink are transferred from cage to cage or transported to other facilities in wire transfer cages (Fig. 23.24).

Chemical restraint of mink has become a standard practice and may produce less stress for the animal than manual restraint. Ketamine hydrochloride (5.0–10.0 mg/kg) is used.

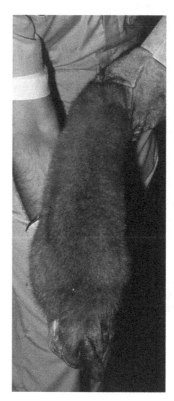
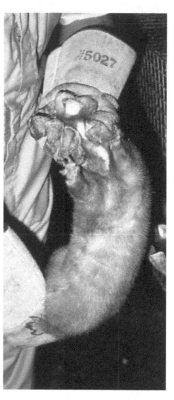

FIG. 23.22.   Once the head and tail are secure, the mink may be manipulated into various positions.

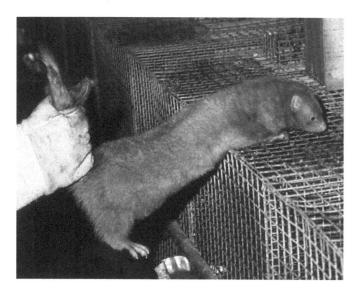

FIG. 23.20.   Handling a ranch-raised mink: Remove mink from cage by grasping the tail.

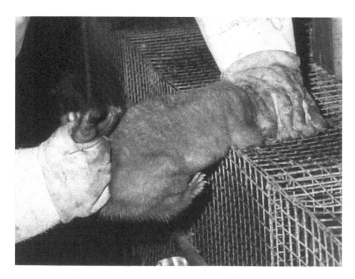

FIG. 23.21.   While it clings to the wire, pin the head.

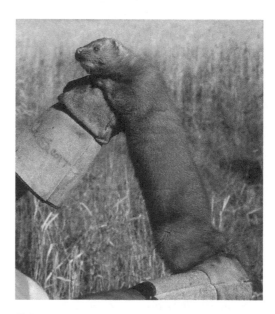

FIG. 23.23.   Ranch-raised mink are usually docile enough to allow manual handling. Wild mink would be likely to bite through these gloves.

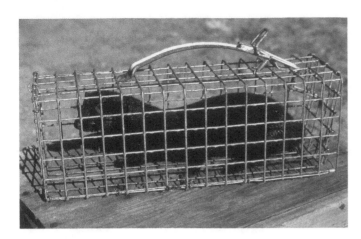

FIG. 23.24. Mink transfer cage.

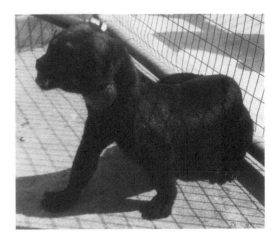

FIG. 23.26. Tayra captured with a snare.

The wolverine is the largest mustelid, weighing up to 18 kg (30 lb), and is about 38 cm (15 in.) high at the shoulder.

The wolverine assumes a defensive posture by rolling over on its back, preparing to scratch and bite. If tethered it will continuously spin, necessitating a handler to constantly untwist the leash or snare to prevent strangulation. The wolverine may be placed in a squeeze cage for intramuscular injection of ketamine hydrochloride (10.0 mg/kg). A pole syringe is also effective for administering ketamine if the animal is confined in a limited space.

River otters and tayras may be handled with nets or snares (Figs. 23.25, 23.26). Sea otters require specialized handling techniques. Divers trap them from the wild in a basket net from beneath while the otters float on the surface of the sea. The net is closed with a drawstring to keep the otter inside and immediately lifted out of the water.

Sea otters are extremely susceptible to stress caused by handling and transporting. This unique marine mammal

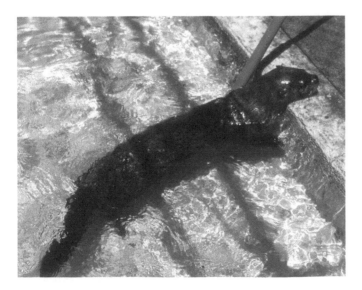

FIG. 23.25. River otter captured with a snare.

has no insulating blubber layer. Protection against hypothermia is provided by the dense coat of fur. The underlying fine silky fibers next to the skin are kept dry by the perfectly groomed outer fibers. If the fur is soiled with feces, urine, or any other material during caging, the fur will mat and lose its water-resistance and hence its insulating qualities. Once the fur is matted, the entire coat becomes wet, heat is lost, and the animal becomes chilled. Seemingly irreversible pneumonia is the result. Great care must be taken to prevent soiling of the coat during any procedure involving sea otters.

VIVERRIDAE—MONGOOSE, CIVET CAT[8]

Viverrids are similar in body structure, size, and habits to mustelids and may be handled in the same manner.

HYAENIDAE—HYENAS, AARDWOLF[36,38]

Hyenas are efficient scavengers and active predators. Their primary weapons are their strong jaws and teeth. Handling mature hyenas requires the use of squeeze cages or chemical immobilization. They can tear through a net with little difficulty and are usually too strong to handle with a snare. Manual handling of larger than infant animals is unwise.

FELIDAE—CATS[5,20,26,33,34,39,44]

Members of the cat family vary in size from those smaller than the domestic house cat to the Siberian tiger, which may weigh as much as 340 kg (750 lb). Obviously restraint techniques must vary with the size.

All felids have sharpened re-curved claws, capable of lacerating flesh, and they are extremely fast in striking out with the front paws. Some species of cats claw only with their front feet; others, such as the leopard, rake with the hind feet as well. Cats have great mobility of the head, allowing them to slash with the fangs from almost any position.

There is wide variation in behavior among members of the family Felidae. Some of the smaller cats are the most high-strung and vicious. The leopard cat is aggressive, even though it is often kept as a pet. The clouded leopard is one of the more docile species; if raised with human association, it is likely to respond well to mild restraint and may be handled by manual techniques (Fig. 23.27). It is seldom necessary to resort to snares, nets, or squeeze cages to restrain a hand-raised clouded leopard. Most cats will become docile around people if trained properly (Fig. 23.28).

Other species respond to restraint in various manners. Once a cheetah is grasped with a snare and restrained, it usually lies quietly unless intense pain is inflicted. Even hand-raised cats will not tolerate any procedure inflicting pain, however slight. Contrarily, a leopard may fight vigorously the entire time it is being restrained.

Infant felids are easily handled manually (Figs. 23.29, 23.30). They may be wrapped in a towel or canvas (Fig. 23.31, 23.32). More-mature wild felids must be handled more

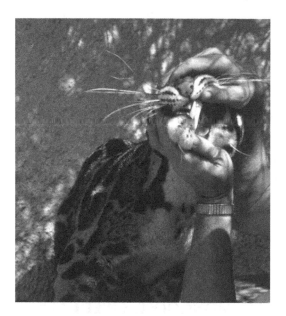

FIG. 23.27. Manual handling of wild felids is usually restricted to those who raised them, such as this clouded leopard.

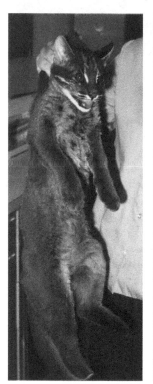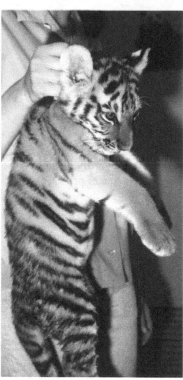

FIG. 23.29. Infant and juvenile felids usually become limp when grasped by the nape of the neck. This method is used by the mother to transport the kitten; thus, relaxation is an expected behavioral pattern.

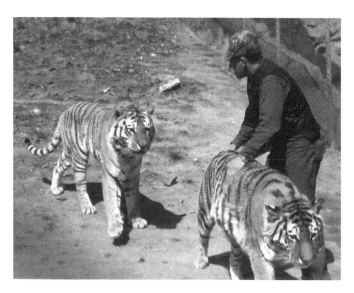

FIG. 23.28. These hand-raised tigers have great rapport with their caregiver.

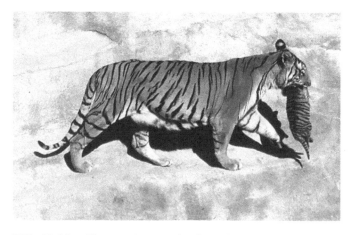

FIG. 23.30. Tiger mother carrying her cub.

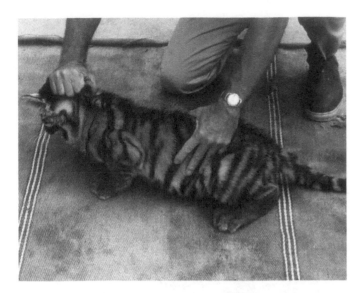

FIG. 23.31. Tiger cub may be wrapped in a towel or piece of canvas to eliminate scratching during examination.

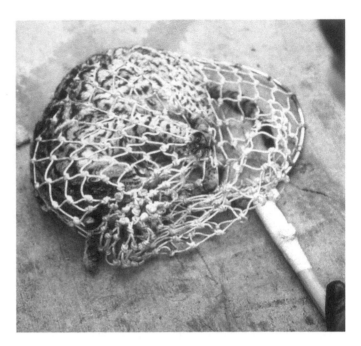

FIG. 23.33. Small- to medium-sized wild felids are easily netted.

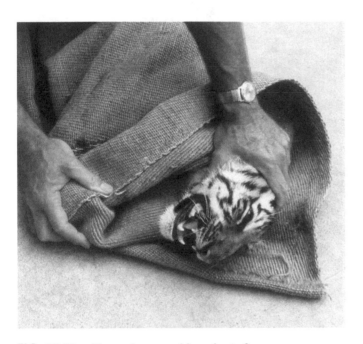

FIG. 23.32. Tiger cub wrapped in a sheet of canvas.

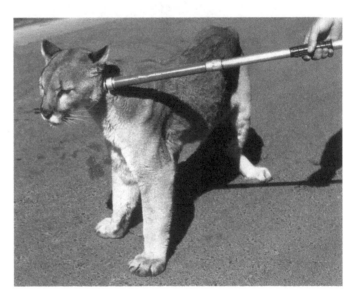

FIG. 23.34. Snare may be used on tame and semi-tame felids.

carefully. Small individuals weighing up to 14 kg (30 lb) may be handled with a net (Fig. 23.33); in some instances, they may be grasped with a snare and then handled with gloved hands. Wide-gauntleted welder's gloves are useful when working with small felids, not so much to prevent biting (most of these animals can bite through the heaviest leather glove) but to protect the handler from severe scratching.

Trained cats are handled in a different fashion than truly wild or zoo cats. The trainer may be able to restrict the activity of even a large cat by the use of a snare (Fig. 23.34) or special chains (Fig. 23.35). These chains may be useful in that the

animal may be snapped or chained to a post and then grasped by the tail to administer a quick intramuscular injection in the hindquarters. The trainer handling an animal in this manner must be fully capable of restricting the animal.

Small cats weighing up to 15 kg may be grasped by a snare. The snare has the advantage of keeping the animal away from the handler as well as serving as an extension of the arm to catch the animal. Once the snare is in place, the tail may be grasped to hold the hindquarters facing toward the restrainer.

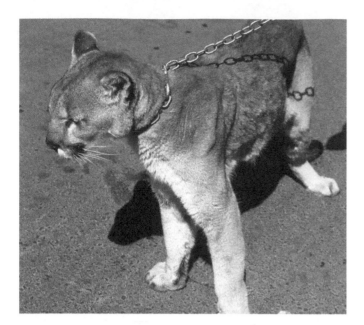

FIG. 23.35. Snap chain used to control a trained cat.

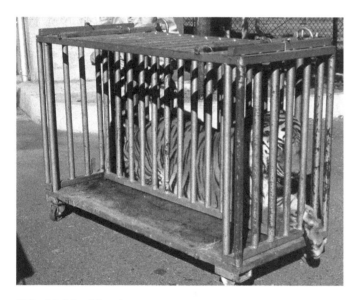

FIG. 23.36. Tiger in a squeeze cage.

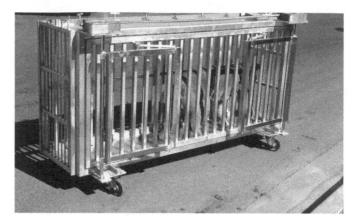

FIG. 23.37. Commercial carnivore squeeze cage.

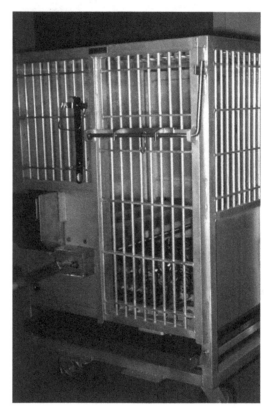

FIG. 23.38. Small felids may be handled in primate squeeze cages.

If a net is used on cats it should be made of mesh fine enough to prevent the animal from poking its head or paw through the holes. The animal may strangle as it fights to extract its head from the mesh; if it puts a paw through the net, someone may be clawed.

Squeeze cages are frequently used for handling large cats. Numerous types and styles have been designed (Figs. 23.36 to 23.39). Restraint cages are available commercially or may be custom-made. Because of the body conformation, large cats such as the tiger, lion, jaguar, or leopard should be squeezed from side to side; smaller species from top to bottom. General manipulation and precautions for the use of squeeze

cages are described in Chapter 2. Felids may reach out through the bars and claw the unwary (Fig. 23.40).

When prolonged treatment is required, it is advisable to strap the immobilized animal to the table (Fig. 23.41) to preclude injuries to the animal (or handler) if it awakens from sedation unexpectedly.

Accessible veins for obtaining blood samples and administering intravenous infusions are both medial and lateral saphenous veins (Fig. 23.42) and the femoral, jugular, and cephalic veins. Felids also have a well-developed lateral tail vein that is easily penetrated (Fig. 23.43).

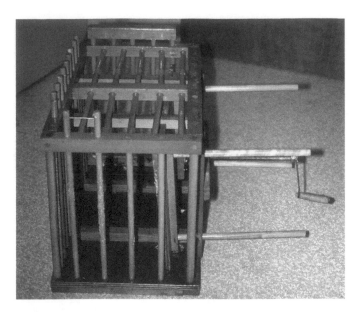

FIG. 23.39. Home-made squeeze cage for an ocelot.

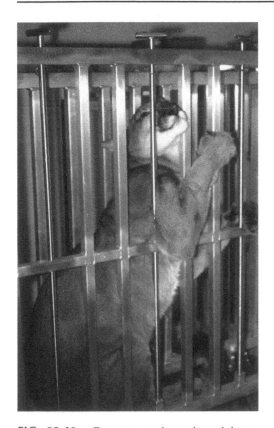

FIG. 23.40. Cats may reach out through bars. (Caution handlers and bystanders.)

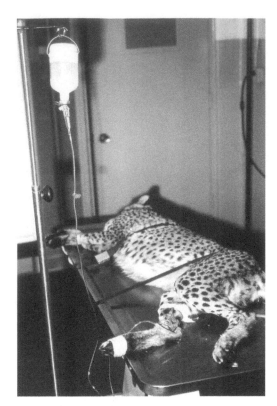

FIG. 23.41. Cheetah strapped to table while undergoing therapy.

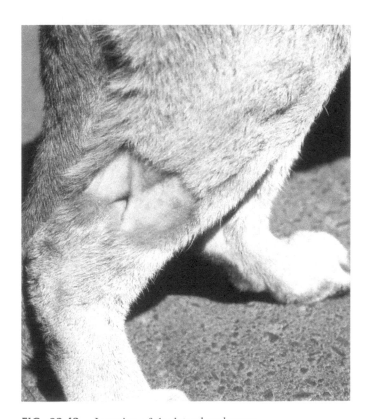

FIG. 23.42. Location of the lateral saphenous vein in a large felid.

The mouth of a felid can be opened for oral examination or surgery by using a commercial or improvised speculum such as a wooden block (Fig. 23.44).

Transport

Small cats may be directed into crates or transfer cages with a shield. Larger cats may be baited into crates with food.

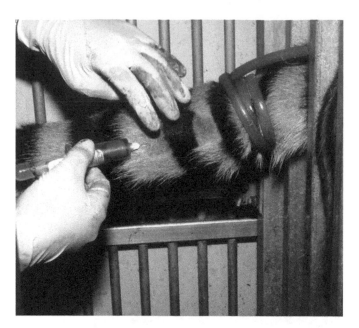

FIG. 23.43.   Collecting blood from the lateral tail vein while the tiger is physically restrained in a squeeze.

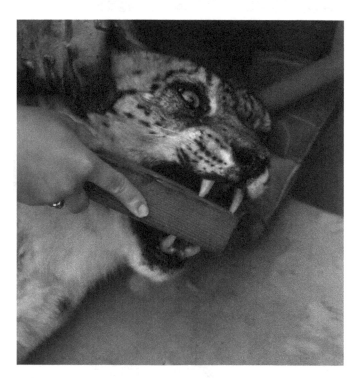

FIG. 23.44.   Wooden block used to hold the mouth open.

Some must be immobilized before they can be crated. A plywood sheet, a human stretcher, or a sheet of canvas (Fig. 23.45) should be used to move an immobilized cat from one spot to another in preference to dragging it along the ground. Shipping crates and transfer cages must suit the size and behavior of the cat and comply with regulations.[2]

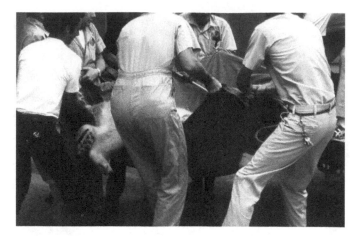

FIG. 23.45.   A sheet of canvas used to transport a large carnivore.

Chemical Restraint

The chemical restraint agents and combinations mentioned in this chapter represent those used by the author or experienced veterinarian with detailed knowledge of carnivores. Other protocols have been used, and no claim is made for including all possible drugs and combinations. For more detailed information, particularly for anesthesia, consult the references.

Small carnivores may be handled by physical restraint, but this is rarely possible with the larger species. Thus, chemical immobilization is frequently necessary to examine, collect laboratory samples, and perform therapy. Carnivores have been immobilized daily for as many as 45 days. The author is aware of a mountain lion, *Felis concolor*, involved in an embryo transfer study that was immobilized over 200 times. Numerous chemical sedative and immobilizing agents or combinations thereof may be used. Table 23.6 lists a few of the agents with suggested dosage, based on the author's experience and reference to the literature, to be used as a guide. Selection may be based on availability of drugs, experience of the operator, cost, and size and species of carnivore. Blank spaces in the table do not mean that the drug or combination has not been used; it may have been tried, but results have not been reported. If in doubt on a species new to the operator, consult a nearby zoo veterinarian for assistance.

It is not the intent of the author to review all aspects of chemical immobilization of carnivores. The references provide adequate depth and breadth of information on the subject and the references found in those publications expand the information pool further. The recent publication, *The Capture and Care Manual*,[10] is a wealth of information on field immobilization, primarily of African species, but with application to animal groups also found on other continents and in zoos.

Carnivores in the free-ranging state may be trapped or treed first or shot from blinds or bait sites. Captive carnivores are usually immobilized with blow darts or powered projectiles. Subtle differences in dosage may exist between captive and free-ranging animals. One tends to use slightly higher doses on free-ranging animals to assure adequate and rapid immobilization. Gender differences may also be a factor, but usually there will be more variation as a result of emotional status.

Most of the drugs used for carnivore immobilization may be administered by any route and some orally. Site selection for intramuscular injection may be critical, particularly in captive animals that may have a tendency toward obesity. For instance, in captive bears, the muscles of the rear limb may be laden with fat and appropriate response to a given dose may not occur because of intra-fat deposition. Thus, in bears, the author prefers the triceps muscle area of the forelimb, dorsal to the elbow and caudal to the humerus and scapula. (See Chapter 19, Fig. 19.23.)

Etorphine is an excellent drug for immobilization of bears. The pharmaceutical companies involved in tranquilizer and neuroleptanalgesic[10] drug development are frequently outside of North America. Thus, North American veterinarians may be the last to benefit from newer agents that come on the market elsewhere. South African wildlife veterinarians have been at the forefront of clinical testing and using new agents. It is recommended to administer atropine sulfate (0.04 mg/kg) subcutaneously or intramuscularly when immobilizing or anesthetizing a carnivore.

When ketamine is administered as the only immobilizing agent in large cats and bears, it may stimulate the development of tonic seizures (Fig. 23.46). Combinations of ketamine with other agents such as xylazine may block the tetanic effects of ketamine. If possible, the xylazine should be administered 15 or 20 minutes before the ketamine to allow time for its taking effect. Ketamine has a shorter induction time and may initiate its tetanic effect before the xylazine has taken

effect. Do not use tranquilizers to counter these tetanic effects. Use diazepam or midazolam.

Orphaned neonate felids may be handled much like a domestic kitten, as shown in Figures 23.47 to 23.49. If bottle feeding is necessary, position the kitten or cub into a natural nursing position (Fig. 25.50), not cradled in one's arms. Supplemental heat may be necessary. Human infant isolettes are excellent (Fig. 25.51).

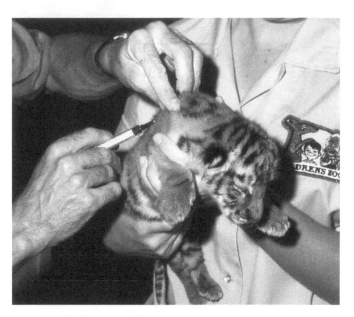

FIG. 23.47. Vaccinating a tiger cub.

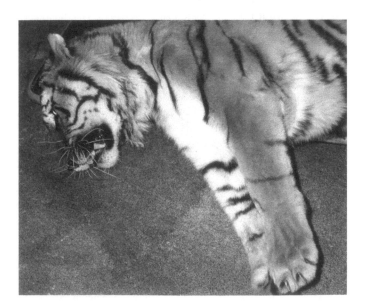

FIG. 23.46. A tiger seizuring from the effects of ketamine.

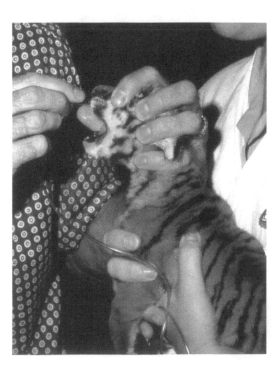

FIG. 23.48. Passing a stomach tube in a tiger cub.

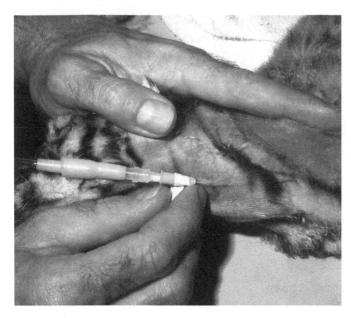

FIG. 23.49. Jugular vein venipuncture in a tiger cub.

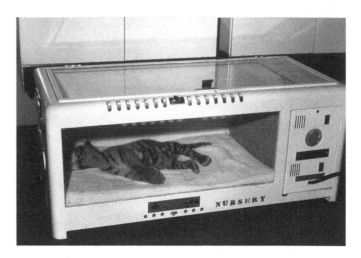

FIG. 23.51. A human isolette used to supply supplemental heat to a neonate felid.

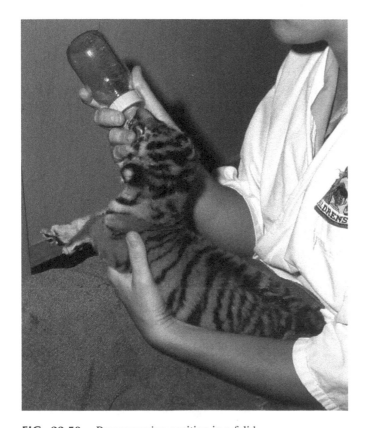

FIG. 23.50. Proper nursing position in a felid kitten or cub.

REFERENCES

1. Adams, W.V., Sanford, G.E., Rott, E.E., and Glasgow, L.L. 1964. Night-time capture of striped skunks in Louisiana. J Wildl Manage 28:368–73.
2. Anonymous. 2007. Live Animal Regulations, 34th Ed. Montreal, Can.: International Air Transport Association.
3. Arnemo, J.M., Moe, R., and Smith, A.J. 1993. Immobilization of captive raccoon dogs with medetomidine-ketamine and remobilization with atipamezole. J Zoo Wildl Med 24:102–08.
4. Brand, D.J. 1993. Physical capture of the black-backed jackal. In: McKenzie, A.A., Ed. The Capture and Care Manual, Pretoria: The South African Veterinary Foundation, pp. 278–85.
5. Brand, D.J. 1993. Physical capture of the caracul. In: McKenzie, A.A., Ed. The Capture and Care Manual, Pretoria: The South African Veterinary Foundation, pp. 255–61.
6. Burroughs, R.E.J., and McKenzie, A.A. 1993. Handling, care, and loading of immobilized carnivores. In: McKenzie, A.A., Ed. The Capture and Care Manual, Pretoria: The South African Veterinary Foundation, pp. 178–83.
7. Bush, M., and Montali, R.J. 1993. Medical management of pandas. In: Fowler, M.E., Ed. Zoo and Wild Animal Medicine, 3rd ed., Philadelphia: W.B. Saunders, pp. 408–11.
8. Denver, M. 2003. Procyonidae and Viverridae. In: Fowler, M.E., and Miller, R.E., Eds. Zoo and Wild Animal Medicine. 5th Ed. St. Louis, Saunders/Elsevier. pp. 516–17.
9. Deresienski, D.T., and Rupprecht, C.E. 1989. Yohimbine reversal of ketamine/xylazine immobilization of raccoons. J Wildl Dis 25:169–74.
10. Ebedes, H. 1993. The use of long-acting tranquilizers in captive wild animals. In: McKenzie, A.A., Ed. The Capture and Care Manual, Pretoria: The South African Veterinary Foundation, pp. 65–70.
11. Espie, I. 1993. Transportation of carnivores. In: McKenzie, A.A., Ed. The Capture and Care Manual, Pretoria: The South African Veterinary Foundation, pp. 286–92.
12. Fernandez-Moran, J. 2003. Mustelidae. In: Fowler, M.E., and Miller, R.E., Eds. Zoo and Wild Animal Medicine. 5th Ed. St. Louis, Saunders/Elsevier. pp. 501–06.
13. Fleming, G., Citino, S.B., and Bush, M. 2006. Reversible anesthetic combination using medetomidine, butorphanol and

midazolam in in-situ African wild dogs *Lycoan pictus*. 2006 Proceedings Am Assoc Zoo Vets. pp. 214–15.

14. Fox, M. W. 1971. Behaviour of Wolves, Dogs and Related Canids. New York: Harper & Row.

15. Gregg, D.A., and Olson, L.D. 1975. The use of ketamine hydrochloride as an anesthetic for raccoons. J Wildl Dis 11:335–37.

16. Haigh, J.C., Lee, L.J., and Schweinsburg, R.E. 1983. Immobilization of polar bears with carfentanil. J Wildl Dis 19:140–44.

17. Haigh, J.C., Stirling, I., and Broughton, E. 1985. Immobilization of polar bears with a mixture of tiletamine hydrochloride and zolazepam hydrochloride. J Wildl Dis 21:43–7.

18. van Heerden, J. 1993. Chemical capture of the wild dog. In: McKenzie, A.A., Ed. The Capture and Care Manual, Pretoria: The South African Veterinary Foundation, pp. 247–50.

19. van Heerden, J., Burroughs, R.E.J., Dauth, J., and Dreyer, M.J. 1991. Immobilization of wild dogs with tiletamine hydrochloride/zolazepam hydrochloride combination and subsequent evaluation of selected blood chemistry parameters. J Wildl Dis 27:225–29.

20. Herbst, L.H., Packer, C., and Seal, U.S. 1985. Immobilization of free-ranging African lions with a combination of xylazine hydrochloride and ketamine hydrochloride. J Wildl Dis 21:401–04.

21. Jacobson, J.O., Meslow, E.C., and Andrews, M.F. 1970. An improved technique for handling striped skunks in disease investigations. J Wildl Dis. 6:510–12.

22. Jalanka, H.H., and Roeken, B.O. 1990. The use of medetomidine, medetomidine-ketamine combinations, and atipamezole in nondomestic mammals: A review. J Zoo Wildl Med 21:259–82.

23. Jalanka, H.H. 1993. New alpha 2 adrenoceptor agonists and antagonists. In: Fowler, M.E., Ed. Zoo and Wild Animal Medicine, 3rd ed., Philadelphia: W.B. Saunders, pp. 477–80.

24. Kennedy-Stoskopf, S. 2003. Canidae. In: Fowler, M.E., and Miller, R.E., Eds. Zoo and Wild Animal Medicine. 5th Ed. St. Louis, Saunders/Elsevier. pp. 482–85.

25. Kirkwood, J K. 1993. Medical management of pandas in Europe. In: Fowler, M.E., Ed. Zoo and Wild Animal Medicine, 3rd ed., Philadelphia: W.B. Saunders, pp. 404–08.

26. Klein, L.V., and Stover, J. 1993. Medetomidine-ketamine isoflurane anesthesia in captive cheetahs and antagonism with atipamezole. Proc Annu Meet Am Assoc Zoo Vet Saint Louis, MO, pp. 144–45.

27. Kollias, G., and Abou-Madi, N. 2007. Procyonids and mustelids. In: West, G., Heard, D., and Caulkett, N., Eds. Zoo Animal and Wildlife Chemical Immobilization and Anesthesia. Ames, Iowa, Blackwell Publishing, pp. 417–28.

28. Kreeger, T.J., Faggella, A.M., Seal, U.S., Mech, L.D., Callahan, M., and Hall, B. 1987. Cardiovascular and behavioral responses of gray wolves to ketamine/xylazine immobilization and antagonism by yohimbine. J Wildl Dis 23:463–70.

29. Kreeger, T.J. 1999. Chemical restraint and immobilization of wild canids. In: Fowler, M.E., and Miller, R.E., Eds. Zoo and Wild Animal Medicine—Current Vet. Therapy. 4th Ed. Philadelphia, WB Saunders. p. 434.

30. Kreeger, T.J., Seal, U.S., and Faggella, A.M. 1986. Xylazine hydrochloride/ketamine hydrochloride immobilization of wolves and its antagonism by tolazoline hydrochloride. J Wildl Dis 22:397–402.

31. Kreeger, T.J., Mandsager, R.E., Seal, U S., Callahan, M., and Beckel, M. 1989. Physiological response of gray wolves to butorphanol xylazine immobilization and antagonism by naloxone and yohimbine. J Wildl Dis 25:89–94.

32. Larsen, R.S., and Kreeger, T.J. 2007. Canids. In: West, G., Heard, D., and Caulkett, N., Eds. 2007. Zoo Animal and Wildlife Chemical Immobilization and Anesthesia. Ames, Iowa, Blackwell Publishing, pp. 395–408.

33. Logan, K.A., Thorne, E.T., Irwin, L L., and Skinner, R. 1986. Immobilizing wild mountain lions with ketamine hydrochloride and xylazine hydrochloride. J Wildl Dis 22:97–103.

34. Meltzer, D-G.A. 1999. Medical management of a cheetah breeding facility in South Africa. In: Fowler, M.E., and Miller, R.E., Eds. Zoo and Wild Animal Medicine—Current Vet. Therapy. 4th Ed. Philadelphia, WB Saunders. pp. 415–22.

35. Norwalk, R.M., and Paradiso, T.L. 1983. Walker's Mammals of the World, 4th Ed, Vol. 2, Baltimore, Johns Hopkins Univ. Press, pp. 929–1094.

36. Ramsay, M.A., Stirling, I., Knutsen, L.O., and Broughton, E. 1985. Use of yohimbine hydrochloride to reverse immobilization of polar bears by ketamine hydrochloride and xylazine hydrochloride. J Wildl Dis 21:396–400.

37. Ramsay, E.C. 2003. Ursidae and Hyaenidae. In: Fowler, M.E., and Miller, R.E., Eds. Zoo and Wild Animal Medicine. 5th Ed. St. Louis, Saunders/Elsevier. pp. 523–26.

38. Richardson, P.R.K., and Anderson, M.D. 1993. Chemical capture of the aardwolf. In: McKenzie, A.A., Ed. The Capture and Care Manual, Pretoria: The South African Veterinary Foundation, pp. 244–46.

39. Rogers, P.S. 1992. The immobilization of lions and leopards with Zoletil. In: H. Ebedes, Ed. The Use of Tranquilizers in Wildlife, Pretoria: Department of Agricultural Development, pp. 66–67.

40. Sedgwick, C.J. 1993. Allometric scaling and emergency care: the importance of body size. In: Fowler, M.E., Ed. Zoo and Wild Animal Medicine, 3rd ed., Philadelphia: W.B. Saunders, pp. 34–37.

41. Spelman, L.H., Sumner, P.W., Levine, J.F., and Stoskopf, M.K. 1993. Field anesthesia in the North American river otter. J Zoo Wildl Med 24:19–27.

42. Spelman, L.H. 1999. Otter Anesthesia. In: Fowler, M.E., and Miller, R.E., Eds. Zoo and Wild Animal Medicine—Current Vet. Therapy. 4th Ed. Philadelphia, W.B. Saunders.

43. Stirling, I., Spencer, C., and Andriashek, D. 1989. Immobilization of polar bears with Telazol in the Canadian Arctic. J Wildl Dis 25:159–68.

44. Wack, R.F. 2003. Felidae. In: Fowler, M.E., and Miller, R.E., Eds., St Louis, Elsevier, pp. 491–500.

45. de Wet, T. 1993. The capture of large carnivores using orally administered drugs. In: McKenzie, A.A., Ed. The Capture and Care Manual, Pretoria: The South African Veterinary Foundation, pp. 251–54.

46. Williams, T.D. 1993. Rehabilitation of sea otters. In: Fowler, M.E., Ed. Zoo and Wild Animal Medicine, 3rd ed., Philadelphia, W.B. Saunders, p. 434.

CHAPTER 24

Nonhuman Primates

CLASSIFICATION (NUMBERS IN PARENTHESES DENOTE NUMBER OF KNOWN SPECIES)

Order Primates
  Suborder Prosimii (prosimians): tree shrew, lemur, loris, bush baby, tarsier (51)
  Suborder Anthropoidea: monkeys, apes
    Family Cebidae: New World monkey (37)
    Family Callithricidae: marmoset, tamarin (33)
    Family Cercopithecidae: Old World monkey (58)
    Family Pongidae: ape (11)
Family Hominidae: man (1)

Adults are called males and females. Newborn and young are called infants, youngsters, or juveniles.

Primates vary in size from a 60-g (0.15-1b) pygmy marmoset to a 275-kg (605-lb) gorilla (Table 24.1).

TABLE 24.1. Weights of primates

Animal	Kilograms
Tree shrew	0.1–0.2
Slow loris	0.5–1.5
Tarsier	0.08–0.15
Squirrel monkey	0.75–1.1
Capuchin	1.65–4
Spider monkey	6–8
Woolly monkey	5.5–6
Pygmy marmoset	0.06–0.07
Marmoset	0.1–1
Green monkey	7
Colobus monkey	12
Rhesus macaque	4.5–13
Baboon	14–41
White-handed gibbon	5–8
Chimpanzee	
male	56–80
female	45–68
Orangutan	
male	75–100
female	<40–150
Gorilla	<275

DANGER POTENTIAL

All species defend themselves by biting (Fig. 24.1). All primates have large teeth and strong jaws with well-developed canine teeth. In gibbons and langurs—particularly the adult males—the canine teeth are vicious weapons, but the animals are by no means helpless without them. Owners of pet monkeys often have the canine teeth extracted, under the mistaken belief that this removes the danger of injury from biting. This is far from the fact. Even with the canines

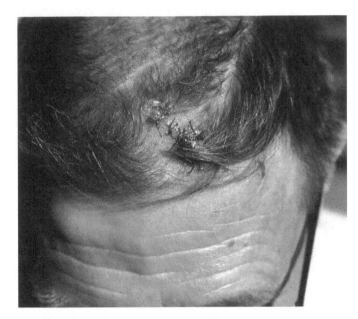

FIG. 24.1. Wound inflicted while attempting to net a primate.

removed, a 20-kg macaque is capable of biting the finger from an adult person with one snap. Baboons and apes are particularly dangerous to handle because of their exceptionally large canine teeth and their extreme aggressiveness. Research facilities housing such animals use special cages with a movable wall for animal restraint.

A secondary defense is scratching. Primate hands are able to grasp with strong fingers and hard fingernails, and scratches may be deep and painful. Medium-sized and large primates can also severely pinch and contuse any tissue within reach.

When working around primates, handlers should wear clothing that is neat and trim, with no pockets to provide a fingerhold and no full-length necktie; a primate may grab the tie and choke the handler. Primates also snatch glasses, pencils, or any other available object.

Unless one has had some experience working with primates, it is difficult to appreciate their tremendous strength. I recall a partially tamed 20-kg chimpanzee that could jerk its arm away from a man exerting the full strength of both hands on its arm. To subdue this same animal required four adult men, one gripping each limb to stretch and hold it for examination.

The larger apes can maintain a grip on a hand or a limb that is impossible for a person to break. You cannot pull your hand away from the one-finger grip of an orangutan or gorilla. With a full handhold, such animals can crush hands and dislocate joints with little effort. It is extremely important when working with primates that the animal is not allowed to grab any part of the clothing or the body.

Primates are also able to throw objects at the handler, a trait possessed by no other group of animals, often resulting in significant injuries to people. Great apes have been known to pull hypodermic darts from their bodies and throw them back at the marksman with tremendous force. When excited, a chimpanzee or a gorilla may pick up dirt, feces, water, stones, plant debris, or anything else handy and throw it at the handler.

Primates can remember and identify persons for whom they have conceived a dislike. Restrainers are most likely to be remembered. When I enter the enclosure to examine a chimpanzee at a nearby zoo, I must don a special raincoat and use a garbage can lid as a shield to deflect the bombardment of debris.

Some New World species of primates possess a prehensile tail. Although the tail is unlikely to harm a captor, it complicates restraint because it is used almost like another limb.

Nonhuman primates may be the source of infectious diseases in humans and vice versa.[8] Greater attention is now being given to quarantine procedures and protecting keepers and the public from potential zoonoses. Many zoos have strict protocols for handling nonhuman primates, including the use of protective outer clothing, masks, and rubber gloves when direct handling is necessary.

ANATOMY, PHYSIOLOGY, AND BEHAVIOR

The anatomical characteristic most important in restraint is the dexterity of the animal's hands and arms. A primate can prevent capture with a net by pushing away the hoop, or ensnarement by throwing off the loop. Primate hands may also grasp the handler to prevent him or her from carrying out the contemplated procedure and can seriously injure the handler as well.

All primates have tremendous relative strength compared to human beings, and this must be taken into account when selecting a restraint procedure. Most primates have short necks and relatively long limbs, allowing them to reach great distances. Nonhuman primates lack a human's highly developed ability to dissipate heat by sweating, so provision must be made for temperature control when restraining these animals.

Many Old World primate species have cheek pouches that are used to temporarily store gathered food. Caution is advised when restraining animals with bulged cheeks, for the food material may be dislodged and inhaled during manipulation.

Gibbons, siamangs, and great apes have laryngeal air sacs that are used to modulate vocalization. In gibbons, sia-

mangs, orangutans, and gorillas, the air sacs extend ventrally from the larynx over the front of the thorax. The orangutan has the most extensive arrangement, with the air sac reaching to the waist and around the mandible toward the ears.[6] These air sacs may become infected, and purulent exudate may flow into the larynx when immobilized animals are in a prone position and aspiration may ensue. Respiration must be monitored in any sedated animal, but great apes are especially vulnerable to malpositioning.

In nature most primates live either in family groups or in larger social units. A troop of baboons may include 40 to 70 individuals. Groups have a definitive hierarchical social structure. The dominant individual is usually a male, but in some societies it is a female. The alpha animal is the most difficult to subdue and restrain and may interfere with the restraint of subordinates. In addition, the whole troop may attack, especially if one is attempting to separate out an infant or remove a dead infant.

A primate that has previously been restrained will be extremely difficult to approach a second time. Primates have excellent powers of recall, which make them wary of unpleasant experiences; a successful ruse can almost never be repeated.

When an individual is removed from a group of primates for examination, surgery, or other activities, the social structure is altered; reestablishment may require some time. During the interim, conflict is relative to the status of the individual who was removed. If it was the alpha animal, the subordinate animals will vie with one another to determine a new dominant individual. When the removed animal is replaced, it may find it impossible to reestablish itself at the previous level in the social structure. An individual can usually be safely reintroduced within 3 days of the removal; after that, success will be questionable. After a week, the "newcomer" will almost certainly be attacked and possibly killed unless special techniques are used to disguise the introduction. One way to do this is to move the whole group into a new area and, during the confusion, introduce the newcomer. Another technique is to place the newcomer into the enclosure at night. Some feel that it is important to remove medicinal odors before reintroducing the animal.

It is essential for those who maintain captive populations of primates to understand these behavioral characteristics. The restrainer must be aware of and prepared to deal with the consequences of removing individuals from a social group.

PHYSICAL RESTRAINT[6,7,9,15–17]
Prosimians

Small tarsiers and similar species may be grasped barehanded (Figs. 24.2, 24.3). Usually, however, the initial contact is made while wearing leather gloves (Fig. 24.4). Nets are universal tools. The animal may be extricated from the net and held bare-handed (Fig. 24.5).

Keepers of colonies of small primates (marmosets, tamarins) develop techniques for routine handling. One such

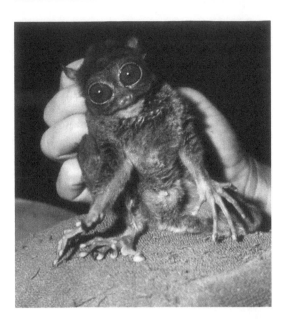

FIG. 24.2. Grasping a small tarsier bare-handed.

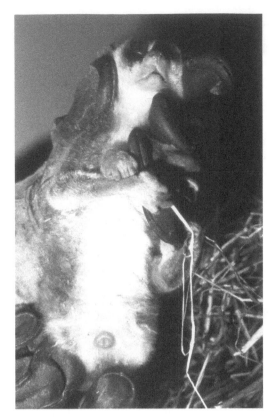

FIG. 24.4. Grasping a galago with gloved hands.

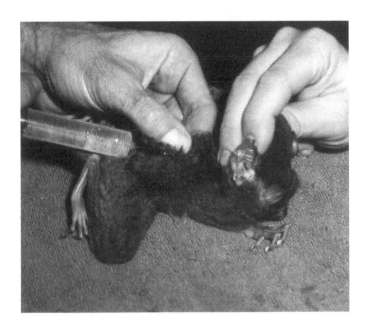

FIG. 24.3. Administering fluids to a tarsier.

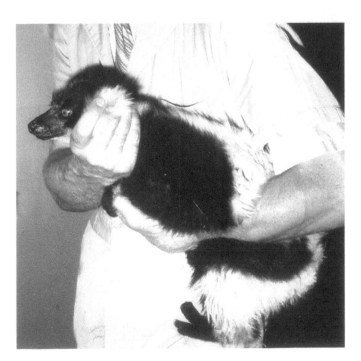

FIG. 24.5. Proper method for holding a lemur following net capture.

technique incorporates a special night box with a sliding trap door. A hoop covered with a stockinette is placed over the opening (Fig. 24.6). When the night box is opened, the animal can be frightened into the stockinette (Fig. 24.7). A net may be used as well. Once in the stockinette, it can be weighed or restrained and handled in any desired manner (Fig. 24.8). To remove the animal, grasp it through the stockinette behind the head at the nape of the neck, taking care to avoid the mouth. Slowly work the stockinette off, regrabbing the animal beneath the stockinette. The animal may then be manipulated bare-handed. Do not disregard the sharpness of the teeth or the

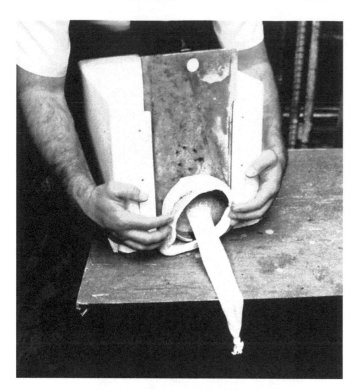

FIG. 24.6. Marmosets and tamarins may be captured from their night boxes by placing a segment of stockinette or a net over the door and encouraging the animal to crawl into it.

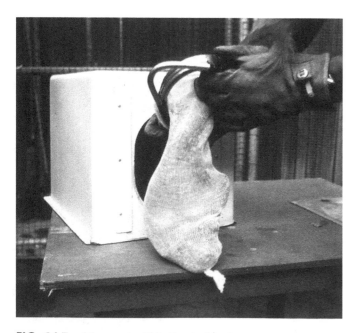

FIG. 24.7. Marmoset within the stockinette.

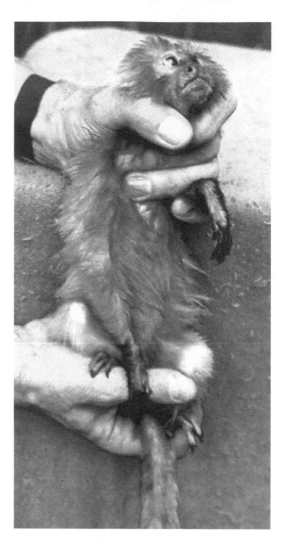

FIG. 24.8. A. Marmoset may be removed from the stockinette and held bare-handed.

Simians—Small- to Medium-Sized

Nets are commonly used to capture primates weighing up to 15 kg (33 lb). The diameter of the hoop and the size of the mesh are determined by the species to be captured. Mobile fingers and hands will entangle themselves if the mesh is too large. In no case should the animal be able to stick its head through the mesh, and preferably it should be unable to put a limb through the mesh.

Special precautions must be taken when entering a cage containing a group of monkeys, because the alpha male may attack. It is desirable to have a backup handler present, armed with a broom to ward off attack. In group cages, it is not unusual for one or more monkeys to jump directly at the handler. This may be a defensive or an offensive maneuver, or the monkey may merely use the head or body of the handler as a springboard en route to some other vantage point. When entering a cage of animals known to jump at the handler, wear a face mask similar to those used by fencers (Fig. 24.11).

quickness of movement of these animals (Fig. 24.9). Hands should be kept away from the animal's face.

Chemical immobilization and medication of small species of primates should be preceded by accurate weight determination (Fig. 24.10).

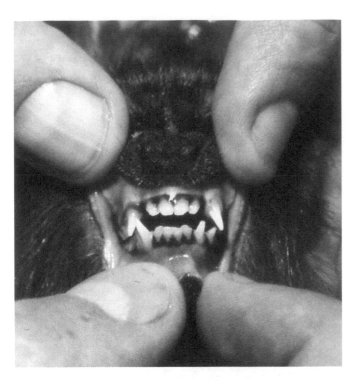

FIG. 24.9.   **B.** Teeth of a golden marmoset.

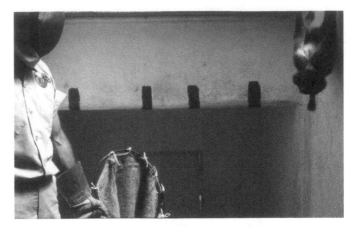

FIG. 24.11.   A fencer's face mask should be worn when attempting to capture primates that may jump at the handler.

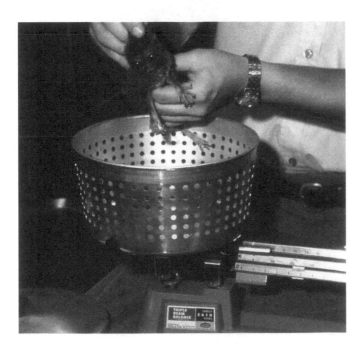

FIG. 24.10.   Small species such as the tarsier must be weighed to accurately determine dosage for chemical immobilization or for medication.

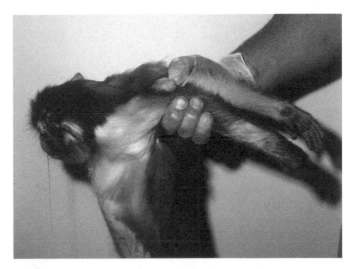

FIG. 24.12.   Recommended method for handling a primate weighing up to 10 kg. Note that a finger is kept between the arms of the monkey.

A small monkey (up to 5.0 kg [11.0 lb]) that has been netted may be grasped behind the head at the nape. This manipulation must be carried out swiftly to prevent the animal from turning its head to bite the handler. The arms of a larger monkey may be gripped above the elbows and pulled behind the back (Fig. 24.12).

Some simple examinations and medications may be given with the monkey held in the net; if more complex procedures are required, it must be removed. This may be an arduous task, because the monkey will cling to the net with its mouth, all four feet, and its tail, if prehensile. Patience is required of all primate handlers. Once the monkey is out of the net, hold it as illustrated in Figures 24.12 to 24.15.

Gloves are an important tool for working with primates. Special double-thickness heavy leather gloves are made to help prevent mutilation of the handler's hands (Fig. 24.16). The extra thumb or mitten is offered to the animal to chew on while the other hand grasps the head. Some handlers prefer to wear gloves; others feel that bare hands are desirable because tactile discrimination and grip are enhanced.

Macaques and baboons can crush the fingers even through a heavy leather glove. Some handlers use chain-mail butcher's gloves for added protection (Fig. 24.17).

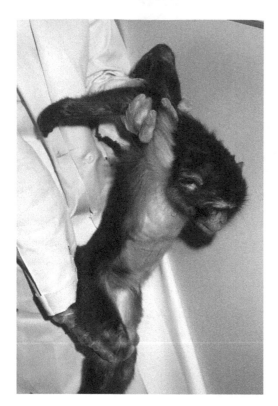

FIG. 24.13. Further restraint may be obtained by grasping the legs.

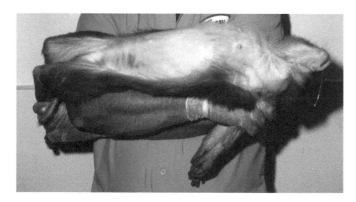

FIG. 24.14. Abdomen of a primate is exposed for examination or tattooing.

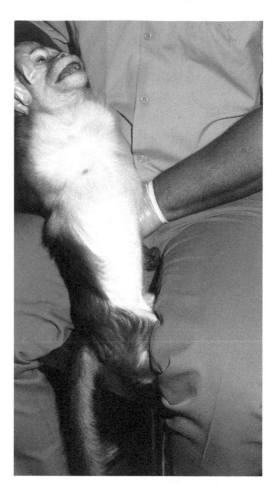

FIG. 24.15. Medium-sized primate, firmly secured.

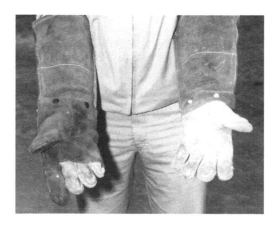

FIG. 24.16. Gauntleted, double-layered heavy leather gloves for working with primates.

Troops of nonhuman primates maintained in large enclosures must be restricted to a smaller enclosure such as a night house or a holding pen (Fig. 24.18). Animals may be netted from the smaller holding area (Fig. 24.19), or special funnels and runways constructed to catch the animals in a squeeze cage (Figs. 24.20 to 24.22).

Large primates should be handled in squeeze cages or by chemical restraint. Many types of squeeze cages have been designed for working with primates. It is not the purpose of this presentation to analyze and rate the myriad cages that can be fabricated; however, two are illustrated (Figs. 24.23 to 24.25; see also Chapter 2). To remove an unsedated monkey

from a squeeze cage, position the animal with its back to the door so it cannot bite the handler (Fig. 24.23). Then pull the arms behind the monkey's back as previously described (Fig. 24.24).

Figure 24.26 illustrates a method of passing a stomach tube in a physically restrained animal. The head is grasped as

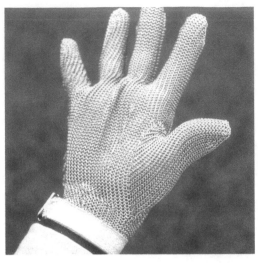

FIG. 24.17. Chain-mail (butcher's) glove to prevent serious injury from primate canine teeth.

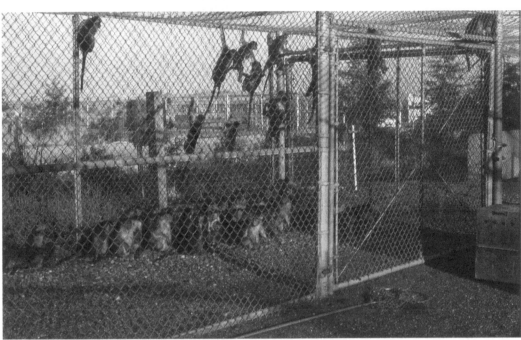

FIG. 24.18. Macaques in a small holding area within a larger enclosure.

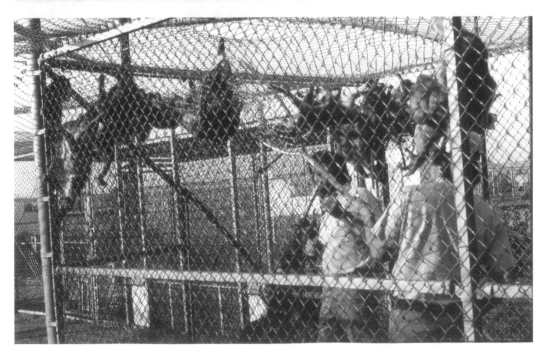

FIG. 24.19. Macaques being netted in a holding pen.

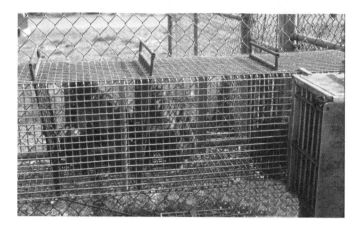

FIG. 24.20. Runway from a holding pen to a squeeze cage.

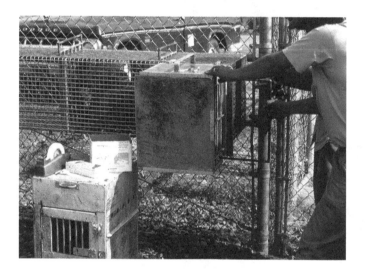

FIG. 24.21. Catching a macaque in a squeeze cage at the end of a runway.

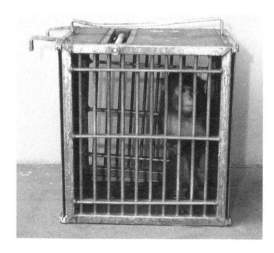

FIG. 24.22. Squeeze cage to allow chemical immobilization.

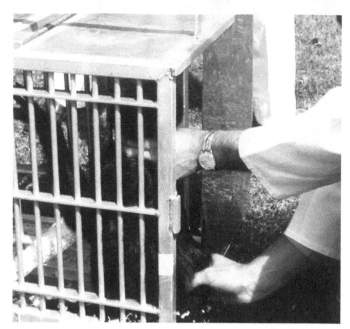

FIG. 24.23. Removing a primate from a transfer cage.

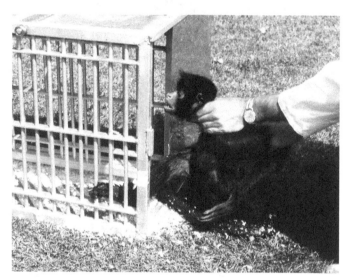

FIG. 24.24. Grasping a primate from a transfer cage.

indicated and a piece of wooden doweling is inserted in the mouth. An appropriately sized stomach tube can be inserted over the top of the doweling or through a hole drilled in the doweling. The tube should be large enough to inhibit its passage into the trachea. The stomach tube is lubricated and inserted into the mouth. Gentle pressure on the tube will induce the animal to swallow it. After the tube has been inserted, the placement should be checked by immersing the other end of the tube in a pan of water. If the tube has been misplaced into the trachea, bubbles will be emitted with each expiration. A few bubbles may issue even though the tube is

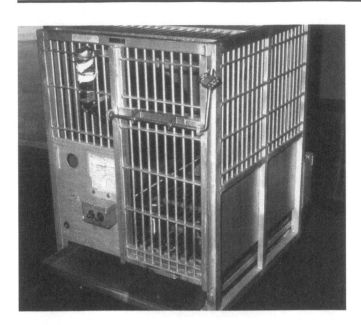

FIG. 24.25. Commercial primate squeeze cage for animals up to 25 kg.

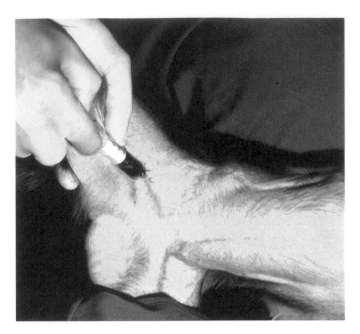

FIG. 24.27. Venipuncture of the femoral vein.

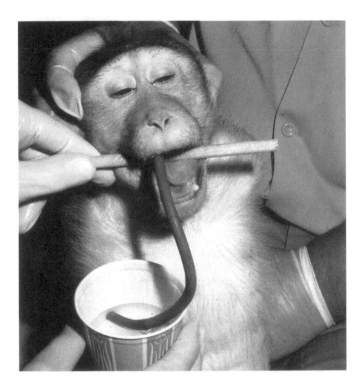

FIG. 24.26. Passage of an intragastric tube using a dowel as a speculum.

in the stomach, because of pressure on the stomach or perhaps some gas in the stomach. However, air bubbles from the stomach should not coincide with expiration. After proper placement has been assured, medication may be placed into the stomach.

Blood samples from primates may be collected from numerous superficial vessels. The cephalic vessels of the arms are similar to those of human beings and dogs. In small to medium-sized New World monkeys, the saphenous vein on the posterior aspect of the calf is an excellent vessel from which to obtain samples. In small animals or in moribund animals with low blood pressure, it is necessary to cut alongside the vessel to see it and direct the needle into it. When large quantities of blood are required, the femoral vein is penetrated just prior to the point of entrance into the pelvis (Fig. 24.27). It is desirable to slightly sedate the animal in order to avoid movement while the needle is in the vessel.

Apes

In nearly all instances the manipulation of gorillas, chimpanzees, and orangutans requires chemical immobilization. Some zoos have constructed massive squeeze cages for apes, but most of these become inoperable or are not sufficiently adaptable for universal use. I do not recommend that squeeze cages be built into new facilities. The chemical immobilization agents currently available are generally safe, efficient preparations and impose much less stress and harm on the animals than any method of physical restraint adequate to hold them.

Special Procedures and Techniques

Tuberculin testing is an absolutely essential program for the management of captive primates. The preferred sites for intradermal injections of tuberculin are the eyelid, the abdomen, or the areola. For the eyelid site, the animal is restrained in a suitable manner, the upper lid is stretched, and the material is injected with a fine 26-gauge short beveled needle (Fig. 24.28).

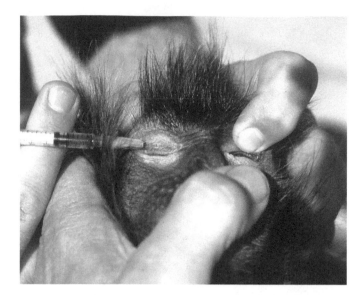

FIG. 24.28. Tuberculin testing using the eyelid.

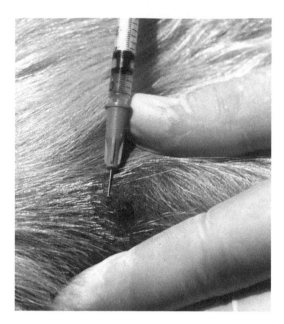

FIG. 24.30. Tuberculin testing on the areola.

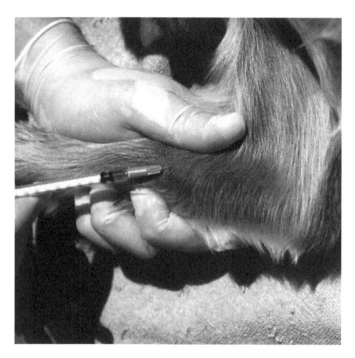

FIG. 24.29. Tuberculin testing on the forearm.

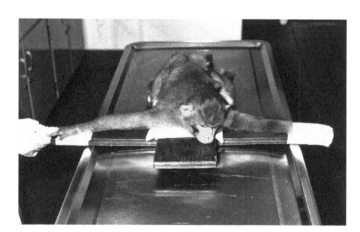

FIG. 24.31. Primate being secured on a plywood cross (used for continuous medication or other treatment).

Any relatively hairless area can be used, such as the forearm (Fig. 24.29) or the areola around the nipple (Fig. 24.30), or the hair may be carefully clipped from a chosen site on the abdomen. Palpation is required to read the test at all sites other than the eyelid. Results of injecting the eyelid can be seen. The test site should be inspected at 24, 48, and 72 hours.

To transfer a small primate from one swinging-door cage to another, use the technique described in Chapter 2.

Primates have become important as laboratory animals. Large colonies of various species are maintained in primate centers of university and other research laboratories through-out the world. A great deal of experience relating to the care and handling of animals has been gained in such institutions, but many of the techniques practiced are not really desirable for general primate restraint. An acceptable special restraint device used in primate centers and veterinary hospitals is the wooden cross (Figs. 24.31, 24.32).

One particularly perplexing problem faces the veterinarian who must handle a pet primate. The pet may arrive in the arms of its owner, but when it becomes necessary for the veterinarian to grasp the animal, the owner is completely incapable of assisting in the operation. Attempts to take the animal or initiate restraint while the animal is held in the arms of the owner may result in the owner being bitten. If at all possible, the animal should be transferred to a squeeze cage and quickly immobilized with a chemical restraint agent.

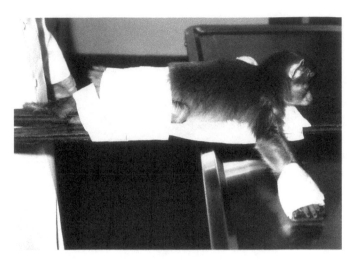

FIG. 24.32. Primate taped to a cross.

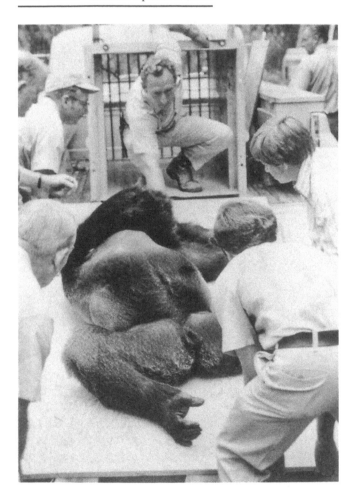

FIG. 24.33. Sheet of plywood used as a stretcher for a large gorilla.

Alternatively the animal should be handed to a third party who is capable of handling it. In nearly all instances pet primates have been fed a deficient diet and are likely to suffer from demineralization of the bone, predisposing them to fractures; extraordinary care must be taken to avoid injuring them by the restraint procedure.

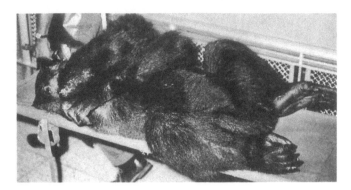

FIG. 24.34. Transporting gorilla on a human stretcher.

TRANSPORT[3]

Small to medium-sized primates may be placed in small cages and easily moved from one place to another. Large animals such as the gorilla may be transported on heavy plywood sheets or human stretchers following chemical immobilization (Figs. 24.33, 24.34).

CHEMICAL RESTRAINT[1,2,4–8,10,12–14]

The chemical restraint agents and combinations mentioned in this chapter represent those used by the author or experienced veterinarians with detailed knowledge of primates. Other protocols have been used, and no claim is made for including all possible drugs and combinations. For more detailed information, particularly for anesthesia, consult the references.

Primates are easily handled with chemical agents now available. Fortunately the dosage levels of each drug are essentially the same throughout the order.

Ketamine is used at 8.0–15.0 mg/kg depending on the duration of the intended procedure or size of the species (smaller individuals require a higher dose). The combination of tiletamine/zolazepam is used extensively in immobilizing nonhuman primates. Dosage in the smaller species (bush babies, marmosets) is 7.0–8.0 mg/kg; in medium-sized animals (vervets, spider monkeys, capuchins), 4.0–6.0 mg/kg; larger animals (baboons, macaques), 3.0–4.0 mg/kg; and in great apes, 2.0–3.0 mg/kg. Recovery time from tiletamine/zolazepam immobilization is dose dependant. Use low doses for quick procedures. See Table 24.2 for selected chemical restraint agents for primates.

TABLE 24.2. Selected chemical restraint agents for immobilization of primates[15]

Agent	Dose (mg/kg), IM
Isoflurane	5% induction, 2.5% maintenance, face mask
Ketamine	5.0–10.0
Ketamine/medetomidine	5.0/0.05
Tiletamine/zolazepam	1.5–3.6

Caution is advisable when administering chemical immobilizing drugs to Old World nonhuman primates that are in estrus. The tumescent area is highly friable, and severe hemorrhage may result from accidental injection. When the sex skin area is quiescent, the subcutaneous tissue is highly fibrous and absorption from the area is prolonged.

When immobilizing a nonhuman primate within an enclosure with multiple animals, be aware that other members of the troop may attack a partially immobilized animal. Be prepared to protect the immobilized individual (use a stream of water or broom to frighten others away).

Allow immobilized animals to recover in isolation. If the procedure has lasted for only a few minutes to hours, return to a group may be uneventful. When an animal must be separated for days to weeks, behavioral problems may ensue with reintroduction.

The chemical restraint of a primate in a large open cage is difficult. Small species have limited muscular areas available as injection sites. Even the chimpanzee or orangutan may provide a small target for the dart. Apes are extremely wary, especially if they have been previously immobilized. They will create a violent disturbance when anyone attempts to point a gun or blowgun at them. The animals may charge the bars, reaching out and grabbing at the shooter (Fig. 24.35). They may spit or throw feces, debris, or water. They may keep running about the cage, preventing a stationary target; or they may station themselves in a corner, folding their arms and legs into positions that leave essentially no muscle mass visible as a target site. Patience, experience, and readiness to take advantage of fleeting opportunities are necessary to achieve success in such cases.

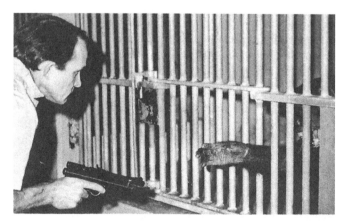

FIG. 24.35. Chemical immobilization of large apes is difficult. Here, the animal is close to the bars, grabbing at the handler.

Use the least traumatic projection system possible when immobilizing nonhuman primates. Any blow dart or Telinject system is excellent in most captive situations, although powered weapons may be necessary for immobilizing the great apes.

The author was involved in an immobilizing program in a troop of human-habituated yellow baboons in Africa.

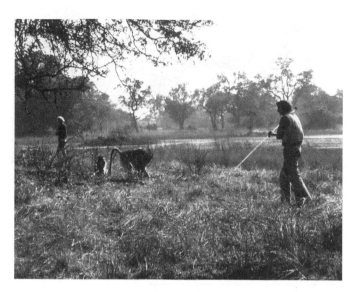

FIG. 24.36. Field immobilization of baboons using a blowgun and ketamine.

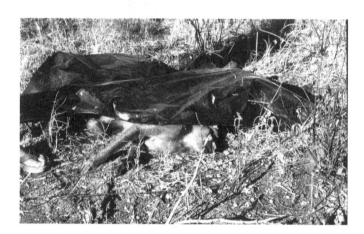

FIG. 24.37. Covering an immobilized baboon with plastic to block the view of other baboons, rendering it a nonentity.

Researchers could approach within 2–5 m with a blowgun (Fig. 24.36). Most of the injected baboons climbed a nearby tree. As immobilization progressed, they began to slip down the tree from one branch to another. Ultimately, they fell from the tree (no injuries resulted). Generally, other members of the troop ignored the immobile baboon and wandered off to feed. However, the beta male soon began to stay nearby and make threatening gestures as the handlers approached. It became necessary to walk past the immobile animal and drop a black plastic sheet over it (Fig. 24.37). Then the beta male would join the rest of the troop in foraging.

In field immobilization situations, it is important for someone to stay with the animal until it is fully recovered and help to guide it in the direction taken by the rest of the troop. Other troops foraging through the area would attack and kill an isolated and weakened animal.

Isoflurane inhalation anesthesia is used as an alternative to injectable ketamine or tiletamine/zolazepam sedation. A

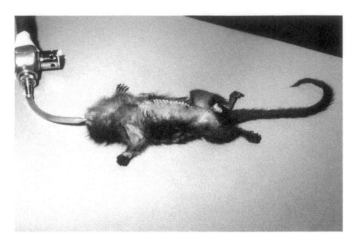

FIG. 24.38. It is difficult to intubate tiny primates, but Cole endotracheal tubes may be used effectively.

small transfer cage may be placed within a closed clear plastic bag or an anesthesia chamber. A 4% flow rate should be selected. When relaxation is sufficient, the animal may be changed to a face mask or intubated and the flow rate reduced to 1–2%. When a nonhuman primate weighing less than 1 kg is intubated (Fig. 24.38), injudicious manipulation of the endotracheal tube may traumatize the mucous membrane and cause sufficient swelling to obstruct airflow following extubation.

Small nonhuman primates require supplemental heat during recovery from anesthesia. A circulating warm-water pad or a human infant incubator is useful for this purpose (Fig. 24.39).

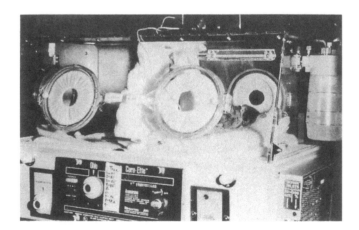

FIG. 24.39. Human infant incubator.

REFERENCES

1. Bonner, W.B., Keeling, M.E., Van Ormer, E.T., and Haynie, J.E. 1972. Ketamine anesthesia in chimpanzees and other great ape species. In: Bourne, G.H., Ed. The Chimpanzee, vol. 5, Baltimore: University Park Press, Basel, Karger, pp. 255–68.
2. Burroughs, R.E.J. 1993. Chemical capture of primates. In: McKenzie, A.A., Ed. The Capture and Care Manual, Pretoria: The South African Veterinary Foundation, pp. 328–31.
3. Espie, I. 1993. Transportation of primates. In: McKenzie, A.A., Ed. The Capture and Care Manual, Pretoria: The South African Veterinary Foundation, pp. 334–35.
4. Foster, P.A. 1973. Immobilization and anesthesia of primates. In: Young, E., Ed. The Capture and Care of Wild Animals, Capetown, South Africa: Human and Rousseau, pp. 69–76.
5. Harris, J.M. 1974. Restraint and physical examination of monkeys and primates. In: Kirk, R.W., Ed. Current Veterinary Therapy V, Philadelphia, W.B. Saunders, pp. 586–88.
6. Janssen, D L. 1993. Diseases of great apes. In: Fowler, M.E., Ed. Zoo and Wild Animal Medicine, 3rd ed., Philadelphia, W.B. Saunders, p. 334.
7. Joslin, J.O. 2003. Other primates excluding great apes. In: Fowler, M.E., and Miller, R.E., Eds. Zoo and Wild Animal Medicine. 5th Ed. St. Louis, Saunders/Elsevier. pp. 346–80.
8. Joslin, J.E. 1993. Zoonotic diseases of nonhuman primates. In: Fowler, M.E., Ed. Zoo and Wild Animal Medicine, 3rd ed., Philadelphia, W.B. Saunders, pp. 358–73.
9. Junge, P.E. 2003. Prosimians. In: Fowler, M.E., and Miller, R.E., Eds. Zoo and Wild Animal Medicine. 5th Ed. St. Louis, Saunders/Elsevier. pp. 334–37.
10. Kearns, K.S., Swenson, B., and Ramsay, E.C. 2000. Oral induction of anesthesia with droperidol and transmucosal carfentanil citrate in chimpanzees. J Zoo An Med 31(1):185–89.
11. Loomis, M.R. 2003. Great apes. In: Fowler, M.E., and Miller, R.E., Eds. Zoo and Wild Animal Medicine. 5th Ed. St. Louis, Saunders/Elsevier. pp. 381–96.
12. Olberg, R-A. 2007. Monkeys and gibbons. In: West, G., Heard, D., and Caulkett, N. 2007. Zoo Animal and Wildlife Immobilization and Anesthesia. Ames, Iowa, Blackwell Publishing, pp. 375–86.
13. Sleeman, J. 2007. Great apes. In: West, G., Heard, D., and Caulkett, N. 2007. Zoo Animal and Wildlife Immobilization and Anesthesia. Ames, Iowa, Blackwell Publishing, pp. 387–94.
14. Sleeman, J.M., Cameron, K., Mudakikwa, A.B., Nizeyi, J-B, Anderson, S., Cooper, J.E., Richardson, H.M., Macfie, E.J., Hastings, B., and Foster, J.W. 2000. Field Anesthesia of free-ranging mountain gorillas from the Virunga Volcano Region of Central Africa J Zoo An Med 31(1):9–14.
15. de Wet, T. 1993. Physical capture of primates. In: McKenzie, A.A., Ed. The Capture and Care Manual, Pretoria: The South African Veterinary Foundation, pp. 332–33.
16. Whittingham, R.A. 1971. Trapping and shipping baboons. J Inst Anim Tech 22:66–82.
17. Williams, C.V., and Junge, R.E. 2007. Prosimians. In: West, G., Heard, D., and Caulkett, N. 2007. Zoo Animal and Wildlife Immobilization and Anesthesia. Ames, Iowa, Blackwell Publishing, pp. 367–74.

CHAPTER 25
Marine Mammals

CLASSIFICATION (NUMBERS IN PARENTHESES DENOTE NUMBER OF KNOWN SPECIES)

Order Cetacea: whales
    Suborder Odontoceti: toothed whale, dolphin (80)
    Suborder Mysticeti: baleen whale (12)
Order Pinnipedia
    Family Otariidae: eared seal, sea lion (13)
    Family Odobenidae: walrus (1)
    Family Phocidae: seal (18)
Order Sirenia: dugong, manatee (4)

The polar bear and the sea otter[33] are also marine mammals, but they are discussed in the chapter on carnivores.

Marine mammals are adapted to an aquatic habitat and present special problems to the animal restrainer. In the United States they are all under the regulations of three agencies of the federal government:[33]

1. U.S. Department of Commerce, National Marine Fisheries Service (the Marine Mammal Protection Act, 1972).
2. U.S. Department of the Interior, United States Fish and Wildlife Service (The Endangered Species Act, 1973). This act regulates those animals that are listed as endangered species or are threatened with extinction without due care. Many marine mammals are in this category.
3. The U.S. Department of Agriculture, Animal and Plant Health Inspection Service (Animal Welfare Act and Animal Welfare Regulations). This is codified in the Code of Federal Regulations Title 9 (animals), Chapter 1 (animal welfare), Part 3 (standards), Subpart E (marine mammals). The act regulates marine mammals that are used in research and those being exhibited.

Marine mammals are high profile animals and are on the radar screen of animal rights activists and animal rights extremists groups. (See Chapter 8 for more details.)

Marine mammals vary in length from 1.0–30.0 m (3.0–100.0 ft) and may weigh up to 81,000 kg (89 t) (blue whales). Names of gender are listed in Table 25.1.

TABLE 25.1. Names of gender of marine mammals

	Adult Male	Adult Female	Newborn/Young	Group Name
Animal	Male	Female		
Whales	Bull	Cow	Calf	Pod
Dolphin	Bull	Cow	Calf	
Sea lion	Bull	Cow	Pup	Herd
Walrus	Bull	Cow	Pup	
Seals	Bull	Cow	Pup	

DANGER POTENTIAL[26,27]

Toothed whales are carnivorous. Large species, such as the killer whale, may be dangerous. Pools are usually cleaned with the animals in another pool. Dolphins are usually safe for divers to be with, but they may play roughly.

A dolphin may throw its head about and smash it into a handler. Dolphins often bump objects with their large and powerful mandibles and can easily break the arm of a person.

All cetaceans flip the flukes up and down. A large killer or pilot whale could crush a person with a slap of the tail. Baleen whales do not bite, but the tail fluke may injure a handler.

The dugong and the manatee are mild-mannered herbivorous animals that are unlikely to bite, but a person may be injured by being pressed against a wall of a tank or hit with the extremely strong tail.

Seals and sea lions are efficient carnivorous predators. They have strong teeth capable of tearing flesh. The large bulls of various species are able to badly bruise or crush an individual who approaches too closely or becomes pressed against a wall during a restraint procedure. Walrus tusks may impale careless handlers, but more commonly the head becomes a battering ram.

ANATOMY AND PHYSIOLOGY

Marine mammals lack readily accessible limbs that can be grasped for restraint. Just beneath the skin of most species is a blubber layer of insulation that must be considered during restraint procedures. Marine mammals have a highly specialized thermoregulatory system, eliminating heat by conduction from the appendages as they swim through the water. The single most important precaution to take for the safety of a captive animal is to make sure it does not overheat. A continual spray of water should be played on restrained animals. Ice should always be available if a cetacean is to be out of a pool for more than a few minutes. A towel should be placed over the skin of the appendages, then ice placed on the towel.

The massive bodies of large marine mammals are buoyantly supported by water displacement in their oceanic habitat. When they are "dry-docked" or beached for examination or treatment, tremendous pressures are exerted on anatomical systems, particularly on the flexible thorax. Such burdens may embarrass respiration if the animals are kept out of water too long.

Cetaceans breathe through a blowhole on the top of their head. Never obstruct this orifice.[26,27] The breath-holding reflex is necessary for marine mammals to remain submerged for many minutes when diving. Bradycardia may accompany the breath holding particularly in pinnipeds. The significance of this reflex action is that such breath holding may occur during restraint and anesthesia procedures. It is desirable that an endotracheal tube be placed to provide positive pressure respiration during prolonged chemical restraint and anesthesia.

Marine mammals are able to maintain normal internal body temperature either by an insulation layer (blubber or fat) or by a special hair coat that prevents penetration of cold water to the surface of the skin (polar bears, sea otters). The limbs, flippers, and flukes are aided by a countercurrent circulatory arrangement. See Chapter 4 for more details. In either case, caution must be exercised to prevent hyperthermia when restraining.

PHYSICAL RESTRAINT

Cetaceans—Whales and Dolphins[6,8,23,25]

Pinnipeds and cetaceans are popular attractions in zoos and oceanaria (Fig. 25.1), where trained veterinarians look after the animals. However, pinnipeds and cetaceans may be encountered on coastal shores and beaches when they strand themselves or haul out because of weakness or illness.

The general public may respond quickly to a stranded cetacean or other marine mammals of any age, and in some instances, harm is inflicted because of ignorance of proper procedures. The public should be discouraged from doing anything but first aid, which consists of clearing water, sand, and seaweed from the blowhole; keeping the animal cool by pouring water over the flippers; providing shade if possible (cover with towels or sheeting); keeping the animal upright and digging trenches around the appendages to relieve pressure.[23] Pinnipeds may bite if approached too closely.

Further manipulation should be performed only by trained personnel associated with a marine mammal rescue and rehabilitation center that may be contacted through www.marinemammalcenter.org. A northern California rescue center may be contacted at www.tmmc.org with links to the National Marine Fisheries Service's marine mammal health and stranding program.

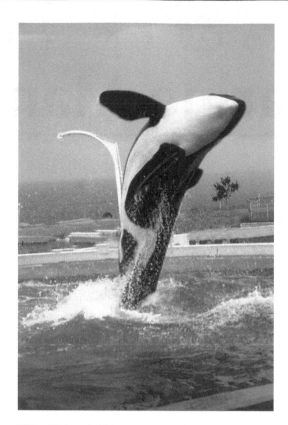

FIG. 25.1. A killer whale jumping at an oceanarium.

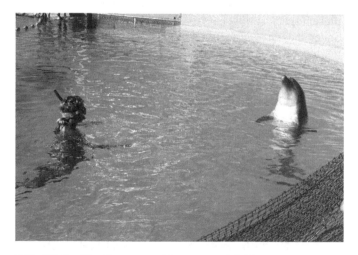

FIG. 25.2. Handler approaching a tame dolphin in a pool.

A calm dolphin may be removed from a tank by first isolating it using nets (Figs. 25.2, 25.3). The top of the net should have floats and the bottom of the net should be weighted with lead weights to ensure containment of the animal. Then the dolphin is maneuvered into position so that a stretcher-sling may be placed beneath the animal (Fig. 25.4) and lifted out of the pool. If the animal must be dry-docked for more than a few minutes, it should be placed on a foam rubber pad

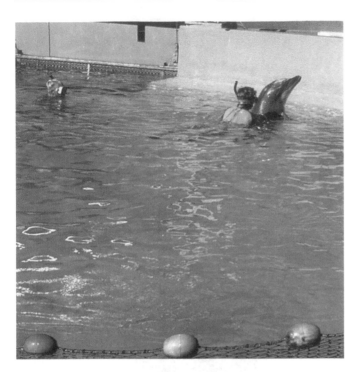

FIG. 25.3. Catching a dolphin after isolating it with a net.

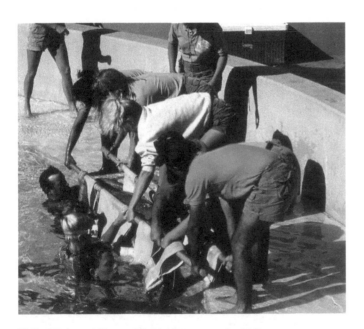

FIG. 25.4. Lifting a dolphin from a pool with a stretcher.

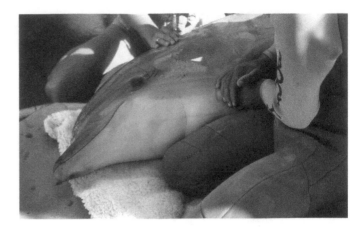

FIG. 25.5. Examination and treatment is carried out quickly to minimize over-heating and stress.

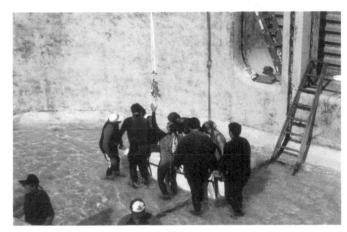

FIG. 25.6. Lowering the water in a pool to allow for separation of an individual and subsequent placement in a sling.

or a mattress. A cetacean may be examined while lying on its abdomen, or it may be gently rolled over onto its side (Fig. 25.5). Be certain to pull the flipper back against the body before rolling it, to preclude injury to the forelimb as the posture change is made.[13] No marine animal should be left unattended while out of the water. Watch carefully for signs of heat stress and possible injury from flipping over or flopping into dangerous positions.

If a dolphin or whale is difficult to catch, the pool may be drained, leaving only a few inches of water (Fig. 25.6). The selected dolphin is separated, using baffle boards and positioning the stretcher beneath the dolphin. A crane is employed to lift the dolphin out of the pool (Figs. 25.7, 25.8).

Sunlight and wind are added hazards to beached cetaceans. The skin is highly susceptible to sunburn, and the eyes can be damaged as well. Water sprayed over the body continually is helpful in preventing hyperthermia (Fig. 25.9), or the animal may be covered with a wet sheet that is re-wet as necessary. Blindfolding may minimize danger to a handler (Fig. 25.10). If a cetacean is to be out of water for an extended period, zinc oxide ointment or anhydrous lanolin should be applied to the skin around the blowhole or any part of the skin not covered by the wet sheet.

If a cetacean is to be beached for an elective procedure, it is recommended that it be done early in the morning or late in the evening to minimize elevated ambient temperatures. Ice should always be available.

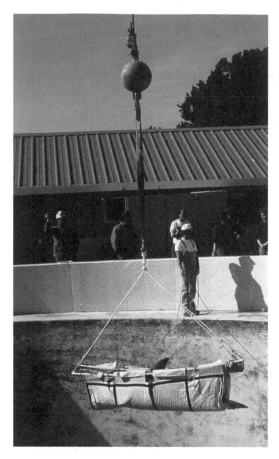

FIG. 25.7. Lifting a dolphin from a pool with a crane.

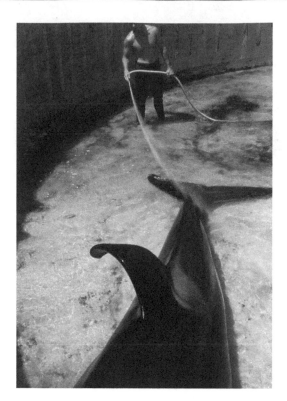

FIG. 25.9. Hosing down a beached cetacean.

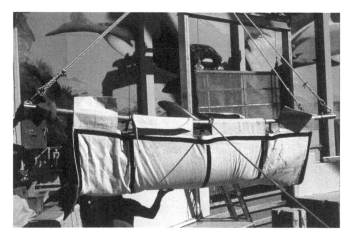

FIG. 25.8. Dolphin in a sling.

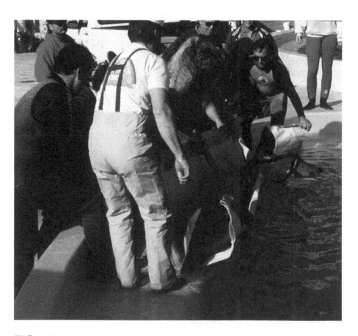

FIG. 25.10. Release of a beached dolphin by slipping from a stretcher.

These air-breathing mammals can stay submerged for only a limited time.

The release of a restrained dolphin should be as painstaking as the capture. Replace the animal on the sling and lower it gently into the water. When the animal is buoyant, free it from the sling. An attendant should be in the water to head the animal toward the center of the pool, never toward the periphery. As soon as the animal is released from the sling

and has taken one complete breath, it may be allowed its freedom. Alternatively, if the cetacean is trained, it may be rested on the edge of the pool, cued to take a breath, then gently rolled into the water (Fig. 25.11), or slipped from a stretcher (Fig. 25.12).

Generally large cetaceans are captured by emptying the tank. Attendants should stay beyond the arc of the tail fluke

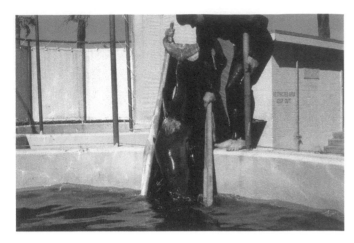

FIG. 25.11. Release of a restrained dolphin by rolling it into the pool.

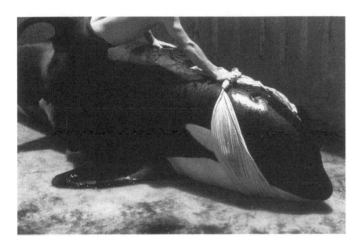

FIG. 25.12. Blinding a killer whale.

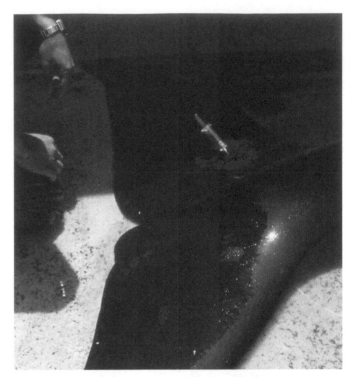

FIG. 25.13. Blood sample collection from the fluke vein.

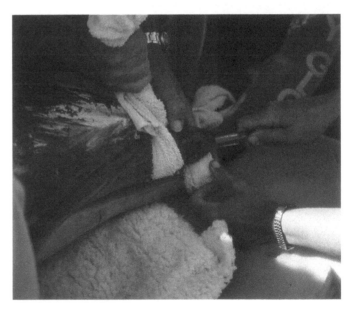

FIG. 25.14. Using towels to hold the mouth open while inserting a stomach tube.

to avoid serious injury. Blindfolding the animal reduces activity, although this does not guarantee that the animal will not flip around and bite. Close to the side of the animal at midbody is likely to be the safest place to stand.

Blood samples for laboratory evaluation may be withdrawn from the tail fluke (Figs. 25.12, 25.13). Captive killer whales and dolphins are usually trained to present the tail fluke at the bank of the pool and allow blood to be collected. The vessels are located approximately one-third of the way posterior to the leading edge of the fluke. A groove indicates the site location on both dorsal and ventral surfaces, but the ventral vein is usually used. These animals are also trained to lie in various positions for ultrasonography or radiography. Some institutions perform routine intragastric intubation (stomach tubing) weekly. A stomach tube is inserted through the mouth after towels are wrapped around the upper and lower jaws to hold the mouth open (Fig. 25.14).

A urine sample is easily collected from a cetacean that has been trained to urinate on command. Otherwise, a catheter

may be inserted into the urethral orifice via the anogenital slit.

Animals may also be trained to beach themselves and to breathe on command.[27] A waterproofed stethoscope facilitates auscultation at poolside while the animal is in the water.

Intramuscular injections are given in the large muscle mass just ahead or on either side of the dorsal fin (Fig. 25.15).

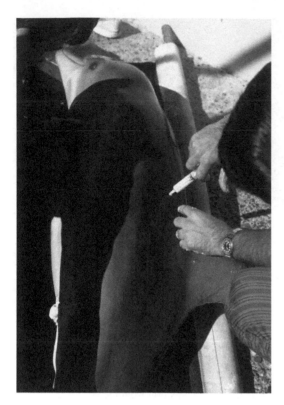

FIG. 25.15. Administering an intramuscular injection on the side of the dorsal fin.

In a dolphin weighing less than 100 kg (220 pounds), use an 18-gauge, 4.0 cm (1.5 in.) needle. In animals over 100 kg, use an 18-gauge spinal needle that is 6.5–9.0 cm (2.5–3.5 in.) long. An adult killer whale may require a 10.0- to 15.0-cm (4.0- to 6.0-in.) needle. Avoid intra-blubber injections. See Table 25.2 for selected chemical restraint agents for cetaceans.

TABLE 25.2. Selected chemical restraint agents for cetaceans

Agent	Sedation (mg/kg)	Immobilization (mg/kg)	Comments and references
Diazepam	B.N. dolphin 0.1–.02, IM K. whale 0.2		6
Midazoloam	B.N. dolphin 0.05–0.15 IM K whale 0.025–0.05		6
Butorphanol	0.05–0.15 IM		6
Ketamine/medetomidine		1.75/0.01–0.04	6

Sirenians—Manatees, Dugongs

Sirenians are aquatic and basically nonoffensive, docile herbivores (Figs. 25.16, 25.17).[2,4,22,31] However, one should avoid the powerful tail that may move up and down or sideways. Physical restraint is usually sufficient for handling these animals. Small manatees may be gently grasped around the

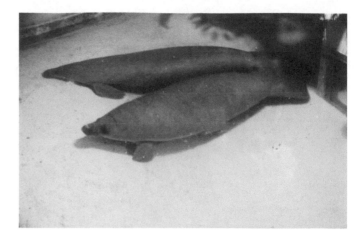

FIG. 25.16. Florida manatee *Trichechus manatus latirostris*.

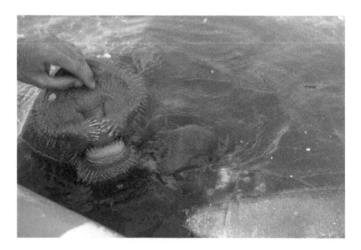

FIG. 25.17. West Indian manatee *Trichechus manatus*.

thorax while in the water, taking care not to inhibit respiration. The infant may then be lifted out of the pool and placed on a sponge rubber mat during examination or treatment. Adults may be lifted out of a pool on a stretcher and then placed on a foam rubber mat. Press the head and tail to the padded surface. This may be facilitated by a rectangular piece of closed-cell foam padding over the back. The restrainer may then lie over the pad and animal.[22]

The venipuncture site for a neonate manatee is from the ventral midline tail vein. In unsedated adult manatees, the venipuncture site is the brachial vessels between the radius and ulna. Use a 20-gauge 38-mm (1.5-in) needle.[22] Intramuscular injections are administered in the musculature over the shoulder area. See Table 25.3 for selected chemical restraint agents for dugong and manatees.

Pinnipeds—Seals, Sea Lions, Walrus[5,7,10–12,16,24,28]

Pinnipeds are amphibious. It is virtually impossible to capture a sea lion in a pool; it can elude or jump over nets.

TABLE 25.3.   Selected chemical restraint agents for dugong and manatees[2,4,22,31]

Agent	Dose (mg/kg), IM
Midazolam	0.02–0.05, IM
Diazepam	0.01–0.035, IV
Xylazine	0.05–0.1, IM
Butorphanol	0.01–0.025, IM
Detomidine	0.005–0.01, IM

The animal should be enticed onto the bank with food, or the pool should be drained before attempting capture.

The sea lion's head is extremely mobile; it can reach out effortlessly to the side and to the back. Handlers should be cautious when working with these animals, because their bite wounds may be severe.

For small sea lions and seals, a handler covers the animal's head with a towel, then presses the neck just behind the head and holds the head to the ground while straddling the body and keeping the flippers pressed against the side of the body (Fig. 25.18). Larger sea lions and seals require two (Fig. 25.19) or three persons (Fig. 25.20); one on the head and astraddle the body while the others hold the flippers against the sides and the hind flippers pulled back. Blood samples from seals may be obtained from the epidural intervertebral sinus between the lumbar vertebrae (Fig. 25.21).[12]

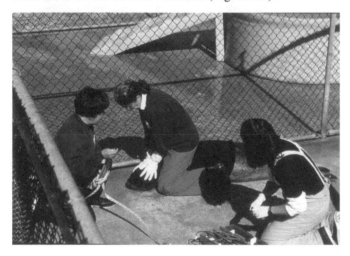

FIG. 25.18. Capturing a pinniped by covering the head with a towel, then by straddling and holding the neck with both hands.

Pinnipeds may also be captured with a neck strap (Figs. 25.22, 25.23) or a bull-pole (Fig. 25.24). The loop of the bull-pole is placed over the head, then the handle is twisted to take up the slack. A shield or herding board may be used to approach a pinniped or direct its movements (Fig. 25.25). Small to large seals and sea lions may also be captured in nets for examination or intramuscular injection (Fig. 25.26 to 25.28).

A special heavy mesh net on a 2.5-cm (1-in.) pipe hoop is effective for handling small pinnipeds (Fig. 25.29). I have netted adult female California sea lions as they rushed from their night quarters when the door was opened.

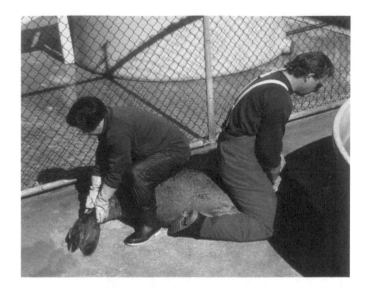

FIG. 25.19. Two people astraddle a pinniped.

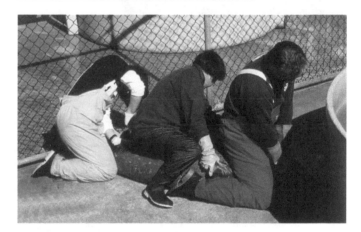

FIG. 25.20. Three people may be required to hold a medium-sized pinniped.

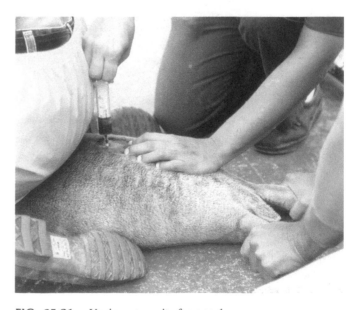

FIG. 25.21. Venipuncture site for a seal.

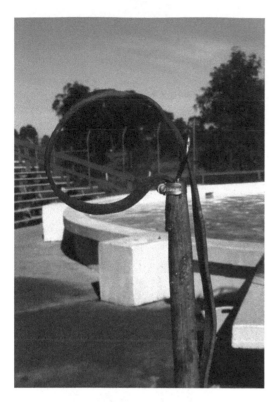

FIG. 25.22. Close-up of a pinniped neck strap.

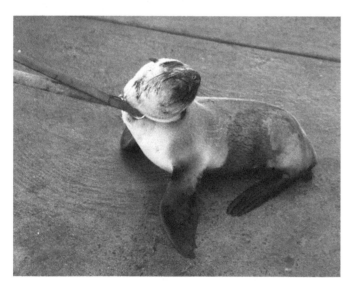

FIG. 25.23. Restraining a sea lion with a neck strap.

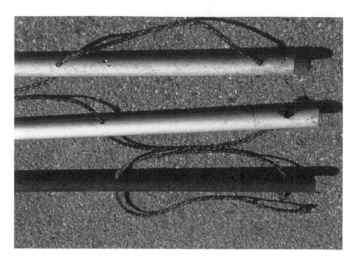

FIG. 25.24. Close-up of a bull-pole used to handle small to large pinnipeds.

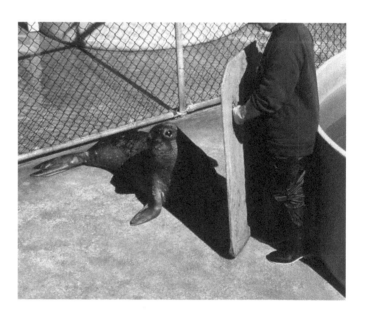

FIG. 25.25. A shield may be used to closely approach a juvenile pinniped.

Walruses may appear to be slow and lumbering, but they are agile in water. Restraint should be attempted only in a dry area or at the bottom of a drained pool. Small- to medium-sized walruses may be netted, keeping in mind the need to stay away from the head. Adults may be herded onto a cargo net that has been spread out on the floor then lifted with a crane to expose the ventral aspect of the flippers, a site for venipuncture.

Special squeeze cages have been designed for handling pinnipeds (Figs. 25.30, 25.31, 25.32). The cage may be lowered into a pool and baited with fish to entice the animal inside. The cage is then lifted to the pool edge, and the squeeze is applied. The animal may be strapped to the board on the floor of the cage and removed.

Usually a pinniped under 100 kg may be physically restrained for blood collection, either by controlling the head with a bull-pole or snare, or by placing them in a squeeze cage. The selection of a site for venipuncture depends on the experience of the handler and the size and species of pinniped.

Blood vessels are deep to preclude excessive cooling in the oceanic environment. Three locations permit access to veins. In sea lions the caudal gluteal vein is penetrated on either side of the coccygeal vertebrae through the notch formed where

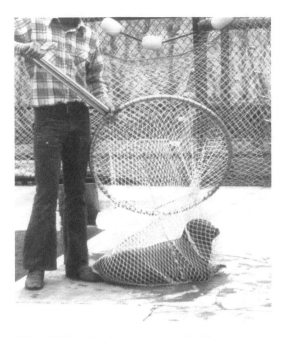

FIG. 25.26. Netting a harbor seal. (Photo courtesy of J. Sweeny.)

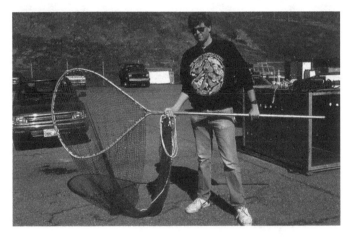

FIG. 25.27. Open-ended net, used to capture and contain pinnipeds.

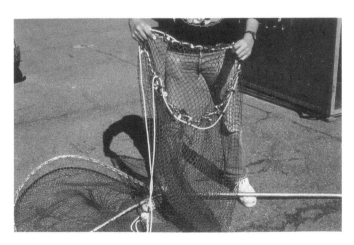

FIG. 25.28. The end may be opened to release the animal once in a cage.

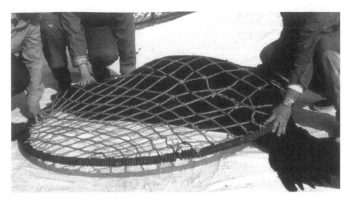

FIG. 25.29. Special hoop net used to restrict movement of a small sea lion.

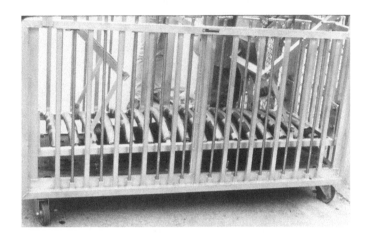

FIG. 25.30. Commercial pinniped squeeze cage. (Photo courtesy of Research Equipment Co., Bryan, Texas.)

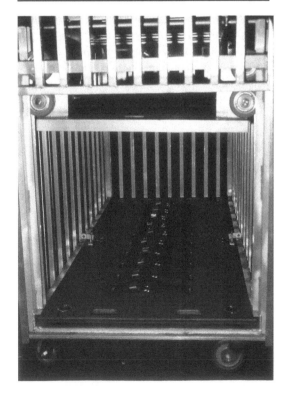

FIG. 25.31. Interior of a commercial pinniped squeeze cage.

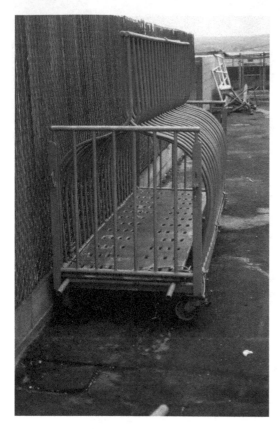

FIG. 25.32. Another commercial sea lion squeeze cage. (Photo courtesy of J. Sweeny.)

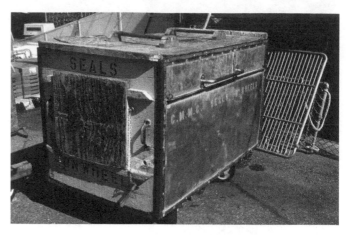

FIG. 25.33. Nebulization or misting chamber for treating respiratory disorders in pinnipeds, closed.

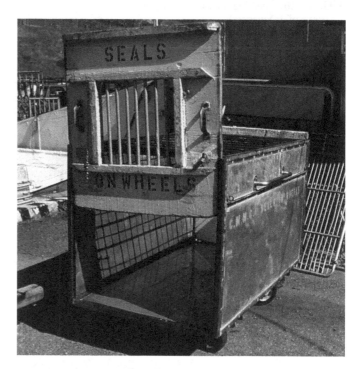

FIG. 25.34. Nebulization or misting chamber for treating respiratory disorders in pinnipeds, open.

the ileum and sacrum unite. Blood specimens may be obtained from a venous sinus formed by the confluence of the internal and external jugular veins and the internal thoracic vein.[9] Sedate the sea lion and place it in dorsal recumbency. Extend the head. Establish a line from the manubrium of the sternum (forward end) to the point of the shoulder. Insert an 18- to 20-gauge 3.5- to 5-cm (1.5- to 2-in.) needle at a site 1.9-cm (0.75-in.) lateral to the sternum on the previously described line. Insert the needle downward in front of the first rib. Maintain a negative pressure on the syringe while inserting the needle.

The intravertebral vein is frequently used for venipuncture in phocids (seals) and otobenids (walrus). Insert the needle on the dorsal midline between the dorsal spines of the lumbar vertebrae from L4 to L7. Needle sizes are as follows: <10 kg, 20 gauge, 2.5 cm; 10–50 kg, 20 gauge, 4 cm; 50–200 kg, 18 gauge, 9.0 cm. Blood may also be obtained from the interdigital veins on the hind flipper. Some clinicians prefer to collect blood from the jugular vein, particularly when a large volume of blood is required. In sea lions less than 45 kg, use a 20-gauge 2.2-cm (1-in.) needle. Occlude the vein distally in the jugular furrow area near the midline and in the upper third of the neck. Sea lions over 180 kg (400 lb) usually require sedation and a 3.8-cm (1.5-in.) needle.

Young sea lions, susceptible to verminous pneumonia, may be nebulized in a combination therapy-transport cart (Figs. 25.33, 25.34). See Table 25.4 for selected chemical restraint agents for immobilization of pinnipeds.

TABLE 25.4. Selected chemical restraint agents for immobilization of pinnipeds, general[9,18,21]

Agent	Dose (mg/kg), IM
Isoflurane	5% induction, 2.5% maintenance With a face mask
Tiletamine/zolazepam	1.0–1.7*
Ketamine/medetomidine	2.5/0.14
Ketamine/diazepam	3.0/0.2
Ketamine/midazolam	1.0/0.1
Ketamine/xylazine	5.6–7.8/0.5–1.3
Midazolam/merperidine	0.1/2.2
Carfentanil	0.003–0.0054
Carfentanil/xylazine	0.006–0.018/0.5–1.3

*Be prepared to deal with apnea.

TRANSPORT[1,19,33]

The transportation of marine mammals has become an art during recent years because of the popularity of commercial oceanaria.[1] Marine mammals are difficult to obtain and expensive to purchase and maintain. Although general principles are outlined here, no one should attempt to transport one of these valuable animals without qualified assistance and appropriate equipment.

Dolphins and whales may be lifted from the water and transported in special stretchers (Fig. 25.35). Stretchers for cetaceans must be constructed with attention to detail. The stretchers should be long enough to support the flukes or such that the flukes just clear the end of the stretcher.[13] If the tarp is short and the animal small, fold the flippers back alongside the body. Protect the eyes from exposure to straps, buckles, netting, or anything else that might injure them.

For long-distance transport, a cetacean should be floated on foam rubber cushions whenever possible. Thick layers of foam should be placed on the stretcher before placement of the animal. The stretcher should be anchored to the walls of a cradle, and the cradle should be filled with water. The foam acts like a sponge to keep the appendages moist and cool. If ice is to be added, towels should separate the skin from direct contact with ice. A special Santini box with a double-padded floor has been successfully used for shipping dolphins.[1]

Marine mammals are high-profile species in the eyes of the public and regulatory officials. The Marine Mammal Protection Act requires safe, humane care. The equipment and facilities for transport of the larger cetaceans are highly sophisticated and expensive. These animals should not be moved without the benefit of the expertise of those trained to move these animals, using state-of-the-art stretchers and cradles. Joseph and others provide details for transport of all marine mammals.[19]

Overheating is an ever-present hazard for marine mammals during transport. The skin must be constantly moistened and the body temperature monitored throughout the voyage. Ice may be added to shipping cradles to retard overheating.

Individual variations in animal behavior will greatly affect the success of transport. If the animal continually thrashes about during the journey, abrasions and/or pressure sores are almost sure to occur. The flippers are also susceptible to damage. An improperly designed stretcher or a thrashing animal may traumatize the base of the flipper or impair circulation by continued pressure.

Pinnipeds may be shipped in rather simple crates (Figs. 25.36, 25.37) or large fiberglass shipping crates for dogs. However, they also must be carefully monitored to prevent hyperthermia.

Sirenians are transported by much the same methods as cetaceans.

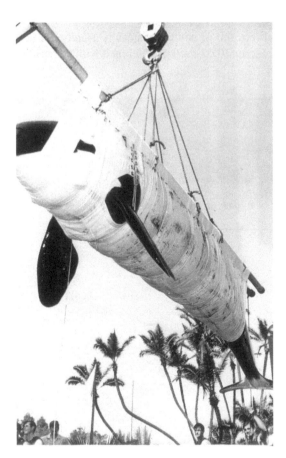

FIG. 25.35. Lifting killer whale in a stretcher. (Photo courtesy of L. Cornell.)

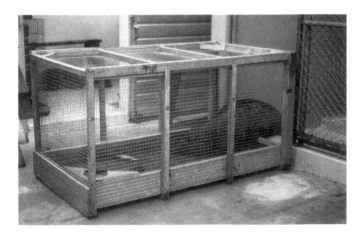

FIG. 25.36. An elephant seal being enticed with fish into a crate.

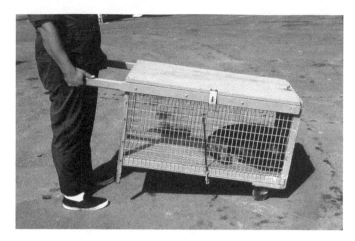

FIG. 25.37. Wheeled crate for moving small pinnipeds within a facility.

CHEMICAL RESTRAINT[7,9,13–16,18,20,21,24]

Chemical restraint of marine mammals should not be attempted without consultation with a veterinarian experienced in marine mammal medicine. The chemical restraint agents and combinations mentioned in this chapter represent those used by experienced veterinarians with detailed knowledge of marine mammals. Other protocols have been used, and no claim is made for including all possible drugs and combinations. For more detailed information, particularly for anesthesia, consult Williams and others[31], Lynch and Brodley,[21] or Chittick and Walsh.[4]

It is difficult to generalize about the application of chemical restraint to marine mammals. Reactions to restraint drugs are extremely variable. Their unique cardiovascular and pulmonary physiology makes it difficult to accurately predict drug effects. Numerous drugs and combinations have been used to sedate, chemically immobilize, and anesthetize marine mammals.[32] Following are some general statements and a few recommendations (Tables 25.1 to 25.4).

Breath holding (apnea) is absolutely necessary when a marine mammal dives and stays under water for several minutes. Bradycardia may accompany the breath holding, particularly in pinnipeds. The significance of this reflex action in restraint and anesthesia is that apnea may occur during restraint procedures. Prolonged procedures should include endotracheal intubation, in the event that positive pressure respiration is necessary.

Cetaceans

Captive cetaceans are usually trained to allow collection of laboratory specimens. More prolonged procedures may require chemical immobilization or a pre-anesthesia sedation prior to inhalation anesthesia. The agents and dosage for chemical restraint of selected cetaceans are listed in Table 25.2.[25]

Endotracheal intubation is accomplished by oral insertion of a hand to dislocate the arytenoidoepiglotal tube (modified larynx) from the nasopharyngeal sphincter of the blowhole. The trachea of cetaceans is large to accommodate inhalation of a large quantity of air quickly. Large endotracheal tubes for horse are employed for larger cetaceans.[25]

Pinnipeds

Most pinnipeds may be trained to allow diagnostic procedures with minimal physical restraint. In untrained animals it may be necessary to use chemical restraint. Many agents have been used (Table 25.4), but diazepam is recommended at 0.1–0.2 mg/kg IM.[12] The preferred intramuscular injection site is in the pelvic region because this area has the least covering of blubber. Use a 4.5-cm (2.0-in.) needle.[12] Small pinnipeds may be anesthetized by pinning the head as described previously and placing a cone over the nose (Fig. 25.38). Either isoflurane or halothane in oxygen at a flow rate of 4–5% is satisfactory, but marine mammals are capable of holding their breath for a number of minutes. Larger animals should be sedated and the facemask applied. As soon as relaxation occurs, the trachea should be intubated to provide respiratory assistance during periods of apnea. The mobility of the larynx may necessitate manual placement (Fig. 25.39). Tracheal bifurcation occurs cranially to the thoracic inlet, so the tube should not be inserted to the point where a single bronchus is intubated. A positive pressure respirator may prevent apnea and allow x-raying of the expanded thorax (Figs. 25.40, 25.41).

Chemical restraint of adult manatees is usually not necessary, but diazepam (0.02 mg/kg) combined with meperidine

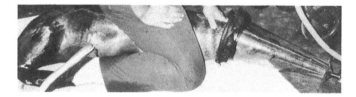

FIG. 25.38. Isoflurane or halothane anesthesia via face mask.

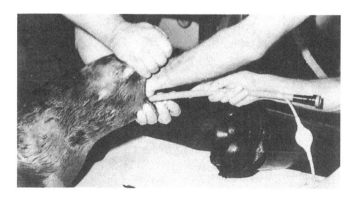

FIG. 25.39. Manual insertion of endotracheal tube after anesthetizing animal with isoflurane or halothane.

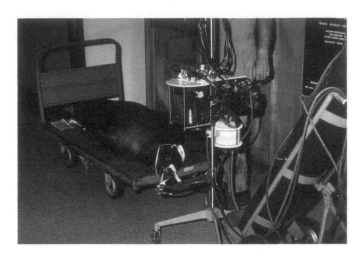

FIG. 25.40. Sea lion anesthetized and using a positive pressure respirator.

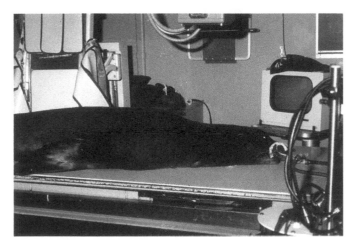

FIG. 25.41. X-raying a sea lion while under anesthesia.

(Demerol) (1.65 mg/kg) IM has provided sufficient sedation for minor surgical procedures, especially with local anesthesia.[30] Dosages of restraint agents are generally lower than for terrestrial mammals, perhaps because of their lower metabolic rate. Table 25.3 lists agents and dosages that have been used.[22]

REFERENCES

1. Antrim, J., and McBain, J.F. 2001. Marine mammal transport. In: Dierauf, L., and Gulland, F.M.D., Eds. CRC Handbook of Marine Mammal Medicine, 2nd Ed. Boca Raton, Florida, CRC Press, pp. 881–91.
2. Bossart, G.D. 2001. Manatees. In: Dierauf, L., and Gulland, F.M.D., Eds. CRC Handbook of Marine Mammal Medicine, 2nd Ed. Boca Raton, Florida, CRC Press, pp. 939–60.
3. Brunson, D.B. 2007. Aquatic mammals. In: Tranquilli, W.J., Thurman, J.C., and Grimm, K.A., Eds. Lumb and Jones' Veterinary Anesthesia and Analgesia, 4th Ed. Ames, Iowa, Wiley-Blackwell Publishing, pp. 832–40.
4. Chittick, E.J., and Walsh, M.T. 2007. Sirenians (manatee and Dugong). In: West, G., Heard, D., and Caulkett, N., Eds. Zoo Animal and Wildlife Chemical Immobilization and Anesthesia. Ames, Iowa, Blackwell Publishing, pp. 497–506.
5. Dierauf, L.A. 1990. Pinniped husbandry. In: Dierauf, L.A., Ed. CRC Handbook of Marine Mammal Medicine: Health, Disease, and Rehabilitation, Boca Raton, Florida, CRC Press, pp. 563–72.
6. Dold, C., and Ridgway, S. 2007. Cetaceans. In: West, G., Heard, D., and Caulkett, N., Eds. Zoo Animal and Wildlife Chemical Immobilization and Anesthesia. Ames, Iowa, Blackwell Publishing, pp. 485–96.
7. Duerr, R. 2002. Harbor seals and northern elephant seals. In: Gage, L.J., Ed. Handrearing wild and domestic animals. Ames, Iowa State University Press. pp. 132–42.
8. Gage, L.J. 1990. Rescue and rehabilitation of cetaceans. In: Dierauf, L.A., Ed. CRC Handbook of Marine Mammal Medicine. Boca, Raton, Florida, CRC Press, pp. 685–92.
9. Gage, L.J. 1993. Pinniped anesthesia. In: Fowler, M.E., Ed. Zoo and Wild Animal Medicine, 3rd ed., Philadelphia: W.B. Saunders. pp. 412–13.
10. Gage, L.J. 2002. Handrearing sea lions and fur seals. In: Gage, L.J., Ed. Handrearing wild and domestic animals. Ames, Iowa State University Press. pp. 143.
11. Gage, L.J., and Samansky, T.S. 2002. Handrearing walruses. In: Gage, L.J., Ed. Handrearing wild and domestic animals. Ames, Iowa State University Press. pp. 150–57.
12. Gage, L.J. 2003. Pinnipedia (seals, sea lions, walrus). In: Fowler, M.E., and Miller, R.E., Eds. Zoo and Wild Animal Medicine, 5th Ed., St. Louis, MO, Saunders/Elsevier, pp. 459–63.
13. Gales, N.J., and Burton, H.R. 1987. Prolonged and multiple immobilizations of the southern elephant seal using ketamine hydrochloride-xylazine hydrochloride or ketamine hydrochloride-diazepam combinations. J Wildl Dis 23:614–18.
14. Geraci, J.R. 1973. An appraisal of ketamine as an immobilizing agent in wild and captive pinnipeds. J Am Vet Med Assoc 163:574–77.
15. Geraci, J.R., Skirnisson, K., and St. Aubin, D.J. 1981. A safe method for repeatedly immobilizing seals. J Am Vet Med Assoc 179:1192–93.
16. Gulland, F.M.D. 2001. Seals and Sea lions. In: Dierauf, L., and Gulland, F.M.D., Eds. CRC Handbook of Marine Mammal Medicine, 2nd Ed. Boca Raton, Florida, CRC Press, pp. 907–26.
17. Haulena, M., and Heath, R.B. 2001. Marine mammal anesthesia. In: Dierauf, L., and Gulland, F.M.D., Eds. CRC Handbook of Marine Mammal Medicine, 2nd Ed. Boca Raton, Florida, CRC Press, pp. 655–88.
18. Haulena, M. 2007. Otariid seals. In: West, G., Heard, D., and Caulkett, N., Eds. Zoo Animal and Wildlife Chemical Immobilization and Anesthesia. Ames, Iowa, Blackwell Publishing, pp. 469–78.
19. Joseph, B.E., Asper, E.D., Antrim, J., and Pearson, J.C. 1990. Marine mammal transport. In: Dierauf, L.A., Ed. CRC Handbook of Marine Mammal Medicine: Health, Disease, and Rehabilitation. Boca Raton, Florida, CRC Press, pp. 543–52.
20. Loughlin, T.R., and Spraker, T. 1989. Use of telazol to immobilize female northern sea lions in Alaska. J Wildl Dis 25:353–58.
21. Lynch, M., and Bodley, K. 2007. Pocid seals. In: West, G., Heard, D., and Caulkett, N., Eds. Zoo Animal and Wildlife Chemical Immobilization and Anesthesia. Ames, Iowa, Blackwell Publishing, pp. 459–68.
22. Murphy, D. 2003. Sirenia. In: Fowler, M.E., and Miller, R.E., Eds. Zoo and Wild Animal Medicine, 5th Ed., St Louis, MO, Elsevier, pp. 476–82.

23. Needham, D.J. 1993. Cetacean stranding. In: Fowler, M.E., Ed. Zoo and Wild Animal Medicine, 3rd ed., Philadelphia: W.B. Saunders. pp. 415–25.

24. Paras, A. 2008. Capture and anesthesia of otariids in the wild. In: Fowler, M.E., and Miller, R.E., Eds. Zoo and Wild Animal Medicine, 6th Ed. St Louis, Saunders/Elsevier, pp. 312–18.

25. Reidarson, T.H. 2003. Cetacea (Whales, dolphins, porpoises). In: Fowler, M.E., and Miller, R.E., Eds. Zoo and Wild Animal Medicine, 5th Ed., St Louis, MO, Elsevier, pp. 442–59.

26. Ridgeway, S.H. 1972. Homeostasis in the aquatic environment. In: Ridgeway, S.H., Ed. Mammals of the Sea, Springfield, Illinois, Charles C. Thomas, pp. 689–94.

27. Sweeney, J.C. 1993. Blood sampling and other collection techniques in marine mammals. In: Fowler, M.E., Ed. Zoo and Wild Animal Medicine, 3rd ed., Philadelphia, W.B. Saunders, pp. 425–28.

28. Walsh, M.T., Asper, E.D., Andrews, B., and Antrim, J. 1990. Walrus biology and medicine. In: Dierauf, L.A., Ed. CRC Handbook of Marine Mammal Medicine: Health, Disease, and Rehabilitation. Boca Raton, Florida, CRC Press, pp. 593–94.

29. Walsh, M.T., Reidarson, T., McBain, J., Dalton, L., Gearhart, S., Chittick, E., Shmitt, T., and Dold, C. 2006. Sedation and anesthesia techniques in cetaceans. 2006 Proceedings Am Assoc Zoo Vets. pp. 237–39.

30. White, J.R., and Francis-Floyd, R. 1990. Manatee biology and medicine. In: Dierauf, L.A., Ed. CRC Handbook of Marine Mammal Medicine: Health, Disease, and Rehabilitation. Boca Raton, Florida, CRC Press, pp. 603–09.

31. Williams, T.D., Williams, A.L., and Stoskopf, M.K. 1990. Marine mammal anesthesia. In: Dierauf, L.A., Ed. CRC Handbook of Marine Mammal Medicine: Health, Disease, and Rehabilitation. Boca Raton, Florida, CRC Press, pp. 175–92.

32. Williams, T.D. 1993. Rehabilitation of sea otters. In: Fowler, M.E., ed. Zoo and Wild Animal Medicine, 3rd ed. Philadelphia, W.B. Saunders, pp. 432–35.

33. Young, N.M., and Shapiro, S.L. 2001. U.S. Federal Legislation governing marine mammals. In: Dierauf, L., and Gulland, F.M.D. Eds. CRC Handbook of Marine Mammal Medicine, 2nd Ed. Boca Raton, Florida, CRC Press, pp. 741–66.

CHAPTER 26
Elephants

CLASSIFICATION

Order Proboscidea
Family Elephantidae: Asian elephant, African elephant

The elephant has captured attention since prehistoric eras. The caveman drew pictures of extinct elephant relatives on the walls of his home, and undoubtedly used the flesh of the animals for food.

The Asian elephant (Fig. 26.1, left) is one of the oldest animals in domesticity. Both Asian and African species have carried human beings and moved their heavy loads for hundreds of years. The African elephant (Fig. 26.1, right) is much less tractable than the Asian and thus has not been as extensively used as a beast of burden.

A mature male elephant is called a bull, the female a cow. Newborn and young are called calves.

UNIQUE ANATOMY AND PHYSIOLOGY

Table 26.1 lists some approximate sizes of elephants.

The respiratory apparatus of the elephant is unique. In most mammals the lungs are situated within the chest cavity in a vacuum, as illustrated on the right side of Figure 26.2. Air is pressed out of the lungs by respiratory muscles, and negative pressure in the chest refills the lungs with air.

In elephants, the lung is adhered to the chest wall by fibrous tissue and there is no pleural space to establish a vacuum (Fig. 26.3). Respiration depends on the free lateral movement of the chest wall and contraction of the diaphragm in a bellows-like action. This fact must be taken into consideration when the elephant is cast or put into positions that may inhibit respiration. When an elephant is viewed in profile, the lowest point on the body is the abdomen. If the elephant lies down in sternal recumbency, pressure is exerted dorsally, compressing the abdominal viscera (Fig. 26.4). This places extra pressure on the diaphragm, possibly preventing its full excursion to help draw air into the lungs. If the elephant is conscious, it can compensate and maintain respiratory exchange. If the elephant has been chemically immobilized, it may be incapable of compensating, and hypoxemia may result.

Some scientists working with elephants feel that having the animal in lateral recumbency is also hazardous because

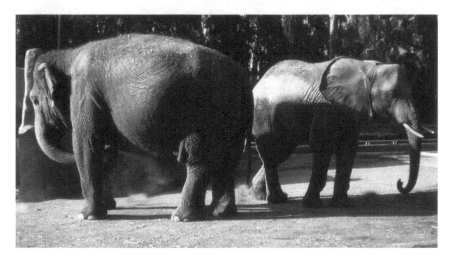

FIG. 26.1. Elephants: Asian female, left. African female, right.

TABLE 26.1. Elephant size

| | Approximate Weight | | | | | | | |
| | Newborn | | Adult female | | Adult male | | Height | |
Animal	(lb)	(kg)	(lb)	(kg)	(lb)	(kg)	(ft)	(m)
Asian elephant	198	90	7,920	3,600	9,900	4,500	8.2–10	2.5–3.0
African elephant	220	100	11,000	5,000	13,200	6,000	9.8–13	3.0–4.0

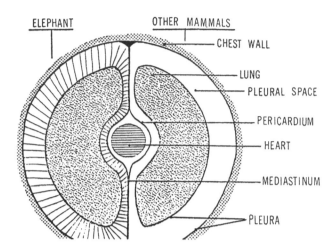

FIG. 26.2. Diagram of the pleural cavity of elephants.

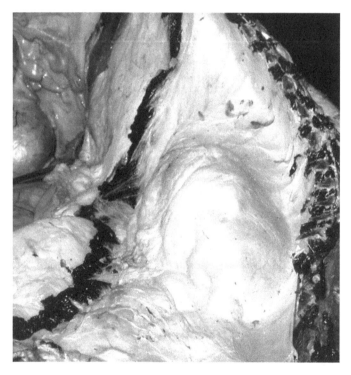

FIG. 26.3. Pleural adhesions in an elephant.

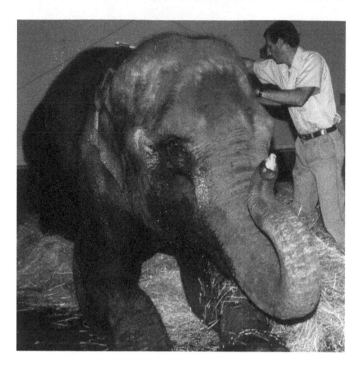

FIG. 26.4. An elephant should not be allowed to remain in sternal recumbency for extended periods; respiration may be compromised and elbows and knees suffer excessive straining and contusion.

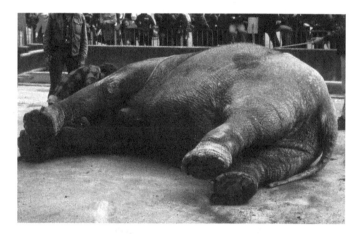

FIG. 26.5. Elephant may remain in lateral recumbency under chemical immobilization and anesthesia for up to 5 hours and maintain normal respiratory function.

the weight of the body may prevent full excursion of the chest wall (Fig. 26.5). However, I have maintained elephants in lateral recumbency for as long as 5 hours during surgical procedures without seeing a change in the arterial oxygen saturation.

If prolonged surgery is anticipated, the site where the elephant is to lie should be well padded. A heavily constructed waterbed mattress was used successfully in repeated surgeries of a large Asian cow (Fig. 26.6).

The elephant trunk is a vital organ (Fig. 26.7). An injured or paralyzed trunk is a serious problem; if it cannot be corrected, the elephant may starve. The tip of the trunk is an extremely delicate prehensile organ. A tiny peanut may be grasped with ease. The trunk also places food into the mouth. Water is drawn up into the tip of the trunk and blown into the mouth. The trunk is involved in almost every activity of the elephant.

Seventy percent of the airflow into the lungs is via the nares in the trunk. At the approximate location where the nares enter the bony skull, there is a sigmoid flexure and a sphincter arrangement that allows the elephant to pull water and dirt up into the nares but prevents inhalation into the lungs. The trunk hangs limp at birth, and the calf nurses with

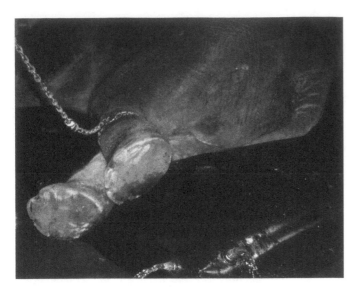

FIG. 26.6. Extended recumbency is better carried out with adequate padding, such as a specially constructed waterbed mattress.

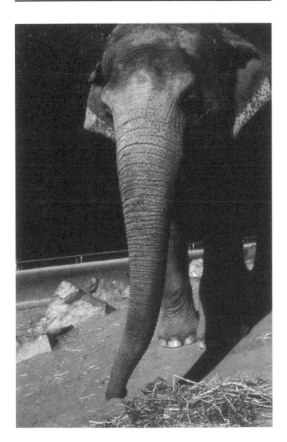

FIG. 26.7. Elephant trunk.

its mouth as other mammals do. Within a few weeks the calf begins to develop dexterity with the trunk.

The tusks of the elephant are modified incisor teeth, not canines. Ivory is a unique form of dentine. When casting or restraining elephants, consider the position of the tusks and what they may strike against or drive through.

Tusks are present in both male and female African elephants, but they grow larger and longer in the male. In the Asian elephant the female may either lack tusks or have small, underdeveloped tusks. The tusks continue to grow throughout life. The tusk is hollow at the base, which is the pulp cavity, containing nerves and blood vessels, and is the growing point. The pulp cavity ends approximately at the point where the tusk passes the trunk. A broken tusk is likely to abscess if the pulp cavity is exposed. Fortunately ivory usually breaks diagonally across the tusk, minimizing the chance of opening the pulp cavity. An elephant suffering from the pain associated with an abscessed tusk is extremely dangerous.

Elephants have highly vascularized ears, which are an organ of heat regulation. An elephant customarily stands flapping its ears on a warm day. During immobilization the elephant is incapable of moving its ears, and hyperthermia may develop with prolonged restraint when the ambient temperature is high.

Elephants are called "pachyderms" because the skin is thick. They share this characteristic with some other large herbivores such as the rhinoceros and hippopotamus. The thickness of the skin is primarily a result of thickened dermis. The epidermal layer is approximately the same thickness as that of horses or cattle and is extremely sensitive. Insects such as flies or mosquitoes annoy elephants and cause them to blow dirt or mud over their backs to protect the delicate epithelial surfaces.

The elephant is subject to scratches or cuts through the epidermis into the dermis. These bleed as readily as those of other mammalian species. The epidermal surface of the elephant is also susceptible to abrasion, so ropes pulled beneath or around the animal in restraint must be moved slowly to prevent burns.

BEHAVIOR

The elephant is intelligent and sensitive. It is highly responsive to a trainer who exercises proper judgment in working with it. One who works around these animals must have confidence and be capable of providing consistent discipline without inflicting prolonged discomfort. Otherwise the elephant will become either belligerent or unreliable, seeking occasions to catch the handler off guard. A belligerent elephant may inflict serious or fatal injury. The elephant is quick to pick up voice tones indicating that a handler is confident or, conversely, is frightened or uncertain.

Particular attention should be paid to the ears and trunk to assess the mood of an elephant. Following are behaviors to be aware of:

Alert: The elephant stands facing a person with the head raised, ears spread, tail elevated, as shown in Figure 26.8.
Kick: An elephant may strike forward with a forelimb or toward the side or rearward with a hind limb.

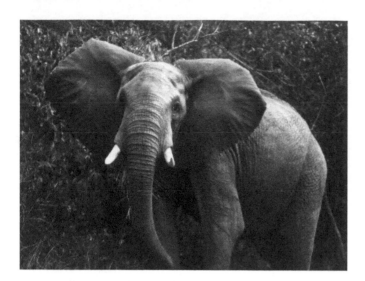

FIG. 26.8. Alert behavior.

Mock charge: The elephant runs toward another elephant or a person with ears extended, head and tusks held high. The tail may or may not be elevated, and the trunk extended. The charging elephant stops before reaching the target and usually trumpets.

Real charge: The trunk is tucked under the head, the head is up and attempts to contact the target. The ears are usually close to the head and usually there is no trumpeting.

Slap: An elephant strikes another elephant or a person with the trunk.

Sniff: The trunk is extended down and forward in a "J" shape, with the tip out horizontally to sniff another elephant, or person, as shown in Figure 26.9.

It is important to be aware of an elephant's mood and take special precautions when it is annoyed or excited. The

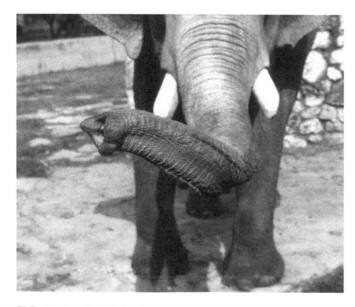

FIG. 26.9. Sniff behavior.

position of the ears is an important indicator of mood. When an elephant is excited, its ears are brought forward and extend out from the head; the trunk is curled upward.

As with most animals, elephants develop likes and dislikes for those who work with them. An elephant's dislike for an individual is difficult to overcome. Usually it is necessary to assign another person to care for that particular animal. Physical examination of an elephant may prove frustrating because elephants are unlikely to stand still. Even though gentle and unconcerned about the manipulations in progress, these animals constantly shift weight from one leg to another. At the same time, the trunk moves about, investigating the examiner's body, extremities, and anything else within reach. They are particularly fond of removing objects from pockets. Trained animals may allow a rectal examination with only a handler controlling the head (Fig. 26.10).

Sexually mature male elephants are unpredictable and may be aggressive, particularly when in musth. Musth is a normal physiologic and behavioral phenomenon of male elephants, usually beginning at 10–15 years of age. It is not a rut period, as is typical of cervids. Studies have shown that serum

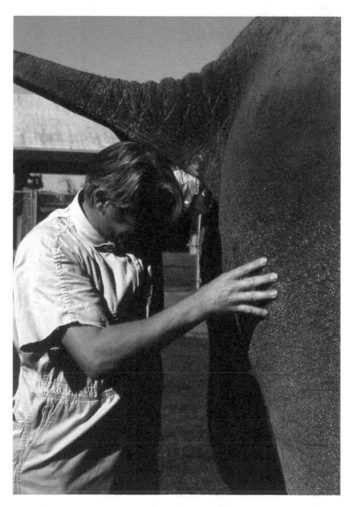

FIG. 26.10. Rectal examination of a trained elephant.

testosterone levels are elevated during musth, and the secretion from the temporal gland also contains testosterone, but successful breeding may take place outside the musth period. In fact, bulls in musth may be aggressive to cows as well as to personnel who are handling the elephant.

Musth is characterized by aggressive behavior, drainage of fluid from the temporal glands, dribbling of urine from the prepuce, anorexia, dehydration, somnolence, and unusual vocalization. Musth usually lasts 6–12 weeks, but instances of it lasting up to a year have been recorded.[57] Bulls in musth may be extremely dangerous and several handlers have been killed. Institutions that maintain adult bulls must have an elephant restraint device to allow handling of the bull without direct contact by the keepers.

Training

Modern elephant management programs emphasize training based on positive reinforcement that makes the elephant a willing participant in the handling procedures.

Training an elephant is challenging, as it relies completely on effective communication between the elephant and the trainer, using the language of actions and consequences. It is highly recommended that one handler only be given the responsibility of training a new behavior. Using more than one handler to train may introduce inconsistencies in the training process, which may cause confusion and anxiety on the part of the elephant. Each elephant facility should have a written elephant training protocol under the direct supervision of the elephant manager.

DANGER POTENTIAL

When watching elephants lumber around in a zoo, one may receive the impression that an elephant is slow, but such is not the case. Elephants are able to move swiftly.

Elephants use several methods for offense and defense including biting, slapping with the trunk, grasping with the trunk and pulling, pushing, or throwing. Elephants may purposely step on a person's foot, and they are adept at kicking and can easily balance on one front and one hind leg.[34] Extreme aggression may be exhibited by the elephant kneeling and head-pressing upon what they perceive as a threat, inconvenience, or a toy. Even an elephant in an elephant restraint device (ERD) or on tethers may injure a person unfamiliar with an elephant's reach or its signals of aggressive intent.

In addition to direct contact, the trunk may be used to throw objects such as feces, straw, dirt, pieces of wood, rocks, or other missiles at a handler. Also the elephant may draw water up into the trunk and spray it at any individual to whom it takes a dislike.

Some elephants may acquire the bad habit of slapping people with the trunk. They become very clever and bait an individual into moving closer by extending the trunk for petting. A certain curve is left in the trunk; when the person moves closer, the trunk is flipped out. The force may fracture facial bones or ribs or knock a person over.

The tusks are an obvious hazard. Elephants have gored unwary victims and have also been known to crush people against walls with the tusks. The vast bulk of the elephant may also injure by pressing people against solid objects.

Those who work around elephants should be extremely careful; the elephant continually moves from one foot to another, and if due caution is not exercised, a person may be stepped on—either by accident or on purpose.

Some elephants are adept at kicking with the hind legs. The kick is usually directed backward. The speed with which a kick is administered will astound persons who believe that the elephant is slow moving.

While the swinging tail is usually not considered an offensive weapon, it must be considered when administering medication in the rear quarters or when tethering a hind leg. Being soundly struck hurts, and a blow to the face or head could be injurious (Fig. 26.11).

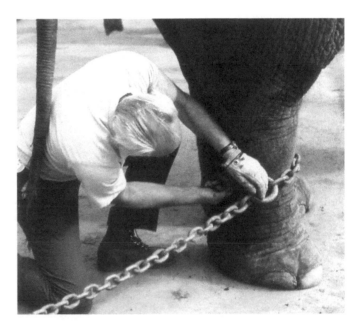

FIG. 26.11. A flailing tail may inflict injury.

It is unwise for anyone to work on an elephant alone. Some elephants become adept at maneuvering a person into a position where he or she cannot get free. The regular attendant should be present to control the head and command the elephant to move into positions suitable for examination and/or treatment. Even the presence of the keeper is sometimes insufficient to control an animal that is really annoyed or intent on injuring a person. The handler must be constantly aware of the position and activity of the elephant and must always have a planned escape route.

PHYSICAL RESTRAINT[19,20]

Elephants should be taught to respond to voice (Fig. 26.12), visual, and pressure commands and cues. Minimal

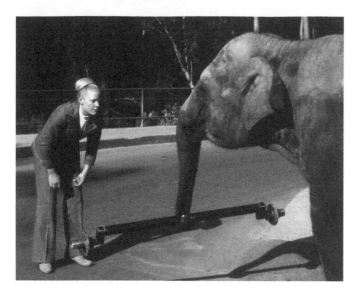

FIG. 26.12. Elephant responding to visual and verbal commands.

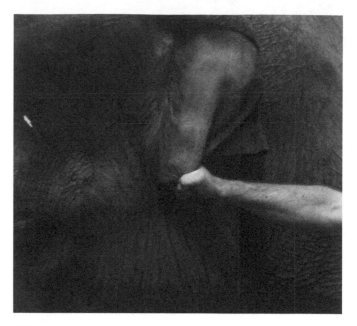

FIG. 26.14. Grasping the ear of a mature elephant.

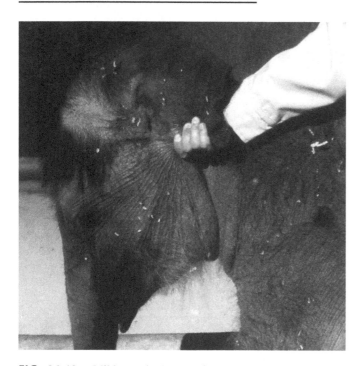

FIG. 26.13. Mild restraint by grasping an ear.

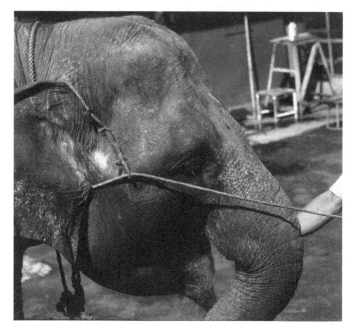

FIG. 26.15. Leading a young elephant with a loop of rope around the ear.

restraint may be applied to a calf or juvenile by grasping the ear (Fig. 26.13 to 26.15). An elephant may be trained to place a foot on a spindle or tub (Fig. 26.16), and to lift and hold a foot (Fig. 26.17). It is obvious that a handler cannot keep an elephant's leg in the air without its consent. It is important that no painful procedures be carried out when the elephant is in this position, since it would then step down quickly, possibly injuring the attendant. In addition, it is highly unlikely that anyone would be able to induce that elephant to lift the foot again, for fear that additional pain might be inflicted.

An elephant may be trained to open the mouth (Fig. 26.18) or lie down (Fig. 26.19).

The guide (inappropriately called a bull hook or ankus) is an indispensable tool for working with elephants (Figs. 26.20, 26.21). The tip of the guide is made of a metal rod (preferably stainless steel) or cut from a metal sheet approximately 1 cm (3/8 in) thick. The straight prong has a side arm that makes it possible to either give a push or pull cue. The prongs are tapered to a narrow point, but should not be so sharp as to easily penetrate or lacerate the skin. The metal tip is attached to a wooden, fiberglass, nylon, or metal handle 30–90 cm (12–36 in.) long.

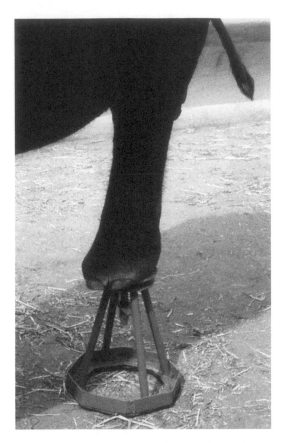

FIG. 26.16.   An elephant trained to place a foot on a spindle.

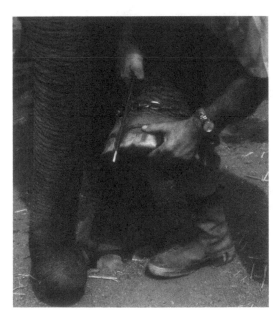

FIG. 26.17.   An elephant trained to lift and hold a foot on a knee for rasping toenails.

The primary purpose of the guide is to exert pressure to sensitive spots on the body, inducing the elephant to move away from the source of the pressure. Thus by pushing or pulling at various sites on the body, such as behind the ear or

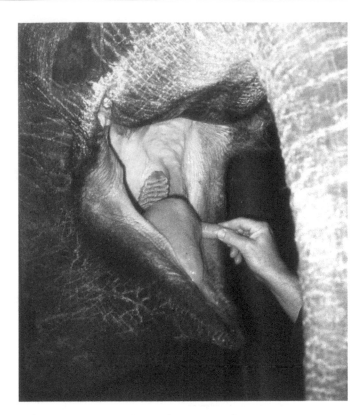

FIG. 26.18.   An elephant trained to open its mouth for inspection.

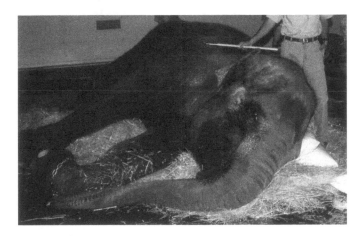

FIG. 26.19.   An elephant trained to lie down on cue.

behind the front leg, one encourages the animal to move in a specific direction. Immature elephants may be handled entirely by use of a guide if properly trained.

The guide may be used to encourage an elephant to move a rear limb (Fig. 26.22) or a forelimb (Fig. 26.23).

Elaborate maps of sensitive sites have been worked out by those who use the elephant daily as a beast of burden. A modified location map is illustrated in Figure 26.24. The handler of an individual elephant soon discovers where the animal can be touched to elicit the most satisfactory responses.

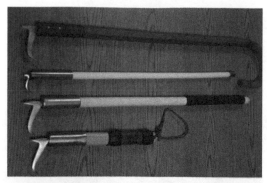

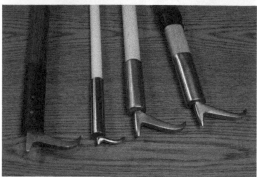

FIG. 26.20.   Elephant guides.

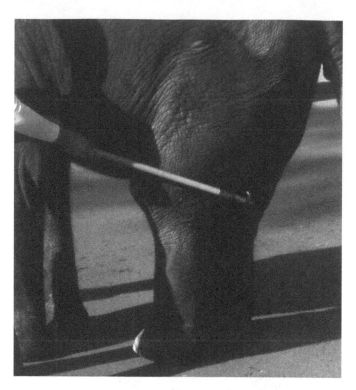

FIG. 26.22.   Moving a hind limb by cueing with a guide.

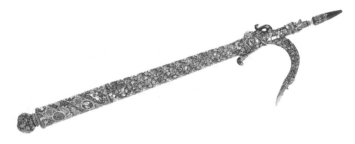

FIG. 26.21.   A jeweled elephant guide used on royal elephants in India.

The guide handle should not be used indiscriminately as a club; an elephant resents harsh discipline. Not only is it inhumane, but it is not effective.

The guide may be used on mature adult elephants, but if the elephant chooses not to obey, there is little the handler can do. Uncooperative elephants must be chained or shackled to be examined or treated.

Tethering

A tether is a tool used to confine an elephant, serving the same purpose as for a horse in a box stall, a pet dog or cat confined to a cage or room of a home, or a dog tethered to a doghouse. Tethering keeps the elephant from wandering, provides security for other animals and people, and provides order and routine for elephants. It provides a special space for the elephant and enables conducting routine procedures such as toenail trimming, administration of medication, and cleaning the area.

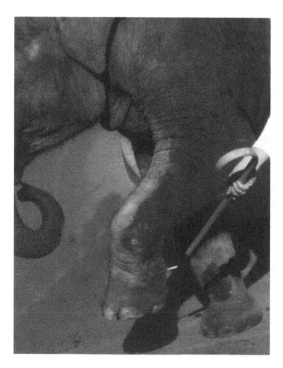

FIG. 26.23.   Lifting a forelimb by cueing with a guide.

Elephants have become a cause célèbre for animal activists who feel that elephants are being mistreated in captivity. Great exception is taken to tethering as a means of confinement and management of elephants. Sufficient pressures have

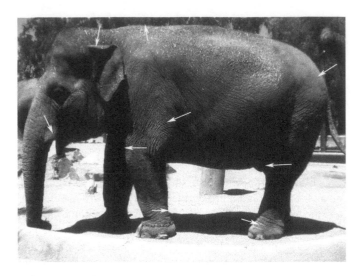

FIG. 26.24. Pressure sensitive sites on an elephant.

been exerted on legislators in some states to result in the enactment of laws to define just how an elephant may be handled. Bowing to public pressures, the American Zoo and Aquarium Association (AZA) has established an elephant management policy encouraging zoos that maintain elephants to have a restricted hands-off protocol for handling their animals. A chain is often used for a tether instead of rope or cable because a chain is less easily tangled, is stronger and thus better for use with elephants, doesn't collect moisture (urine) as a rope or even a cable would do, and is more flexible. The desirable diameter of the metal rod used to construct a chain for elephant confinement is 5/16 to 1/2 inch. The chain links are welded. Chain size is important; 7.9 mm (5/16 in.) or larger should be used on adult elephants (Table 26.2).

TABLE 26.2. Chain size and strength

| Diameter of Rod | | Length of Link | | Working Load* | | | |
| | | | | Proof coil | | High test | |
(mm)	(in.)	(mm)	(in.)	(kg)	(lb)	(kg)	(lb)
4.8	3/16	31.7	1.25	341	750	. . .	. .
6.4	1/4	38.1	1.5	568	1,250	1,136	2,500
7.9	5/16	44.4	1.75	852	1,875	1,818	4,000
9.4	3/8	50.8	2.0	1,193	2,625	2,318	5,100

*Working load is approximately one-half the breaking strength.

Chains used to restrict movement in a male in musth should be heavier. Chains are only as strong as their weakest link, which are usually the swivels, snap hooks, Brummel hooks, and slot links, so the connections should be checked daily (Table 26.3).

Routine tethering consists of one front leg and the opposite hind leg tethered. Front leg tethers are attached to the lower leg between the foot and the carpus (wrist). Frequently an anklet or bracelet is placed on the leg and the tether is attached to the anklet (Figs. 26.25, 26.26). The different shape of the hind foot allows a tether to slip off the foot; therefore,

TABLE 26.3. Brummel hook specifications

| Size and Material | Bail Diameter | | Length of Hook | | Safe Load | |
	(mm)	(in.)	(mm)	(in.)	(kg)	(lb)
Aluminum alloy (00)	10	0.42	37.44	1.56	227	500
Manganese, bronze (0)	10	0.42	37.44	1.56	454	1,000
Manganese, bronze (1)	13	0.56	48.72	2.03	909	2,000
Manganese, bronze (2)	15	0.69	63.12	2.63	1,818	4,000

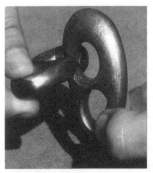
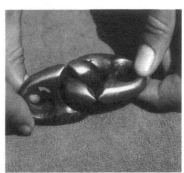
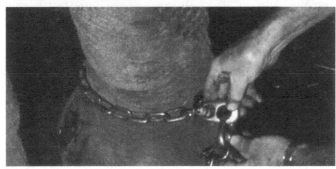

FIG. 26.25. Using Brummel hooks to attach a tether to the leg.

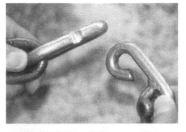
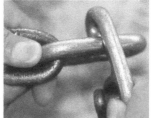
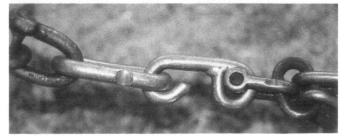

FIG. 26.26. An alternate hook to attach a tether to a leg.

the hind leg tether is attached above the hock (tarsus) and around the tibia. Alternate legs should be tethered routinely.

Tethers should be long enough to allow the elephant to lie down and rise to its feet easily, but not so long as to allow the elephant to turn around and become entangled. Swivels should be used minimally on front leg tethers to prevent the tether from binding as the elephant moves. Bolt cutters should be readily available to free the elephant quickly in case of an emergency.

All captive elephants should be trained to accept tethers on all four legs, whether or not the animal is routinely tethered. The chaining procedure should begin in infancy so that the elephant becomes accustomed to standing quietly when chained. It is imperative that an adult elephant be fully accustomed to the use of chains so that, if manipulative procedures must be carried out to administer medication or treatment, the animal can be adequately controlled by leg chains.

Numerous methods are used for attaching chains to the leg. Chains on the hind legs must be placed above the hock, lest they slip off. The bell shape of the front feet permits chaining just above the foot. Some handlers attach a short length of chain around the leg as a permanent bracelet or anklet. A clevis is used to attach the bracelet to the tethering chain. Another method is to wrap the end of the chain around the leg and clevis it to an appropriate link.

A rope loop is sometimes used for temporary restraint while the chain is being attached. Dangerous animals should be chained from behind a fence separating the handler and the animal. The fastest method of attaching the chain to the elephant's foot is with the use of Brummel hooks (Fig. 26.25). Brummel hooks may be obtained in various sizes (Table 26.3) and function in pairs. Stainless steel Brummel hooks are stronger and more rigid than those made of bronze and thus are preferable (Table 26.3). Bronze is weaker and softer. Another type of hook is illustrated in Figure 26.26.

When Brummel hooks are used, a permanent anklet is attached to the elephant's lower leg with one Brummel hook as part of the anklet chain. The tethering chain, which is permanently attached to a post or ring, includes a Brummel hook as the end link. When the elephant is brought into position, these two hooks can be joined rapidly since the hooks have no moving parts. The Brummel hooks are secure since it is unlikely that the elephant can shake the chain or manipulate it in such a way that the hooks line up in the proper position for disengagement.

Tethering is neither inherently evil nor necessarily injurious to elephants. To prevent chafing of the skin in the area of the leg encircled, the anklet (bracelet) may be enclosed in a segment of discarded canvas fire hose.

Elephant tethers should not be too long. In one instance an elephant was tethered inside a truck with the tether sufficiently long that the elephant could move partially out the door. An attendant mistakenly left the door ajar. As the elephant tried to exit the door, it fell, fracturing a leg.

Animals unaccustomed to chains may strain or jerk so hard on a leg chain that tendons, ligaments, or joints are injured. Training at an early age will obviate this.

If the skin of an elephant tends to abrade under the chain encircling the leg, the chain may be covered with a length of canvas or rubber hose.

Physical Restraint Behind a Barrier (Protected Contact)[19]

Many North American zoos have begun managing elephants from behind a protective barrier, wherein the elephant and the handler do not occupy the same space and the elephant is free to move away from an activity at any time. Training involves giving rewards for appropriate behavior, which may involve placing a foot through a portal for inspection or nail trimming or presenting some other part of the body (Fig. 26.27). Handling in this method is not entirely risk free, since the trunk may be extended between the bars of a protective barrier. Hands and arms extended through a barrier may be grasped or pressed against the barrier.

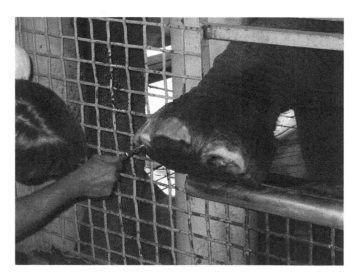

FIG. 26.27. Trimming an elephant foot behind a protective barrier.

Elephants may be trained to target. The handler uses a long pole to touch a place to where the elephant should go or an area of the body that should be presented to the protective barrier for inspection or a procedure. Whistles or clickers may be used as a bridge for reinforcement.

Handling an elephant in a restraint device prevents the elephant from moving away from the activity. There are many varieties of elephant restraint devices (ERD), from simple narrow aisles that limit side-to-side movement to elaborate units with movable walls and gates controlled manually, electrically, or by hydraulics (Figs. 26.28 to 26.31). The pipes and bars, in fact the entire construction, must be designed for the largest elephant that may be anticipated using the ERD. The AZA encourages any zoo that maintains elephants to have an ERD. If mature bulls are to be exhibited, an ERD is a requirement. As of 2006, more than 50 North American zoos have ERDs.

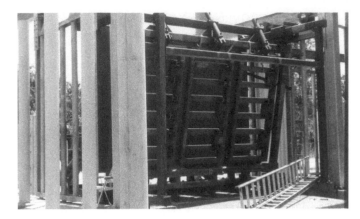

FIG. 26.30. ERD at a Florida zoo.

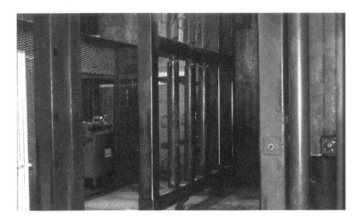

FIG. 26.28. Original elephant restraint device built at the Portland zoo.

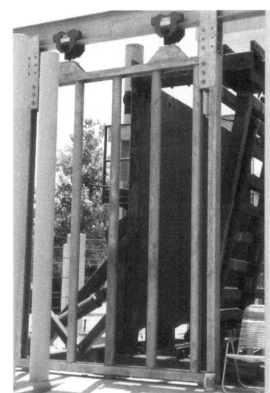

FIG. 26.31. Rear view of an ERD at a Florida zoo.

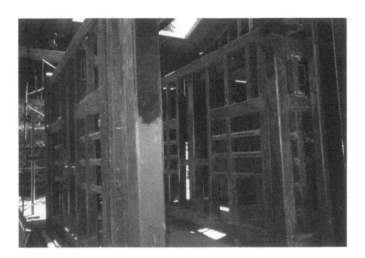

FIG. 26.29. Another view of the original ERD.

and heavy horizontal logs all lashed together and the whole anchored to a large tree.

Although there are many variations and designs of ERDs, all should have the following certain basic elements:

Some ERDs are capable of restricting lateral movement only; others are designed to tilt the elephant onto its side. It is important that the elephant is properly trained to enter the ERD and that the experience is positive or it may refuse to re-enter the device. The concept of an ERD has been utilized in Asia for more than one thousand years, and is still being used today. Instead of metal pipe, the Asian chute is constructed of upright poles buried in the ground like a fence post

1. They should allow access to all four feet and legs, tusks, trunk, face, ears, both sides, hind quarters, and back.
2. The ERD must be easily and quickly opened to free an elephant that has collapsed or has tried to lie down.

3. The ERD should be able to comfortably contain an elephant for an extended time for prolonged medical or husbandry procedures.
4. It should be able to safely accommodate the largest or smallest elephant in the facility.

Additionally the ERD should be placed in an aisle so all elephants must pass through the ERD as a part of the daily routine. It is important that an elephant is not confined in an ERD to undergo only unpleasant experiences. The ERD should be located in an area of the holding facility where it can be used any day and in any kind of weather. While an elephant is confined in the ERD, a bypass to yards and enclosures is needed for other elephants.

Accustoming elephants to accept an ERD requires considerable training. The trainer/handlers must know each individual elephant and the operation of the ERD. The ERD is a tool used to complement a sound elephant management program, and should never be used as substitute by a poor management program or poorly trained staff.[25]

No Contact

Not making contact with elephants is not an acceptable management strategy. Untrained elephants may resist any type of handling and must be sedated or anesthetized to conduct even the smallest non-painful procedure. See Chapter 20, Chemical Restraint.

An elephant's feet frequently require manicuring and/or examination to remove foreign objects, to check for excessive wear of the footpads, or to trim nails or hangnails. A wise keeper or handler will work continually with the elephant so it becomes accustomed to lifting the feet. If toenails are rasped frequently there is no need to cut them too short; thus the best interests of both animal and handler are served.

Designers of facilities for elephants should remember that the trunk has extensive reach. All electrical fixtures, water pipes, and other loose objects must be kept well beyond trunk distance. When an elephant must be moved to new quarters or into a hospital area, attendants frequently overlook the fact that, though items are out of reach of other animals, they are within range of the extended trunk. There is not only danger for the attendant when water pipes burst or electrical wires are torn loose, but the elephant may likewise be electrocuted in the process.

The animal's reaching ability creates other hazards, because elephants continually investigate; anything hanging loose or in the pockets of the examiner may be grasped and swallowed. This includes stethoscopes, thermometers, and other diagnostic equipment.

An elephant that was being treated for an abscess grasped the protective plastic sleeve the examiner was wearing. The plastic sleeve was torn off the examiner's arm and swallowed immediately. This represented a serious hazard for the elephant since it could have produced an obstruction within the intestinal tract. Fortunately the plastic was passed in the feces without incident.

On one occasion, I had driven a university hospital vehicle to a nearby zoo. When it came time to leave, the keys to the vehicle could not be found. Five days later the keys appeared in the stool of an elephant that had been examined the day of the loss. Elephants are notorious for snatching purses, glasses, or other objects from patrons of zoos who are unwise enough to allow such items within reach of the highly prehensile trunks.

An elephant in sternal recumbency may be pulled on to its side by placing a rope on the tusk or around the front leg. The rope is then passed up over the head or body and the animal pulled over. A truck or small tractor may be required to pull over a large elephant. The head rope must not pass over the eye or ear. The legs should be positioned before turning to minimize twisting.

COLLECTION OF BLOOD SAMPLES

Venipuncture may be performed on one of the large veins on the caudal aspect of the ear. Either digital pressure (Fig. 26.32) or an inflatable cuff (Fig. 26.33) may be used to raise the vein. Another accessible vein is the medial saphenous vein on the rear lower leg (Fig. 26.34).

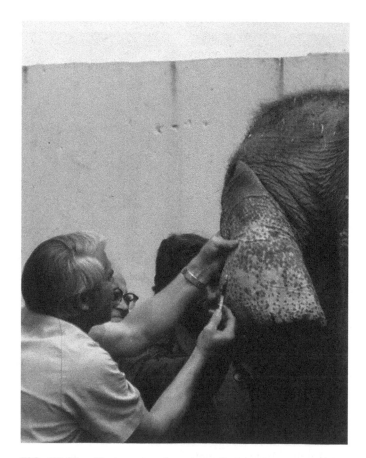

FIG. 26.32. Venipuncture from an auricular vein.

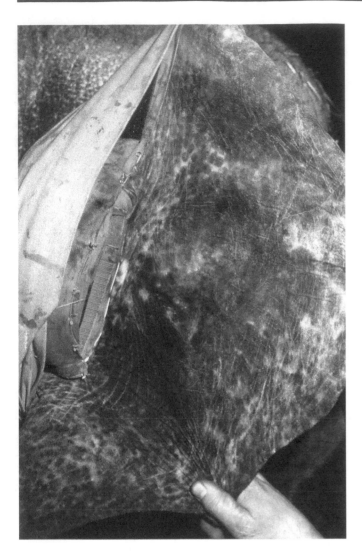

FIG. 26.33. Venipuncture using an inflatable cuff to distend the vein.

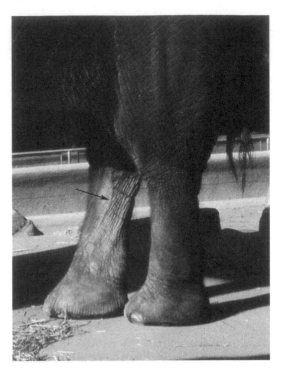

FIG. 26.34. The medial saphenous vein.

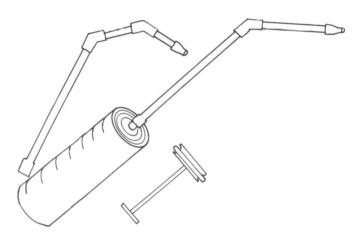

FIG. 26.35. A home-constructed dose syringe fashioned from a calibrated plastic cylinder and metal tubing (8 mm [1/4 in.]) with 45° couplers. The total length of the tubing must be at least 40 cm (16 in.) The tip should be plastic or rubber to avoid trauma to the pharynx. The plunger is fabricated with an "O" ring for the necessary seal.

Oral Medication

Administering oral medication to an elephant may be difficult, especially if the medication must be repeated for several days. Elephants have a keen sense of taste and odor perception, so some method of masking a bitter taste must be found. Many methods to encourage an elephant to accept medication have been tried. One method may work on a given elephant but be unsuccessful on another. Relatively bland medication may be mixed with a sweet feed such as that fed to horses. Others melt milk chocolate and while the chocolate is liquid stir in the medicine; then the liquid is frozen and fed to the elephant. Many elephants enjoy sweet foods. Training is the key to success. The most plausible method of ensuring swallowing is to use a liquid suspension in a dose syringe. Large syringes are available commercially, but the tip must be modified to provide an angle to reach over the base of the tongue (Fig. 26.35). It is necessary to use a mouth gag or bite block to hold the mouth open and prevent crushing

the nozzle (Fig. 26.36). The elephant should be trained to swallow on command.

Slinging

A crane is required to lift an elephant in a sling. If it is necessary to place a sling on a recumbent elephant, a length of iron reinforcing rod used in construction may be pushed beneath the animal just behind the foreleg and just in front of the rear leg. Then a small rope is attached to the rod, pulled

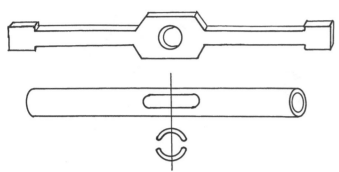

FIG. 26.36. Mouth gags to hold the mouth open. Top: a wooden block constructed of 5.0 cm (2.0 in.) hard wood. The length should be approximately 0.6 m (2.0 ft) and the hole 5.0 cm in diameter. Bottom: an 8.0 cm (3.0 in.) metal pipe covered with duct tape. The slot is 2.5 cm (1.0 in.).

back in the opposite direction, attached to the appropriate sling straps (cargo bands) and pulled through. One strap behind the front limbs and another in front of the hind limbs provides adequate lift.

A safety strap should unite the front strap on one side around the chest to the other side (Figs. 26.37 to 26.39). Similarly, a butt strap should connect the rear straps. These may be anchored with ropes. They are used in case the elephant struggles or is tilted, creating a risk of the elephant slipping out of the sling. Both the front and rear sling straps should be attached to a crane hook, or an appropriate spacer may be used to keep the front and rear straps apart. The crane operator should be provided with the weight of the elephant so the maximum angle can be calculated for the boom of the crane to lift the elephant safely. Sling straps are usually provided by the crane company.

A COMMERCIAL SLING FOR ELEPHANTS. An elephant weighing 2,817 kg (6,210 lb) required surgery on a foot, but couldn't be laid down to administer an anesthetics agent or be chemically immobilized without causing potential damage to an arthritic elbow. A special sling and hoisting system were developed for this elephant so that she could be anesthetized while standing and then gently lowered to the floor (Figs. 26.40, 26.41). It was not possible to move a crane of sufficient capacity into the elephant house to support her. A suspension system and a hoist were designed and installed by local firms. Columbia Wire and Iron Works (555 N. Channel, Portland, Oregon) designed the suspension system.[1,2] Allied Power Products, Inc., of Beaverton, Oregon (Robert Peterson, owner) designed the hoist.

The suspension system consisted of two steel "I" beams braced on the top with right angle and diagonal steel strips bolted to the "I" beams. The beams spanned a distance of 9.8 meters (32.2 feet) and were set on brackets anchored to solid concrete walls with multiple 19 mm by 150 mm (3/4 in. by 6 in.) epoxy anchor bolts.

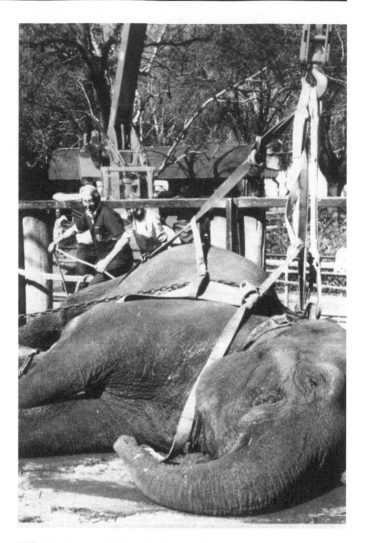

FIG. 26.37. A fashioned sling to lift an elephant.

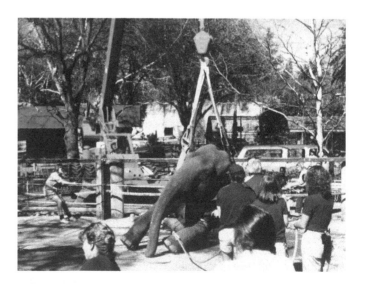

FIG. 26.38. An elephant being lifted.

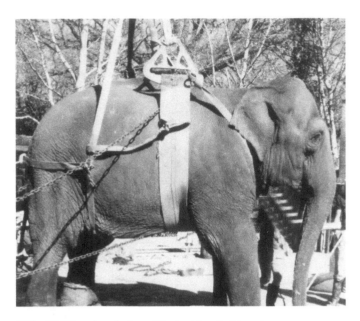

FIG. 26.39. An elephant lifted with a fashioned sling.

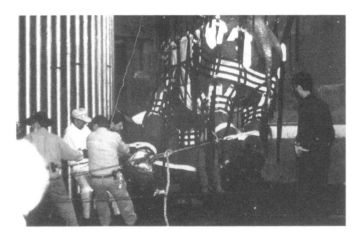

FIG. 26.40. A commercial elephant sling.

The hoist system was powered by the hydraulic pump used to operate the door system in the elephant house. The hoist was designed to move horizontally on a "hammerhead" trolley, rolling on the suspension system's "I" beams. A continuous loop of wire cable extended from one wall to the other, under the control of an electro/hydraulic diverter valve.

Vertical movement was achieved by a swivel hook/load block (with two sheaves), having a lifting capacity at the hook of 9,072 kg (20,000 lb). The vertical speed of the hoist, under load, was 0.3 m (one ft) per 3 seconds. Thus, it required approximately 1 minute to lower the elephant from the standing position to lateral recumbency.

Speed of descent and lifting was an important issue. Once the elephant had collapsed into the sling, it was imperative that she be lowered into lateral recumbency as quickly as possible. An elephant has a unique thoracic anatomy. The

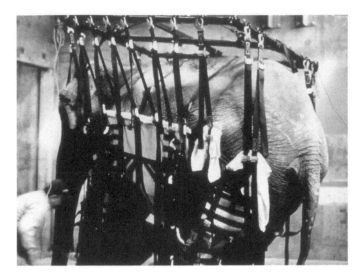

FIG. 26.41. An elephant sling used to lower an anesthetized elephant to the floor.

plcural space is obliterated by fibrous tissue, thus, no negative pressure is possible. Inspiration is accomplished by flattening the dome of the diaphragm and by lateral movement of the rib cage. The lowest point on the ventral abdomen is caudal to the rib cage. When pressure is exerted on the abdomen, such as in a sling or sternal recumbency, the abdominal viscera are deflected cranially, putting pressure on the diaphragm. The sling also restricts lateral movement of the rib cage.

The sling design was adapted from a sling used to support horses with orthopedic challenges or rescuing horses by means of a helicopter. The sling bed (heavy nylon fabric) was supported by twelve 2-in. (5.08 cm) nylon straps, each having a breaking strength of over 12,000 pounds (5,443.2 kilograms). The frame superstructure of the sling was constructed of square, metal-welded tubing with a wall thickness of 1/4 inch (0.64 cm) and outside dimension of 2 in. (5 cm).

The sling was designed for use with four hydraulic rams to adjust the fit of the sling to the animal. The frame was 44 in. (1.12 m) long and 29 in. (0.74 m) wide, with 22 eye rings to attach straps. Because of restricted lifting clearance in the elephant barn, it was not possible to use the hydraulic rams. Four choker cables were used to attach the metal frame to the hook on the hoist.

CHEMICAL RESTRAINT[3,9,14,17–19,22,31,37–40,44,48,50,54,63]

The chemical restraint agents and combinations mentioned in this chapter represent those used by the author or an experienced veterinarian with detailed knowledge of elephants. Other protocols have been used, and no claim is made for including all possible drugs and combinations. For more detailed information, particularly for anesthesia, consult Horne[31] or Fowler.[19]

Both Asian and African elephants are on the list of endangered species. Circuses and zoos that have skilled keepers/handlers are able to accomplish much by physical restraint, but animals accustomed to little human interaction require sedation or chemical immobilization before even minor procedures can be performed. The use of a squeeze helps to alleviate part of the problem, but does not solve it. Table 26.4 lists drugs that have been used in elephants. Free-ranging elephants may require a higher dose than a docile captive animal, and Asian elephants may require more than for comparably sized Africans.

A number of studies have been conducted in recent years and different dosages have been reported. This may be the result of differences in the environment or age of the animal. The dosages listed should be considered only as a guide. No inexperienced person should attempt to sedate or immobilize an elephant without prior consultation with an experienced veterinarian. The author's primary experience in immobilizing elephants has been with the use of etorphine, but carfentanil, an even more potent opiate, may be used in place of etorphine.[19,35,58]

Etorphine hydrochloride (M99) is valuable when it is necessary to obtain complete control of an elephant. It is a marvel of biology that a total of 5.0 mg of a drug given to an elephant weighing 5,000 kg can immobilize it within 15–30 minutes.

The dose is 0.0022–0.004 mg/kg for the Asian elephant and 0.0015–0.003 mg/kg for the African. Prolonged immobilization and anesthesia may be accomplished by repeated administration of etorphine. The induction time for field immobilization may be shortened by including hyaluronidase in the mixture.[26,42,43]

In two separate instances with the same elephant, anesthesia was prolonged up to 4 hours by intravenous administration of etorphine.[17] After initial immobilization, 1 mg of etorphine was given every 15 minutes. It was found to be most satisfactory to administer this as a continuous drip in physiological saline solution.

In a zoo the procedure for immobilizing an elephant should include draining of any pools in the enclosure and tethering the elephant so it does not fall into a moat or empty pool. If the elephant is tractable, the drug can be administered

TABLE 26.4. Chemical restraint agents for elephants[a,19,31,36,37]

Agent	Standing Sedation (mg/kg)	Immobilization (mg/kg)	Comments and references
Xylazine			Best in combinations
Asian	0.04–0.08		1, 5, 6, 32, 51, 53, 57, 64
African	0.08–0.10		
Butorphanol	0.01–0.03		
Etorphine		0.002–0.004, adult Asian	7, 17, 18, 23, 24, 28, 29, 34, 36, 43, 58, 60
		0.0015–0.003, African	
Diazepam	400.0–800.0 TD		To control seizures, 20
Acepromazine	0.004–0.06		20
Azaperone			20, 56
Asian	0.024–0.038		
African	0.056–0.107		
Haloperidol lactate			20
Asian	40.0–100.0 mg TD		
African	40.0–120.0 mg TD		
General	0.025–0.046 mg/kg		
Perphenazine enanthate (Trilafon)			4, 12, 16, 20
Asian	200.0–250.0 mg TD		
African	100.0–300.0 mg TD		
Detomidine	0.0055		20
Medetomidine	0.04–0.08		55
Carfentanil		0.002–0.004	35, 58
Thiafentanil (A3080)			13
Succinylcholine Chloride		0.65	19, 25, 26, 27, 45, 46
Combinations			
Xylazine/ketamine		0.12/0.12, Asian	2, 33
		0.20/1.0–1.5, African	
Xylazine/azaperone		10.0–20.0/40.0–60.0 mg TD	Adult African bull, 56, 62
		12.0/50.0 mg TD	Adult African cow
		5.0–9.0/40.0–70.0 mg TD	Calves, juveniles
Carfentanil/azaperone		12.0/50.0 mg TD	Adult African bull
			Adult African cow
		10.0/50.0 mg TD	Calves, juveniles
		3.0–7.0/40.0–70.0 mg TD	20
Etorphine/Azaperone		Free-ranging Africans	62
		10–20/40–60 mg TD adult male	
		20–15/0.0 adult female	
Reversal Agents			
Naltrexone (Trexan, naltrexone)		50–100 mg TD per 1.0 mg of narcotic	20
Naloxone (Narcan)		1.0 mg Narcan per 1.0 mg of Xylazine	20, 59
Atipamezole (Antesedan)		1.0 mg Ati per 10.0 mg of xylazine	51
Tolazoline		10.0–50.0 mg TD or 0.004 mg/kg	20

[a] Use a long needle, 60.0–80.0 mm (2.35–3.15 in.) with a midshaft collar.

by a handheld syringe. If not, a projectile syringe may be used.

Effects of etorphine will be observed within 10–15 minutes. The trunk hangs limp or loses some of its investigativeness. The animal will start to sway back and forth. Keepers or handlers must stay away from the animal from this point on because the elephant may fall suddenly. A nearby attendant may be fatally crushed if the elephant falls on him. Recumbency occurs within 20–30 minutes (Fig. 26.42).

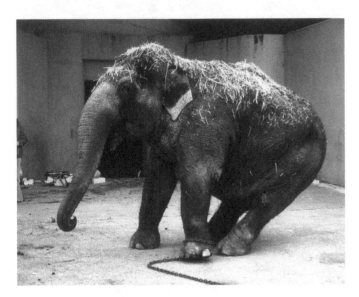

FIG. 26.42. An elephant becoming recumbent following etorphine administration.

Special needles are required for injecting elephants. Needles should be 6.0–8.0 cm long with an outside diameter of 3.0 mm (15 gauge). Opinion varies as to whether or not the tip should be plugged and holes bored on the sides of the needle, to prevent the needle from cutting skin plugs. A special needle can be constructed by plugging the end with solder, filing it to produce a symmetrical tip, and boring tiny holes behind the plug to disperse medication laterally into the tissue. Barbed needles should not be used on captive elephants because of the trauma associated with removal. Collared needles will remain in place sufficiently long to disperse the drug.

If the elephant must fall on a specific side, take appropriate steps before induction to guide the fall (Figs. 26.43, 26.44). An elephant that has fallen on the wrong side may be turned with ropes, using the parbuckle principles (Fig. 26.45).[20] This device was used by the lumber industry to move huge logs in an era before modern equipment was available.

At the conclusion of the necessary period of immobilization, the reversal agent is administered. Although diprenorphine (M50-50) was developed specifically to reverse the effects of etorphine, naltrexone has become the drug of choice for reversal of opiate chemical restraint agents. There are fewer problems of renarcotization. Naltrexone should be

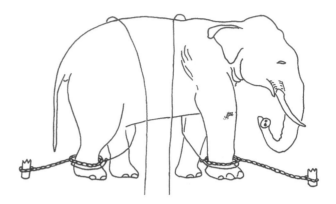

FIG. 26.43. Ropes used to ensure that elephant falls on the correct side when chemically immobilized (side view).

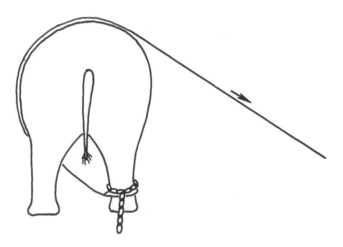

FIG. 26.44. Casting method (end view).

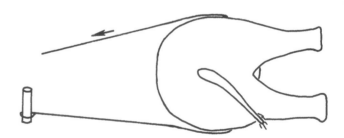

FIG. 26.45. Parbuckle principle used to turn large animals such as elephants and rhinos from one side to the other.

administered intravenously in an ear vein. The elephant will begin to investigate with its trunk within 1–2 minutes. Shortly thereafter it will begin rocking the body and roll into the sternal position. The front legs are placed in front of the animal and the forequarters are raised. Slowly the elephant will rise all the way. This should occur within 2–15 minutes.

Although etorphine and carfentanil are the drugs of choice when immobilizing elephants, other drugs may be used for standing sedation and immobilization (Table 26.4). Standing sedation may be accomplished using acepromazine; dosage of 0.04–0.06 mg/kg are highly effective. Xylazine in dosages of 0.08–0.14 mg/kg has been used (Fig. 26.46). This type of sedation is not suitable for working on the feet. One must always be aware that an elephant may lie down and appear to be sleeping.

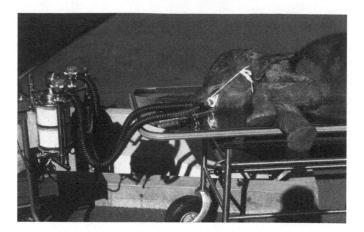

FIG. 26.47.   An elephant calf under inhalant anesthesia.

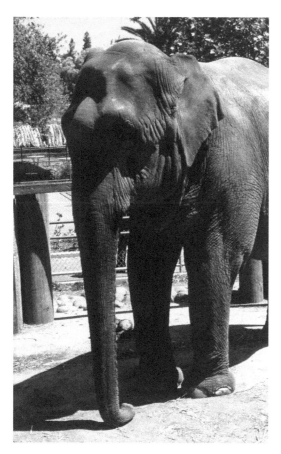

FIG. 26.46.   An elephant under the sedative effects of xylazine hydrochloride.

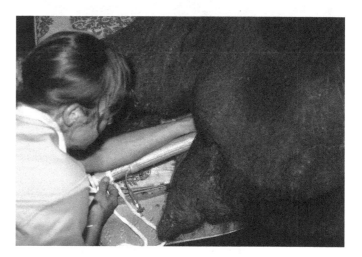

FIG. 26.48.   Endotracheal intubation of an adult elephant.

Various combinations of etorphine, carfentanil, butorphanol, azaperone, xylazine, medetomidine, and acepromazine are used in practice by experienced clinicians. Inexperienced persons should not use any immobilizing agent without first consulting someone experienced in its use.

Etorphine is used both as an immobilizing and an anesthetizing agent; however, major surgery should be done under inhalation anesthesia. Isoflurane is the inhalant agent of choice.[19] Inhalation anesthesia may be performed in elephant calves using the same techniques as in livestock species (Fig. 26.47). Endotracheal intubation also may be accomplished in adult elephants. The animal must be immobilized and a wooden block placed between the upper and lower teeth on one side to hold the mouth open. A person with a small hand then carries a sterilized equine stomach tube into the mouth and inserts it into the trachea. The hand is withdrawn and a large (30.0–40.0 mm inside diameter) equine endotracheal tube is passed over the stomach tube and on into the trachea using the stomach tube as a guide (Fig. 26.48).

Miscellaneous Considerations

Assisted respiration may be accomplished using nasal insufflation or a modified leaf blower.[30]

Injection sites should be cleansed and antibiotic mastitis ointment infused into the needle tract. If this is not done, abscesses following darting may be seen.

Adverse reactions to chemical immobilizing agents have been reported.[4,8,41,52]

PINK FOAM SYNDROME.   Opiates cause hypertension when used alone. This may cause extravasation of plasma and blood into the pulmonary alveoli resulting in a pink froth. This is a serious complication, and when it occurs, the animal should be reversed as soon as possible. Hypertension may be minimized if azaperone is administered along with the opiate, or is administered as soon as the elephant becomes immobilized.

TRANSPORT[10,11,15,47,49]

Circuses have been transporting trained performing elephants for decades. Special railroad cars (Fig. 26.49) or trailers (Fig. 26.50) are employed. Although ramps are usually used to load and offload, adult elephants are capable of stepping down from a bed that is 0.8 m above the ground. Transporting untrained zoo elephants may be an entirely different story.

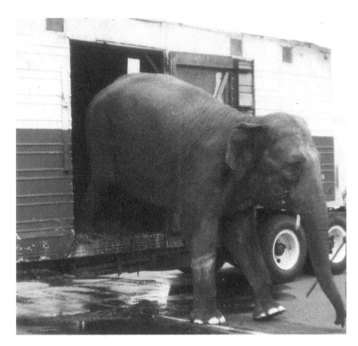

FIG. 26.50. An elephant stepping down from a semi-tractor trailer.

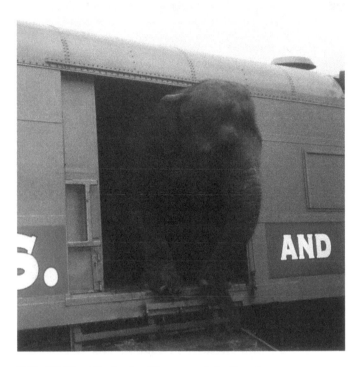

FIG. 26.49. Elephant exiting a special railroad car.

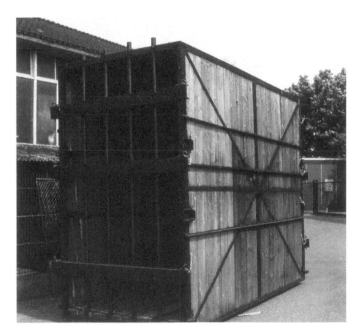

FIG. 26.51. An elephant crate.

Elephants may be crated and moved via truck, airplane, or ship if the crates are adequately constructed (Fig. 26.51). Adult elephants require special facilities. Semi-trailer or railroad cars must be reinforced inside with 6.4 mm (34 in.) sheet iron to withstand the tusks and butting of elephants. Rings must be provided to secure both front and hind legs.

Chains must be kept short, and access must be provided for handlers to chain and unchain the elephant. Normally elephants are removed from trucks on short ramps or at docks where the elephant can walk out at truck-bed level. They can climb or step down a few feet if trained to do so.

Following is an example of the challenge of transporting an adult zoo elephant. Arrangements had been made to move a docile adult female to another zoo. She could be chained, but was not reliable outside her enclosure. A semi-trailer that was used by a professional elephant trainer was positioned near the gate of the enclosure, and chains extended through the trailer and were anchored so that as she moved forward into the truck the slack could be taken up. Once inside the trailer, she was chained by all four feet to rings in the floor. The floor of the trailer was constructed of 5.0-cm (2.0-in.) solid oak decking.

The loading was uneventful and the 450-mile journey began. Approximately 24 km (15 miles) into the journey, a keeper following the truck in another vehicle noticed the elephant's trunk protruding from the floor of the trailer. The elephant had broken the flooring by repeatedly dropping to her knees. A metal plate was welded to the under-frame of the trailer to prevent her from falling through the floor. The elephant was returned to the zoo and off-loaded.

Ultimately, arrangements were made to move this single female to another zoo across the country. Considerable time and effort was expended to train the elephant to accept the novel environment of a trailer. An elephant crate was placed next to the enclosure and the animal was fed in the crate. When accustomed to the crate, the doors were closed and ultimately she was chained inside the crate. This became routine for her.

When the day of the move arrived, the elephant was placed in the crate, then the trailer was positioned in front of the crate. The front door of the crate was opened and the elephant moved into the trailer with minimal hesitation. The trip was uneventful. The key to the successful move was the training that had prepared her for a new experience.

To move elephants within a zoo, chain difficult elephants between two docile animals. This technique may also be used with two pieces of heavy machinery such as large tractors, by attaching chains in front of and behind the elephant as depicted in Fig. 26.52.

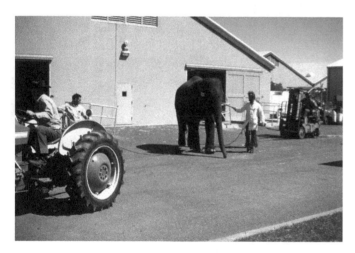

FIG. 26.52.   Moving an elephant by tethering between vehicles.

REFERENCES

The literature of the chemical immobilization of elephants is voluminous. For an extensive bibliography see Fowler and Mikiota,[19] Chapter 9, Chemical Restraint and Anesthesia. In: Fowler, M.E., and Mikota, S.K. The Biology, Medicine and Surgery of Elephants. St. Louis, Elsevier, pp. 91–110.

1. Aik, S.S. 1992. Preliminary observations on the training of Burmese elephants using xylazine. New Zealand Vet J 40(2):81–84.

2. Allen, J.L. 1986. Use of tolazoline as an antagonist to xylazine-ketamine-induced immobilization in African elephants. Am J Vet Res 47(4):781–83.

3. Appayya, M.K., and Khadri, S.S.M.S. 1992. Chemical capture of wild elephants and their translocation carried out in Karnataka state. In: Silas, E.G., Nair, M.K., and Nirmalan, G., Eds. The Asian Elephant: Ecology, Biology, Diseases, Conservation and Management (Proceedings of the National Symposium on the Asian Elephant held at the Kerala Agricultural University), Trichur, India, pp. 107–12.

4. Blumer, E.S. 1991. A review of the use of selected neuroleptic drugs in the management of non-domestic hoofstock. Proc Am Assoc Zoo Vet, pp. 326–32.

5. Bongso, T.A. 1979. Sedation of the Asian elephant (*Elephas maximus*) with xylazine. Vet Rec 105(19):442–43.

6. Bongso, T.A. 1980. Use of xylazine for the transport of elephants by air. Vet Rec 107(21):492.

7. Bongso, T.A. and Perera, B.M.A.O. 1978. Observations on the use of etorphine alone and in combination with acepromazine maleate for immobilization of aggressive Asian elephants (*Elephas maximus*). Vet Rec 102(15):339–40.

8. Cheeran, J. 2002. Adverse drug experiences in elephants. J Indian Vet Assoc Kerala 7(3):61.

9. Cheeran, J.V., Chandrasekharan, K., and Radhakrishnan, K. 1992a. Tranquilization and translocation of elephants. In: Silas, E.G., Nair, M.K., and Nirmalan, G., Eds. The Asian Elephant: Ecology, Biology, Diseases, Conservation and Management. (Proceedings of the National Symposium on the Asian Elephant held at the Kerala Agricultural University), pp. 176.

10. Cheeran, J.V., Chandrasekharan, K., and Radhakrishnan, K. 1992b. Transportation of elephants by rail. In: Silas, E.G., Nair, M.K., and Nirmalan, G., Eds. The Asian Elephant: Ecology, Biology, Diseases, Conservation and Management (Proceedings of the National Symposium on the Asian Elephant held at the Kerala Agricultural University, Trichur, India, January 1989), pp. 120–22.

11. Cheeran, J.V., Chandrasekharan, K., and Radhakrishnan, K. 2002. Tranquilization and translocation of elephants. J Indian Vet Assoc Kerala 7(3):42–46.

12. Dangolla, A., Silva, I., and Kuruwita, V.Y. 2004. Neuroleptanalgesia in wild Asian elephants (*Elaphas maximus maximus*). Vet Anaesthesia and Analgesia 31:276–79.

13. de Vos, V. 1978. Immobilization of free-ranging wild animals using a new drug. Vet Rec 103(4):64–68.

14. de Vos, V. 1985. Immobilization of the African elephant. Proc 2nd Int Congr Vet Anesth, pp. 142–43.

15. Dublin, H.T. and Niskanen, L.S., Ed. 2003. IUCN/SSC AFESG Guidelines for the in situ Translocation of the African Elephant for Conservation Purposes. http://www.save-the-elephants.org/elereflib.htm.

16. Ebedes, H. 1993. The use of long acting tranquilizers in captive wild animals. In: McKenzie, A.A., Ed. The Capture and Care Manual. Pretoria, Wildlife Division Support Services: South African Veterinary Foundation, pp. 71–99.

17. Fowler, M.E., and Hart, R. 1973. Castration of an Asian elephant using etorphine (M99) anesthesia. J Am Vet Med. Assoc 163:539–43.

18. Fowler, M.E. 1995. Chemical restraint. In: Fowler, M.E. Restraint and Handling of Wild and Domestic Animals, 2nd Ed. Ames, Iowa State University Press, pp. 36–56.

19. Fowler, M.E., and Mikota, S.K. 2006. Chemical restraint and general anesthesia. In: Fowler, M.E., and Mikota, S.D., Eds. Biology, Medicine and Surgery of Elephants. Ames, Iowa, Blackwell Publishing, pp. 91–109.

20. Fowler, M.E. 2006. Physical restraint and handling. In: Fowler, M.E. and Mikota, S.K., Eds. Biology, Medicine and Surgery of Elephants. Ames, Iowa, Blackwell Publishing, pp. 75–90.

21. Gross, M.E., Clifford, C.A., and Hardy, D.A. 1994. Excitement in an elephant after intravenous administration of atropine. J Am Vet Med Assoc 205(10):1437–38.

22. Harthoorn, A.M. 1973. Drug immobilization of large wild herbivores other than antelopes. In: Young, E., Ed. The Capture and Care of Wild Animals, Cape Town, Human and Rousseau, pp. 51–53.

23. Harthoorn, A.M., and Bligh, J. 1965. The use of a new oripavine derivative with potent morphine-like activity for the restraint of hoofed wild animals. Res Vet Sci 6:290–99.

24. Hattingh, J., Knox, C.M., and Raath, J.P. 1994. Arterial blood pressure of the African elephant (*Loxodonta africana*) under etorphine anesthesia and after remobilisation with diprenorphine. Vet Rec 135(19):458–59.

25. Hattingh, J., Pitts, N.I., De-Vos, N.I., Moyes, D.G., and Ganhao, M.F. 1991. The response of animals to suxamethonium (succinyldicholine) and succinylmonocholine. J South African Vet Assoc 62(3):126–29.

26. Hattingh, J., Pitts, N.I., Ganhao, M.F,. Moyes, D.G., and de Vos, V. 1990. Blood constituent responses of animals culled with succinyldicholine and hexamethonium. S Afr Vet Assoc 61:117–18.

27. Hattingh, J., Wright, P.G., de Vos, V., McNairn, I.S., Ganhao, M.F., Silove, M., Wolverson, G., and Cornelius, S.T. 1984. Blood composition in culled elephants and buffaloes. J S Afr Vet Assoc 55(4):157–64.

28. Heard, D.J., Jacobson, E.R., and Brock, K.A. 1986. Effects of oxygen supplementation on blood gas values in chemically restrained juvenile African elephants. J Am Vet Med Assoc 189(9):1071–74.

29. Honeyman, V.L., Cooper, R.M., and Black, S.R. 1998. A protected contact approach to anesthesia and medical management of an Asian elephant (*Elephas maximus*). Proc Am Assoc Zoo, pp. 338–41.

30. Horne, W.A., Tchamba, M.N., and Loomis, M.R. 2001. A simple method of providing intermittent positive-pressure ventilation to etorphine-immobilized elephants (Loxodonta africana) in the field. Journal of Zoo and Wildlife Medicine 32(4):519–22.

31. Horne, W.A., and Loomis, M.R. 2007. Elephants and Hyrax. In: West, G., Heard, D., and Caulkett, N. Zoo Animal and Wildlife immobilization and Anesthesia. Ames, Iowa, Blackwell Publishing, pp. 507–22.

32. Jacob, V., Cheeran, K., Chandrasekharan, K., and Radhakrishnan, K. 1983. Immobilization of elephant in musth using xylazine hydrochloride. 7th Annual Symposium of the Indian Society of Veterinary Surgeons, p. 62.

33. Jacobson, E.R., Allen, J., Martin, H., and Kollias, G.V. 1985. Effects of yohimbine on combined xylazine-ketamine-induced sedation and immobilization in juvenile African elephants. J Am Vet Med Assoc 187(11):1195–98.

34. Jacobson, E.R., Chen, C. L., Gronwall, R., and Tiller, A. 1986. Serum concentrations of etorphine in juvenile African elephants. J Am Vet Med Assoc 189(9):1079–81.

35. Jacobson, E.R., Kollias, G.V., Heard, D.J., and Caligiuri, R. 1988. Immobilization of African elephants with carfentanil and antagonism with nalmefene and diprenorphine. J Zoo An Med 19:1–7.

36. Kock, M.D., Martin, R.B., and Kock, N. 1993. Chemical immobilization of free-ranging African elephants in Zimbabwe, using etorphine mixed with hyaluronidase and evaluation of biological data collected soon after immobilization. J Zoo Wildl Med 24:1–10.

37. Kock, R.A., Morkel, P., and Kock, M. D. 1993. Current immobilization procedures used in elephants. In: Fowler, M.E., Ed. Zoo and Wild Animal Medicine, 3rd ed. pp. 436–40. Philadelphia: W.B. Saunders.

38. Kreeger, T.J., Arnemo, J.M., and Raath, J.P. 2002. Handbook of wildlife chemical immobilization. Wildlife Pharmaceuticals Inc. Fort Collins, Colorado, U.S.A. 412 pages.

39. Manna, S. 1996. Chemical immobilization and treatment of a wild elephant. Indian Vet J 73(12):1260–61.

40. Mikota, S.K., and Page, C.D. 1994. Anesthesia and chemical restraint. In: Mikota, S.K., Sargent, E.L., and Ranglack, G.S., Eds. Medical Management of the Elephant. West Bloomfield, Michigan, Indira Publishing House, pp. 41–49.

41. Morton, D.J., Kock, M.D., and Miller, R.M. 1977. Segmental gangrene and sloughing of elephant's ears after intravenous injection of phenylbutazone. Vet Med Small Animal Clinician 72(4):633–37.

42. Morton, D.J., and Kock, M. 1991. Stability of hyaluronidase in solution with etorphine and xylazine. J Zoo Wildl Med 22(3):345–47.

43. Osofsky, S.A. 1995. Pulse oximetry monitoring of free-ranging African elephants (*Loxodonta africana*) immobilized with an etorphine/hyaluronidase combination antagonized with diprenorphine. Proc Am Assoc Zoo Vet, East Lansing, Michigan, pp. 241–45.

44. Osofsky, S.A. 1997. A practical anesthesia monitoring protocol for free-ranging adult African elephants (*Loxodonta africana*). J Wildl Dis 33(1):72–77.

45. Pitts, N.I., and Mitchell, G. 2002. Pharmacokinetics and effects of succinylcholine in African elephant (*Loxodonta africana*) and impala (*Aepyceros melampus*). Eur J Pharm Sci 15(3):251–60.

46. Pitts, N.I., and Mitchell, G. 2003. In vitro succinylcholine hydrolysis in plasma of the African elephant (*Loxodonta africana*) and impala (*Aepyceros melampus*). Comp Biochem Physiol C Toxicol Pharmacol 134(1):123–29.

47. Raath, J.P. 1993. Transportation of the African elephant. In: McKenzie, A.A., Ed. The Capture and Care Manual Pretoria: The South African Veterinary Foundation, pp. 493–97.

48. Raath, J.P. 1993. Chemical capture of the African elephant. In: McKenzie, A.A., Ed. 1993. The Capture and Care Manual. Pretoria Wildlife Division Support Services: South African Veterinary Foundation, pp. 484–511.

49. Raath, J.P. 1999. Relocation of African elephants. In: Fowler, M.E., and Miller, R.E., Eds. Zoo and Wild Animal Medicine: Current Therapy 4. W.B. Saunders, Philadelphia, PA, USA pp. 525–33.

50. Ramsay, E. 2000. Standing sedation and tranquilization in captive African elephants (*Loxodonta africana*). Proc Am Assoc Zoo Vet New Orleans, Louisiana, pp. 111–14.

51. Rietschel, W., Hildebrandt, T., Goritz, F., and Ratanakorn, P. 2001. Sedation of Thai Working Elephants with Xylazine and Atipamezole as a Reversal. A Research Update on Elephants and Rhinos; Proceedings of the International Elephant and Rhino Research Symposium, Vienna, pp. 121–23.

52. Sarma, K.K. 1999. Bizarre behaviour of an elephant during xylazine anesthesia. Indian Vet J 76(11):1018–19.

53. Sarma, K.K., and Pathak, S.C. 2001. Cardiovascular response to xylazine and Hellabrunn mixture with Yohimbine as reversal agent in Asian elephants. Indian Vet J 78(5):400–92.

54. Schmitt, D.L. 2003. Proboscidea (elephants). In: Fowler, M.E., and Miller, R.E., Eds. Zoo and Wild Animal Medicine. 5th Ed. St. Louis, Saunders/Elsevier. pp. 541–44.

55. Sarma, B., Pathak, S.C., and Sarma, K.K. 2002. Medetomidine a novel immobilizing agent for the elephant (*Elephas maximus*). Res Vet Sci 73(3):315–17.

56. Schmitt, D., Bradford, J., and Hardy, D.A. 1996. Azaperone for standing sedation in Asian elephants (*Elephas maximus*). Proc Am Assoc Zoo Vet, Puerto Vallarta, Mexico, pp. 48–51.

57. Schmidt, M.J. 1983. Antagonism of xylazine sedation by yohimbine and 4-aminopyridine in an adult Asian elephant (*Elephas maximus*). J Zoo An Med 14:94–97.

58. Schumacher, J., Heard, D.J., Caligiuri, R., Norton T., and Jacobson, E.R. 1995. Comparative effects of etorphine and carfentanil on cardiopulmonary parameters in juvenile African elephants (*Loxodonta africana*). J Zoo Wildl Med 26(4):503–07.

59. Smuts, G.L. 1975. An appraisal of naloxone hydrochloride as a narcotic antagonist in the capture and release of wild herbivores. J Am Vet Med Assoc 167(7):559–61.

60. Stegmann, G.F. 1999. Etorphine-halothane anesthesia in two five-year-old African elephants (*Loxodonta africana*). J South African Vet Med Assoc 70:(4):164–66

61. Still, J. Raath, J.P., and Matzner, L. 1996. Respiratory and circulatory parameters of African elephants (*Loxodonta africana*) anesthetized with etorphine and azaperone. J South African Vet Med Assoc 67:(3):123–27.

62. Still, J. 1993. Etorphine-azaperone anesthesia in an African elephant (*Loxodonta africana*). J Vet Anaes 20:54–55.

63. Swan, G.E. 1993. Drugs used for the immobilization, capture, and translocation of wildlife. In: McKenzie, A.A. Ed. The Capture and Care Manual. Pretoria Wildlife Division Support Services, South African Veterinary Foundation, pp. 2–64.

64. Thakuria, D.B., and Barthakur, T. 1996. The management of musth in a male African elephant by chemical sedatives in Assam state zoo, Guwhati. Indian Vet J 73(3):339–40.

CHAPTER 28

Hoofed Stock (Other than the Megavertebrates)

CLASSIFICATION

Suborder: Suiformes
    Family: Suidae (pigs and swine)
    Family: Tayassuidae (peccaries)
Suborder: Ruminantia
    Family: Cervidae (deer, moose and wapiti)
    Family: Bovidae (cattle, antelope, goats and sheep)

Names of genders are listed in Table 28.1; weights of representative species are listed in Table 28.2.

TABLE 28.1. Names of gender of hoofed stock

Animal	Mature Male	Mature Female	Newborn and Young
Peccary	Boar	Sow	Piglet
Deer	Buck, stag, hart	Doe, hind	Fawn
Elk	Bull	Cow	Calf
Moose	Bull	Cow	Calf
Reindeer	Buck	Doe	Fawn
Pronghorn	Buck	Doe	Kid
Cattle	Bull	Cow	Calf
Antelope	Buck	Doe	Kid, lamb
Water buffalo	Bul	Cow	Calf
Cape buffalo	Bull	Cow	Calf
Yak	Bull	Cow	Calf
Bison Rocky	Bull	Cow	Calf
Mountain goat	Buck	Doe	Kid
Musk-ox	Bull	Cow	Calf
Goat	Buck	Doe, nanny	Kid
Ibex	Buck	Doe	Kid
Aoudad	Buck	Doe	Kid
Sheep	Ram, buck	Ewe	Lamb
Mouflon	Buck, ram	Ewe	Lamb
Bighorn sheep	Buck, ram	Ewe	Lamb

TABLE 28.2. Weights of representative hoofed stock

Animal	Kilograms	Pounds
Warthog	75–100	165–220
Babirusa	40–100	88–220
Giant forest pig	100–275	220–606
Peccary, collared	15–35	33–77
Peccary, Chacoan	30–45	66–99
Caribou	318	700
Wapiti	200–350	440–770
Moose	825	1,815
Deer		
Fallow	40–80	88–176
Sika	25–110	55–242
White-tailed	22–205	48–451
Mule	50–215	110–471
Pronghorn	36–60	79–132
Eland	900	1,980
American bison	1,000	2,200
Antelope		
Roan	240	528
Sable	214	471
Saiga	23–40	51–88
Buffalo		
African	600–900	1,320–1,980
Water	1,000	2,200
Impala	99	218
Gazelle (Thompson)	40	88
Gnu	180	396
Sheep		
Mouflon	70–150	154–330
Aoudad	50–115	110–253
(Barbary)		

GENERAL CONSIDERATIONS
Physical Restraint

Although chemical restraint is heavily relied upon for examination, loading for transportation, and other situations that require hands on the animal, there remains a need for

355

understanding the basic principles of physical restraint. The routine handling of large numbers of wild ungulates in game farming operations necessitates some form of alleyways, collecting areas, runways, chutes, squeezes, and holding pens. Many new enclosures in zoos likewise have facilities for containment of ungulates for close inspection, immobilization, or loading into crates.

Hoofed animals may not recognize a chain link or wire net fence as a barrier, especially when newly placed in such an enclosure. Fences should be draped with plastic sheeting or burlap sacking until the animals are accustomed to the fence (Fig. 28.1).

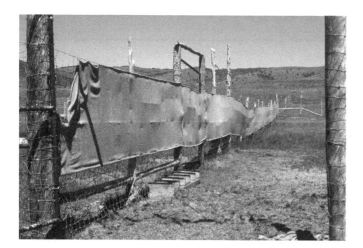

FIG. 28.1. Visual barrier over the wire for introducing ungulates into a new fenced-in enclosure.

Although difficult to herd otherwise (Fig. 28.2), hoofed animals may be moved effectively and efficiently by manipulating opaque plastic sheeting (Figs. 28.3, 28.4, 28.5). The technique was first described by Oelofse in 1970 (see Chapter

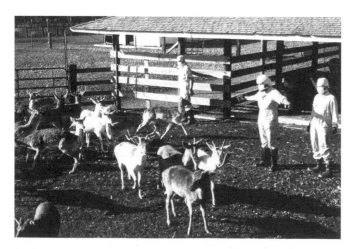

FIG. 28.2. Attempting to herd deer may be a frustrating experience.

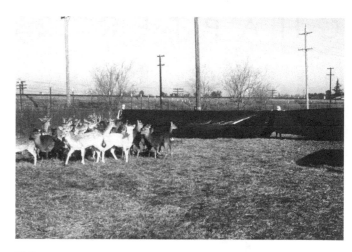

FIG. 28.3. Opaque plastic sheeting used for directing hoofed animals.

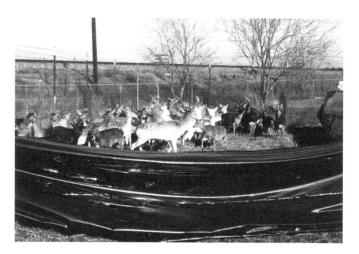

FIG. 28.4. Plastic sheeting used to temporarily confine a herd of deer into a small area for close inspection.

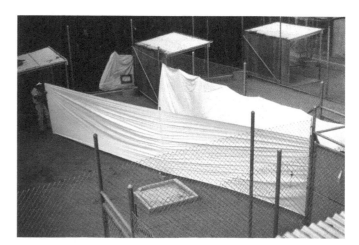

FIG. 28.5. Plastic sheeting used to load an antelope into a crate from a zoo enclosure.

23, Restraint and Handling of Wild and Domestic Animals, Second Edition) and subsequently has been used in numerous instances to capture and retain wild animals in an enclosed area. Hoofed animals recognize the sheeting as a barrier and can be persuaded to move through gates, into shipping crates, or into alleyways by judicious manipulation of this material.

This technique is effective with cervids, antelope, zebra, and rhinoceros, but dorcas gazelle and giraffe do not respond well. Gazelles reach their heads under and flip up the plastic sheeting, and obviously it is difficult to obtain a sheet of plastic wide enough to prevent a giraffe from seeing over it.

If an enclosure is too small to admit a truck or trailer, remove downed, sick, or injured animals by dragging them on a large 1.22×2.44 m (4×8 ft) piece of plywood sheeting 15 mm (5/8 in.) thick, with holes drilled approximately 4 in. from the forward corners. (See Chapter 14, Camelids.) Thread wire or chain loops through the holes and attach a chain. Lay the plywood sheeting next to the animal and carefully lift or pull the injured animal onto the sheet. The plywood sheet can be dragged from the pen by the use of snatch blocks. Canvas tarp may be used similarly, but if the animal must be dragged some distance, the musculature, ribs, and bones may be bruised through the canvas.

Do not use whips or clubs when working with any animal. A swat from a household broom or a flat scoop shovel is more effective, producing noise to scare the animal and encourage it to move rather than simply inflicting pain. When animals are excited by the stress of moving or during the alarm stage, pain perception is lessened. Mild pain will not be felt; if intense pain is inflicted, hostile reactions may ensue.

Transport

The critical time for injuries during transport operations is at the time the animal is loaded into or released from the crate. Lack of preparation is the prime cause of failure when loading, unloading, or conducting capture operations of hoofed stock. Too often insufficient thought is given to the needs of the animal and the specific behavioral characteristics that must be accommodated to achieve the desired end with as little fuss as possible.

Most operations are carried out much too rapidly. The animals should be fed in open crates or capture pens over a period of several days to allow them to become accustomed to confined areas. Special chutes may be arranged to guide the animals into a new enclosure, or ramps may be constructed in alleyways or alongside a familiar barn or shed so animals do not feel harassed. It is possible to arrange the chutes to funnel an animal to a crate, chase it in, and close the door behind it. Other alternatives are to immobilize the animal and allow it to recover in the crate; or immobilize it, give an antidote, and as the animal regains mobility direct it into the crate.

Each group of animals has its own set of requirements for crating. Unfortunately there is no single source of information on crating for all species. The International Air Transport Association (IATA) has published a manual describing a variety of crates and cages.[2]

It is important to select a crate or cage suited to the biological requirements of the animal.[21] The floor area should be based on that required by the animal when resting and recumbent and its special needs for space to lie down or arise. For instance, an antelope or gazelle can lie down and get up in a space the length and width of its body. In this case a suitable crate need not be much wider or longer than the body. If a crate is too long, the animal may charge the door, causing injury to the head and neck. If a crate is too wide, the animal may attempt to turn around and get stuck in a dangerous position. The height of a crate for a horned animal should allow the animal to stand with its head in a normal position. If the height of the crate permits the animal to jump up, it may fall over backward.

Many deaths have been caused by animals having too much room. In one instance a fringe-eared oryx walked into a too-large crate, the door was closed behind her, and she became frightened and tried to turn around. In the ensuing struggle she tipped herself upside down with her head pinned beneath her body. Fortunately the crate could be opened quickly and the animal pulled out; if the incident had occurred en route, no one could have saved her.

It is vital that crate construction provide for adequate air exchange, not only to supply sufficient oxygen for respiration, but to remove odors and noxious gases such as ammonia. A black buck, 130 cm long and 80 cm high at the shoulder, placed in a crate with inside dimensions of 180×35 cm high would occupy 25–35% of the volume of the crate, leaving approximately 595 L of air space. If the resting black buck needs 15 L of air per minute at an ambient temperature of 18–21°C, the air in the crate would be exhausted in 39 minutes. If the animal is excited or the temperature is raised, the air may be exhausted in 10–15 minutes. Elevated ambient temperatures increase the air requirement, because the animal breathes more rapidly to assist in cooling.

Ventilation ports should be provided near the floor above the bedding and also near the top of the crate to provide a draught effect, drawing air into and out of the crate. However, any opening through which a foot or horn could protrude must be screened. Ventilation ports have the added advantage of permitting visual access to the animal. All openings should be closed with sliding panels rather than hinged doors. Since animals are susceptible to carbon monoxide poisoning, crates should not be placed near exhaust fumes from internal combustion engines. The floors of crates for ungulates are frequently cleated to prevent slipping; this is acceptable if the cleats are short (8 mm high). Higher cleats cause discomfort to a recumbent animal and also have detrimental effects; uneven pressure may inflict trauma on localized areas of the limbs or body, especially if the animal becomes weakened and lies down for a long time.

Most hoofed animals should be shipped in individual crates. This is of prime importance if the animals are horned. Members of a group may have been companions for a long time, but when they are placed in close confinement, aggressiveness may develop which may result in fatalities to subordinates. The behavior of animals under stress or confined in close quarters is unpredictable.

At no time should animals of varying sizes be placed in the same shipping crate—even mothers and offspring. A smaller animal is apt to be trampled by the larger. If transporting cannot be delayed until after weaning, the young must be separated by a partition or put into a separate crate. An infant that has been kept away from its mother for an extended period may engorge on milk when they are reunited. If manual handling of the female is possible, it is desirable to partially milk the female before permitting the infant to nurse, so it cannot overeat.

When crates containing large hoofed animals are loaded, they should be oriented with the hind end facing the front of the vehicle. Smaller species will be more comfortable if the crate is loaded sideways. This orientation may prevent serious damage from jolting stops and starts.

The release of an animal from a crate may also be dangerous. Some animals bolt from the crate immediately upon seeing the open door. Others, especially if the interior is dark, accept the crate as a haven and refuse to leave it. The least stressful method of release is to place the crate within an enclosure or in the doorway of the enclosure, open the crate, and let the animal come out on its own to investigate the new surroundings.

ARTIODACTYLA (ORDER)

Suborder Suiformes
    Superfamily Suoidea
        Family Suidae: warthog (Fig. 28.6), babirusa (Fig. 28.7), bushpig (Fig. 28.8), giant forest hog

Family Tayassuidae: peccaries, collared (Fig. 28.9), white-lipped (Fig. 28.10), and Chacoan (Fig. 28.11).

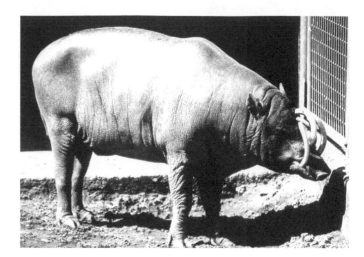

FIG. 28.7. Babirusa, *Babyrousa babyrussa.*

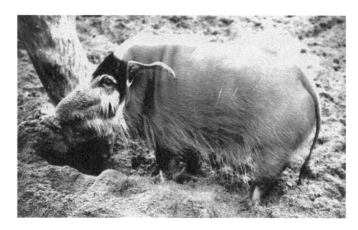

FIG. 28.8. Red river hog (bush pig), *Potamochoerus porcus.*

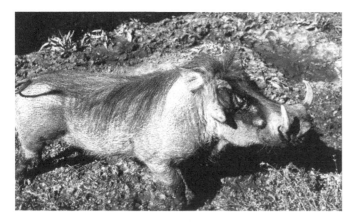

FIG. 28.6. Wart hog, *Phacochoerus aethiopicus.*

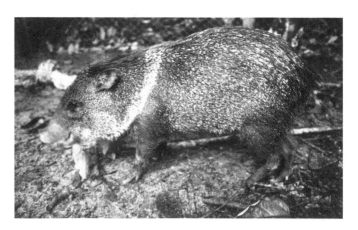

FIG. 28.9. Collared peccary, *Tayassu tajacu.*

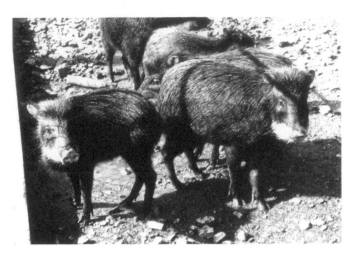

FIG. 28.10. White-lipped peccary, *Tayassu pecari*.

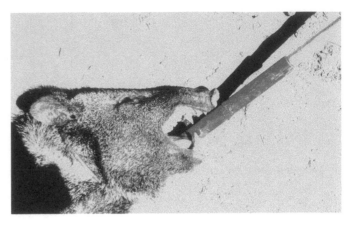

FIG. 28.12. Collared peccary biting a come-along.

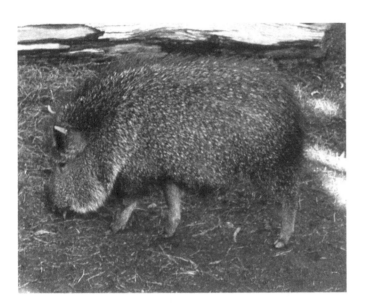

FIG. 28.11. Chacoan peccary, *Catagonus wagneri*.

Wild Pig, Peccary

DANGER POTENTIAL. Members of these two families bite and gore. They neither kick nor strike, and most of them are not heavy enough to crush or trample. They possess sharp teeth, with the canine teeth elongated to form tusks, particularly in the male (Fig. 28.12). These tusks are formidable weapons, used to rend and disembowel opponents. Wild pigs may be aggressive. Do not enter an enclosure confining them without protection.

The peccary is a small ferocious animal with a vicious disposition. It can inflict serious or fatal injury with its tusks and needle-sharp teeth, which can easily penetrate heavy leather gloves. Peccaries are fast and agile and are quick to resent restraint. Even small piglets are obstreperous and hard to subdue.

ANATOMY AND PHYSIOLOGY. Wild pigs and peccaries are heavy-bodied, short-necked, short-legged animals. Physically they resemble domestic pigs. Both have the thick layer of insulating fat common to all species of swine, predisposing them to overheating when subjected to restraint.

The canine teeth of all species are razor sharp, but vary in morphology from species to species. In peccaries, the canines are elongated, and the arrangement is much like that of a carnivore. Each canine tooth is sharpened by abrasion against the canine in the opposite jaw. In African suids, the maxillary canine is directed laterally, then turns dorsally and slightly caudally to become a formidable tusk, especially in the male. The mandibular canine is directed dorsally, then slightly caudally. The canine teeth of the babirusa are unique in that the maxillary set begins development in the usual ventral direction but the entire alveolar unit turns 180° and the tooth projects dorsally through the nasal bones and skin (Fig. 28.7).

PHYSICAL RESTRAINT.[2,5,27,50,53,54] Wild swine and peccaries do not tolerate snout snares. If panels are used, take care that the animals don't push their snouts under the panel and escape or attack. A technique used in Brazil to handle peccaries is to direct the animals into a small covered enclosure. A nylon-mesh net cone is placed over an exit and the door opened (Figs. 28.13, 28.14). The animal makes a dash for freedom but is caught in the narrow tip of the cone. A large, heavy-duty fish-landing net may also be used to catch small pigs. Pigs and peccaries may then be snared singly, grasped by the hind legs, and stretched. A snare must be tightly secured so it does not slip over the narrow head. Gloves offer some protection from teeth.

Peccaries are more agile and aggressive than wild pigs and consequently must be handled with greater care. Peccary piglets must also be snared and stretched, though newborn wild pigs can be handled manually in the same manner as domestic piglets. Large members of this group must be run

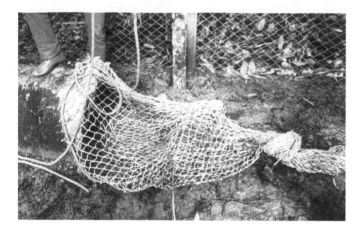

FIG. 28.13. Cone net used to capture a peccary.

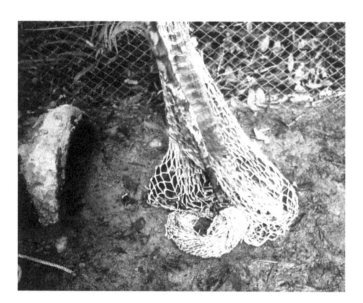

FIG. 28.14. Peccary in a net.

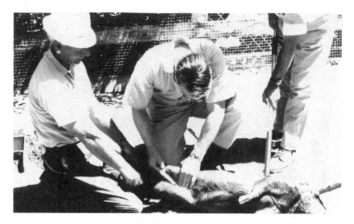

FIG. 28.15. Blood collection from the femoral vein.

TABLE 28.3. Selected chemical restraint agents for wild suids and tayassuids[50]

Agent	Dose (mg/kg), IM
Tiletamine/zolazepam	2.18
Midazolam/butorphanol/medetomidine	0.3/0.3/0.07
Midazolam/butorphanol/detomidine	0.3/0.3/0.12
Midazolam/butorphanol/xylazine	0.3/0.3/3.0
Butorphanol/tiletamine/zolazepam (telazol)	0.3/0.6
Ketamine/xylazine	3.5/0.2
Ketamine/medetomidine	3.5/0.07

ARTIODACTYLA (ORDER)

Suborder Ruminantia
    Family Tragulidae: chevrotain
    Family Cervidae: deer, wapiti, moose, caribou
    Family Antilocapridae: pronghorn
    Family Bovidae: all remaining ruminants
        Subfamily Bovinae: cattle-like, yak, bison, gaur (Fig. 28.16), bongo (Fig. 28.17)
        Subfamily Cephalophinae: duiker (Fig. 28.18)
        Subfamily Hippotraginae: waterbuck, oryx (Fig. 28.19), kob
        Subfamily Alcelaphinae: gnu (Fig. 28.20), hartebeest
        Subfamily Antilopinae: gazelle, impala, klipspringer (Fig. 28.21)
        Subfamily Caprinae: Rocky Mountain goat (Fig. 28.22), ibex (Fig. 28.23), and aoudad (Fig. 28.24)

Deer, Elk, Moose

DANGER POTENTIAL. Small members of these groups bite. The enlarged canine teeth, protruding from the mouth as tusks, are formidable and must be reckoned with during restraint. Other cervids seldom bite. The primary weapons of most cervids are the antlers, used both in display and as weapons. All members of this group strike with their front feet and are capable of inflicting serious wounds with the sharp hoofs.

through a chute or put into a squeeze cage to make examinations, give injections, or obtain laboratory samples. Blood samples may be collected from the femoral vein (Fig. 28.15) or the precava as in domestic swine.

CHEMICAL RESTRAINT.[11,27,34,50] The chemical restraint agents and combinations mentioned in this chapter represent those used by the author or experienced veterinarians with detailed knowledge of hoofstock. Other protocols have been used, and no claim is made for including all possible drugs and combinations. For more detailed information, particularly for anesthesia, consult the references.

Table 28.3 provides the dosage of drugs used to sedate and chemically immobilize suids. When administering drugs intramuscularly, try to avoid intra-fat injections by selecting a needle long enough to penetrate to the muscle underlying the fat layer.

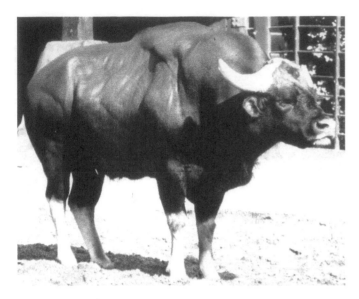

FIG. 28.16. Gaur, *Bos gaurus*.

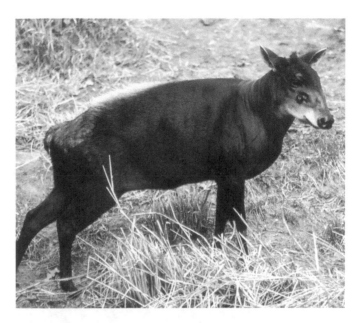

FIG. 28.18. Yellow-backed duiker, *Cephalophus* sp.

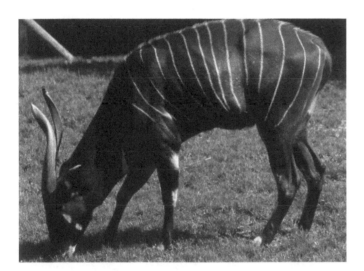

FIG. 28.17. Bongo, *Tragelaphus euryceros*.

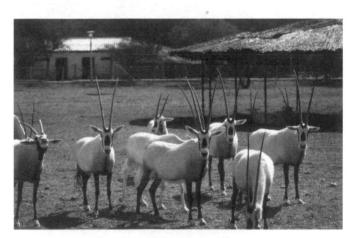

FIG. 28.19. Arabian oryx, *Oryx leucoryx*.

ANATOMY AND PHYSIOLOGY. Antlers are normally shed and regrown annually. They are specialized bony protuberances stemming from a pedicle on the poll. As antlers develop, they are covered by a highly vascularized velvet. During this period of time, the bone is relatively soft and easily broken. Velveted antlers should not be grasped during restraint. An antler fractured while in velvet will bleed profusely. When the antler matures, the velvet dries and is rubbed off until the antler is highly polished. At this point, the rut begins and the animal becomes more aggressive.

A rutting animal is dangerous not only to other cervids but also to keepers who must enter the enclosure. It may be necessary to amputate the antlers of a rutting buck. Leave approximately 4–6 in. of the stump on the skull for a fulcrum against which the animal can rub to remove the base. If it is cut too far distally, the purpose of removing the antler is

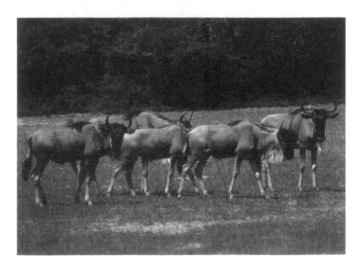

FIG. 28.20. Gnu (wildebeest), *Connochaetus* sp.

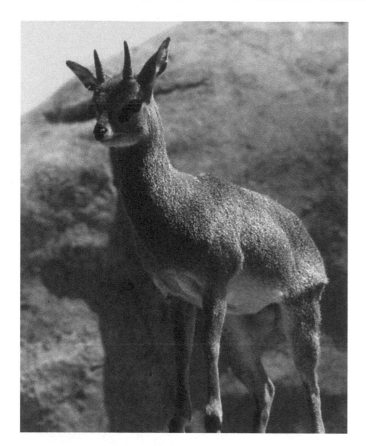

FIG. 28.21.   Klipspringer, *Oreotragus oreotragus.*

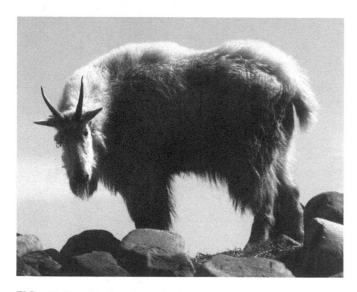

FIG. 28.22.   Rocky Mountain goat.

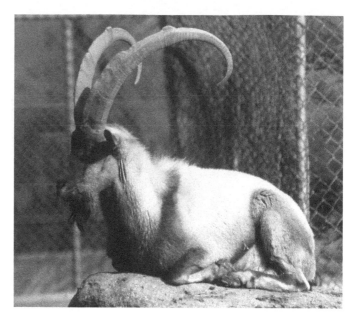

FIG. 28.23.   Ibex, *Capra ibex.*

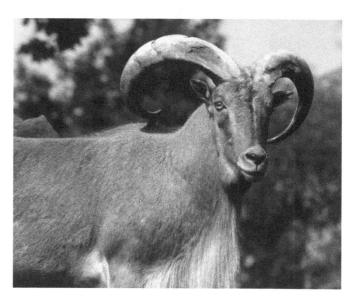

FIG. 28.24.   Aoudad, *Ammotragus lervia.*

defeated; if it is cut too close to the head, the stag will fail to shed the small scur, causing abnormal antler growth around the scur the next year. Antlers are limited to the male of the species except for caribou (reindeer), in which both sexes grow antlers.

Reindeer have been domesticated and utilized for milk and meat in the northern latitudes for many centuries. Their wild counterpart, the caribou, is a relatively calm, phlegmatic animal and can be handled manually. Caribou may be held by the antlers or placed in crates or squeeze cages for manipulation.

Physical Restraint[31,32]

Special chutes may be constructed for handling free-ranging, farm, or ranch-raised cervids.[36,37] The designs employed are nearly as numerous as the managers/owners who build them. Some are elaborate and fully enclosed for all-weather working of the animals. North American managers have copied from their counterparts in New Zealand and Australia, who have more experience in game ranching.

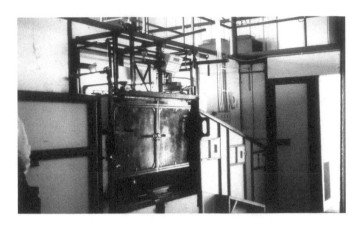

FIG. 28.25. Hydraulically operated, drop-floor chute for handling large numbers of farmed deer.

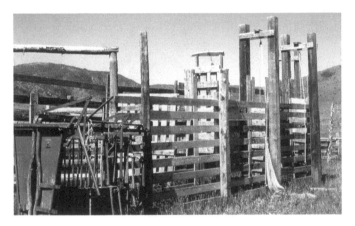

FIG. 28.26. Commercial cattle chute modified to accommodate wapiti (elk). *Cervus elaphus canadensis.*

Hydraulically operated squeeze chutes may be incorporated into the system (Fig. 28.25).

Figure 28.26 illustrates a chute arrangement used to handle elk (*Cervus elaphus canadensis*) that congregate at the same location year after year during the winter months. Either cow elk or de-antlered bulls may be herded into the chute area and gradually moved into a funnel-shaped arrangement that leads to a narrow channel, admitting animals to the chute in single file. A circular chute arrangement is also used (Fig. 28.27). The animals are herded to the periphery of the corral to begin their movement through the funnel. The sides of the enclosure and chute should be high. The inside of the chute should be smooth, covered with plywood or a similar material so animals cannot gain a footing to climb the walls. As the animals progress along the channel, doors can be closed at intervals to separate individuals. A special cattle chute is placed at the end of the channel. A loading ramp leading from an enclosed sorting facility is illustrated in Figure 28.28.

Temporary, but still elaborate, facilities may be located in a strategic site where free-ranging elk may be herded by helicopter to enter an extended funnel (Fig. 28.29). Once contained in the central holding area, the elk may be moved

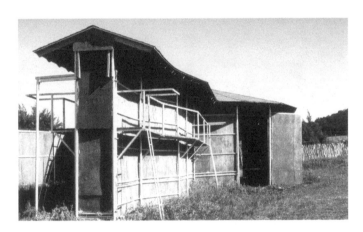

FIG. 28.28. Loading facility for handling hoofed stock.

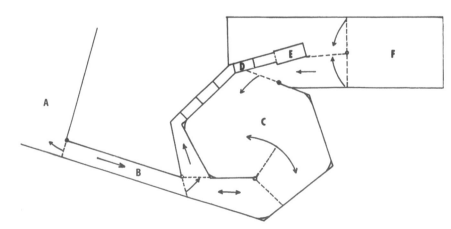

FIG. 28.27. Diagram of a holding area and approach to a chute for handling hoofed animals. **A.** general enclosure; **B.** alley to chute area; **C.** inner court; **D.** compartmentalized chute area; **E.** squeeze chute; **F.** release area.

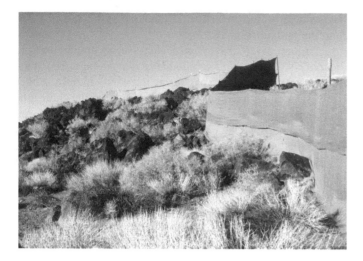

FIG. 28.29. Wing of a funnel to direct elk into a central area with a helicopter.

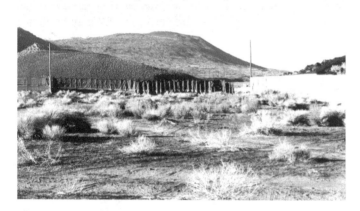

FIG. 28.30. View across a central area toward a liftable fence. When the elk are driven into the central area the fence is down, giving the elk the feeling that they are able to escape. As soon as the elk are in the central area the fence is lifted and the gate behind them is closed.

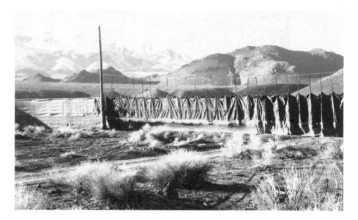

FIG. 28.31. The fence is lifted into place remotely.

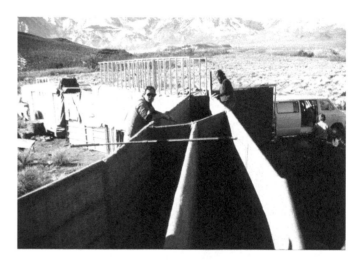

FIG. 28.32. The elk are then directed into chutes where they can be handled and loaded into trucks or trailers.

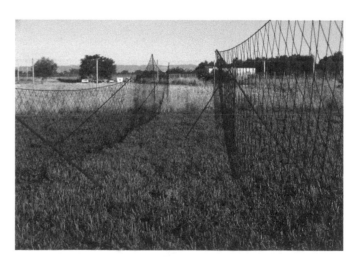

FIG. 28.33. Collapsible net for capturing deer.

through a series of gates into alleyways and a squeeze chute to collect samples or perform other diagnostic procedures, or they may be shifted to a loading ramp and moved into a truck or trailer for translocation to another area (Figs. 28.29 to 28.32).

Smaller cervids have been captured by driving them into a collapsible net, after which they are physically restrained or chemically immobilized (Fig. 28.33). An alternative net capture technique is to lay the net in a path that is likely to be traveled by a group of animals. One end of the net should be anchored to a fence or tree, and the other end held by one of the handlers. As the animals are carefully hazed to pass over the collapsed net, the selected individual is watched. As it approaches the net, the handler jerks the net taut, and the animal will run into the net. As soon as the animal becomes

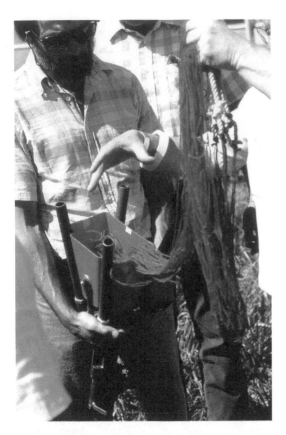

FIG. 28.34.   Loading a net into the canister.

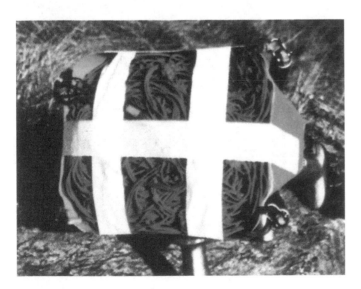

FIG. 28.35.   Net gun loaded.

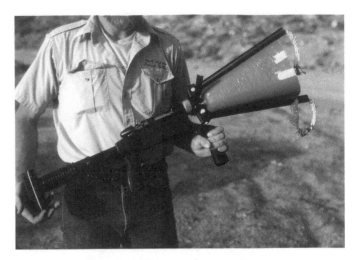

FIG. 28.36.   Net gun loaded and ready to fire.

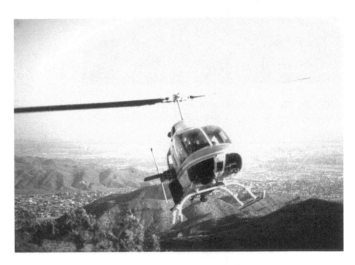

FIG. 28.37.   Net gun ready to be fired from a helicopter.

entangled, the handlers can subdue it by grasping the front and hind legs and stretching it.

Special devices have been designed to project a net over an animal (Figs. 28.34, 28.35, 28.36). Loaded weights are attached to the corners of the net, and charges propel the weights outward. The device may be fired from the ground, from a helicopter (Fig. 28.37), or from the skid of a snowmobile.

The polished antlers may be used as leverage for restraint if the handler is strong enough to hold the animal. When cervid antlers are in velvet, this procedure is not suitable because the antlers are sensitive, highly vascular, and easily fractured. Antlered animals may require chemical immobilization for restraint.

Small cervids without antlers may be handled manually. Figure 28.38 illustrates one method of holding a small mule deer (*Odocoileus hemionus*). When grasped in this position, the animal will usually relax, entering a trancelike state. If additional restraint is required, the animal may be placed in lateral recumbency and held as shown in Figure 28.39, or it may be held with the forelimbs brought up behind the head and the hind legs stretched out. Sometimes several people are needed to restrain a cervid. Padding beneath the animal prevents trauma.

TRANSPORT.   Moving large immobilized cervids such as elk and moose is a major project. The same procedures

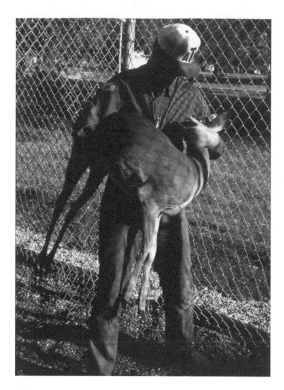

FIG. 28.38. Restraint of a small mule deer, *Odocoileus hemionus*. Legs are directed away from handler.

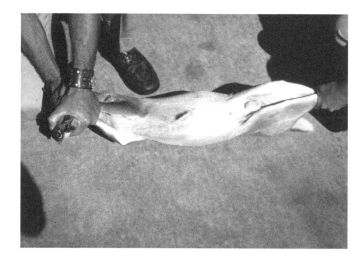

FIG. 28.39. Stretching and holding a muntjac deer, *Muntiacus muntjak*, in lateral recumbency.

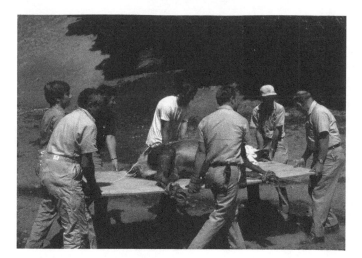

FIG. 28.40. Chemically immobilized wapiti lashed to sheet of plywood.

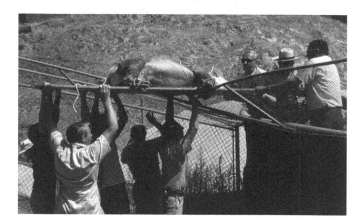

FIG. 28.41. Plywood stretcher being lifted out of a moated enclosure.

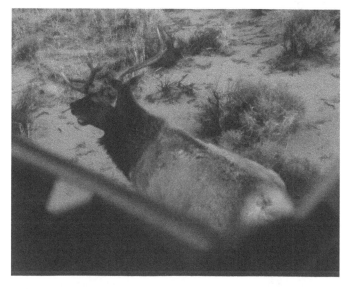

FIG. 28.42. Immobilizing a bull elk from a helicopter.

described for camelids are appropriate. (See Chapter 14, Camelids.) Figure 28.40 shows an immobilized wapiti secured to a plywood sheet. The animal was then lifted out of a moated enclosure (Fig. 28.41).

Figures 28.42 to 28.45 illustrate the handling of a bull elk from immobilization to reaching a staging area.

Individual crates are usually used to transport cervids. Cervids may be loaded into crates and lifted into trucks or trailers if appropriate facilities are available in the zoo. A

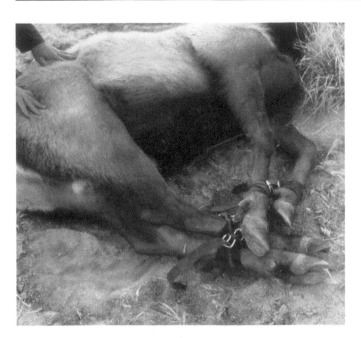

FIG. 28.43. Hobbling an elk preparatory to lifting in a sling.

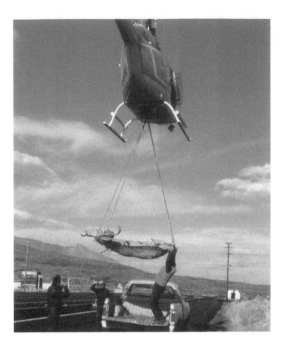

FIG. 28.45. Moving an elk to a waiting vehicle.

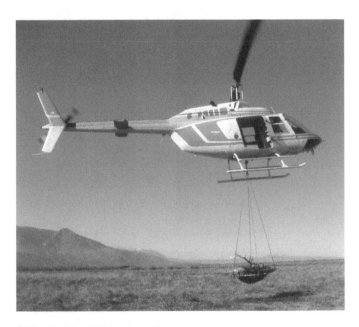

FIG. 28.44. Lifting in a sling.

group of animals may be shipped together in a truck if sizes and sexes are segregated.

CHEMICAL RESTRAINT.[12,14,18–22,28–31,33,44,46–48,52,55] Numerous drugs have been employed for sedation and immobilization of cervids (Table 28.4). When immobilizing or physically restraining cervids, it is desirable to diminish visual sensations by blindfolding. A combination of butorphanol, azaperone, and medetomidine (BAM, Wildlife Pharmaceuticals, Fort Collins, Colorado) has been found to be a safe and effective immobilizing cocktail for use in cervids. A stock solution

TABLE 28.4. Selected chemical restraint agents for cervid immobilization[12,14]

Agent	Dosage for immobilization (mg/kg)
Xylazine/tiletamine/zolazepam*	1.0–3.0/2.0–3.0
Medetomidine/ketamine	0.1–0.2/2.5
Thiafentanil	0.05–0.1
Butorphanol/azaperone/medetomidine**	See discussion

* Telazol.
** BAM.

is made by mixing 28.0 mg of butorphanol, 18.0 mg of azaperone, and 11.0 mg of medetomidine per 1.0 ml of the solution. The dosage for North American mule and white-tailed deer is 1.0 ml of the combined ingredients per 45.4 kg (100 lb) of animal IM.

The intranasal administration of xylazine at a dose of 1.5–2.0 mg/kg has been used to provide rapid and effective sedation for deer and sheep that have been physically captured in a net.[14]

Free-ranging bull elk may be chemically immobilized by darting them from a helicopter. While immobilized, the animal may be secured on a special sling and airlifted by helicopter to a staging area or an awaiting vehicle.

Cattle-type Animals, Antelope, Sheep, Goat, Pronghorn

DANGER POTENTIAL. Horns are formidable weapons possessed by many members of the Bovidae family. They are found on both sexes, but males have larger horns and are usually more likely to fight than females. The horns may be massive structures such as those of the bighorn sheep or African buffalo or fine and fragile, or any gradation between.

The horns may be used strictly for display or continually in mock or serious battle.

In addition to the horns, many members of this family have sharp hoofs. Wild species are particularly likely to lash out with the feet and may cause fractures or other severe injuries with a kick.

ANATOMY AND PHYSIOLOGY. Horns are modified epidermal structures consisting of a cornified outer layer covering a bony core. Horns are permanent, not shed annually like antlers. They are used for display and fighting and in some species function in a thermoregulatory capacity. The horns of some species may be grasped as handles for controlling the head. Horns are easily damaged during restraint, particularly those of young animals in which the bony core has not yet permanently fused to the skull.

BEHAVIOR. There are widely separated extremes of behavior within this group—from docile animals, such as some of the sheep that are rarely aggressive, to fierce animals like the gnu, which may attack without provocation.

Introducing a new animal into an established hoofed stock exhibit is dangerous and must be done gradually and carefully. These animals form social groups with hierarchical status. The newly introduced animal is likely to be aggressively harassed. To prevent harassment, the animal should first be released into a small box stall or pen near the other animals, permitting them to become acquainted as they nose each other over gates or through fences. Adequate sight and physical barriers should be provided within the enclosure to allow the new animal to find a refuge.

PHYSICAL RESTRAINT.[5,26,49,51] Smaller members of this family may be manually restrained. The animals should be restricted to a small enclosure, grasped, and the legs stretched and held. Ropes are sometimes used to capture these animals. Once the animal is caught, assistants must quickly grasp the animal, lest it jump toward the roper or injure itself by struggling. A tarp or blanket may prevent injury from flailing feet. Sufficient restraint is usually achieved by grasping both front and hind feet, controlling the head at the same time.

Fences adequate to contain quiet hoofed animals may not prevent excited animals from jumping out of an enclosure. Furthermore, when frightened, some hoofed animals may actually climb fences—an act they would probably not attempt if undisturbed. The escape response is intense in these animals, and they will extend themselves to achieve escape in manners beyond general comprehension. I have seen a bison jump or climb a 2.5-m (8-ft) chain-link fence to escape capture.

When individuals must be captured from herds of ungulates, it is desirable to restrict the herd to a small enclosure such as a box stall before beginning capture operations. Sometimes it is necessary to construct such a confining area out of plywood sheeting and temporary poles. Even temporary construction should be substantial, because the animals will likely bump against it or charge it; if it is flimsy, it

will break and cause more serious injuries than may be imagined.

Once an animal group is inside a shed or a small enclosure, rope loops may be tossed onto the heads of selected individuals so they can be dragged out and grasped without alarming others of the herd. I have handled mouflon and aoudad sheep on numerous occasions in this manner without serious injury to animals or staff.

Nets are used to handle a wide variety of hoofed animals; even the lordly musk ox can be captured with a heavy cargo net.

Most wild bovids will flee on the approach of a person. However, some species such as the gnu, particularly the males, may become aggressive when approached. When cornered and unable to escape, many otherwise docile animals turn and attack. Plywood shields offer some protection to the person who must enter an enclosure to direct a single animal into another area (Figs. 28.46, 28.47). Metal or wooden

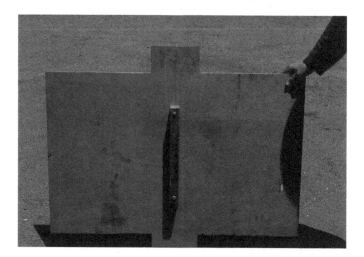

FIG. 28.46.   Plywood shield with handhold on the back.

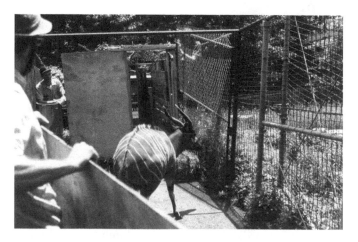

FIG. 28.47.   Bongo being directed into a trailer with plywood shields. Individuals within a species vary greatly as to the degree they will tolerate such manipulation.

handles may be attached to the reverse side of the shield for either one or two men to grasp. Shields may be attached to the front of a vehicle if the pen is large enough to allow the operation of a tractor, a skip loader, a truck, or other motorized equipment. If any young animals are in the herd, they should be captured quickly, or the large rams should be removed as rapidly as possible.

Squeeze cages and chutes have been designed for use with hoofed animals. Figure 28.48 shows a squeeze cage used at a California zoo. It is adjustable to fit a wide variety of hoofed animals. Extreme caution must be used when putting horned animals into such a device. In many instances, it is wiser to use chemical immobilization on these to preclude possible injury to the horns.

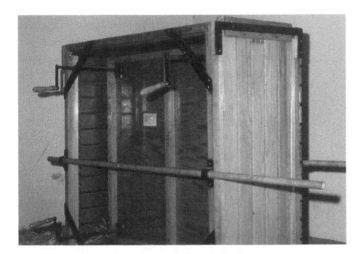

FIG. 28.48. An excellent portable squeeze chute and transfer crate for hoofed animals.

Occasionally tuberculin testing programs or other activities necessitate the handling of large numbers of hoofed stock. Chutes may be improvised. Railroad ties or other timbers can be sunk into the ground and plywood sheeting applied to the inside, forming a chute. The inside of the chute must be smooth to prevent animals from gaining a foothold to climb out.

In one instance a chute built to handle bison was unsatisfactory because the animals were able to catch their hoofs in the planking on the inside of the 8-foot chute and climb out. When the inside planking was covered with plywood, climbing was minimized. Some of the bison tore off the outer shell of the horn by rubbing their heads up and down against the inside of the chute. Fortunately the horny shells grew back within a few months. However, the shape of the damaged horn was not as symmetrical as the original.

Confining animals in close quarters stimulates aggressive tendencies, and the animals may fight. Time spent on any procedure requiring close confinement should be kept to a minimum.

Attempting to drive animals into a chute area or box stall or enclosed pen is a frustrating experience. The animals sense a change and are not easily herded into a new enclosure.

Sheep will follow a leader, and it may be possible to rope the dominant animal and pull it into the enclosure. The other animals will then follow it in. A usually successful technique is to feed the animals inside the restraining enclosure for a few days before the procedure is scheduled. Plastic sheeting has been an important contribution to the art of persuading animals to enter a new area.

Most ungulates are diurnal and have limited night vision. If these animals can be confined inside a darkened stall, it is often possible for a keeper or handler to enter such an enclosure, grab a selected individual, and carry it outside without alarming the group. Obviously this may be dangerous if the group includes horned individuals.

If animals in a darkened stall or enclosure can be shifted into a darkened funnel leading into a chute arrangement with doors that can be closed behind each individual, animals of hoofed species can be handled more easily and with little stress.

Commercial cattle chutes may be modified to use with some wild species (Figs. 28.49, 28.50, 28.51). Musk oxen or other cattle-type wild animals may be directed through alleyways into one of the squeeze chutes. Commercial chutes frequently must be modified (e.g., lined with plywood) to prevent wild animals from climbing up the inside.

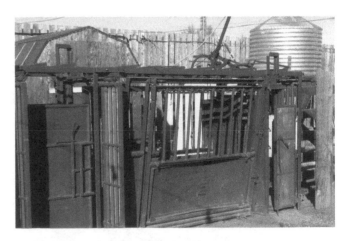

FIG. 28.49. Custom-designed squeeze chute for handling farmed musk oxen.

Use only those chutes that permit the animal to move its head down if it falls or throws itself in the chute. Chutes must open from the front to allow aid to be given to an animal that falls. The upright posts of the front gate may be padded to minimize trauma to the shoulders of the animal if it lunges against the semi-opened gate to escape.

Many wild animal facilities now have built-in chutes or semi-squeeze cages to assist in the management of bovids.

Most people who have dealt with a large variety of hoofed animals have used rope as a tool of restraint. Although proficiency with a rope may be an invaluable asset, it must be recognized that rope is of limited value for capturing most wild ungulates. The commotion generated by swinging or

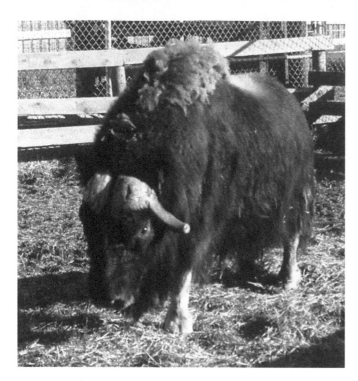

FIG. 28.50. Musk ox, *Ovibos moschatus*.

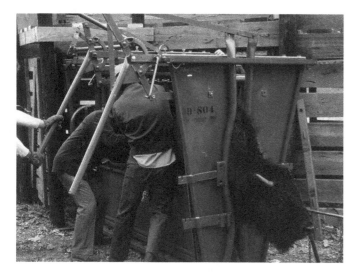

FIG. 28.51. Bison cow, *Bison bison*, being handled in a cattle chute.

tossing the rope is much more threatening than the typical wild ungulate can tolerate. It will usually bolt and run headlong and may injure itself.

Several factors should be kept in mind when using ropes on wild ungulates:

1. Consider the general temperament of the animal. The extremely nervous, flighty gazelle and antelope species are likely to be injured during such a capture operation. Wild sheep, on the other hand, frequently may be caught with a rope if necessary.

2. Decide how to control the animal immediately after capture. Many a roper has gloated over a successful catch, only to find the captured animal to be uncontrollable. Instead of the typical pullback response exhibited by a domestic cow, sheep, or goat, many wild animals attack the roper or lunge wildly in every direction, making it impossible to grasp the animal. This is particularly dangerous with animals that have heavy or sharp horns. If roping is used to capture these animals, a dally post is needed to restrict the animal's subsequent activity; otherwise, assistants attempting to grasp the animal may be injured. Large species such as bison, yak, or water buffalo are so strong that even two or three people may be unable to slow or stop them sufficiently to take a dally around a post or a tree. More phlegmatic bovid species such as the yak usually may be roped by the horns, tied or dallied to a post, and pulled into lateral recumbency by another rope tied to the hind legs.

3. Consider whether or not the rope can be quickly released after the manipulation has been completed. Ropes equipped with quick-release hondas may be used, but they lack balance for throwing and are not likely to be the rope of choice for such operations. It may be necessary to tie a small rope to the honda of the lariat so the lariat can be easily pulled free when the animal is released. Keep in mind that the animal may be highly agitated and apt to attack the handlers as it is released. Be sure handlers are protected when working with ropes on wild animals. Keep a sharp knife readily available at all times to cut the rope. Unforeseen circumstances frequently develop that necessitate quick release of an animal.

Even a skilled calf roper may be humiliated when attempting to rope an antelope. The speed and dodging ability of antelope is phenomenal. Tossing a loop is not a usable approach except in a massed group of animals. This technique is simply not fast enough to ensnare an animal that can jump and dodge as rapidly as an antelope. A swing toss must be used. One must use a small loop and give ample lead to the animal; otherwise it will jump completely through or past the loop.

Any roping operation carried out in the midst of a group of animals is fraught with danger to both roper and animal. The normal flight response sends animals jumping and scurrying here and there throughout the pen or enclosure. The heights to which frightened animals can jump is astounding. I have seen mouflon sheep standing 62.5 cm high at the shoulder jump over the head of an adult man. The behavior of excited and/or cornered animals is totally unpredictable. If sufficient numbers of animals are panicked, they may run over or jump on the roper.

On one occasion when roping mouflon sheep, one ewe attempted to jump over an assistant. The ewe did not quite make it and placed all four feet on the person's forehead to ricochet. Needless to say, this was rather traumatic to the individual involved.

Hoofed animals that have been in captivity for a long time have not been able to maintain their wild athletic condition. When they become excited and run around the pen as a roper attempts to capture one of them, great harm can be done. The animals may overheat or become exhausted. They may injure themselves or others by jumping on top of one another, especially when there are young members in the herd. The young are particularly subject to trampling and exhaustion. I have seen animals drop from exhaustion during such maneuvers and die from pulmonary edema brought on by severe exertion. Such chases may also be the inciting cause for capture myopathy. (See Chapter 9.)

When shipping horned animals, protect the horns from trauma. The heavy horns of animals like buffalo or eland may shred the inside of a crate. Pieces of hose applied to the tip of the horn can prevent this (Fig. 28.52). Tape the hose onto the horns, bending the tip of the hose over and taping it to protect the tip of the horn and the inside of the crate. Hose applied to an overly aggressive animal will also protect others from injury. Rubber balls were placed on the tips of the horns of an exceptionally aggressive saiga antelope male to prevent him from traumatizing cage-mates (Fig. 28.53).

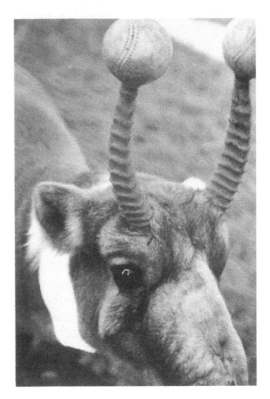

FIG. 28.53. Rubber balls placed on horns prevent aggressive saiga antelope, *Saiga tataric*, from goring pen-mates.

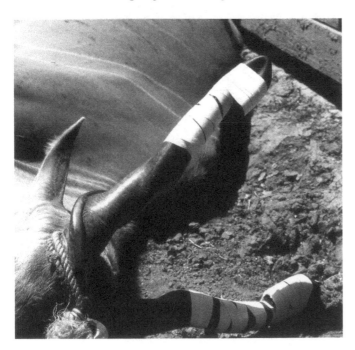

FIG. 28.52. An eland ready for crating. Horns are protected by placing rubber hosing over the tips.

It may be necessary to dehorn or tip the horns of extremely and continuously aggressive animals. The horns of most species can be tipped without causing significant hemorrhage if no more than 1 or 2 in. of the sharp point is removed. Removing more than this will cut the bony core, causing hemorrhage. Cauterizing will stop hemorrhage. Complete dehorning is a surgical procedure that requires anesthesia and hemorrhage control. Dehorning an adult animal will open the cornual sinus, requiring special care to prevent infection and/or fly infestation.

CHEMICAL RESTRAINT.[3,9,10,13,15–17,23–26,35–41,43,45,56,57] Numerous chemical restraint agents have been employed, either singly or in combinations, for immobilizing wild ruminants. The dosage regimens reported vary markedly. No attempt is made by the author to list all the regimens used. When faced with an unfamiliar situation or species, the reader should consult the references[15,23,44,56], a zoo veterinarian, or wildlife researcher with recent experiences in dealing with that particular species to ascertain current recommendation. Under field conditions, response to a drug or combination of drugs and dosage may be highly variable depending on the ambient temperature, humidity, body condition of the animal(s), nutritional status, and whether darting from a blind versus a vehicle or helicopter chase. A few drugs and dosages are listed in Tables 28.5 to 28.7.

All precautions mentioned for other species are applicable. It is important to fast an adult ruminant for 36–48 hours and restrict water intake for 12 hours before beginning elective procedures, to minimize the risk of regurgitation. Other precautions are illustrated in Figures 28.54 to 28.57.

Proper positioning following immobilization is important to prevent passive regurgitation (Fig. 28.58). Keep the

TABLE 28.5. Selected tranquilizers (standing sedation) for hoofed stock[17,23,24]

Agent	Dose (mg/kg)	Induction/duration of sedation
Azaperone	0.5–2.0	15.0–30.0/3.0–6.0 hours
Haloperidol	0.05–0.1	3.0–4.0 Min/16.0 hours
Perphenazine enanthate	0.4–1.2	1.0–6.0 hours/7.0–10.0 days

TABLE 28.6. Selected chemical restraint agents for ruminant type animals (yak, gaur, banteng, bongo, African buffalo)[17]

Agent	Immobilization dose (mg/kg)
Cattle type (yak, gaur, bongo, African buffalo)	
Etorphine/xylazine	0.012–0.038/0.1–0.7
Carfentanil/xylazine	0.01–0.03/0.05–0.25
Thiafentanil/xylazine	0.011–0.018/0.05–0.25
Medetomidine/ketamine	0.025–0.1/0.05–3.0
African antelope (impala, eland, gnu)	
Medetomidine/tiletamine/zolazepam	0.1/1.0
Etorphine/azaperone	Adult male impala
	4.0–5.0/100.0 mg TD
	Adult female impala
	3.0–5.0/100.0 mg TD
	Adult male eland
	10.0–12.0/180.0–200.0 mg TD
	Adult female eland
	6.0–8.0/180.0–200.0 mg TD
Gazelles	
Carfentanil/xylazine	0.02/0.2–0.5
Ketamine/medetomidine	4.0/0.05
Tiletamine/zolazepam	2.0–4.0
Medetomidine/ketamine/butorphanol	0.04–0.07/2.0–4.0/0.02–0.04

TD = total dose.

TABLE 28.7. Selected chemical restraint agents for wild sheep and goats[13,42]

Agents	Dose
Etorphine/acepromazine	2.5–4.0/10.0 mg TD IM
Carfentanil/xylazine	0.044/0.2 mg/kg IM
Carfentanil	0.035 mg/kg IM
Ketamine/medetomidine	1.5–2.0/0.06–0.08 mg/kg

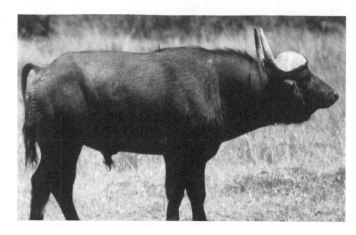

FIG. 28.55. Cape Buffalo, *Syncerus caffer*.

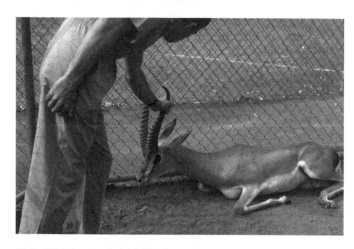

FIG. 28.56. An immobilized antelope must be approached slowly and steadily, with as little noise as possible and no sudden or jerky movement.

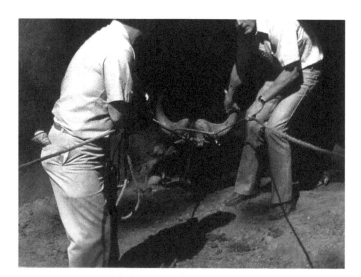

FIG. 28.54. Immobilized African buffalo being moved to a shipping crate.

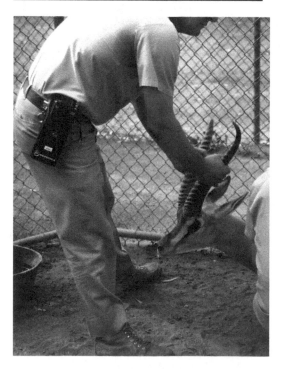

FIG. 28.57. Controlling the head while working on partially immobilized ungulate.

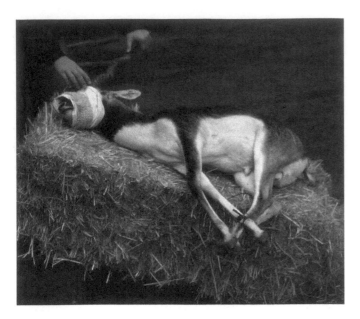

FIG. 28.58. Moving a black buck, *Antilope cervicapra*. Visual stimulation is blocked and head is elevated to reduce chances of regurgitation.

neck straight with the head elevated and on the right side if possible.

It is usually not recommended to use xylazine alone for immobilization. An eland may appear to be sedated, but is easily aroused and any manipulation of the legs will result in a swift kick response (Fig. 28.59).

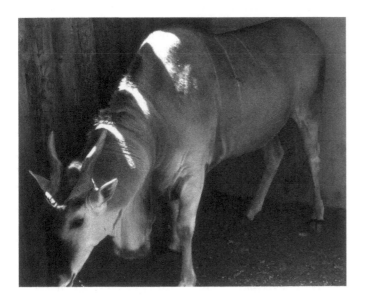

FIG. 28.59. An eland under partial sedation with xylazine.

Caprinids (goats, goat-like animals and sheep) may require chemical immobilization, but the capture of multiple individuals is usually accomplished using nets of various types. Figures 28.60 and 28.61 illustrate a drop net erected to entice bighorn sheep (*Ovis canadensis*) under a net by baiting

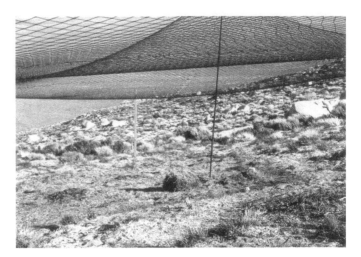

FIG. 28.60. A baited drop net for bighorn sheep, *Ovis canadensis*.

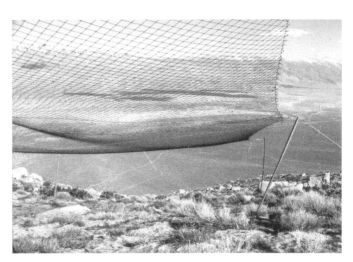

FIG. 28.61. Guy ties containing a charge that severs the rope, allowing the net to fall.

them with apple pumice or alfalfa hay. Once a group congregates under the net, a person observing from a remote location detonates charges that drop the net onto the sheep. Then handlers physically extract the animals from beneath the net and either physically restrain them or administer an immobilizing agent.

A drive net may be used to capture bighorn sheep that are driven over a pass by helicopter (Figs. 28.62 to 28.65). The collapsible net is placed in a location frequently used by the sheep. Handlers are secreted at the ends of the net. A helicopter slowly drives a herd toward the pass and then speeds up as they come near the net. As the sheep hit the net, it collapses and handlers rush in to do whatever is necessary.

CHEMICAL RESTRAINT.[11,28–30,34–36] See Table 28.7 for restraint agents used for sheep and goats.

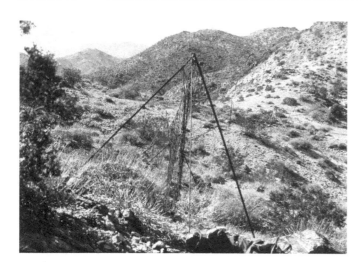

FIG. 28.62. Net placed at a pass.

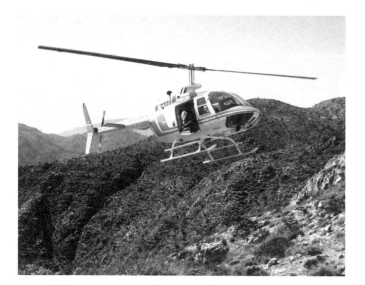

FIG. 28.63. A helicopter brings a herd to the net.

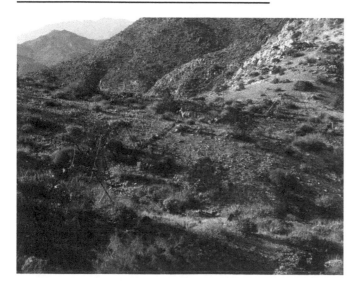

FIG. 28.64. The sheep don't perceive the net as a barrier and rush into it.

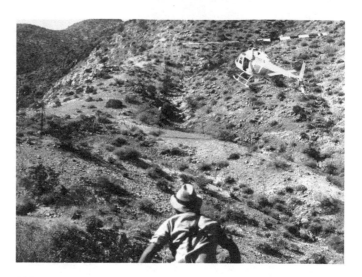

FIG. 28.65. Handlers rush out to restrain the sheep before they are able extricate themselves from the net.

REFERENCES

1. Allen, J.L. 1989. Renarcotization following carfentanil immobilization of nondomestic ungulates. J Zoo Wildl Med 20:423–26.
2. Anonymous. 2007. Live Animal Regulations, 34th Ed., Montreal, International Air Transport Association.
3. Ball, R.L. 2007. Antelope. In: West, G., Heard, D., and Caulkett, N., Eds. Zoo Animal and Wildlife Immobilization and Anesthesia, Ames, Iowa, Blackwell Publishing, pp. 613–21.
4. Bengis, R. 1993. Hand capture of impala. In: McKenzie, A.A., Ed. The Capture and Care Manual, Pretoria: The South African Veterinary Foundation, pp. 404–06.
5. Bengis, R. 1993. Chemical capture of the African buffalo. In: McKenzie, A.A., Ed. The Capture and Care Manual, Pretoria: The South African Veterinary Foundation, pp. 583–89.
6. Blumer, E.S. 1991. A review of the use of selected neuroleptic drugs in the management of nondomestic hoofstock. Proceeding Amer Assoc Zoo Vet, Calgary, Canada, pp. 333–39.
7. Burroughs, R.E.J. 1993. Principles of darting antelope and other herbivores. In: McKenzie, A.A., Ed. The Capture and Care Manual, Pretoria: The South African Veterinary Foundation, pp. 131–37.
8. Burroughs, R.E.J. 1993. A summary of the practical aspects of drugs commonly used for the restraint of wild animals. In: McKenzie, A.A. Ed. The Capture and Care Manual, Pretoria: The South African Veterinary Foundation, pp. 65–70.
9. Burroughs, R.E.J. 1993. Chemical capture of antelope. In: McKenzie, A.A., Ed. The Capture and Care Manual, Pretoria: The South African Veterinary Foundation, pp. 348–80.
10. Burroughs, R.E.J., and McKenzie, A.A. 1993. Handling, care, and loading of immobilized herbivores. In: McKenzie, A.A., Ed. The Capture and Care Manual, Pretoria: The South African Veterinary Foundation, pp. 184–92.
11. Burroughs, R.E.J. 1993. Chemical capture of the warthog. In: McKenzie, A.A., Ed. The Capture and Care Manual, Pretoria: The South African Veterinary Foundation, pp. 621–22.
12. Caulkett, N., and Haigh, J.C. 2004. Anesthesia of North American deer. Ithaca, New York, International Veterinary Information Service (www.ivis.org).

13. Caulkett, N., and Haigh, J.C. 2007. Wild sheep and goats. In: West, G., Heard, D., and Caulkett, N., Eds. Zoo Animal and Wildlife Immobilization and Anesthesia, Ames, Iowa, Blackwell Publishing, pp. 629–33.

14. Caulkett, N., and Haigh, J.C. 2007. Deer (Cervids). In: West, G., Heard, D., and Caulkett, N., Eds. Zoo Animal and Wildlife Immobilization and Anesthesia, Ames, Iowa, Blackwell Publishing, pp. 607–12.

15. Caulkett, N., and Haigh, J.C. 2007. Bison. In: West, G., Heard, D., and Caulkett, N., Eds. Zoo Animal and Wildlife Immobilization and Anesthesia, Ames, Iowa, Blackwell Publishing, pp. 643–46.

16. Clausen, B., Hjort, P., Strandgaard, H., and Soerensen, P.L. 1984. Immobilization and tagging of muskoxen in Jaameson Land, Northeastern Greenland. J Wildl Dis 20:141–45.

17. Curro, T.G. 2007. Non-domestic cattle. In: West, G., Heard, D., and Caulkett, N., Eds. Zoo Animal and Wildlife Immobilization and Anesthesia, Ames, Iowa, Blackwell Publishing, pp. 635–42.

18. DeGiudice, G.D., Seal, U.S., and Kreeger, T.J. 1988. Xylazine and ketamine-induced glycosuria in white-tailed deer. J Wildl Dis 24:317–21.

19. Del Giudice, G.D., Krausman, P.R., Bellantoni, E.E., Etchberger, R.C., and Seal, U.S. 1989. Reversal by tolazoline hydrochloride of xylazine hydrochloride/ketamine hydrochloride immobilizations in free-ranging desert mule deer. J Wildl Dis 25:347–52.

20. Dew, T.L. 1988. Use of tolazoline hydrochloride to reverse multiple anesthetic episodes induced with xylazine hydrochloride and ketamine hydrochloride in white-tailed deer and goats. J Zoo Wildl Med 19:8–13.

21. Dieterich, R.A. 1993. Medical aspects of reindeer farming. In: Fowler, M.E., Ed. Zoo and Wild Animal Medicine, 3rd ed., Philadelphia: W.B. Saunders, pp. 123–28.

22. Doherty, T.J., and Tweedie, D.P.R. 1989. Evaluation of xylazine hydrochloride as the sole immobilizing agent in moose and caribou—and its subsequent reversal with idazoxan. J Wildl Dis 25:95–98.

23. Ebedes, H. 1993. The use of long-acting tranquilizers in captive wild animals. In: McKenzie, A.A., Ed. The Capture and Care Manual, Pretoria: The South African Veterinary Foundation, pp. 65–70.

23. Ebedes, H., and Raath, J.P. 1999. Use of tranquilizers in wild herbivores. In: Fowler, M.E., and Miller, R.E., Eds. Zoo and Wild Animal Medicine-Current Vet. Therapy, 4th Ed. Philadelphia, W.B. Saunders, pp. 575–84.

25. Espie, I. 1993. Transportation of the warthog. In: McKenzie, A.A., Ed. The Capture and Care Manual, Pretoria: The South African Veterinary Foundation, p. 623.

26. Flamand, J.R.B. 1999. Medical aspects of Arabian oryx reintroduction. In: Fowler, M.E., and Miller, R.E., Eds. Zoo and Wild Animal Medicine-Current Vet. Therapy, 4th Ed. Philadelphia, W.B. Saunders, pp. 687–90.

27. Fowler, M.E. 1993. Wild swine and peccaries. In: Fowler, M.E., Ed. Zoo and Wild Animal Medicine, 3rd ed., Philadelphia: W.B. Saunders, pp. 513–21.

28. Gibson, D.F., Scanlon, P.F., and Warren, R.J. 1982. Xylazine hydrochloride for immobilizing captive white-tailed deer. Zoo Biol 1:311–22.

29. Green, M.J.B. 1986. Immobilization of Himalayan musk deer in captivity using ketamine and xylazine. J Zoo An Med 17:56–58.

30. Haigh, J.C., and Hudson, R.J. 1991. Farming Wapiti and Red Deer in North America, Saint Louis, Ill., C.V. Mosbey.

31. Haigh, J.C. 1993. Game farming with emphasis on North America. In: Fowler, M.E., Ed. Zoo and Wild Animal Medicine, 3rd ed., Philadelphia: W.B. Saunders, pp. 87–101.

32. Haigh, J.C. 1999. The use of chutes for ungulate restraint. In: Fowler, M.E., Ed. Zoo and Wild Animal Medicine, 4th Ed., Philadelphia: W.B. Saunders, pp. 657–62.

33. Hastings, B.E., Stadler, S.G., and Kock, R.A. 1989. Reversible immobilization of Chinese water deer with ketamine and xylazine. J Zoo Wildl Med 20:427–31.

34. Hellgren, E.C., Lochmiller, R.L., Amoss, M.S., and Grant, W.E. 1985. Endocrine and metabolic responses of the collared peccary to immobilization with ketamine hydrochloride. J Wildl Dis 21:417–25.

35. Jalanka, H.H. 1989. Chemical restraint and reversal in captive markhors, A comparison of two methods. J Zoo Wildl Med 20:413–22.

36. Jalanka, H.H. 1988. Evaluation of medetomidine- and ketamine-induced immobilization in markhors and its reversal by atipamezole. J Zoo Wildl Med 19:95–105.

37. Jalanka, H.H. 1993. New alpha2 adrenoceptor agonists and antagonists. In: Fowler, M.E., Ed. Zoo and Wild Animal Medicine, 3rd ed., Philadelphia: W.B. Saunders, pp. 477–80.

38. Jalanka, H.H., and Roeken, B.O. 1990. The use of medetomidine, medetomidine-ketamine combinations, and atipamezole in nondomestic mammals: A review. J Zoo Wildl Med 21:259–82.

39. Janssen, D.L., Rath, J.P., de Vos, V., Allen, H.A., Swan, G.E., Jessup, D., and Stanley, T. 1991. Field studies with the narcotic immobilizing agent A3080. Proceedings of the American Association of Zoo Veterinarians, Calgary, Canada, pp. 340–41.

40. Janssen, D.L., Swan, G.E., Raath, J.P., McJames, S.W., Allen, J.L., de Vos, V., Williams, K.E., Anderson, J.M., and Stanley, T.H. 1993. Immobilization and physiologic effects of the narcotic A-3080 in impala. J Zoo Wildl Med 24:11–18.

41. Jessup, D.A. 1993. Translocation of wildlife. In: Fowler, M.E., Ed. Zoo and Wild Animal Medicine, 3rd ed., Philadelphia: W.B. Saunders, pp. 493–98.

42. Jessup, D.A. 1999. Capture and handling of mountain sheep and goats. In: Fowler, M.E., and Miller, R.E., Eds. 1999. Zoo and Wild Animal Medicine—Current Vet. Therapy, 4th Ed. Philadelphia, W.B. Saunders, pp. 481–87.

43. Jorgenson, J.T., Samson, J., and Festa-Bianchet, M. 1990. Field immobilization of bighorn sheep with xylazine hydrochloride and antagonism with idazoxan. J Wildl Dis 26:522–27.

44. Karesh, W.B., Janssen, D.L., and Oosterhuis, J.E. 1986. A comparison of carfentanil and etorphine/xylazine immobilization of axis deer. J Zoo Anim Med 17:58–61.

45. Kock, M.D., and Berger, J. 1987. Chemical immobilization of free-ranging North American bison in Badlands National Park, South Dakota. J Wildl Dis 23:625–33.

46. Kreeger, T.J., Plotka, E.D., and Seal, U.S. 1987. Immobilization of white-tailed deer by etorphine and xylazine and its antagonism by nalmefene and yohimbine. J Wildl Dis 23:619–24.

47. Kreeger, T.J., Del Giudice, G.D., Seal, U.S., and Karns, P.D. 1986. Immobilization of white-tailed deer with xylazine hydrochloride and ketamine hydrochloride and antagonism by tolazoline hydrochloride. J Wildl Dis 22:407–12.

48. Mech, D., Del Giudice, G.D., Karns, P.D., and Seal, U.S. 1985. Yohimbine hydrochloride as an antagonist to xylazine hydrochloride—ketamine hydrochloride immobilization of white-tailed deer. J Wildl Dis 21:405–10.

49. Morkel, P., and La Grange, M. 1993. Capture of antelope using the netgun. In: McKenzie, A.A., Ed. The Capture and Care Manual, Pretoria: The South African Veterinary Foundation, pp. 393–403.

50. Padilla, L.R., and Ko, J.C.H. 2007. Non-domestic suids. In: West, G., Heard, D., and Caulkett, N., Eds. Zoo Animal and Wildlife Immobilization and Anesthesia, Ames, Iowa, Blackwell Publishing, pp. 567–77.

51. Raath, J.P. 1993. Transportation of the African buffalo. In: McKenzie, A.A., Ed. The Capture and Care Manual, Pretoria: The South African Veterinary Foundation, pp. 590–94.

52. Renecker, L.A., and Olsen, C.D. 1986. Antagonism of xylazine hydrochloride with yohimbine hydrochloride and 4-aminopyridine in captive wapiti. J Wildl Dis 22:91–96.

53. van Rensburg, P.J.J. 1993. Physical capture of the bushpig. In: McKenzie, A.A., Ed. The Capture and Care Manual, Pretoria: The South African Veterinary Foundation, pp. 617–20.

54. van Rensburg, P.J.J. 1993. Chemical capture of the bushpig. In: McKenzie, A.A., Ed. The Capture and Care Manual, Pretoria: The South African Veterinary Foundation, pp. 615–16.

55. Seal, U.S., Schmitt, S.M., and Peterson, R.O. 1985. Carfentanil and xylazine for immobilization of moose on Isle Royale. J Wildl Dis 21:48–51.

56. West, G. 2007. Gazelles. In: West, G., Heard, D., and Caulkett, N., Eds. Zoo Animal and Wildlife Immobilization and Anesthesia, Ames, Iowa, Blackwell Publishing, pp. 623–28.

57. Wilson, S.C., Armstrong, D.L., Simmons, L.G., Morris, D.J., and Gross, T.S. 1993. A clinical trial using three regimens for immobilizing Gaur. J Zoo Wildl Med 24:93–101.

CHAPTER 29

Birds

CLASSIFICATION

Flightless Birds
Order Sphenisciformes: penguin
Superorder Ratitae
Order Struthioniformes: ostrich
Order Casuariiformes: cassowary
Order Apterygiformes: kiwi
Order Rheiformes: rhea
Water Birds
Order Anseriformes: duck, goose
Order Gaviiformes: loon
Order Podicipediformes: grebe
Order Pelecaniformes: pelican, cormorant
Shore and Gull-like Birds
Order Charadriiformes: plover, gull
Order Procellariiformes: albatross, petrel
Raptors
Order Falconiformes: hawk, eagle
Order Strigiformes: owl
Galliformlike Birds
Order Galliformes: pheasant, grouse
Order Tinamiformes: tinamou
Long-billed, Long-legged Birds
Order Ciconiiformes: heron, stork, flamingo
Order Gruiformes: crane, rail
Large-billed Birds
Order Coraciiformes: kingfisher, roller, hornbill
Order Piciformes: woodpecker, toucan
Order Cuculiformes: cuckoo
Pigeons and Doves
Order Columbiformes
Psittacine Birds
Order Psittaciformes: parrot
Hummingbirds and Swifts
Order Apodiformes
Song, Perching, and Miscellaneous Birds
Order Caprimulgiformes: frog mouth
Order Coliiformes: coly
Order Trogoniformes: trogon
Order Passeriformes: finch, warbler, crow

Generally the male is called a male, a cock, or rooster; the female is a hen. Newly hatched birds are called chicks. The male falcon is called a tiercel; the female is the falcon. Newly

hatched pigeons are squabs. Waterfowl names are the same as those designating domestic species.

Approximately 8,600 species of birds, grouped in 27 orders, are distributed throughout the world. Birds vary in size from a 2-g hummingbird to an ostrich weighing 136 kg (300 lb). Aviculture is a popular hobby and/or serious pursuit of many persons. Husbandry practices necessary to maintain birds in an aviary are well known for some species. Most species of birds have been maintained in either public or private aviaries at one time or another.

It would be impossible to discuss every species or even every family of birds in a book of this type. Fortunately groups of birds with like anatomical or behavioral traits respond similarly to certain types of restraint practices.

ANATOMY AND PHYSIOLOGY

Certain aspects of the avian circulatory system have a bearing on restraint, particularly as it relates to injectable chemical restraint. In mammals, the venous drainage from the hindquarters and the tail is via the iliac veins to the caudal vena cava, and back to the heart. In birds and reptiles, venous return is via a renal portal drainage system. In this system in birds, a valve in the iliac vein, which drains the hindquarters, may shunt blood through the kidneys before it reaches the renal vein; blood then passes on to the caudal vena cava.

Some drugs, notably ketamine hydrochloride, are excreted from the body via the kidneys. Therefore, if an injection of ketamine is administered in the thigh muscle, blood draining that area may carry the drug to the kidney where it may be partially excreted before it reaches the brain to exert its sedative effect. The bird's autonomic nervous system controls the valve, but the person administering the drug is unable to determine whether the valve is closed or open. The safest route of administration is into the breast muscles.

Respiratory function in birds is unique. The lungs are assisted in respiration by a series of air sacs. Birds lack a complete diaphragm, and the lungs are intimately associated with the chest wall. Thus inspiration and expiration are dependent on a bellows system to pull air into the lungs and push it back out. On inspiration the sternum moves downward and forward, expanding the chest and abdominal cavities, drawing air into the abdominal and caudal thoracic air sacs (Fig.29.1A). On expiration, the sternum moves backward and upward,

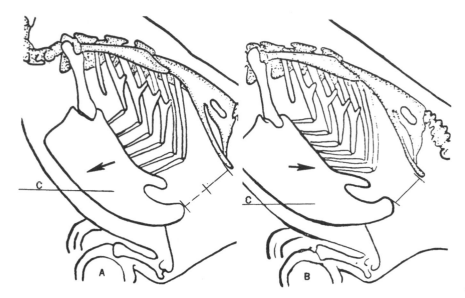

FIG. 29.1. Diagram showing movement of sternum and ribs during respiration. **A.** Inspiration. **B.** Expiration. Note: **C.** is the sternum, or keel.

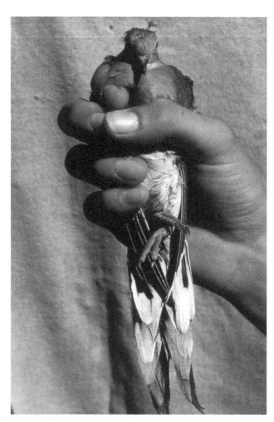

FIG. 29.2. Poor restraint: Hand completely encircling the body may inhibit respiration.

compressing the structures and driving air through the secondary and tertiary bronchi, the lung, and out the trachea (Fig. 29.1B). Any manipulation that prevents the proper excursion of the sternum will interfere with respiration. Hands and fingers must not completely encircle the thoracic cavity and immobilize the sternum (Fig. 29.2), and the sternum must be able to move freely when a bird is placed into a plastic tube or encircled with a stockinette.

Cartilaginous rings completely encircle the trachea of birds, minimizing the danger of tracheal collapse during manipulation. However, the extreme mobility of the neck and trachea makes it possible to kink the trachea and inhibit the free flow of air.

The location of the nostrils varies from species to species. Some species are capable of breathing through the mouth; others are not. Before instituting any restraint practice that would cover or interfere with the nostrils, ascertain the specific type of breathing required by that species. Also examine the nares to make certain they are not plugged by feed or exudate.

The bones of the wings and legs of birds are constructed for lightness. Some bones are pneumatized, being connected to the air sac system of the respiratory tract; others are hollow. The cortex of the humerus and femur are thin. These modifications assist flight but increase fragility. Fractures are easily induced by rough manipulation.

Both the upper and lower jaws of psittacine birds have movable articulation with the skull.

Feathers cover the entire surface of the body of a bird, forming an efficient insulating layer. The presence of this insulating layer may be detrimental to a bird under restraint. Muscular activity increases heat production, which, coupled with inability to dissipate heat from the body surface, may produce hyperthermia. Many birds normally maintain body temperatures up to 41–42°C (105.8–107.6°F), higher than those of mammals. Cellular necrosis of all animal tissue begins at body temperatures of 45°C (113.0°F), leaving a bird little margin for increase from normal.

DANGER POTENTIAL

Birds possess four structures that are used in defense and offense: the beak, the wings, the feet, and the legs. Beaks of birds are highly varied, adapted for the food-gathering habits of individual species. Feet also are adapted for various food-gathering or defensive habits. Only large birds defend themselves with wings or legs. More details on defense and offense are found with specific groups.

PHYSICAL RESTRAINT[3,9]

Some general procedures are applicable for the handling of all types of birds. The head must be controlled. This is accomplished by grasping the bird at the nape. A variety of handholds may be used to control the head, varying with the size or strength of the bird and the procedure to be carried out. For small birds, the author prefers to place the thumb and forefinger on the sides of the lower jaw (Fig. 29.3). Some clinicians place the thumb beneath the lower jaw and exert pressure upward (Fig. 29.4). In either case, the neck is not completely encircled. For small passerine and psittacine birds that are to be bled from the jugular vein, the head and neck are held between the index and middle fingers. Restraint of most birds is accomplished by approaching the bird from behind, grasping the head and the body, and holding the legs together.

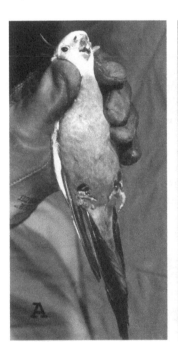
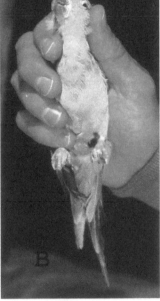

FIG. 29.3.   **A.** Correct hold for small psittacine birds. **B.** Handling a cockatiel may require gloves as protection from a stronger beak.

A net is the common tool used in capturing birds from large cages or aviaries (Fig. 29.5). Many birds are extraordinarily fragile, and a careless handler may easily fracture wings and legs if the hoop of the net is slammed onto the bird or if the bird is removed from the net in a rough manner. Once the bird is captured, the basic procedure is to grasp the bird by the head at the nape of the neck or by the beak, depending on the species, and carefully remove the net. The legs of raptors must be grasped first, then the head, as described.

Birds in a small cage are usually approached with a towel to block the bird's vision of an approaching hand (Figs. 29.6, 29.7). Gloves may be worn, but birds tend to recognize a

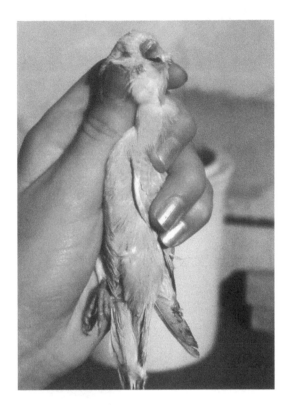

FIG. 29.4.   Holding a budgerigar.

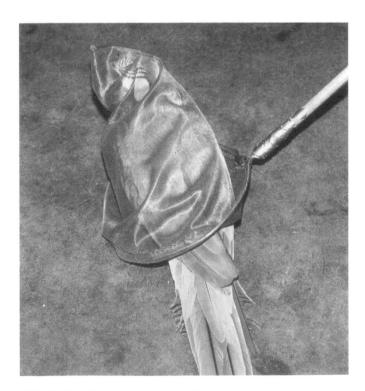

FIG. 29.5.   Capturing a bird in a hoop net.

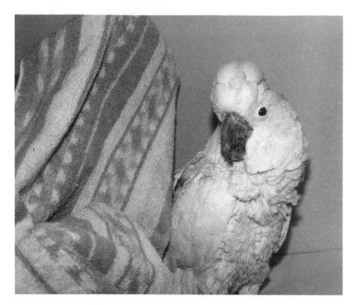

FIG. 29.6. Approaching a cockatoo with a towel.

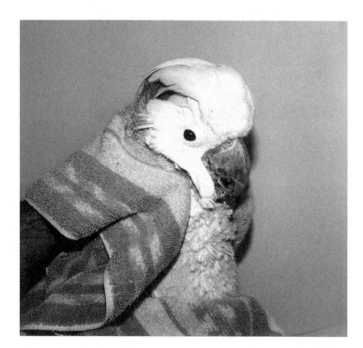

FIG. 29.7. Holding with a towel.

gloved hand as a hand and will peck at the glove or flit around more vigorously than when a towel is used.

The safe release of birds following restraint requires care and attention. To release a bird, turn it right side up and allow it to sit on the floor. Make certain that none of the talons or claws are enmeshed in clothing or gloves and that the bill is free; then give the bird a slight push to release it. Be especially wary of the talons of raptors. Pull the hands back quickly after release.

Do not release a bird in midair. The bird has been disoriented during the period of restraint and may have been kept in an abnormal position for a long time. It may need a moment or two to regain its balance and composure.

TRANSPORT

Many specialized crates and cages are used for shipping and moving birds. Hummingbirds may be placed in individual stockings or fabric jackets in front of a source of liquid diet. Antarctic penguins must be kept cool. Heavy-gauge wire must be used for caging large macaws to preclude their chewing their way out. Unique requirements must be met when transporting each group of birds. Handlers with no experience in transporting birds should contact a private or public aviary or zoo for information.

CHEMICAL RESTRAINT[3,9,16]

The chemical restraint agents and combinations mentioned in this chapter represent those used by the author or experienced veterinarians with detailed knowledge of birds. Other protocols have been used, and no claim is made for including all possible drugs and combinations. For more detailed information, particularly for anesthesia, consult Hawkins[3] or Siegel-Willcot.[15]

Many procedures may be carried out without sedation or anesthesia. The art of avian anesthesia has become sophisticated and is beyond the scope of this book. Veterinarians who use isoflurane find that this is the safest and most efficient agent for immobilizing small- to medium-sized birds for diagnostic and therapeutic procedures. Small birds may be placed directly inside a face mask used for a large dog. A variety of plastic containers may be modified to serve as face masks. The bottom of the container is replaced with a segment of a rubber glove, stretched and taped to the container to serve as a diaphragm (Fig. 29.8). The bird's head is inserted through a small hole cut in the stretched rubber.

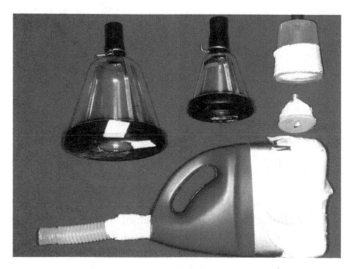

FIG. 29.8. Face masks: Fashioned from plastic bottle, left, and small animal mask, right.

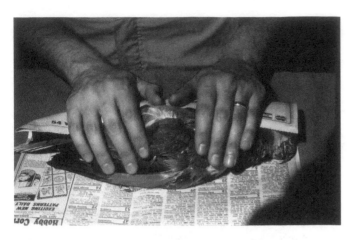

FIG. 29.9. Wrapping a bird in a newspaper roll.

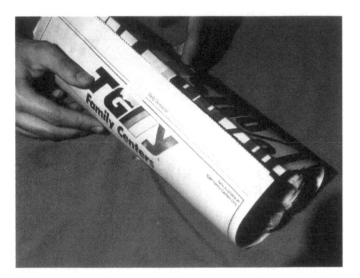

FIG. 29.10. A bird wrapped up in newspaper.

The flow of isoflurane in oxygen should be 4–5% until the bird relaxes, then be reduced to 1–2%. If the procedure is short, anesthesia is maintained via the face mask. For longer procedures the trachea should be intubated for more controlled respiration.

Recovery from isoflurane immobilization is rapid. The bird need be held only for a few minutes and then is usually able to stand.

Without access to a vaporizer or appropriate inhalation agents, injectable immobilization may be used. Ketamine hydrochloride (25–50 mg/kg) is the standard injectable immobilizing and anesthetic agent for use in birds.[1–3,6,7,9,11,14–16,18] One milligram will sedate a 50-g budgerigar for conducting radiographic examinations and minor surgery. Recovery is usually more prolonged than with isoflurane or methoxyflurane. If desired, the bird may be wrapped in a section of newspaper to keep it from flapping its wings or falling over as it recovers (Figs. 29.9, 29.10).

Various agents have been incorporated into baits for the capture of free-ranging birds.[8] Alpha chloralose and tribromo-ethanol (Avertin) have been effective for capturing seed-eating binds. Non-treated grain is fed for a few days, then the bait is provided. The dose of alpha chloralose is 0.5 mg/250 g (1 cup) of grain. Higher concentrations of the drug may cause mortality. Allow 1–2 hours for development of the maximum effect.

Tribromoethanol is added to the grain at the rate of 3 g/250 g. A combination of alpha chloralose (0.5 g) and tribromoethanol (0.5 g/250 g of grain) has also been used.

PENGUINS

Danger Potential

Penguin wings are modified to form flippers used for swimming. The wings must be adequately controlled, otherwise the penguin may beat a handler and inflict bruises or severe injuries, especially if a wing is flipped into the face. Penguins also have sharp beaks that are used to catch fish, and may seriously tear the flesh of a manipulator.

Physical Restraint

Penguins should be restricted to a dry area without access to a pool. An appropriately sized hoop net may be used to make the initial capture (Figs. 29.11, 29.12), or a small penguin may be approached from behind and grasped firmly at the base of the head (Fig. 29.13) while hoisting it up into the air. The legs may then be grasped and a light stretch applied. If the wings must be restricted in movement, another person must assist. Blood samples may be obtained from a penguin by venipuncture of the brachial vein (Fig. 29.14), tarsal vein, or the jugular vein.

An excellent method for capturing and handling large penguins is to use an appropriately sized plastic garbage can with the bottom cut out. Slowly approach the bird and place

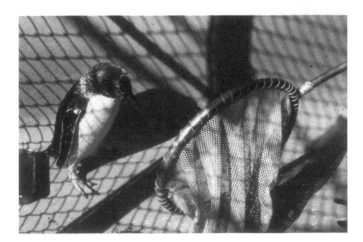

FIG. 29.11. Using a hoop net to capture a small penguin.

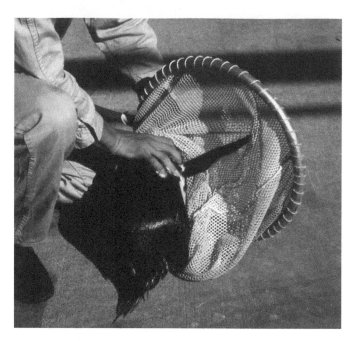

FIG. 29.12. While holding the head through the net, re-grasp the head under the net.

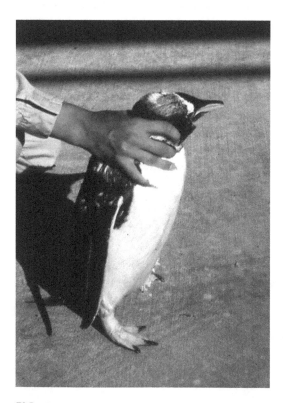

FIG. 29.13. Small birds may be grasped firmly at the base of the head.

the container over it. The bird's movements are restricted without undue trauma, yet many manipulations may be carried out through the open bottom. Large penguins should be hooded, otherwise the hands may be injured.

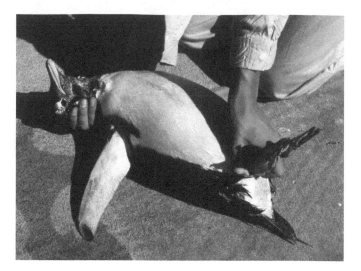

FIG. 29.14. A blood sample from a penguin may be obtained by venipuncture of the brachial vein.

Chemical Restraint

Injectable chemical restraint agents are rarely used in penguins. Isoflurane-induced general anesthesia is fastest and safest.

RATITES (OSTRICH, RHEA, EMU, CASSOWARY, KIWI)

Ratites are flightless birds that originated from flighted ancestors. The term ratite derives from a Latin word, *ratis*, meaning raft-like, referring to the keel-less sternum. These birds have been popular zoo exhibits for hundreds of years, but ostriches, rheas, and emus recently have also become popular in the United States and other countries as farmed birds, with an associated commercial industry planning to utilize the meat, leather, eggs, oil, and feathers. Although some consider farmed ratites as domesticated, that is not so. Domestication is an evolutionary process.

Danger Potential

The primary defensive and offensive structures of large ratites are the feet and legs. Although owners of seemingly docile farmed birds often take great liberties with their birds, it should be kept in mind that these birds may be dangerous, particularly males and especially during the breeding season. Never stand directly in front of one of these birds. An ostrich (Fig. 29.15) or a cassowary is able to disembowel and kill a human with a quick forward thrust of a clawed foot. The toe-nails of emus and cassowaries are sharp, and the medial toe of the cassowary has an elongated nail for raking an enemy (Fig. 29.16). The power of the blow itself may fracture an arm or leg. Even the smaller rhea or emu may inflict a severe contusion with a kick.

An adult male ostrich may be docile until the breeding season begins, at which time he begins to strut and display to

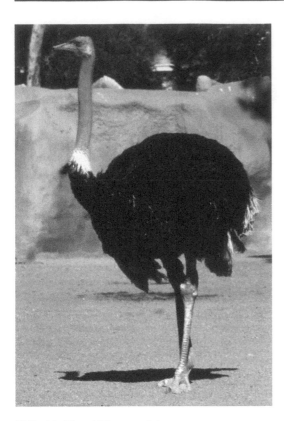

FIG. 29.15.   African ostrich.

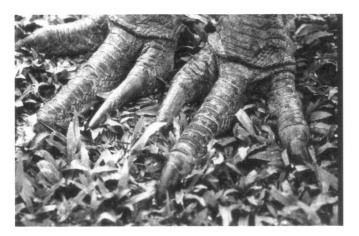

FIG. 29.16.   Medial toenail of a cassowary.

the best defense is to lie flat on the ground, since the forward thrust of the kick is directed 50–80 cm (20–30 inches) above the ground. The bird may trample the victim, but he/she will be spared the potentially lethal blows of kicks. This technique may not work with a cassowary.

Others with more courage or experience suggest that it is possible to stand up to an onrushing ostrich and at the last second, side step while reaching out and catching the bird by the neck and pulling the head down to the ground level. With the head and neck in this position, the ostrich is usually reluctant to kick forward. Additional help would have to be obtained to move the bird to a location where it could be released safely.

As a rule, emus and rheas are not likely to be aggressive, and it is usually safe to enter an enclosure with them. Prolonged chases or exertion should be avoided, particularly when the ambient temperature is over 27°C (80°F). Hyperthermia and exertion may result in sudden death or the development of exertional myopathy (Exertional Stress, capture myopathy), see Chapter 7.

Physical Restraint[6]

Young ratite chicks and juveniles up to 5.0 kg are easily handled by folding the legs and holding the body next to the body of the handler. The chicks may defecate during the process, so direct the vent away from clothing. Avoid forcing the legs of heavier birds into a folded position; the legs may dangle while the body is held.

Adult rheas and emus may be grasped with one arm around the bird's chest and the other arm over the body and grasping the upper leg (Figs. 29.17, 29.18). Lift the bird off

the females. He may begin to fight with other males until a dominance hierarchy is established. When attempting to intimidate a human, he will stand tall, thrust his chest against a fence or gate, fan his wings, and open his mouth and hiss.

It may be dangerous to enter an ostrich or cassowary enclosure without a usual attendant present or without some means of protection; some of these birds may be highly aggressive and may attack, running down and knocking over a handler. An ostrich can run 70 km/hour (40 mph); a human cannot outrun it. Those with more experience than the author suggest that if caught in the open with an attacking ostrich,

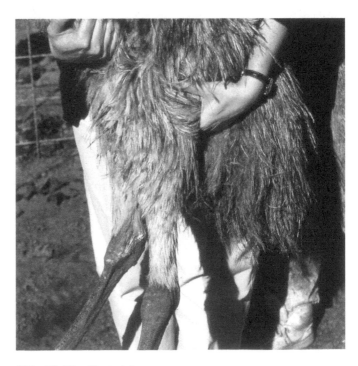

FIG. 29.17.   Restraining an emu.

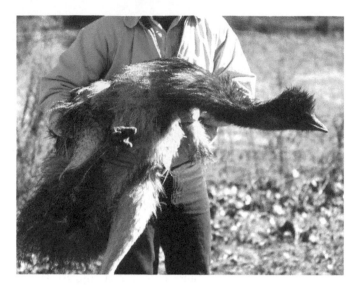

FIG. 29.18.   An alternate method of restraining an emu.

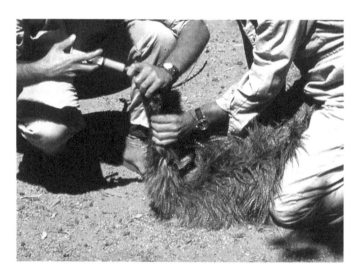

FIG. 29.19.   Straddling an emu when examination or therapy is needed.

its feet quickly and direct the legs slightly away from the handler's body. If prolonged examination or therapy is required, a handler may gently ease the bird to the ground and straddle it in a recumbent position (Fig. 29.19). The handler should be astride over the pelvis (synsacrum) of the bird, and the handler's legs should keep the bird's feet from pushing out to the side. A large emu may lift a person off the ground, so more than one person may be required. Avoid placing an adult rhea or emu on its back because it may be difficult to control flailing legs that may strike the holder in the face or tear clothing.

It takes two people to examine an adult emu and to determine the sex. The handler approaches from behind a bird that has been directed into a corner by a shield. While the bird is standing, the handler grasps the short wing stubs near the

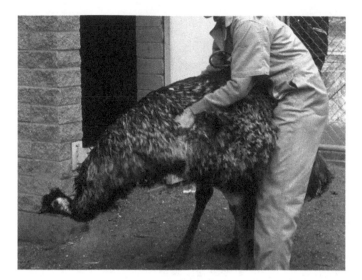

FIG. 29.20.   Standing restraint of an emu.

body and straddles the tail (Fig. 29.20). The person who is to determine the sex then may insert a gloved finger through the vent.

Before hands-on restraint is attempted, adult ostriches should be moved to a smaller holding enclosure, preferably with solid walls. Farms that maintain large numbers of these birds should have alleyways leading to a handling facility, which desirably incorporates a narrow chute to allow close examination of a bird (Fig. 29.21).

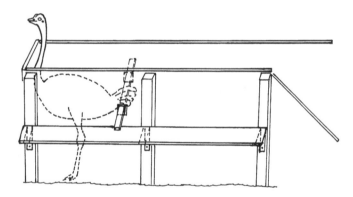

FIG. 29.21.   Permanent narrow alleyway for working with adult ostriches.

A long pole with a branched or forked structure, such as bicycle handlebars, attached to the end may be used to keep an ostrich or cassowary away from a handler in a small enclosure (Fig. 29.22). This device may not be adequate to ward off an attacking ostrich in a large enclosure.

A plywood shield generally offers suitable protection from an ostrich or cassowary, since it may be moved within close proximity to the bird (Figs. 29.23, 29.24). However, these birds can jump considerable heights and may jump over a shield that is too short. To deal with an extremely aggressive cassowary, the shield may be attached to the front of a vehicle,

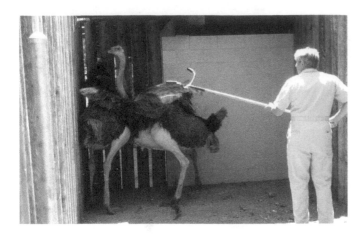

FIG. 29.22. Bicycle handlebars adapted as a keep-away.

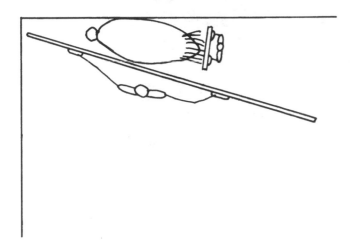

FIG. 29.23. Shields being used to push a bird against a corner and a wall. Someone may push forward from the rear.

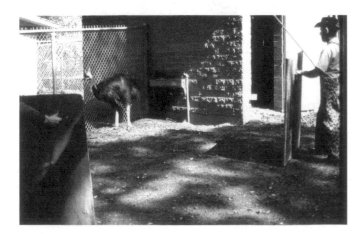

FIG. 29.24. Approaching a cassowary using a shield in order to inject a medication or chemical immobilizing agent.

because a swift kick from one of these birds may knock a person down even though shielded.

A method used to capture an aggressive cock ostrich is for four individuals to coordinate the capture at night. One person approaches the ostrich with a bright spotlight, temporarily blinding the bird. Another handler steps in from the side and grasps the neck near the head and quickly pulls the head down near the ground. The bird will generally take a step or two backward; if so, the handler should follow it. Apply only the minimum pulling force necessary, for if the handler is too aggressive, the neck may be injured. The third handler then moves in quickly and grasps the wings close to the body, while the fourth individual comes up behind the bird and pushes it in the appropriate direction (Fig. 29.25). The ostrich may then be hooded, to avoid having to hold the head near the ground.

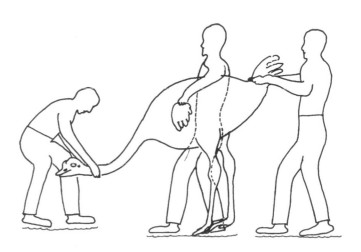

FIG. 29.25. Method of moving an aggressive adult ostrich with three or four people; a fourth person may be needed—one on each side, one behind, and one at the head.

A shepherd's crook (hook) may be used to grasp the neck and pull the head down to lessen the risk to a handler. The crook should have a handle 2.5–3 m long and a hook with an inside diameter of 6–7 cm (2.5–3 inches) (Fig. 29.26). The metal hook may be covered with flexible plastic tubing to minimize contusion of the neck. The crook must be used judiciously and kept straight with the bird at all times (Fig. 29.27). An ostrich will usually pull back from the hook or

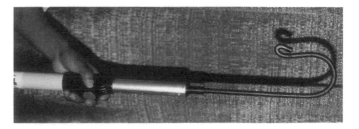

FIG. 29.26. Shepherd's crook.

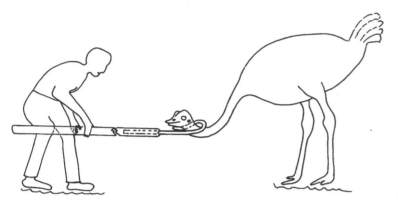

FIG. 29.27. Grasping and holding an ostrich with a shepherd's crook.

may hop in place. It may also become frightened and begin to struggle; if so, it should be instantly released, for struggling with the shepherd's crook in place may result in injury to the bird.

Various stanchions, chutes, or boxes may be employed to restrict the movement of adult ostriches. Some are made commercially; others may be constructed on the farm. (Figs. 29.28, 29.29, 29.30A,B,C,D).

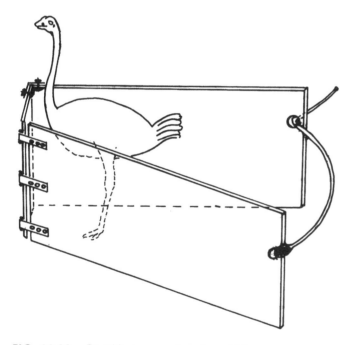

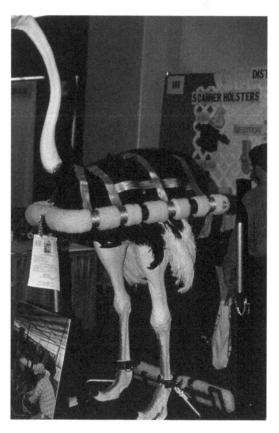

FIG. 29.29. A commercial restraint device.

FIG. 29.28. Portable squeeze chute for ostriches, to be used inside a small enclosure.

Opaque plastic sheeting may be used to form an alley-way or cone to move ostriches from one location to another. Ostriches and cassowaries are much easier to handle if they can be hooded first (Fig. 29.31). The weave of the hood material must exclude all vision, yet allow breathing. Materials used have included coat sleeves, the leg of thermal knit underwear, black stockings, and bags constructed for this purpose, with elastic bands to hold the bag in place when the bird lowers its head.

There are various methods for applying the hood. The hood may be inverted over a hand. A curious ostrich or one in a restricted area may be approached from a safe vantage point. The closed beak is grasped with the inverted hood on the hand and the hood quickly everted over the head. It is critical that the bird be in confinement so that it cannot escape and run away while hooded. The author uses a device for reaching out to place a hood on zoo ostriches (Figs. 29.32, 29.33, 29.34, 29.35). Although the head may bob around to avoid the hood, in a confined area the hood may be placed with safety to both the bird and handler. It is critical that the bird is confined and that everyone involved understands what

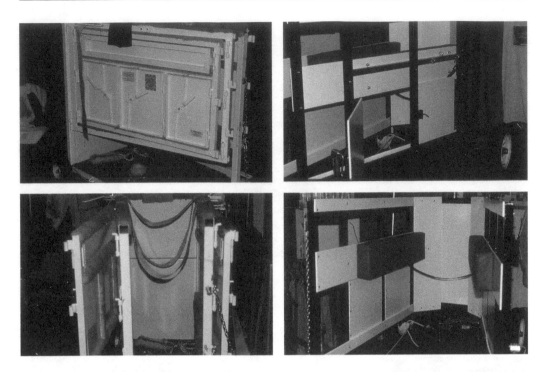

FIG. 29.30. Views of a commercial ostrich restraint chute.

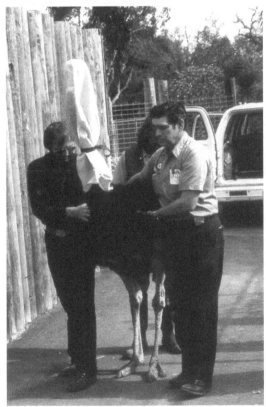

FIG. 29.31. Grasping a hooded ostrich by the base of the wing stubs.

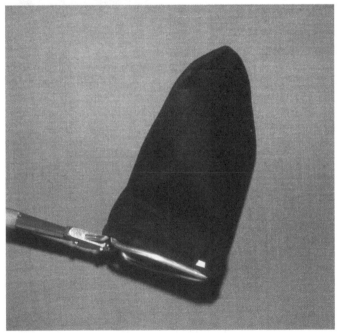

FIG. 29.32. Apparatus for applying hood to an ostrich.

they are to do. If a bird escapes the handlers while hooded, it may begin to run and crash into obstructions, injuring itself.

If a small ostrich is being moved by a single person, the bird may be grasped at the base of the wings from behind,

once the hood is in place. Adult males and females usually require three persons, one on each side grasping a wing and a third behind the bird. Excessive pressure should not be exerted on the wings because the humerus is easily fractured. Emus do not accept hooding, and some rheas also become excited when hooded.

Loading and unloading adult ostriches into trailers or trucks may be dangerous for the safety of the birds. Most desirably, the bed of the trailer should be level with the

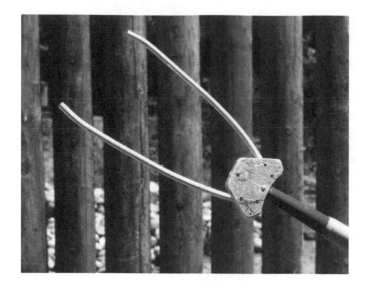

FIG. 29.33. Alternate apparatus for applying hood to an ostrich.

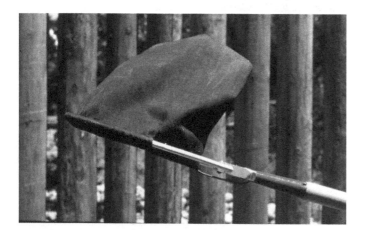

FIG. 29.34. Hood on the device.

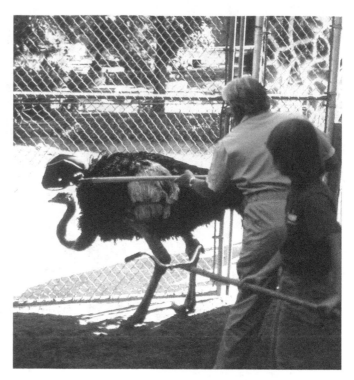

FIG. 29.35. Placing hood on an ostrich.

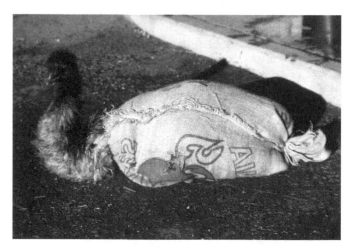

FIG. 29.36. Small emus may be transported a short distance in a burlap sack.

ground, or a gradual ramp should lead to the trailer. The bird may need to be hooded, or it may be driven directly into a trailer, especially if it can exit from a darkened stall into a more brightly lighted area of a trailer.

Step-up trailers used to haul horses are particularly hazardous, because ostriches may slip a foot and lower leg beneath the trailer bed and abrade or even fracture the limb. A sturdy ramp should be constructed, or a trench may be dug under the wheels of the trailer to drop the bed to ground level. Ostriches may stand as high as 3 m. Some horse trailers may not allow an ostrich to stand fully upright. This may be harmless for short distances, but if the bird becomes agitated when it is unloaded, the head and neck may be injured. Unloading is equally dangerous if a bird should bolt from the confinement of a darkened trailer to a lighted open space. It may be wise to rehood a bird upon arrival and physically assist it from the trailer. The hood may then be removed and the bird released. Emus and rheas may be transported individually in crates or in burlap sacks (Fig. 29.36). Groups may be transported in trucks or trailers.

Injuries to the limbs of ratites may necessitate some form of slinging. Figure 29.37 illustrates an improvised sling for an adult emu. Elaborate cradles have been constructed for these birds, but some individuals defy any attempts to help them, constantly struggling against any device.

Kiwis are small inoffensive birds from New Zealand. They are easily handled as illustrated in Figure 29.38.

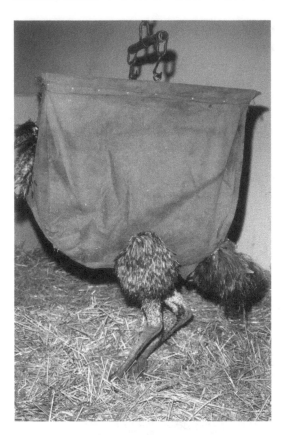

FIG. 29.37. Improvised sling for an emu.

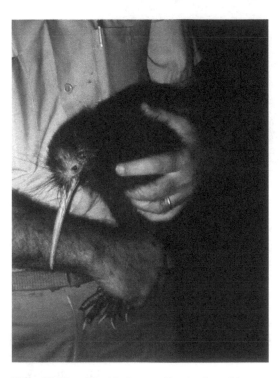

FIG. 29.38. The kiwi, a small ratite from New Zealand, is not aggressive and is easily handled.

Collection of Blood Samples

Venipuncture may be performed via the right jugular vein, the brachial vein on the underside of the wing, or, in an immobilized bird, the medial tarsal vein.

Chemical Restraint[1,2,4,6,12,14,15,18]

Although farmed ratites may respond favorably to the captive environment and may allow physical restraint without undue stress, certain diagnostic procedures and surgery may require immobilization and/or anesthesia. Birds may be immobilized using isoflurane as an inhalant anesthetic via a face mask. This is used for medium-sized birds (rhea, emu) and juveniles of all species and provides rapid induction and rapid recovery. Previous to the advent of recent restraint agents that provide rapid induction, recovery and reversal, immobilization was hazardous to the bird and the restrainer.

See Table 29.1 for weights of adult ratites. Table 29.2 lists selected chemical restraint agents for ostriches and cassowaries.

TABLE 29.1. Body weights of ratites

Species	Adults (kg)
Ostrich	80.0–150.0
Cassowary	29.0–58.0
Emu	30.0–55.0
Rhea	20.0–25.0
Kiwi	1.25–4.0

TABLE 29.2. Selected chemical restraint agents for ratite immobilization[15]

Agent	Ostrich	Cassowary
Sedation		
Azaperone	0.5–2.0	
Diazepam	0.05–0.3	
Immobilization		
Carfentanil/Ketamine	3.0/200.0 mg TD	
Carfentanil/midazolam/ketamine		0.04–0.06/2.5–5.0
Medetomidine/ketamine	0.05–0.15/3.0–7.0	
Etorphine/ketamine		0.1/6.55
Etorphine/acepromazine/xylazine	6.0/25.0/200.0 mg TD	

TD = Total dose.

It may be necessary to use a pole syringe to administer drugs to a cassowary (Fig. 29.39).

Table 29.2 lists agents that have been used in both captive and free-ranging birds. Induction and recovery times are critical. Ostriches tend to lose control of the head and neck early in induction and may injure themselves if they are in a large enclosure. The use of agents for which there are antagonists has made recovery safer.

Ostriches immobilized with tiletamine/zolazepam (Telazol, Zoletil) may experience a rough recovery. Difficulties may be minimized by administering diazepam (5.0 mg) IV when the bird begins to struggle early in the recovery process. The author has recovered small- to medium-sized ratites in a padded box filled with Styrofoam pellets (Fig. 29.40).

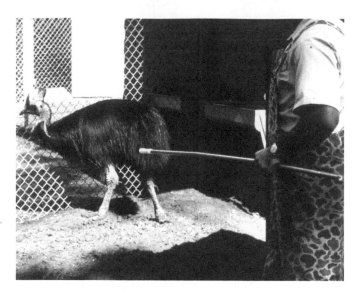

FIG. 29.39. Cassowary being injected with chemical restraint agent via pole syringe. Handler is standing behind a plywood shield.

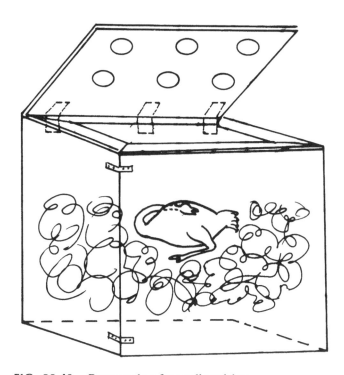

FIG. 29.40. Recovery box for small ostriches.

Chicks and juvenile ratites may be immobilized using isoflurane in oxygen inhalation anesthesia at a flow rate of 5% for induction and 2.5% for maintenance. The head may be placed in a face mask, or the birds may easily be intubated, because the glottis is readily accessible. Be cautious using inflatable cuffs as the cartilaginous tracheal rings are complete in birds, and overinflation may result in ischemic damage to the tracheal mucosa.

WATER BIRDS[5,11,17]
Danger Potential

Ducks, geese, and swans are not innately aggressive. However, large angry geese and swans may attack and inflict significant injuries.

Most waterfowl have dull bills. Although the bills may not be particularly sharp, many are heavy and strong and able to pinch the handler severely if they peck. A few fish-eating species have a sharp hook on the tip and serrations along the margins of the beak to facilitate grasping slippery fish. These structures may tear nasty wounds in the flesh of the unwary handler, particularly if the handler jerks away—a normal response when such a bird grabs hold.

Large geese and swans can beat a handler vigorously with their wings. A large swan male may threaten as illustrated in Fig. 29.41, then follow through by lowering the head, extending the wings, and rushing toward the enemy, hissing loudly. If the attack is pressed, the person may be pecked and beaten.

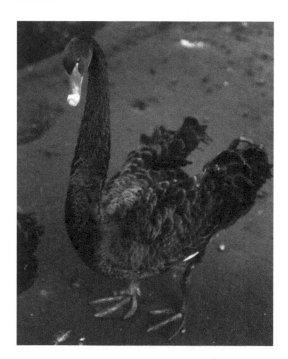

FIG. 29.41. Black swan in threat position.

Both spur-winged geese and screamers have sharp spurs at the carpus of the wing. These may be deliberately and effectively used against an animal handler. When cornered the screamer may fly at a person, flailing its wings. Restrained waterfowl may flail with the feet, but few have long claws. Some tree-nesting species have claws and will scratch a handler if precautions are not taken.

Pelicans are relatively harmless, though a handler should be wary of the sharp hook on the tip of the large beak, since these birds will peck at the eyes. A cornered pelican may fly at a handler, snapping its beak. Grab the beak if threatened. In close quarters the pelican will also beat with its wings.

Grebes and loons have long sharp beaks used for impaling fish. These birds will peck at the face, especially the eyes, of a handler.

Physical Restraint

All waterfowl may be initially captured with nets. The size of the cordage, the mesh, and the hoop should vary according to the size of the bird. Once captured, most species may be extracted from the net and held by the wings and the head in the same manner as domestic waterfowl.

The hook may also be used on captive wild waterfowl, as illustrated in Figure 29.27. A cannon net is used to capture wild ducks and geese. The net is placed in an area where birds can be baited with food. When the birds congregate and are feeding, the net is projected over the top of the birds, incarcerating them. Swans and large geese may be caught initially by hand. The birds are cornered, and the keeper grasps them quickly by the neck and then at the base of the wings. The approach should be from the rear (Figs. 29.42, 29.43). A special restraint jacket may also be used.

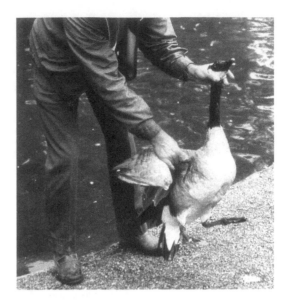

FIG. 29.43. Grasping a goose by the neck and the wings.

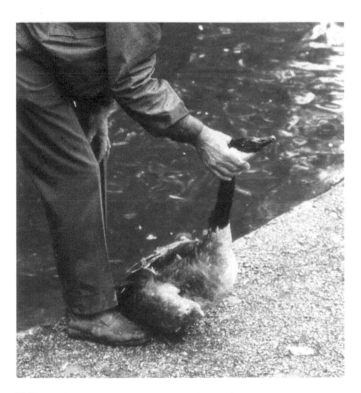

FIG. 29.42. Grasping a goose by the neck.

When attempting to capture a screamer or a spur-winged goose, approach from the rear, using either a net or a broom to ward off the spurred wings. The spurs of birds in an aviary may be dulled or clipped to prevent damage to other birds in the collection or to the keepers. Once captured, these birds are manipulated in the same manner as other waterfowl.

Control the beak at all times when handling grebes and loons or place a cork or other blunt object over the sharp tip of the beak.

SHORE AND GULL-LIKE BIRDS[11]

The numerous species of small- to medium-sized shore birds with long legs and short to long beaks share many characteristics important for restraint. Most of these birds have tiny fragile legs that are easily injured by the hoops of nets or by too severe pressure applied during capturing or handling.

Danger Potential

Some shore birds have long sharp bills, but most are not highly aggressive. Nevertheless, care should be taken in protecting one's face from the beak of any bird. Gulls and terns are equipped with more formidable beaks than other shore birds. The face should be protected when handling these birds, because they often peck at the eyes. Gulls and terns will also peck at the handler's fingers and arms if not prevented.

Physical Restraint

Shore birds are not difficult to handle. All may be captured easily by careful placement of a hoop net. Gently extricate them from the net, holding small species by the body with fingers at the back of the head. Hold larger birds by the body and legs. Place a shore bird in a stockinette or a section of lady's hose for prolonged restraint.

RAPTORS[7,10,13]
Danger Potential

All raptors are carnivorous. The diet of smaller species may consist primarily of insects, but all have beaks and talons adapted for grasping and rending flesh. The sharp tearing beaks are capable of wounding severely. Eagles or large owls can sever a finger from the hand. The claws or talons of raptors are long, strong, and sharp—well adapted for grasping and penetrating prey species.

Vultures employ the beak as a defensive weapon, seldom using talons. Vultures also regurgitate the malodorous crop contents at the slightest provocation during restraint. Other raptorial species rarely defend themselves with the beak, relying on the talons for protection, but hawks and owls will peck when being restrained.

A handler who is grasped by the powerful talons of a large eagle or owl may find it impossible to get free without assistance, unless the bird chooses to let go.

Physical Restraint

It is advisable to wear heavy leather gloves when working with birds of prey even though gloves do not afford full protection because the beaks and talons of raptors can cut through leather without much difficulty.

The tools of the falconer are useful for restraining all raptorial species. The hood is an important tool for decreasing stress and facilitating restraint (Fig. 29.44). If leather hoods are not available, a cloth hood is simple to construct. The falconer places leather bands called jesses around the metatarsi. They are customarily attached to a swivel and thence to a tether, which secures the bird to a perch or a block. It may take some time for the bird to become accustomed to being restrained in this manner. A few birds refuse to accept this type of restraint and continually fly at the falconer or away from the perch to the limit of the tether. This is called "bating." The bird may injure itself if bating behavior is persistent, but

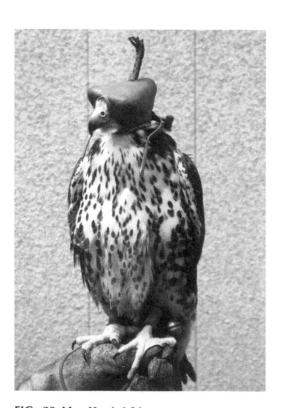

FIG. 29.44. Hooded falcon.

usually after one or two attempts it will not fly from the perch unless frightened.

Vultures are easily captured with a net. Once out of the net, the head must be controlled at all times. The arm of the hand holding the legs should keep the wings folded against the bird's body to obviate flapping. If the wings are free to flap, they may be injured and also would certainly interfere with any procedure.

Tamed captive falcons and hawks are easily handled. To pick up a tame raptor from a perch, first hood the bird. Then approach it from behind and place both hands over the back and wings. Control the feet by clasping the fingers over the legs. For more security separate the little finger from the ring finger, placing them on either side of the legs.

Raptors may be captured by throwing a towel, laboratory coat, or other cloth over them (Fig. 29.45) and wrapping them in the fabric (Fig. 29.46). This technique is most successful if the bird is on the floor of the enclosure when captured.

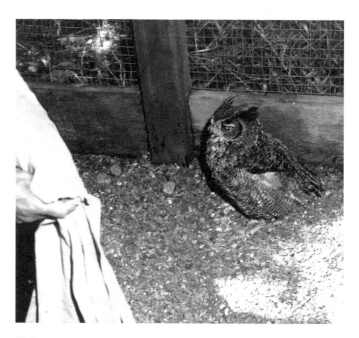

FIG. 29.45. Capturing an owl by throwing a towel over it.

Once the bird is in hand, it may be controlled by grasping the feet and the head in various manners dictated by what is to be done (Figs. 29.47, 29.48). Although gloves are desirable for initial capture, they should be removed when holding the bird to better sense the degree of pressure being applied.

To grasp a bird standing upright in a cardboard box, place both hands on the back over the wings and legs. Press the bird to the floor of the box and direct the fingers of both hands around and underneath the body to grasp the legs and control the feet before lifting the bird.

Owls often throw themselves on their backs and direct a flailing set of formidable talons toward anyone attempting to pick them up (Fig. 29.49). A great horned owl can drive a talon completely through the heaviest leather glove, so

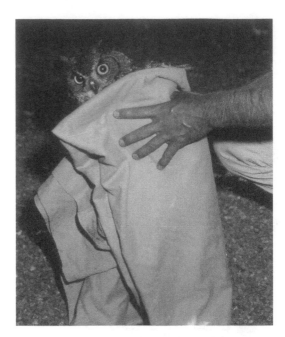

FIG. 29.46. Restraining an owl by wrapping it in a towel.

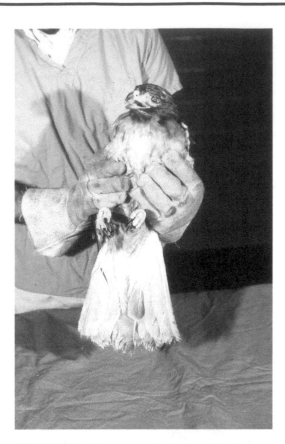

FIG. 29.48. Alternate method of securing feet and wings of a hawk.

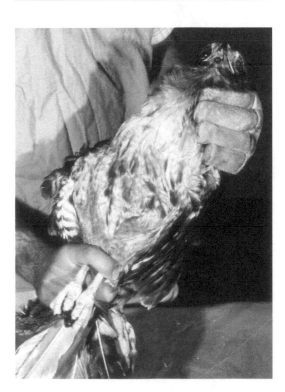

FIG. 29.47. Properly secured hawk.

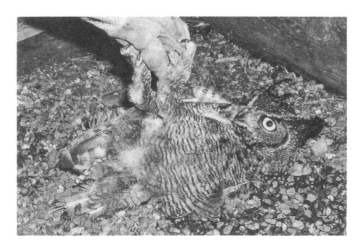

FIG. 29.49. Owl flipped on its back to defend itself with its talons.

approach this bird with caution. Dangle an empty glove above the bird and, while the talons are attached to the glove, grab the legs with the other hand (Fig. 29.50). Young owls may sometimes be captured from this prone position by presenting a towel or small piece of cloth for the talons to grasp. Lift the bird into the air upside down by the towel, reaching beneath it to clutch the legs with the other hand.

If a raptor is perched, the approach may be made from either the back or front. From the back, grasp the wings, body, and legs together (Fig. 29.51A). When approaching from the front, grasp the legs first (Fig. 29.51B).

If a bird impales a handler with a talon during the capturing process, the bird should be released and allowed to move away. If the bird is held and continues to struggle against capture, its grip will be maintained or enhanced. An impaled

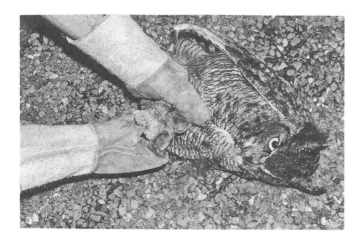

FIG. 29.50.   Owl's legs may be grasped while it is intent on clawing at another object such as a dangling glove or towel.

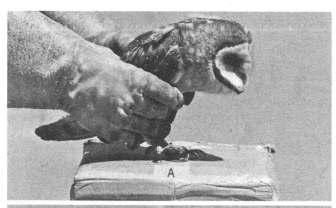

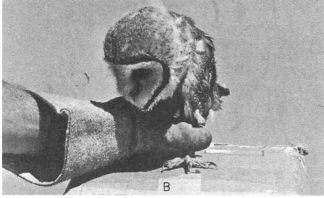

FIG. 29.51.   Approaching a perched raptor. **A.** From the rear. **B.** From the front.

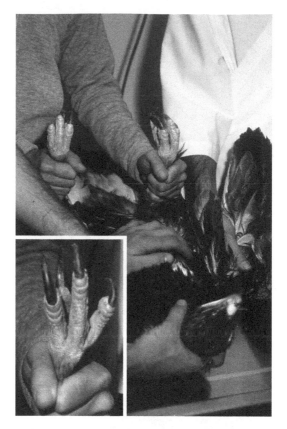

FIG. 29.52.   Golden eagle restrained on a table. Talons must be carefully controlled.

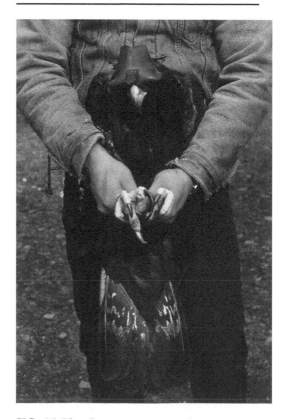

FIG. 29.53.   Proper way to restrain a hooded eagle.

talon may be released by straightening the leg at the tarsal-metatarsal articulation, relaxing the tendon-tightening mechanism that operates to maintain the grip when the leg is flexed. A second person may be needed to force the leg to straighten and release the talons.

It is impossible for an unassisted person to get free from the talons of a bird such as the golden or bald eagle (Figs. 29.52, 29.53) unless the bird is released first. I have

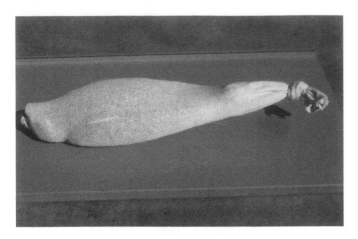

FIG. 29.54. Stockinette restraint.

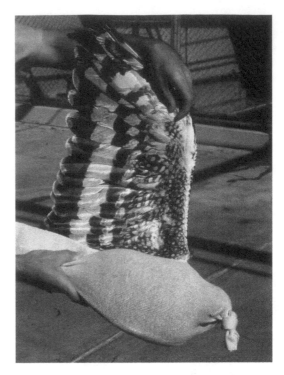

FIG. 29.56. Using a stockinette to control a raptor while exposing a wing for examination.

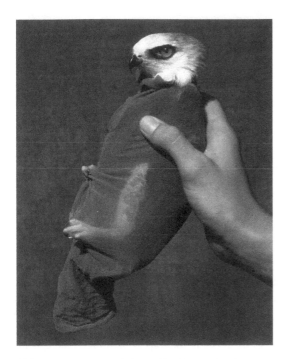

FIG. 29.55. Restraining a kite in a nylon hose.

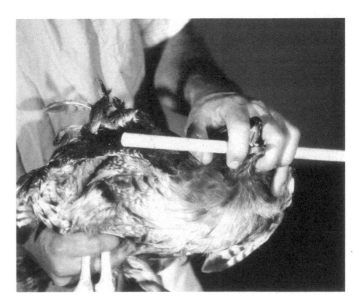

FIG. 29.57. Dowel used as a speculum for a hawk.

attempted to remove a burlap sack from the clutches of a golden eagle. It took one person on each talon to force the bird to relinquish its grip on the sack.

Medium-sized raptors may be effectively restrained after initial capture by placing them in a stockinette or nylon hose (Figs. 29.54, 29.55). The stockinette may serve as a hood to diminish visual stimulation and restrict wing action. To examine a wing or a leg, cut a hole through the stockinette and extract the limb (Fig. 29.56). Birds restrained in nylon hose must be watched carefully, since nylon retains heat to a greater degree than cotton stockinette. Birds have died from hyperthermia as a result of prolonged restraint in nylon hose.

Examination of the mouth of a large raptor may be carried out quite easily with a dowel speculum between the upper and lower beak (Fig. 29.57), or by the use of two tapes. Collars to prevent self-mutilation may be placed on quiet raptors (Fig. 29.58). The bird must not be able to reach the margin of the collar with the tip of its beak.

A raptor may be examined for external parasites as illustrated in Figure 29.59.

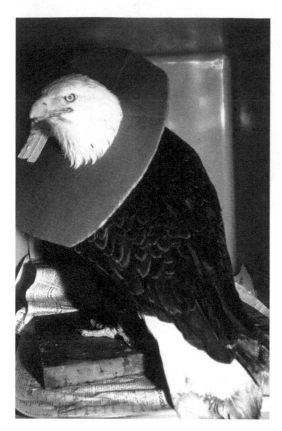

FIG. 29.58. Cardboard collar used to prevent self-mutilation during wound healing.

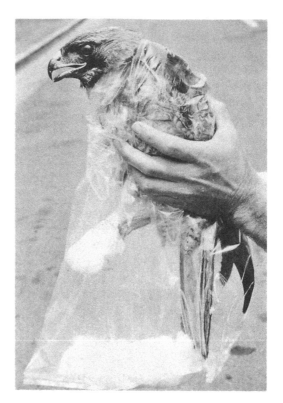

FIG. 29.59. Collecting external parasites from a hawk by placing it in a plastic bag containing chloroform-impregnated pledget of cotton. Make sure the head is kept out of the bag.

Chemical Restraint[7,10,13]

Chemical immobilization may be necessary to perform diagnostic procedures such as radiography. Isoflurane in oxygen (5%), administered via a face mask or endotracheal intubation, provides rapid induction, safety, and rapid recovery. It is the method of choice for those using an appropriate vaporizer.

Ketamine (5–15 mg/kg) and xylazine/ketamine 3/15 mg/kg are acceptable agents for injection. Tiletamine/ zolazepam 10 mg/kg satisfactorily immobilized great horned owls, but not red-tailed hawks. Recovery from injectable sedation may require 1–6 hours.

GALLIFORM BIRDS

Galliforms are heavy-bodied, short-legged, slow-flying birds. These birds spend most of the time on the ground searching for seeds, insects, or herbs.

Danger Potential

Most birds in this group are inoffensive docile birds that can be handled without danger of being pecked or scratched. However, all have claws and may scratch when excited, though none are capable of causing serious injury. Males in this group may exhibit large tarsal spurs, primarily used in fighting among themselves but which may also be used defensively when capture is imminent.

These birds should not be grabbed by the feathers, particularly the tail feathers. Pheasants, crowned pigeons, and turacos release their feathers readily when captured. Although not of long-term significance, lost tail feathers disfigure species in which the tail feathers are important for exhibition. Although generally mild mannered, some pheasant species occasionally become aggressive, particularly during the breeding season. A cock may fly at an intruder with feet outstretched, attacking with tarsal spurs and wings. The face should be protected when attempting to capture male birds.

Physical Restraint

Once the bird is captured, usually by netting, hold the wings close to the bird's body and control the legs (Figs. 29.60, 29.61, 29.62, 29.63). The beak is rarely used for defense.

LONG-BILLED, LONG-LEGGED BIRDS[19,20]
Danger Potential

The primary defense of long-beaked birds is pecking. Herons, storks, cranes, and other birds with large or long sharp-pointed bills may peck at the face and eyes of handlers,

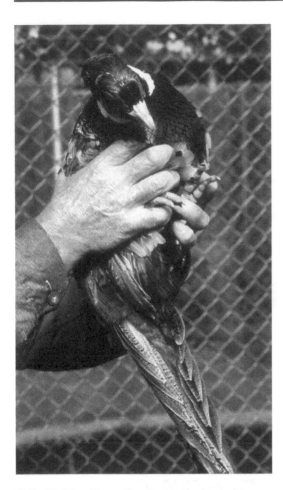

FIG. 29.60. Controlling legs and wings of a pheasant.

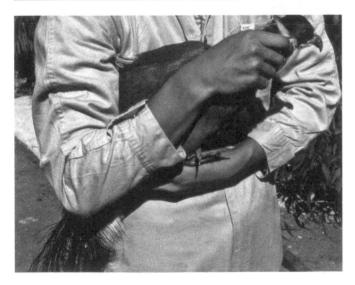

FIG. 29.61. Restraining a pheasant by holding it next to the body.

inflicting serious injury. Flamingos frequently attempt to peck captors and may inflict rather nasty wounds with the serrated margins of the blunt recurved beak. Do not peek into a crate or wire enclosure containing one of these birds, lest it peck at

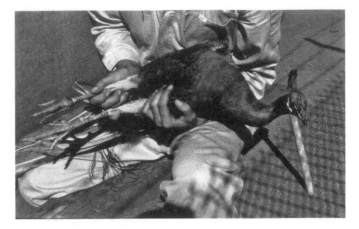

FIG. 29.62. Restraining a peafowl by controlling the legs.

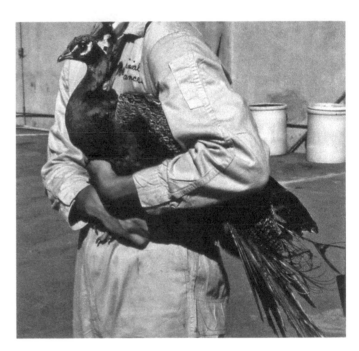

FIG. 29.63. Holding a peafowl for temporary transport.

your eyes. When capturing long-billed birds, control the head first by grasping either the neck or the bill.

Members of this group of birds will attempt to scratch with their long legs, but scratches are seldom severe. The African crowned crane is an exception. This bird will claw much as does a hawk. Guard against injury from the feet, the beating wings, and the beak of this crane.

Physical Restraint

The long thin legs of these birds are easily broken by injudicious handling. Restraint should be applied gently, exerting minimum pressure.

A person should not enter an enclosure confining large cranes without some means of protection such as a broom, a net, or a stick to hold the bird away and keep it from pecking. Cranes may be hooded, as is done with ostriches, to eliminate visual stimuli. A combination hood and net may cover the head of a crane until the neck can be grasped and the wings controlled.

Cranes can usually be herded into a corner with a sheet of plastic, a shield, or a fence panel. If a fence panel is used, the birds may be squeezed into a corner, enabling the handler to grasp an individual by the beak or the neck and wings (Fig. 29.64). Figure 29.65 shows how a crane may be held, but the legs may flail and scratch the handler. When prolonged

restraint of a crane or stork is necessary, tape the bill shut and impale a blunt object such as a cork or rubber stopper on the tip of the beak to prevent jabbing injuries (Fig. 29.66). Large cranes may be moved by placing a soft rope or a sock around the base of both wings and controlling the beak (Fig. 29.67). If cranes and storks must be handled frequently, wear a metal face mask to protect the eyes and face. It is not desirable to capture cranes or storks with a net. The fine bones are fragile

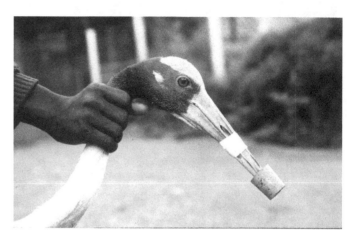

FIG. 29.66. Protecting from sharp bill by placing a cork over the taped beak, leaving nostrils uncovered.

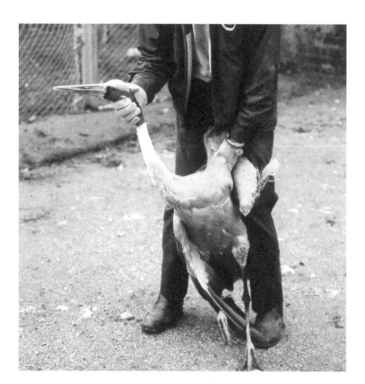

FIG. 29.64. Grasp a crane by the neck first to prevent personal injury from the beak, then grab the wings.

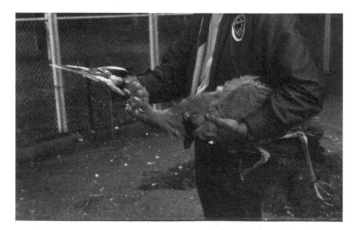

FIG. 29.65. A crane may be held as illustrated, but the legs will flail and may scratch the handler.

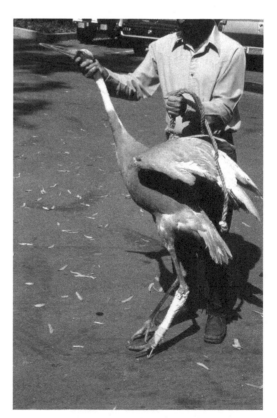

FIG. 29.67. Moving a saurus crane by controlling the head and wings.

and easily fractured or injured if struck with the hoop or entangled in the mesh.

Flamingos can usually be slowly herded into a corner, permitting handlers to enter the enclosure to capture them. Then fasten them by the neck with one hand and quickly grasp the body with the other, lifting the bird off its feet and directing the legs slightly away from the handler. Hold the body of the bird next to the hip of the handler, leaving the legs to move freely. Do not clutch flamingos by their lower legs or attempt to net them, for the long spindly legs may be injured. If it is necessary to restrict the movement of the limbs, do so by grasping the neck with one hand and the base of the legs with the other. (See Fig. 29.68.)

Long-legged birds present special problems during recovery from anesthesia or immobilization. If left to their own devices while awakening, they are likely to stagger and fall, injuring themselves. A satisfactory means of controlling the bird during recovery is to place it in a burlap sack with the head exposed; this prevents it from standing until completely recovered from the effects of the anesthetic (Figs. 29.69, 29.70). Isoflurane inhalation anesthesia eliminates prolonged recovery and risk of injury. These birds are subject to capture myopathy, so leg activity should not be severely restricted.

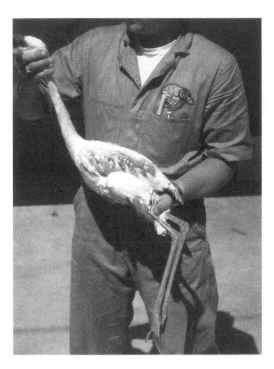

FIG. 29.68. When restraining a flamingo, restrict head movement and grasp the legs close to the bird's body. Alternatively, the left arm could wrap around the body just in front of the legs and allow the legs to remain free.

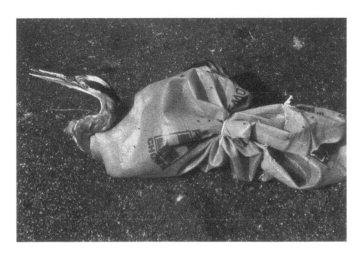

FIG. 29.69. Blue heron in a sack for recovery from anesthesia.

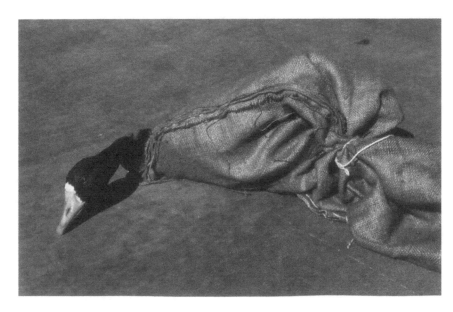

FIG. 29.70. A goose placed in a bag for temporary restraint.

LARGE-BILLED BIRDS

Danger Potential

Toucans, hornbills, and others of this group will peck the face and hands with their massive bills. If you must enter an enclosure with one of these birds, use a mask or a plastic shield (Fig. 29.71).

Physical Restraint

Birds in this group should be initially captured with a net (Fig. 29.72). The bill should be clasped and held shut while the bird is extracted from the net and during subsequent procedures (Fig. 29.73). The bill may be taped shut and a cork impaled on the tip if prolonged restraint is necessary. Once in hand, the beak and wings may be held together close to the

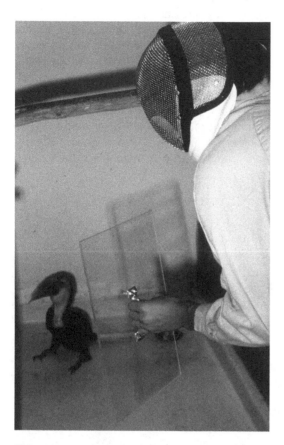

FIG. 29.71. Capturing a hornbill. Handler is protected by fencer's face mask and plastic shield.

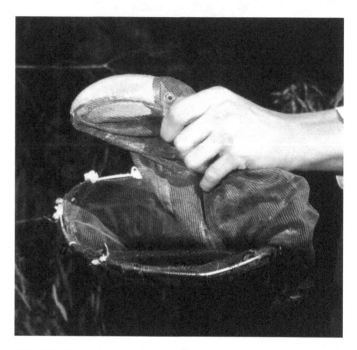

FIG. 29.73. Grasping a toucan through the net.

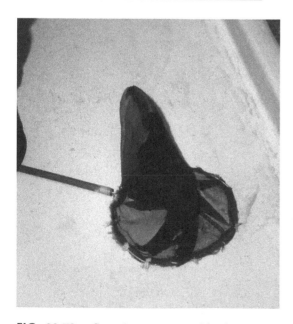

FIG. 29.72. Capturing an toucan with a hoop net.

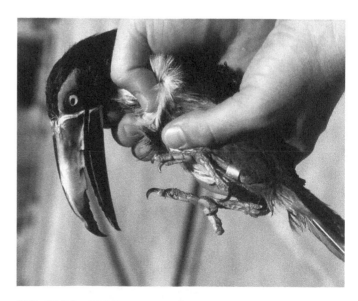

FIG. 29.74. Holding an aracari.

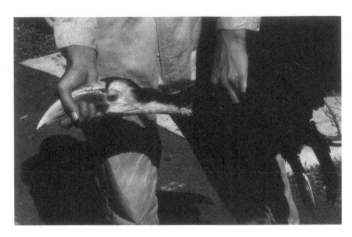

FIG. 29.75. Correct restraint for a hornbill.

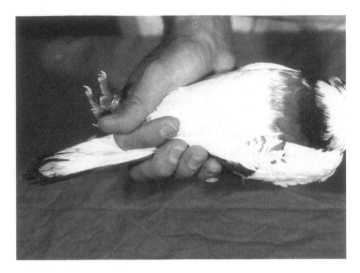

FIG. 29.77. A. Proper pigeon handling.

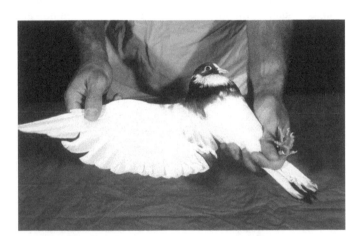

FIG. 29.76. One person may easily restrain and examine a pigeon.

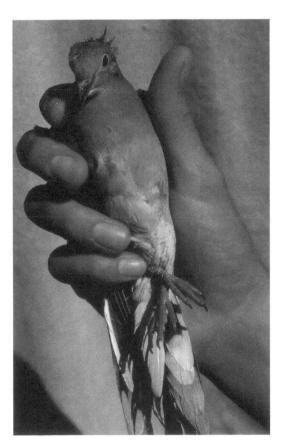

FIG. 29.78. A small dove may be handled like a budgerigar or finch.

body of the bird; or the wings may be grasped as shown in Figures 29.73 and 29.74. Figure 29.75 illustrates how to correctly restrain a hornbill.

PIGEONS AND DOVES

Doves are perhaps the most inoffensive of wild birds to handle. They do not scratch; they are not likely to peck; they have no wing spurs; and they have mild, docile dispositions.

Wild pigeons are handled by the same methods as domestic species. Basic handling procedure is to grasp from above and behind, pressing the wings close to the bird's body. Control of pigeons and doves is shown in Figures 29.76, 29.77, 29.78, and 29.79. Birds of these species are also easily netted.

The large crowned pigeon will shed its feathers if the feathers are grasped improperly during the restraint procedure. Do not grasp the tail, or the tail feathers will pull out.

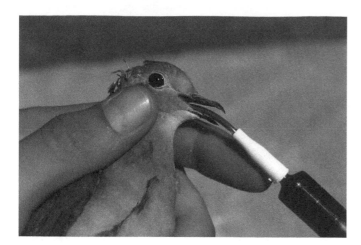

FIG. 29.79. Stomach tube placement in a dove (no speculum is necessary).

PSITTACINE BIRDS—PARROTS, PARAKEETS, LORIES

Danger Potential

Psittacines all have large heavy bills and strong jaws. The diet of these birds consists primarily of nuts and seeds, though some are fruit eaters. The bills of all are capable of seriously injuring an unwary handler. The beak of a large parrot or macaw is a formidable weapon (Fig. 29.80). A large macaw such as a hyacinth can easily crush the bone of a finger. A glove affords little protection from crushing.

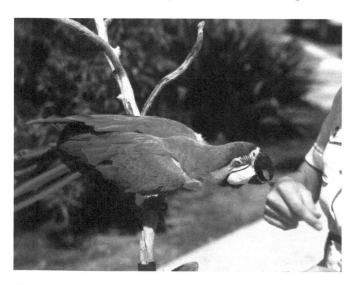

FIG. 29.80. Large macaw pecking a handler.

Some parrots are well adapted to climbing and clinging to branches. These have sharp claws that may injure. However, light gloves afford adequate protection from scratching by the claws of psittacine birds.

The kea parrot is a member of the psittacine group, but its habits resemble those of raptors. It is carnivorous and uses its beak and talons in the same manner and for the same pur-poses as do raptors. It should be handled as if it were a raptor.

Physical Restraint[3]

Darkening the room has a sedative effect on diurnal birds and facilitates capture of psittacines from cages or aviaries. The basic procedure when capturing and handling all psittacine birds is to control the head. Refer to the following discussion in this chapter for head control.

Parakeets (budgerigars) are routinely kept in small cages. If confined in an aviary, they should be captured with a small net. If in a small cage, remove all obstructions such as perches, mirrors, or other dangling objects against which an excited bird may fly and injure itself. Corner the bird against the cage wall or the floor. Approach it from behind and above, placing the thumb and forefinger on each side of the head (Fig. 29.81). Grasp it firmly, but do not crush it. Remove the bird from the cage, fixing the grip to position the bird on its back in the cupped hand with the head controlled by thumb and forefinger.

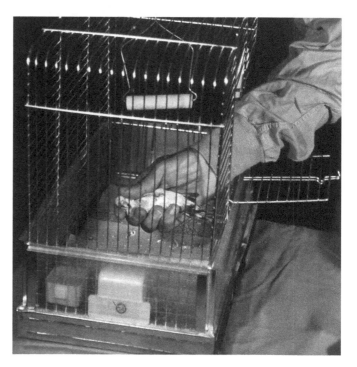

FIG. 29.81. Capturing budgerigar in a cage by grabbing it from behind.

Larger members of this group are handled in much the same manner, but the hands must be protected. The most satisfactory way of approaching a bird in a small cage is to hold a towel between the hands (Figs. 29.82, 29.83). Encourage the bird to begin climbing the side of the cage, then quickly grasp the head and push the body against the cage until a sturdy hold is completed. The towel will partly encircle the bird's wings (Fig. 29.83). Remove the bird from the cage and carefully remove the towel so that the fingers and hand will

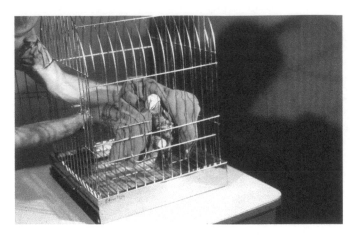

FIG. 29.82. Capturing a parrot by surrounding it with a towel.

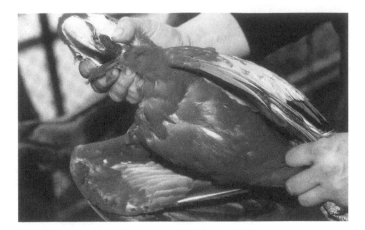

FIG. 29.84. Holding a large macaw with bare hands after initial capture with a towel.

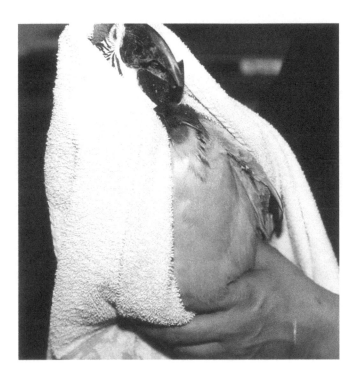

FIG. 29.83. Holding a macaw in a towel.

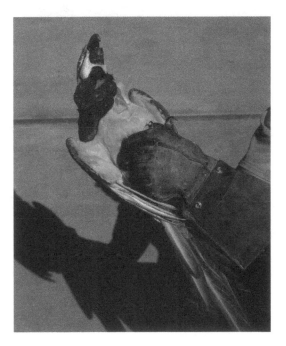

FIG. 29.85. Holding a large macaw with gloves.

have better tactile perception without applying excessive pressure (Fig. 29.84).

Gloves may be worn instead of using a towel, but many birds will be more aggressive toward gloved hands (Fig. 29.85). Large macaws and cockatoos may present a special challenge, especially if they have been repeatedly restrained. A towel or a small rug is the best method for capturing these large birds.

If it is necessary to transfer a captured psittacine bird to another person, the second person places a hand over the hand holding the head, imposing the grip as the first person releases it.

Numerous devices have been used to open a bird's mouth and to hold it open (Fig. 29.86). Speculae made out of metal

or hard plastic may contuse the bars of the jaws. The most satisfactory and least traumatic procedure is to prepare two strips from 2.2-cm (1-in.) adhesive tape. Stretch the strip, and fold it over on itself lengthwise so that the sticky sides adhere to each other. One strip is used to sling the upper jaw and another strip used to sling the lower jaw (Figs. 29.87, 29.88, 29.89). The jaws should be gently, but firmly, parted by fatiguing the muscles rather than by jerking the mouth open. If cultures are to be obtained from the choana, use a tongue depressor stick to press the tongue to the floor of the mouth to prevent it from coming into contact with the swab. In smaller birds the tongue depressor must be split lengthwise.

A budgerigar may be stomach tubed without the use of a speculum by inserting the tube gently through the commissure of the mouth. At the commissure the horny beak cannot

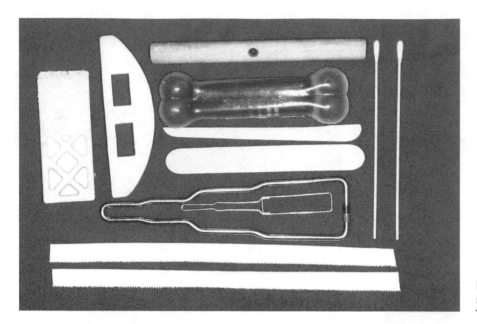

FIG. 29.86. Various devices used for specula to hold the mouth open in birds.

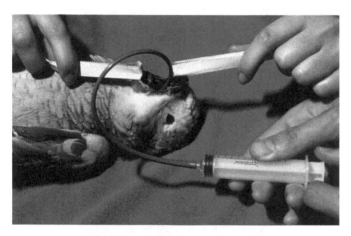

FIG. 29.87. Holding the mouth open with tape strips to obtain a crop sample.

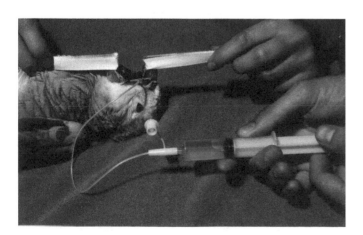

FIG. 29.88. Holding the mouth open with tape speculum to perform a tracheal wash.

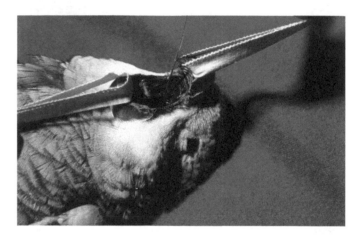

FIG. 29.89. Culturing the choana in a parrot.

cut the tube. The tube can be inserted, held in this position while medication is administered, and withdrawn without causing a great deal of discomfort. A large paper clip may be used for an oral speculum (Fig. 29.90).

Metal feeding tubes or needles are the most common form of intubating the crop. The size and length are determined by the size of the bird.

Small birds may be auscultated directly or with a stethoscope (Fig. 29.91). Blood may be obtained from the right jugular vein, and intramuscular injections may be given into the breast muscle (Fig. 29.92).

When examining small caged birds, it is a good policy to have an anesthetic chamber available to administer oxygen as well as to anesthetize (Fig. 29.93). Birds are easily intubated intratracheally (Fig. 29.94), using a variety of endotracheal tubes (Fig. 29.95). A bird may be taped directly to a radiograph cassette (Figs. 29.96, 29.97) or a restraining board may be used (Fig. 29.98) for radiography.

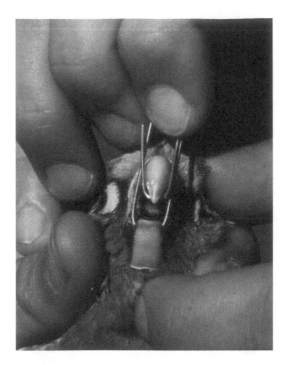

FIG. 29.90. A paper clip used for an oral speculum.

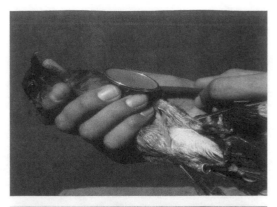

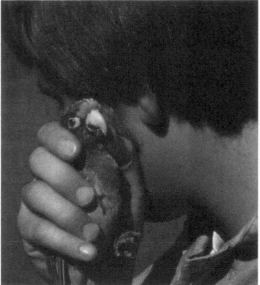

FIG. 29.91. Evaluation of respiratory sounds: Direct listening, lower. Using a stethoscope, upper.

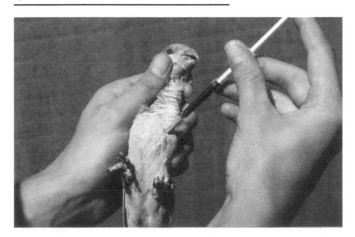

FIG. 29.92. Intramuscular injection into the breast muscle.

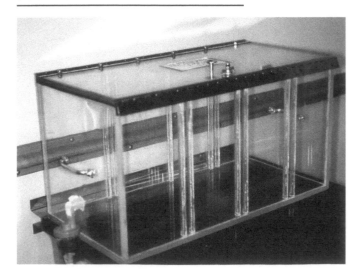

FIG. 29.93. Anesthesia chamber used for birds.

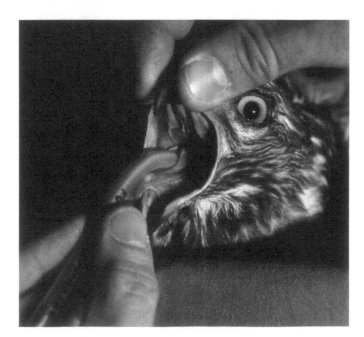

FIG. 29.94. Tracheal intubation of a hawk.

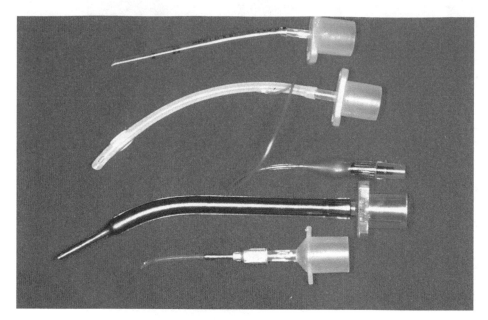

FIG. 29.95. Various types of endotracheal tubes used on birds.

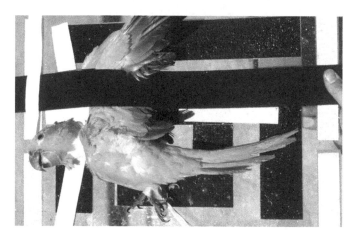

FIG. 29.96. Positioning for lateral avian radiography.

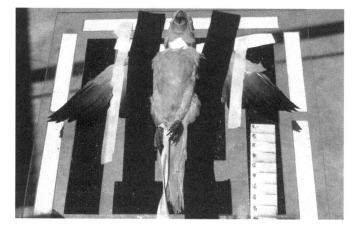

FIG. 29.97. Positioning for dorsoventral radiography.

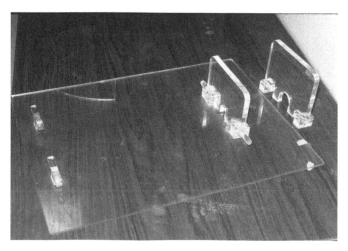

FIG. 29.98. Plastic restraining board for radiography of birds.

Various types of collars may be fashioned for birds, to discourage self-mutilation (Figs. 29.99, 29.100). Appropriately sized Elizabethan collars, like those used for dogs, may be used also.

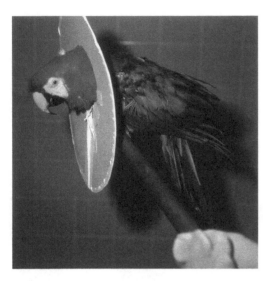

FIG. 29.99. Improvised collar to prevent self-mutilation.

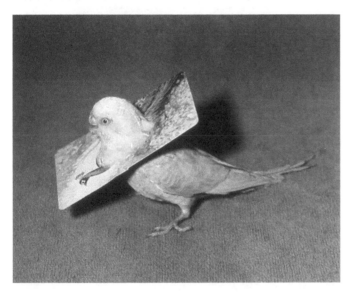

FIG. 29.100. Playing card used as a collar for a budgerigar.

HUMMINGBIRDS AND SWIFTS

It is extremely difficult to capture the rapidly flying hummingbird, which is capable of reversing flight instantaneously. Always work in a darkened room when attempting to capture these birds. Mist nets are used to capture hummingbirds and other small rapidly flying birds.

After initial capture, these birds may be restrained and handled by cupping them gently in the hand (Fig. 29.101). None are aggressive or capable of injuring the handler.

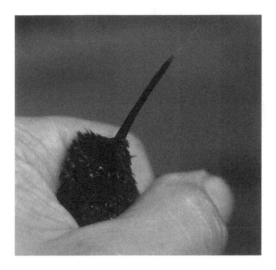

FIG. 29.101. A tiny hummingbird is difficult to hold without crushing it.

SONG, PERCHING, AND MISCELLANEOUS BIRDS[3,9,16]

The small delicate finches and warblers, crows, and hundreds of other species of birds of various sizes are handled in much the same way. Most are inoffensive, and little protection is needed for the hands.

Physical Restraint

In an aviary the birds are captured with a net, carefully removed, and held cupped in the hand with the hand around the base of the head (Fig. 29.102). Small birds rarely injure a handler when they peck, but the habit of securing the head properly should become deeply ingrained. The feet may

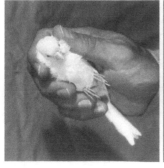
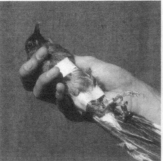
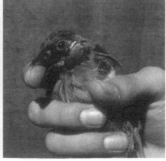

FIG. 29.102. Correct restraint of a canary, left. Correct restraint of a passerine bird, center. A peck from this small bird will not injure the finger, right.

require controlling, though most of these birds will not scratch.

When holding a bird in the cupped hand, do not completely surround the sternum and interfere with respiration. Tiny finches and warblers are extremely difficult to hold safely. Suggested techniques are illustrated in Figure 29.103.

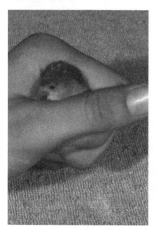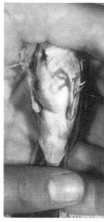

FIG. 29.103. **A.** A tiny finch may require holding as illustrated. **B.** Examination of legs and body may be accomplished as shown.

Darken the room where caged birds are kept to diminish activity and fright before removing them from the cage. Approach birds from behind. A light glove may be required for handling mynah birds and some of the heavier birds such as crows, ravens, and jays, which may resist capture and restraint. Follow the same procedure described for capturing the budgerigar. The beak may be taped shut to eliminate pecking (Fig. 29.104).

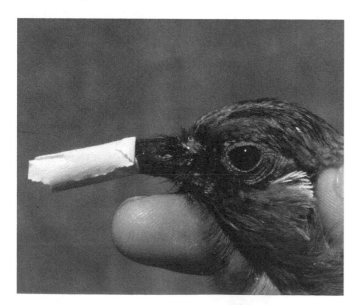

FIG. 29.104. Taping beak to prevent bothersome pecking.

There should be no open windows, open drains, exposed heating elements, or exhaust fans in the examination room. Exhaust fans may suck a small bird into the blades. Small nets should be readily available to capture escaped birds.

Collection of blood from small birds may be challenging, but may be performed at several sites such as the jugular vein (Fig. 29.105); the brachial vein (Figs. 29.106, 29.107, 29.108); and the medial metatarsal vein (Fig. 29.109).

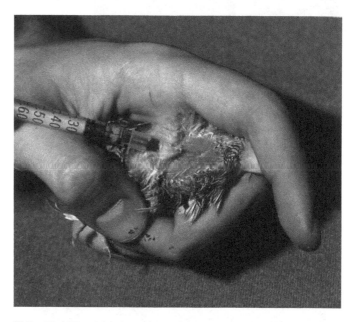

FIG. 29.105. Blood collection from the right jugular vein of a budgerigar.

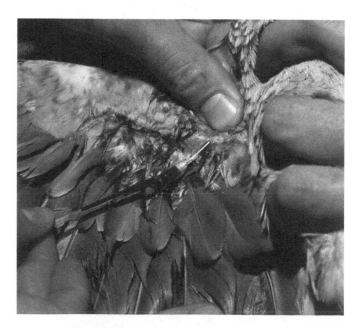

FIG. 29.106. Blood collection from the hub of a needle placed in the brachial vein.

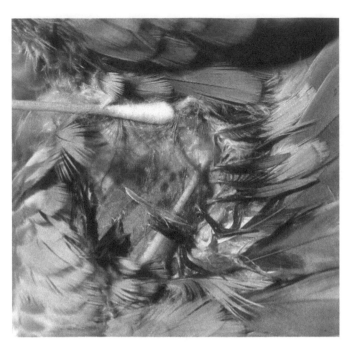

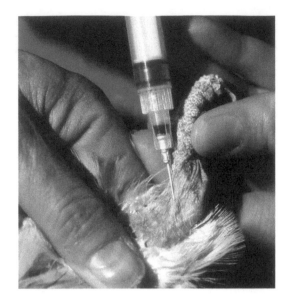

FIG. 29.109. Blood collection from the medial metatarsal vein.

FIG. 29.107. Using a "Q" tip to distend the brachial vein.

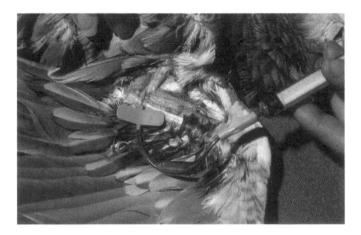

FIG. 29.108. Blood collection from the brachial vein using a butterfly catheter.

REFERENCES

1. Blackshaw, G.D., and Wakeman, B. 1971. Immobilization of an adult ostrich for surgery. J Zoo Anim Med 2:11–12.
2. Cornick-Seahorn, J. 1996. Anesthesiology of ratites. In: Tully, T.N., Jr., and Shane, S.M. Ratite Management, Medicine and Surgery. Malabar, Florida, Krieger Publishing, pp. 79–94.
3. Hawkins, M.G., and Pascoe, P.J. 2007. Cagebirds. In: West, G., Heard, D., and Caulkett, N., Eds. Zoo Animal and Wildlife Chemical Immobilization and Anesthesia. Ames, Iowa, Blackwell Publishing, pp. 269–68.
4. Jensen, J.M. 1993. Ratite restraint and handling. In: Fowler, M.E., Ed. Zoo and Wild Animal Medicine, 3rd ed.,. Philadelphia: W.B. Saunders, pp. 198–200.
5. Jessup, D.A. 1982. Chemical capture of upland game birds and waterfowl: Oral anesthetics. In: Nielsen, L., Haigh, J.C., and Fowler, M.E., Eds. Chemical Immobilization of North American Wildlife, Milwaukee, Wis.: Humane Society, pp. 214–26.
6. Keffen, R.H. 1993. The ostrich: Capture, care, accommodation, and transportation. In: McKenzie, A.A., Ed. The Capture and Care Manual, Pretoria: The South African Veterinary Foundation, pp. 634–52.
7. Kreeger, T.J., Degernes, L.A., Kreeger, J.S., and Redig, P.T. 1993. Immobilization of raptors with tiletamine and zolazepam (Telazol). In: Redig, P.T., Cooper, J.E., Remple, J.D., and Hunter, D.B., Eds. Raptor Biomedicine, Minneapolis: Univ. of Minnesota Press, pp. 141–44.
8. Loibl, M.F., Clutton, R.E., Marx, B.D., and McGrath, C.J. 1988. Alpha-chloralose as a capture and restraint agent of birds: Therapeutic index determination in the chicken. J Wildl Dis 24:684–87.
9. Ludders, J.W., and Matthews, N.S. 2007. Birds. In: Tranquilli, W.J., Thurman, J.C., and Grimm, K.A., Eds. Lumb and Jones' Veterinary Anesthesia and Analgesia, 4th Ed. Ames, Iowa, Wiley-Blackwell Publishing, pp. 841–69.
10. Lumeij, J.T. 1993. Effects of ketamine-xylazine anesthesia on adrenal function and cardiac conduction in goshawks and pigeons. In: Redig, P.T., Cooper, J.E., Remple, J.D., and Hunter, D.B., Eds. Raptor Biomedicine, Minneapolis, Univ. of Minnesota Press, pp. 145–49.
11. Mulcathy, D.M. 2007. Free-living waterfowl and shorebirds. In: West, G., Heard, D., and Caulkett, N., Eds. Zoo Animal and Wildlife Immobilization and Anesthesia, Ames, Iowa, Blackwell Publishing, pp. 299–324.
12. Ostrowski, S., and Ancrenaz, M. 1995. Chemical immobilization of red-necked ostriches under field conditions. Vet Record 136:145–47.
13. Raffe, M.R., Mammel, M., Gordon, M., Duke, G., Redig, P., and Boros, S. 1993. Cardiorespiratory effects of ketamine-xylazine in the great horned owl. In: Redig, P.T., Cooper, J.E., Remple, J.D., and Hunter, D.B., Eds. Raptor Biomedicine, Minneapolis: Univ. of Minnesota Press, pp. 150–53.
14. Raath, J.P., Quandt, S.K., and Malan, J.H. 1992. *Struthio camelus* immobilization using carfentanil and xylazine and reversal with yohimbine and naltrexone. J S African Vet Assoc 62:138–40.

15. Siegal-Willott, J. 2007. Ratites. In: West, G., Heard, D., and Caulkett, N., Eds. Zoo Animal and Wildlife Chemical Immobilization and Anesthesia. Ames, Iowa, Blackwell Publishing, pp. 325–35.

16. Sinn, L.C. 1994. Anesthesiology. In: Ritchie, B.W., Harrison, G.J., and Harrison, L.R. Avian Medicine. Principles and Applications. Lake Worth, Florida, Winger Publishing, pp.1066–80.

17. Stoskopf, M.K., and Kennedy-Stoskopf, S. 1986. Aquatic birds. In: Fowler, M.E., Ed. Zoo and Wild Animal Medicine, 2nd ed., Philadelphia: W.B. Saunders, p. 301.

18. Stoskopf, M.J., Beall, F.B., Ensley, P.K., and Neely, E. 1982. Immobilization of large ratites, with hematologic and serum chemistry data. J Zoo Anim Med 13:160–68.

19. Williams, L.E., and Phillips, R.W. 1973. Capturing sandhill cranes with alpha chloralose. J Wildl Manage 37:94–97.

20. Young, E. 1966. Leg paralysis in the greater flamingo and lesser flamingo following capture and transportation. Int Zoo Yearb 6:226–27.

CHAPTER 30

Reptiles

CLASSIFICATION

Class Reptilia
> Order Crocodilia (2 families, 8 genera, 21 species)
>> Family Gavialidae: gavial
>> Family Crocodilidae: alligator, crocodile, caiman
> Order Chelonia (Testudines) (8 families, 56 genera, 219 species): turtle, tortoise, sea turtle, snapping turtle
> Order Rhynchocephalia (1 family, 1 genus, 1 species)
>> Family Sphenodontidae: tuatara
> Order Squamata
>> Suborder Lacertilia (19 families, 360 genera, 2,839 species): gecko, monitor, iguana, chameleon, Gila monster, legless lizard
>> Suborder Ophidia (9 families, 416 genera, 2,005 species)
>>> Family Boidae: giant constrictor
>>> Family Elapidae: cobra, krait
>>> Family Hydrophidae: sea snake
>>> Family Viperidae: rattlesnake, viper

Family Colubridae: nonpoisonous species

Generally adults are called males and females. A male crocodile is called a bull and the female a cow. Newly hatched or newborns are called hatchlings or juveniles.

Although members of this class share sufficient morphological characteristics to warrant close zoological classification, the requirements for restraint and handling vary widely with the species; therefore, for discussion they will be divided into groups that can be handled with similar techniques.

All reptiles continue to grow throughout life, although the rate of growth slows markedly as they age. Size is an indication of age, but other factors such as nutritional level and environmental temperatures also determine size.

In mammals, the venous drainage from the hindquarters and the tail is via the iliac veins, then to the caudal vena cava, and on to the heart. Reptiles, like birds, have a renal portal system. In reptiles, a valve located in the iliac vein shunts blood through the kidney before it enters the renal vein and continues on to the caudal vena cava. Because of this anatomic characteristic, drugs injected in this area may be partially excreted before they can take effect. Therefore, intramuscular and subcutaneous injections should be given in the cranial half of the body.

The author once reviewed a paper on the use of ketamine in a lizard species, in which a dose of 250 mg/kg was recommended. When questioned about the exorbitant dose, the investigator acknowledged that the drug had been administered in the thigh muscle. Reptiles may be immobilized with less than 80 mg/kg of ketamine if it is administered in the cranial half of the body.

CROCODILIANS

Crocodilians include alligators, crocodiles, gavials, and caimans. Approximately 21 species are scattered throughout tropical and subtropical areas of the world.

Danger Potential

All crocodilians are carnivores, capable of inflicting serious bites even in the newly hatched stage. Crocodilians lurk until a prey species nears, then quickly grasp it and tear off flesh by flinging the head about. They exhibit the same behavior when they bite a person; they grasp and then flip the head, tearing out tissue.

In all crocodilians the muscles that close the mouth are strong, but those that open it are weak, so a person's hands can easily hold the mouth closed.

The tail of crocodilians is used to propel them through the water. During restraint vicious lashing with the tail is a principal method of attack, particularly by larger species.

Physiology and Behavior

Crocodilians are primarily aquatic species that come ashore and bask in the sun to absorb heat. Although they must surface to breathe, they are able to stay submerged for many minutes.

During colder months of the year, some crocodilians become anorectic and enter a torpid state. During this time they subsist on energy reserves stored in the body. Captivity may adversely modify the ability to properly prepare for the torpid state; thus torpid captive animals may be marginally hypoglycemic. Handling one of these animals while it is in the torpid state may send it into hypoglycemic shock by stimulating a too-sudden return to activity, for which the animal is incapable of mobilizing sufficient glucose to meet energy needs. The reaction of torpid crocodilians to chemical restraint agents is extremely unpredictable.

Physical Restraint[3,11]

Small specimens up to 0.6 m (2 ft) in length may be manually handled without difficulty (Figs. 30.1, 30.2). It may

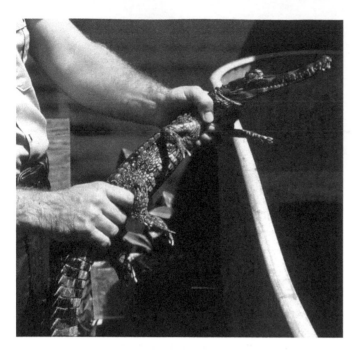

FIG. 30.1.   Grasping a small crocodilian by the neck and tail.

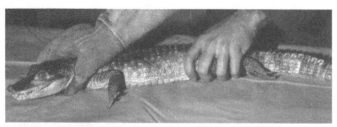

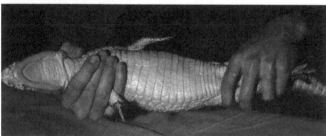

FIG. 30.2.   Holding a small caiman to prevent biting and minimize scratching. Notice that the hind feet are held back against the sides of the tail.

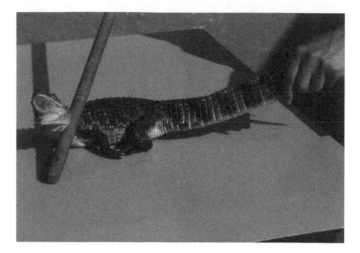

FIG. 30.3.   Controlling a small caiman by partially pinning its head.

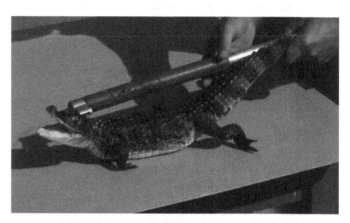

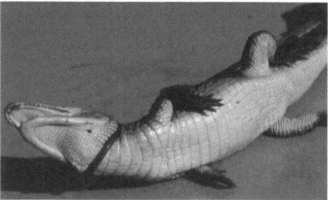

FIG. 30.4.   Controlling a small caiman with a snare.

be necessary to pin the head partially to allow a safe approach (Fig. 30.3). These animals may scratch, so provide suitable protection in the form of gloves or clothing. The tail must be restrained at all times; otherwise even a small animal may slap the handler in the face or injure itself by wildly flailing the tail.

Specimens up to 2 m (6 ft) in length may be handled with a snare. Nooses vary in design from swiveled snares, available commercially, to homemade cable snares. With either type, once the noose is around the neck, the animal is likely to try to twirl on the snare; unless the handler is prepared to twirl the snare with the animal, strangulation or neck injuries may occur. Immediately grasping the tail as soon as a snare is placed around the neck will inhibit twirling on the snare and prevent flailing (Fig. 30.4). Even with a snare around the neck, the head of a crocodile is able to flip rapidly from side to side.

Manual handling of large crocodilians is both difficult and hazardous. Desirable methods of approaching large crocodilians vary with the species. An alligator or caiman can be handled by two or three persons who jump on it simultaneously, one grasping the front legs and controlling the body and another the tail (Fig. 30.5). Speed, agility, and timing are important. Do not attempt this with a crocodile; it is much faster and more aggressive than an alligator or caiman. Nets or special squeeze cages may be used to manipulate any species of crocodile. A large crocodilian may be restrained by the use of heavy cargo nets or by ropes placed around the mouth, legs, and tail. Once the animal is secured, the mouth can be taped shut with electrician's tape or duct tape or tied shut with small ropes (Fig. 30.6).

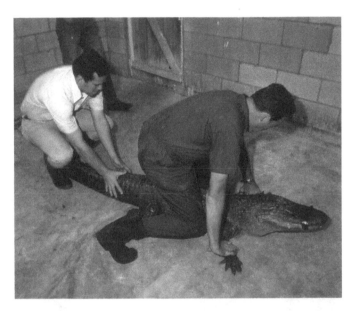

FIG. 30.5. A large alligator may be manually restrained by an experienced, confident team.

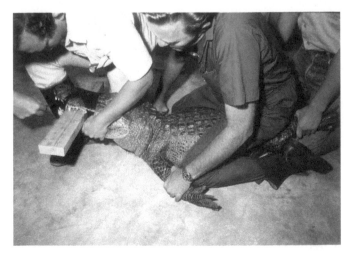

FIG. 30.6. Once an alligator is in hand, the mouth can easily be kept closed by taping it. The board in this instance holds the mouth open for passage of a stomach tube.

Large crocodilians are capable of knocking a person down by merely flipping the head or tail from side to side.

Be cautious. Some species of crocodilians have teeth protruding outside the mouth. If the head is permitted to flail from side to side, these teeth may lacerate anyone nearby. The tail must always be held by one or two individuals or secured by ropes or heavy nets; otherwise the flipping of the tail can inflict lethal injuries. When the animal is under control, it may be turned over or manipulated in any manner necessary for examination, treatment, or obtaining laboratory samples.

A rope noose may be tossed over the head and snout of a crocodilian. If two ropes are used, the animal may be dragged into a crate for shipment. The ropes may be wrapped around the animal to completely truss it up, or it may be lashed to a plank. The plank serves as a stretcher, or a human stretcher may be used to carry specimens up to 2 m long.

The staff at the London Zoo has developed a special funnel bag to control crocodilians. The heavy canvas bag is placed over the jaws and head, and ropes are lashed around the bag to hold the animal's mouth shut.

Crocodilians dissipate heat by evaporation from the mucous membrane of the mouth. A struggling crocodilian with its mouth lashed shut may rapidly overheat. It should be monitored and cooled if necessary.

Persons working in zoos or other exhibit facilities often guide alligators or caimans by grasping the tails. This is not without some danger. It is safer if a colleague keeps the animal from flipping around to the side with a broom or a stick. Both handlers should remain on the same side of the animal.

Squeeze cages for crocodilians are commercially available, or they may be constructed (Fig. 30.7). Squeeze cages should be immersible. The animal may be enticed to enter the submerged cage for food, or the cage may be placed in the area of the pond where the animal habitually lurks.

Blood Collection[10]

Blood samples may be collected by cardiac puncture; by venipuncture of the ventral coccygeal vein (Fig. 30.8) similar to sample collection from a lizard; or from the supravertebral vein(s) dorsal to the vertebrae (Figs. 30.9, 30.10). At the latter site, a 3.75 to 7.6-cm (1.5- to 3.0-in.), 22-gauge needle is inserted through the skin at the midline immediately caudal to the dorsal spine of the atlas, which lies against the occipital crest of the skull. The head should be held in a slightly flexed position (sedation may be necessary). Direct the needle slightly caudal and maintain negative pressure as the needle is advanced. This is also the site recommended for obtaining samples of cerebrospinal fluid, in which case a spinal needle is required and the needle should be inserted deeper.

The heart is located along the ventral midline, approximately 11 scale rows caudal to the forelimbs. For obtaining blood from the heart or the tail vein, the animal should be placed in dorsal recumbency.

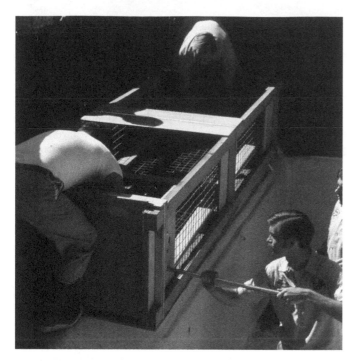

FIG. 30.7.   A portable squeeze cage for capturing and transporting a crocodilian. Cage is lowered into a pool and the animal baited inside. Upon removal, the upper movable wall may be pressed over the animal to restrain it for examination or treatment.

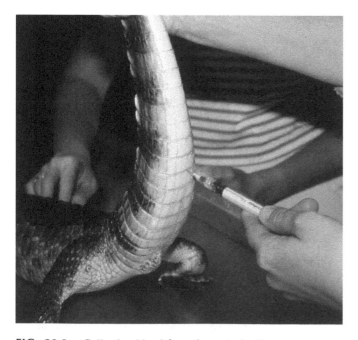

FIG. 30.8.   Collecting blood from the ventral tail vein.

Miscellaneous Clinical Procedures

The stomach of crocodilians may be visualized using endoscopy (Fig. 30.11). Endotracheal intubation is used for administering inhalation anesthesia (Fig. 21.12).

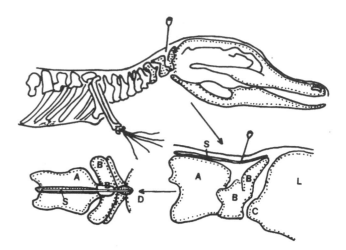

FIG. 30.9.   Schematic diagram of blood collection from the supravertebral plexus of a crocodilian. **A.** axis; **B.** atlas; **C.** occipital condyle; **D.** dorsal view; **L.** lateral view; **S.** supravertebral plexus.

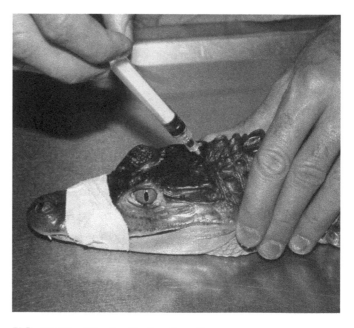

FIG. 30.10.   Blood collection from the supravertebral plexus.

Transport

Crocodilians may be moved or shipped in dog cages, as long as facilities are provided to maintain the proper ambient temperature. They will probably not feed while out of water, but this is of no consequence. Crocodilians may be kept out of water for days.

Chemical Restraint[3,5,11,12]

The chemical restraint agents and combinations mentioned in this chapter represent those used by the author or by experienced veterinarians with detailed knowledge of reptiles. Other protocols have been used, and no claim is made

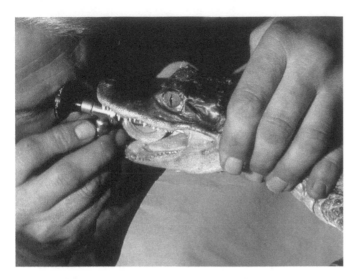

FIG. 30.11. Endoscopy in a small crocodilian.

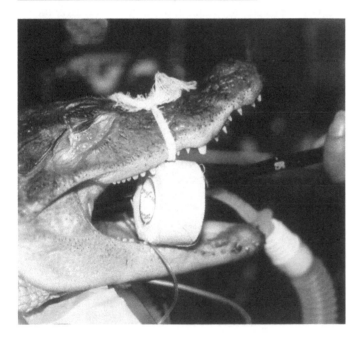

FIG. 30.12. Endotracheal tube fixed in place.

for including all possible drugs and combinations. For more detailed information, particularly for anesthesia, consult the references.[1,5,8,14]

Drug reaction of the poikilothermic crocodilians is variable. Drugs used for chemical sedation or restraint are listed in Table 30.1. Gallamine is a muscle relaxant only and should not be used to replace anesthesia. Tiletamine/zolazepam is an excellent injectable anesthetic agent, keeping in mind that the length of recovery is dose dependant.

CHELONIANS

The terminology used to describe chelonians varies. Generally aquatic species are called "turtles"; "tortoises" are terrestrial species found in arid parts of the world; and "terrapins"

TABLE 30.1. Selected chemical restraint agents for crocodilians[5,11,14]

Agent	Dosage (mg/kg)	Comments
Gallamine triethiodide	1.0–2.0	Reversal, Neostigmine 0.03–0.06. Not an anesthetic. IM
Ketamine/Medetomidine	10.0/0.1	IM, Reversal, Atipamezole
Tiletamine/zolazepam	3.0–15.0	IM, Reversal, Flumazanil
Etorphine	1.3–3.9	American alligator

are species that may have both terrestrial and aquatic phases. However, some freshwater turtles leave the water to bask in the sun and air; other species such as the sea turtles are totally aquatic, living their entire lives in the sea except for short periods when females deposit eggs on sandy beaches.

Danger Potential

The major weapons of turtles and tortoises are the hard bony plates that replace teeth in both upper and lower jaws. There is marked variation in the aggressiveness of different species. Snapping turtles are notorious biters, and occasionally a large tortoise may nip at a person. Some soft-shelled turtles and a few of the side-necked turtles occasionally bite. The side-necked turtle scratches by continually raking with the legs as long as it is grasped, but the wounds inflicted are usually superficial. The western pond turtle and some other species are also persistent scratchers, constantly attempting to win freedom when grasped. Fingers may be pinched if the head and limbs are suddenly withdrawn into the carapace and plastron.

Anatomy

Both turtles and tortoises have an exoskeleton composed of the carapace and the plastron. The carapace supplies a convenient handle for restraint, but it is difficult to examine the animal if the head and limbs are retracted tightly into the shell. In some of the larger species, it is impossible to extract the head and legs without injuring the animal unless chemical immobilizers are administered.

Physical Restraint

To pick up a small- to medium-sized turtle or tortoise, grasp the sides of the carapace (Fig. 30.13). From this position it may be turned over as needed (Fig. 30.14).

When a chelonian is turned over from side to side, there is a slight risk of causing torsion of a segment of the intestine. The animal should be turned slowly. Small- to medium-sized chelonians should be turned over from front to back. This is mechanically difficult with giant tortoises. Return chelonians to the upright position by reversing the direction of the roll.

The animal should not be held with the head down for long periods, since this may interfere with respiration.

If a limb must be examined, grasp the foot and apply gentle, steady traction to withdraw the leg from the protective cover of the carapace and plastron. Do not jerk on the limb, lest injury occur to small bones and other structures of the

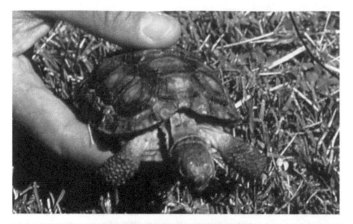

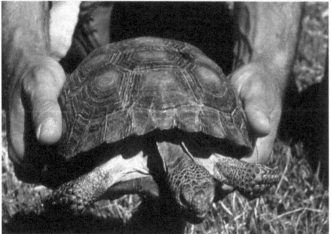

FIG. 30.13. Holding a small tortoise.

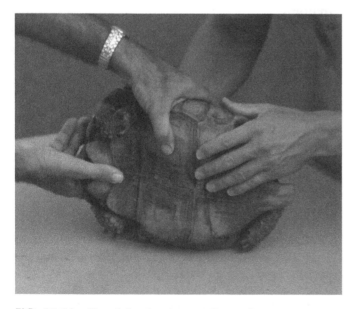

FIG. 30.14. Examining the plastron of a tortoise.

leg. An unsedated large tortoise may be strong enough to defy attempts to pull out the leg.

The head is more difficult to extract, but if you wait until the head is extended voluntarily, you may gently put your

fingers behind the head and hold it out. Considerable effort may be made by the turtle to retract the head, and judgment must be made as to the degree of force that is appropriate to keep the head out.

Soft-shell turtles require careful handling, since they tend to be slightly aggressive and will bite and scratch. The soft carapace makes it difficult to grasp the animal firmly, and heavy-handed restraint practices may impair respiration or damage internal organs. Soft-shells may be netted to lift them out of the water. Wear light gloves to gently grasp the animal.

Snapping turtles may weigh up to 100 kg (220 lb) and are particularly hazardous to handle. They can easily bite off a finger or inflict other serious injury. A small snapper is best handled by grasping the tail and lifting it off the ground or out of the water. Do not allow the head to dangle close to your leg, lest the animal reach out and bite (Fig. 30.15). A medium-sized snapper may require two hands on the carapace (Fig. 30.16). Once the tail has been grasped, a firmer hold may be employed by carefully running the hand closely over the top of the carapace and grasping the carapace just above the head (Fig. 30.17). A large snapper may be lifted by one or two persons grasping the rear and front carapace (Fig. 30.17).

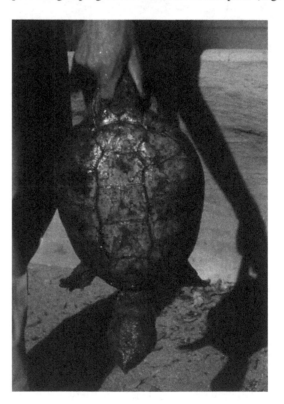

FIG. 30.15. **A.** Holding a small snapping turtle by the tail. **B.** Do not allow the head of a snapper to approach your leg.

Snapping turtles may be turned over onto the carapace. They usually struggle for a moment then relax. Hold the mouth shut by pressing the lower jaw against the upper jaw. Keep the hands in a position that permits quick withdrawal if the turtle should succeed in righting itself.

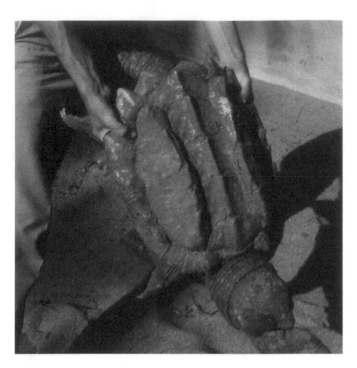

FIG. 30.16. Holding a medium-sized snapper.

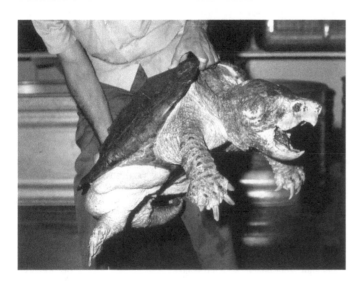

FIG. 30.17. One-person carry for a large snapping turtle. The jaws of this animal are capable of amputating a digit and severely injuring a limb.

Sea turtles weigh up to 600 kg (1,320 lb). They are herbivorous and generally not aggressive. Small specimens may be grasped directly from a tank or netted. Drain the tank to dry-dock large specimens. The flippers are strong and may strike a handler if the turtle is kept right side up. If a turtle is tipped upside down, it tends to relax and quietly allow examination and minor surgery (Fig. 30.18).

Blood Sample Collection[10]

Venipuncture of chelonians may be performed in the jugular vein (Fig. 30.19), cranial vena cava, brachial veins,

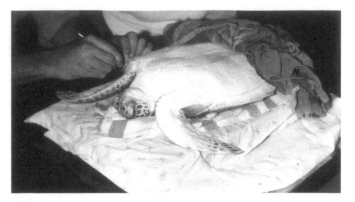

FIG. 30.18. Sea turtle placed in dorsal recumbency for examination or surgery. An automobile inner tube serves as a cradle for his procedure.

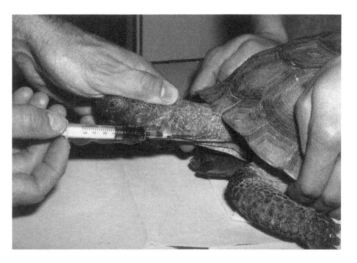

FIG. 30.19. Jugular venipuncture in a sedated tortoise. The vein on the animal's right side may be larger.

and the ventral coccygeal vein. The tail vein is the most accessible site in snapping turtles. To obtain blood from the jugular vein, it may be necessary to sedate the chelonian. Extend the head and apply pressure at the base of the neck. The vein will become visible on the ventrolateral aspect of the neck. The vein is very mobile, so no definite landmarks can be stated. The right jugular vein is the larger.

Direct intracardial penetration can be made through the plastron. Cleanse the tortoise for a sterile puncture. Penetrate on the midline at the junction of the pectoral and abdominal shield (Fig. 30.20).

The mouth of a chelonian may be opened with wooden or plastic wedges. Dowels or sheep and swine specula may be used on large species (Figs. 30.21, 30.22).

Giant tortoises that are weakened or paralyzed may be supported as illustrated in Figure 30.23.

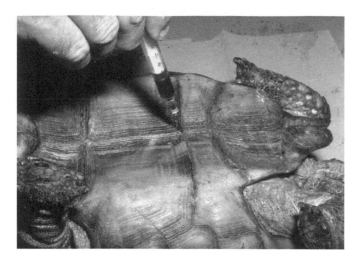

FIG. 30.20. Collecting intracardial blood sample from a tortoise.

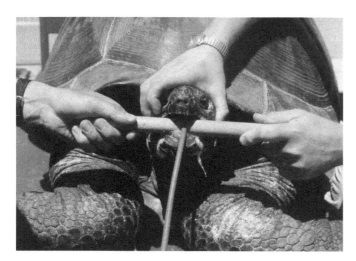

FIG. 30.21. A dowel used to hold the mouth open for stomach intubation.

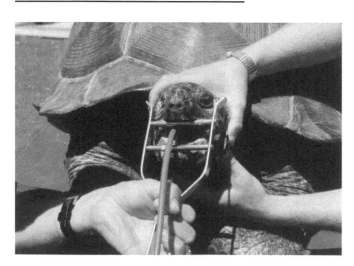

FIG. 30.22. Mouth speculum in place on a giant tortoise. Large animals must be depressed or sedated in order to hold the head out.

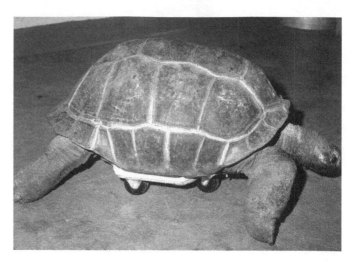

FIG. 30.23. Special dolly allows partially paralyzed tortoise to move about.

Transport

Terrestrial species are easily moved in small cages. Aquatic species must be kept damp but need not be immersed. Even sea turtles can tolerate being out of water for hours if they are kept cool and moist. Foam rubber soaked with water may provide moisture for aquatic turtles or amphibians during transport.

Chemical Restraint[15,17]

Chemical restraint of tortoises and turtles may be carried out using ketamine hydrochloride (15.0–60.0 kg/kg). See Table 30.2 for additional agents. Care should be taken to place chemically immobilized chelonians in a recovery environ-

TABLE 30.2.   Selected chemical restraint agents for chelonians[15]

Agent	Dosage (mg/kg)	Comment
Ketamine/butorphanol/medetomidine	4.0–10.0/0.5–1.0/0.03–0.15	IM
Ketamine/midazolam	20.0–40.0/2.0	IM, Reversal, Flumazanil
Tiletamine/zolazepam	3.0–15.0	IM, Reversal, Flumazanil

ment maintained at a temperature of 27–29°C (80–85°F). If the ambient air temperature is low, the recovery period will be dangerously prolonged. If the temperature is too high, the reptile may develop hyperthermia. Chelonians may be placed in an incubator or on a heating pad if supplemental heat is needed. Make certain that the temperature does not rise above 29°C (85°F). A chemically immobilized tortoise or turtle is incapable of behavioral or physical thermoregulation.

Recovery from chemical immobilization may require several hours, but may be speeded up by administration of appropriate reversal agents. The animal should be carefully monitored until it recovers. Do not allow aquatic species access to water for at least 12 hours after completion of the procedure.

LIZARDS

Lizards vary in size from tiny skinks weighing a few grams to large monitor lizards such as the Komodo dragon weighing 90 kg (200 lb). Restraint techniques suitable for use on such a variety of species differ.

Danger Potential

Lizards may be carnivorous, preying on insects, other reptiles, small mammals, or birds; or they may be herbivorous or both. Dental structures vary from hard bony plates to sharp teeth. The tails of certain species are weapons that can be used as whips. This is particularly true of the common green iguana, in which the tail exceeds 3 feet in length at maturity. This tail may inflict a painful if not serious injury to the unwary handler. Many lizards are agile climbers with long, sharp, grasping claws that may inflict nasty scratches.

There are only two species of poisonous lizards—the Gila monster and the Mexican beaded lizard. Both of these species occur in the arid deserts of southwestern United States and Sonora, Mexico. They are rather phlegmatic lizards, not significantly aggressive unless molested. If annoyed, they are capable of biting firmly and refusing to let go. A continual chewing motion allows venom, extruded onto the teeth of the lower jaw, to work its way into the punctured skin of the victim.

Physical Restraint

Small lizards may be hand held (Fig. 30.24). Some are pugnacious and will attempt to bite. Thin gloves will protect the hands (Fig. 30.25). The scales of some species are rough and may require gloves (Fig. 30.26).

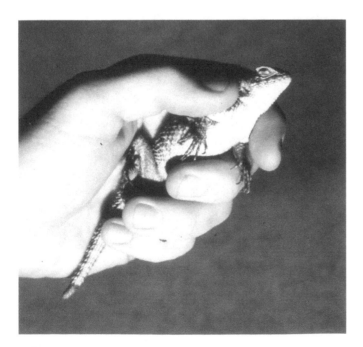

FIG. 30.24. Many small lizards may be manually restrained.

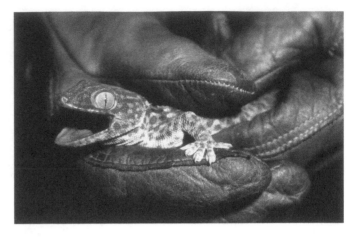

FIG. 30.25. Handling a gecko with gloves.

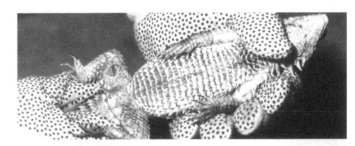

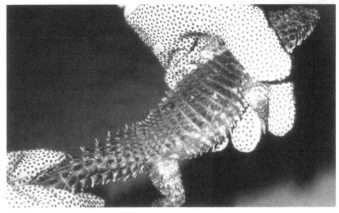

FIG. 30.26. Using gloves to grasp a rough-scaled sungazer lizard.

A lizard should not be caught by the tail. Some species are able to discard the tail as a device to distract predators. Although the tail will eventually regrow, the individual will be a poor exhibit for many weeks to months.

Larger lizards such as iguanas may be presented in a sack for examination. Determine the location of the head and grasp the animal behind the head through the sack, controlling it until it can be regrasped as the sack is carefully removed. Keep the tails of larger species restrained at all times (Fig. 30.27).

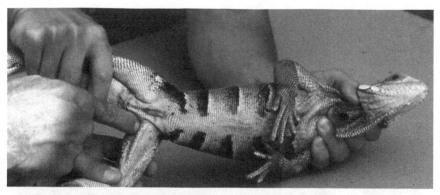

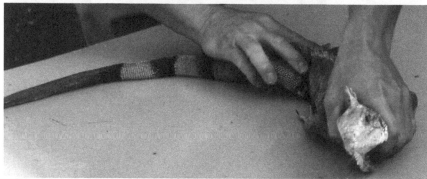

FIG. 30.27. A. An aggressive iguana is grasped from above, securing the head and whiplike tail at the same time. B. Once the animal is grasped, include hind legs in the tail hold to preclude scratching.

If one must handle a lizard to expose the ventral aspect, a long-sleeved shirt or wide-gauntleted gloves should be worn to protect from scratches. Once the animal is in hand, it may be situated in a variety of positions.. The mouth may be opened for examination by pulling on the fold of skin beneath the chin or by pinching and lifting the rostrum (nose). Some lizards resist opening the mouth, and the jaws must be gently pried apart and held open. A wedge-shaped piece of plastic may be used to open the mouth if care is taken to avoid breaking the tiny fragile teeth.

Some large pet iguanas may be held without grasping the nape of the neck (Fig. 30.28). However, they may bite when held in this fashion by a person who manipulates the animal in an unaccustomed manner.

Large lizards must be handled either with nets or snares (Fig. 30.30). Take care to avoid injury to the neck when tightening a snare. Snares, cables, or ropes covered with plastic or rubber tubing are safest. As soon as the snare has been placed on the neck, the tail should be grasped, as with crocodilians. If manipulation is to be prolonged, tape the hind legs to the tail, as shown in Figure 30.30. The ensnared animal may be transported from one place to another with additional support beneath the body. Do not allow the weight to be suspended solely from the neck and tail.

An experienced individual may handle poisonous lizards by grasping them behind the head and neck, as indicated in Figures 30.31, 30.32. They may also be grasped by the tail and lifted with a hook (Fig. 30.33). They are unlikely to climb up their own tails onto the handler's hand.

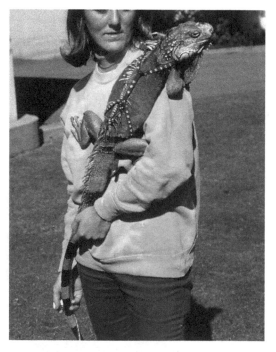

FIG. 30.28. A large pet iguana held by the owner.

Blood Collection[4,10]

Lizards have a vein on the ventral side of the tail. To collect a blood sample, place the lizard on its back (Fig. 30.34). Locate one of the ventral spinous processes; then

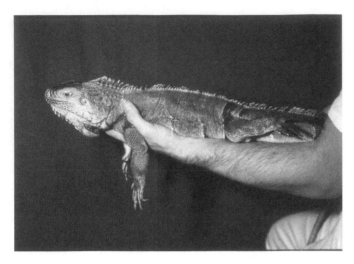

FIG. 30.29. A large pet iguana may be handled by controlling the head and tail.

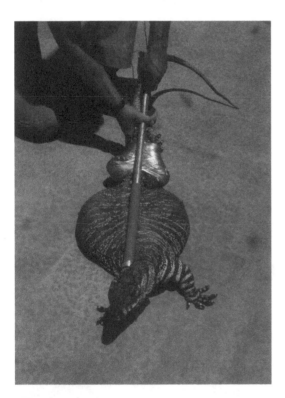

FIG. 30.30. A snare may be used to control large monitors. Note tape on hind legs to prevent scratching.

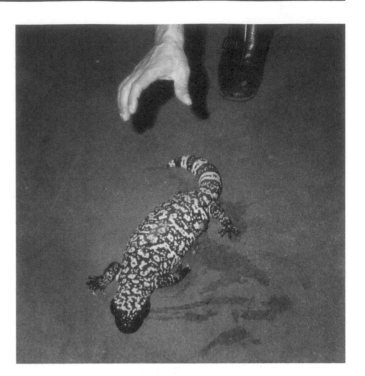

FIG. 30.31. Gila monster approached from above and behind.

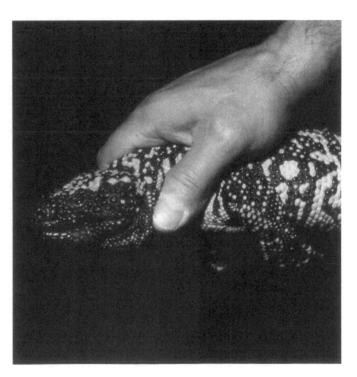

FIG. 30.32. Proper hold for a Gila monster.

insert a 20-gauge needle, directing it forward at a 45-degree angle parallel with the ventral spinous process (Fig. 32.35). Insert the needle until the tip strikes the vertebral body. Withdraw the plunger to establish slight negative pressure in the syringe, and pull the needle slowly back 1–2 mm until blood wells into the syringe. Other accessible veins include the axillary and jugular veins. Cardiac penetration is also appropriate.

Chemical Immobilization

Anesthesia may be induced by inhalation of isoflurane or halothane via a face mask (Fig. 30.36) or by injection (see Table 30.3).

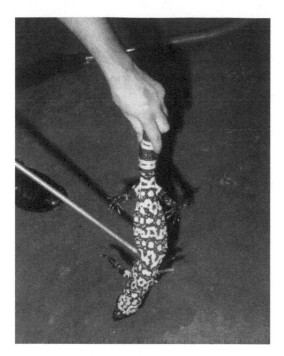

FIG. 30.33. Gila monster handled by the tail; hook gives additional support.

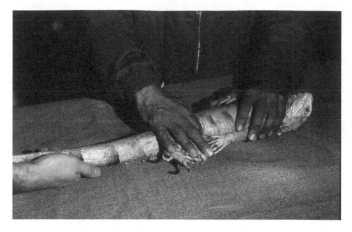

FIG. 30.34. Restraint for an iguana for blood collection from the tail vein.

TABLE 30.3.   Chemical restraint agents for lizards and snakes* (Lloyd[12])

Agent	Sedation, mg/kg	Immobilization, mg/kg	Comments
Medetomidine		0.04–0.15	Reversal, atipamezole
Tiletamine/ zolazepam		2.0–10.0	Recovery may take several hours
Ketamine	10.0–20.0	40.0–80.0	No reversal, may need respiratory assist
Xylazine	0.1	0.5–1.0	Reversal atipamezole, tolazoline
Midazolam		1.0–2.0	
Isoflurane			5.0% for induction, 2.5% for maintenance

* Recovery more rapid if ambient temperature is 30–34°C (86–93°F).

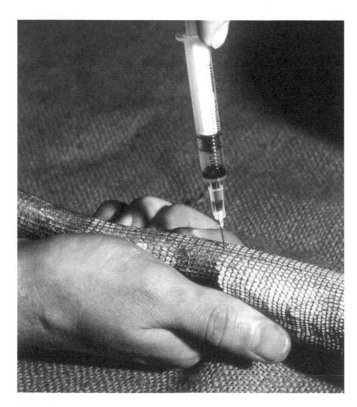

FIG. 30.35. Blood collection from the tail vein.

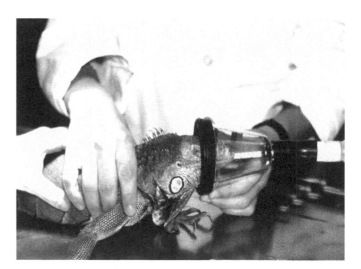

FIG. 30.36. Induction of sedation and anesthesia using a face mask.

SNAKES

Snakes exhibit extreme diversity in morphology, physiology, activity, food habits, and other biological parameters.

Danger Potential

All snakes can bite (Fig. 30.37). Small specimens may be unable to open the mouth widely enough to be a hazard to human beings. Others may inflict serious injury or death. Venomous species require special handling techniques.

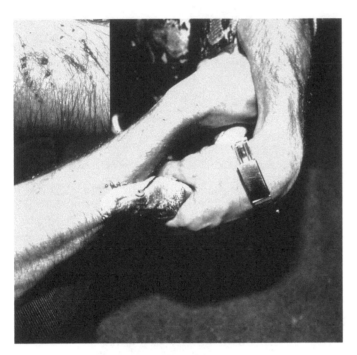

FIG. 30.37. Bite from an owner's python.

Constrictors kill prey by coiling tightly around the body and preventing respiration, thus suffocating the victim. They do not crush the victim's bones. A 3-m (10-ft) boa allowed to completely encircle the body or neck of a restrainer is capable of causing death if assistance is not rendered quickly.

Physical Restraint

NONPOISONOUS SNAKES. Many nonpoisonous snakes (Fig. 30.38) will not bite unless tormented. The head of a large nonpoisonous snake must be controlled, particularly when manipulating for examination (Fig. 30.39). When holding a snake it is important to support the body (Fig. 30.40). An unsupported snake becomes insecure and restless and may thrash about. If the body is left dangling, a vigorous snake may thrash until its neck is dislocated or fractured. One cribo held by the neck thrashed so vigorously that the vertebral column was fractured.

The mouth of a properly held snake may be opened either by pulling on the loose fold of skin between the lower jaws or by gently inserting a plastic spatula, covered forceps, or tongue depressor into the mouth, taking care not to damage the teeth (Figs. 30.41, 30.42, 30.43).

Snake hooks are fundamental tools for working with reptiles (Fig. 30.44). Hooks may be used for directing

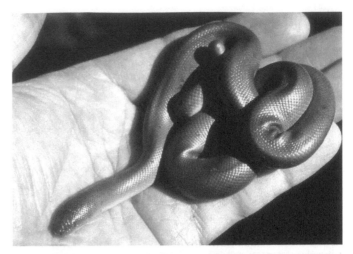

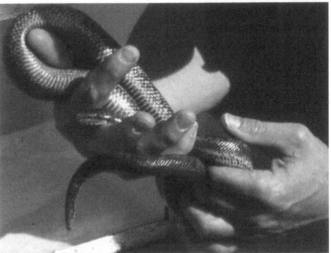

FIG. 30.38. Many nonpoisonous snakes are easily handled manually.

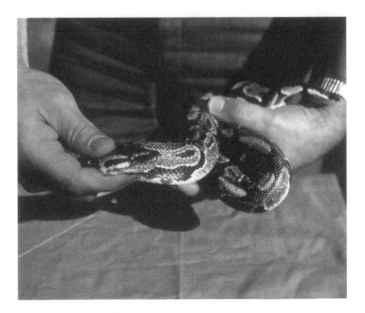

FIG. 30.39. Holding the head and supporting the body.

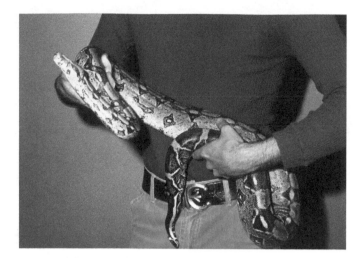

FIG. 30.40.   Proper support of a medium-sized snake.

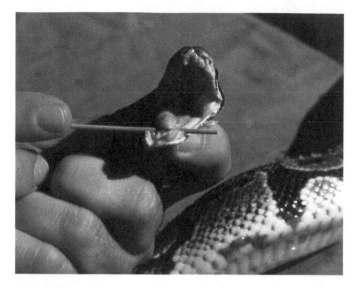

FIG. 30.42.   Opening the mouth of a snake with a plastic wedge.

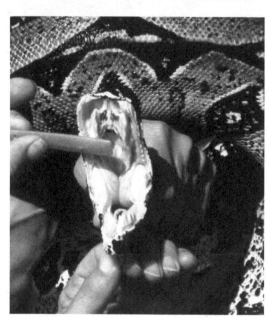

FIG. 30.41.   Opening the mouth of a large snake: Covered thumb forceps.

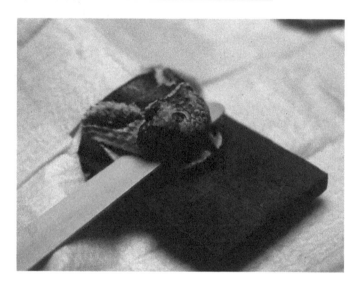

FIG. 30.43.   Opening the mouth with a tongue depressor.

movement, lifting snakes from containers (Fig. 30.45), and a variety of other restraint procedures. A snake hook may be used to pin the head of any snake to the ground, allowing the handler to safely grasp it (Figs. 30.46, 30.47). Only sufficient pressure to hold the snake should be exerted; too much pressure on the neck may seriously injure the spine or dislocate the head. Furthermore, if a manipulation is rough, a snake may subsequently refuse to eat, even to the point of starvation. Grasp the neck and head as illustrated (Figs. 30.48, 30.49).

Be cautious when dealing with large constrictors. They should be removed from a cage with a large hook. If a constrictor is known to be docile, an experienced handler may be able to reach in carefully and grasp the animal (Fig. 30.50). Remember that a snake in its own cage may behave in a ter-

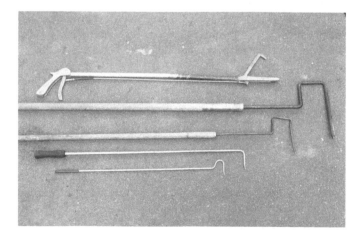

FIG. 30.44.   Pilston snake tong and snake hooks.

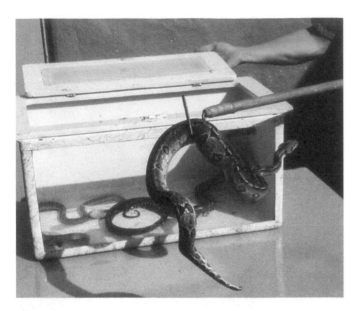

FIG. 30.45. Using a snake hook to remove a snake from a cage.

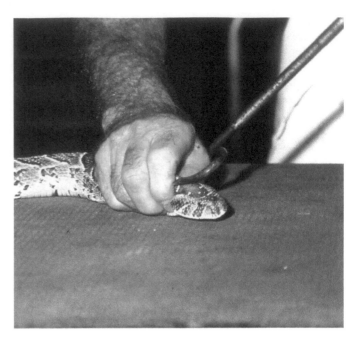

FIG. 30.47. Pinning a poisonous snake. Practice with nonvenomous snakes.

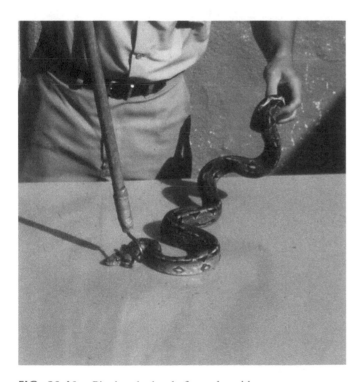

FIG. 30.46. Pinning the head of a snake with a hook.

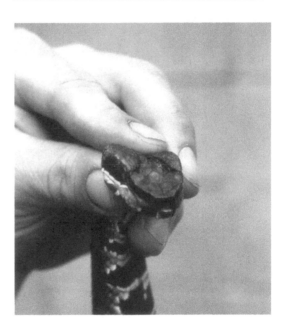

FIG. 30.48. Holding the head of a venomous snake.

ritorial manner and is likely to be more aggressive than if it is removed from the cage into strange territory. Once the animal is out of the cage, it may be placed on the floor and the head gently pinned until it is grasped. Large pythons, anacondas, and boa constrictors may require multiple handlers grasping and holding the snake simultaneously.

A large snake should never be allowed to throw a loop around the neck or body of a handler. It is natural for a snake to coil. A snake coiled around an arm will feel comfortable, and the arm will suffer no harm.

Some agile nonpoisonous snakes are difficult to handle. If pinned, they thrash and often injure themselves. The experienced handler may be able to pin and grab them quickly, but other techniques are more suitable, especially for novices. The snake loop or noose is a more effective tool for these species (Fig. 30.51).

The Pilston snake tong is not a suitable tool for direct handling of snakes, since it is likely to cause injury—

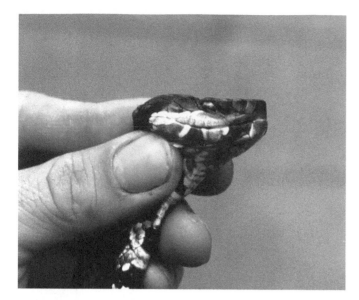

FIG. 30.49.   An alternate method of holding the head.

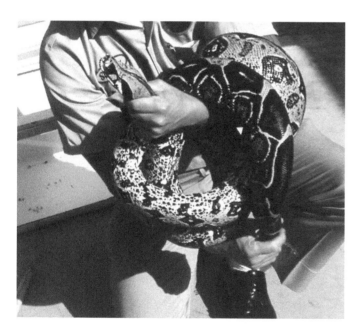

FIG. 30.50.   Supporting a large constrictor snake by coiling it around an arm.

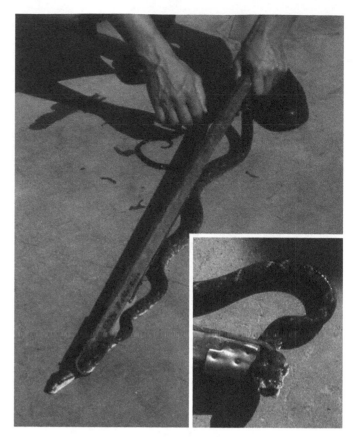

FIG. 30.51.   Strap snake loop.

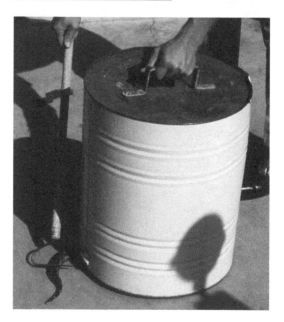

FIG. 30.52.   Large tin can temporarily restricts the activity of a snake.

particularly in the hands of a novice. It is useful for removing dishes, for feeding, or for holding plastic tubes.

The degree of agitation, aggressiveness, or nervousness exhibited by a snake may depend on the temperature at which it is handled and/or the amount of excitement it has experienced immediately prior to the manipulative procedure. An excited snake should be allowed to rest for a time. A can may be put over the snake to allow it to settle in darkness without the stimulation of outside influences (Fig. 30.52).

A small plastic shield, illustrated in Figure 30.53, is used to capture a large, slightly aggressive nonpoisonous snake.

The shield allows constant sight of the head; by applying gentle pressure, the shield can immobilize the snake sufficiently to enable the handler to grasp it behind the head.

Another capture technique is to allow a snake to begin to engulf prey, usually a rodent (Fig. 30.54), grasping the

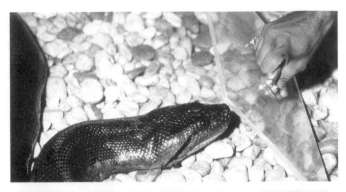

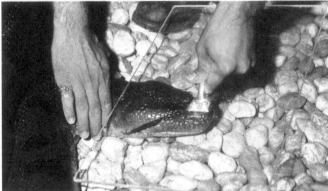

FIG. 32.53. Using a plastic shield to approach and capture an aggressive nonpoisonous snake.

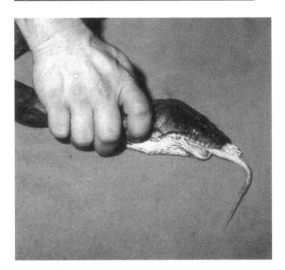

FIG. 30.54. Snake grasped just after it has started to engulf prey.

snake behind the head. This technique is less desirable than others because of the danger of regurgitation if a snake is handled soon after eating. Since regurgitation is undesirable, it is generally wise to refrain from manipulation of snakes other than for emergencies during the first two or three days after consumption of food.

Poisonous Snakes

Many species of poisonous snakes are found throughout the world. Each species has different characteristics, degree of agility, and method of striking, but all are characterized by the presence of sacs from which the venom is extruded into fangs for envenomation of prey species or enemies. It is unwise to restrain any poisonous snake unless antivenin is at hand. Antivenin for a given species of snake must usually be obtained from the native country of the snake. Maintaining a stock of antivenins is costly, but the bite of many of these snakes is lethal unless such protective agents are available within minutes to hours. If a bite occurs during a manipulative procedure and antivenin is unavailable, contact the nearest large reptile collection—either zoo or private facility.

Various groups of poisonous snakes differ in behavioral traits sufficiently to require the development of specialized restraint and handling techniques. No one should handle poisonous snakes without first developing expertise and confidence by practicing the techniques on nonpoisonous snakes. It is important to be confident that you can complete the procedure before beginning it. There may not be a second chance.

Vipers and pit vipers are usually somewhat phlegmatic heavy-bodied snakes. They arrange their bodies into a series of undulating folds from which position they can strike in any direction. The maximum striking distance is approximately two-thirds the length of the body. No snake flies through the air when it strikes. There are nearly as many techniques for handling vipers as there are handlers. Some of the more heroic involve direct catching with the bare hands, a technique that should be left to exhibitionists. Small vipers may be held for intramuscular injections by pressing them with wire screen (Fig. 30.55).

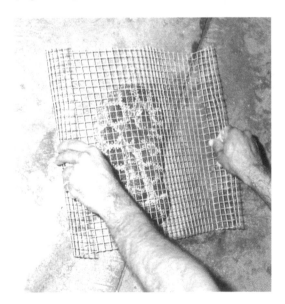

FIG. 30.55. Small vipers may be pressed with a wire screen.

Pinning a snake is a common procedure, but it should be used on venomous species only by the experienced snake handler. Figures 30.46 to 30.49 show the sequence of proper pinning. The hook is gently pressed behind the head; then the thumb and forefinger are used to grasp just behind the jaws. A firm hold must be kept until the snake is released. An alternate hold is with the thumb and second finger, the index finger being placed over the top of the head in the manner illustrated in Figure 30.48.

It is extremely difficult to pin one of the agile elapid snakes without injuring it. Neither is it wise to attempt to pin a massive snake such as a gaboon viper or an African puff adder. The snake noose or loop is more effective to control both types.

Plastic tubes of various sizes make excellent tools for handling many species of poisonous snakes (Fig. 30.56).[12] They are now being used extensively by snake handlers in the United States. The plastic tubes can be capped on one end or left open. Slots in the sides of the tubes permit various procedures to be successfully completed in relative safety for both person and snake.

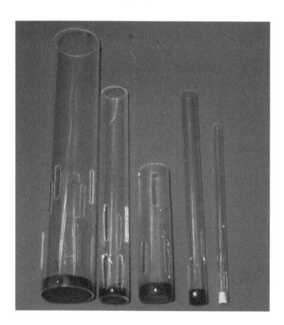

FIG. 30.56. Tubes of various sizes used to restrain snakes.

The plastic tube should be sized so that the thickest portion of the body of the snake can barely pass through it. Otherwise the snake may turn around and come out. To tube the snake, place it on the floor with a hook. Hold the tube with a tong or, with docile or slow-moving species, by hand (Fig. 30.57). When the snake has crawled into the tube one-third of its length, very slowly and deliberately reach down and grasp with one hand both snake and tube at the point they adjoin (Fig. 30.58). Maintain this grasp continually until the snake is released. Never hold the tube with one hand and the snake with the other; the snake might back out of the tube and bite. The tube may also be placed along a wall (Fig. 30.59).

Various manipulative procedures may be carried out with the snake in a tube. Examination of both ventral and dorsal aspects, intramuscular injections, forced sheddings,

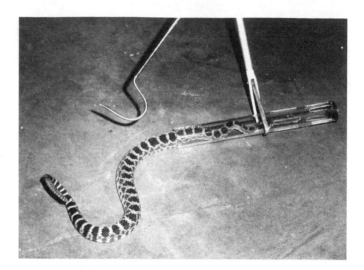

FIG. 30.57. **A.** Guiding a snake into a plastic tube with a hook. **B.** Preparing to grasp a snake and tube at the same point.

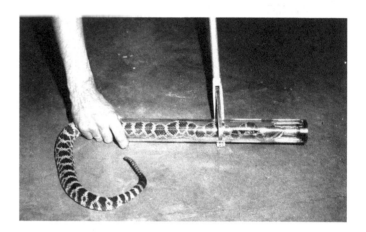

FIG. 30.58. As soon as the snake and tube are grasped, the unit may be manipulated into any position.

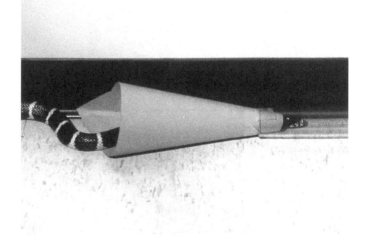

FIG. 30.59. Placing the tube along a wall and using a paper cone to entice the snake to enter the tube.

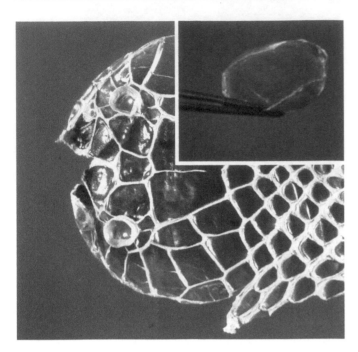

FIG. 30.60. Removing a cap from a snake while in a tube.

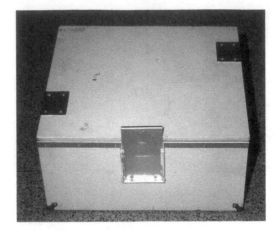

FIG. 30.61. Snake squeeze box.

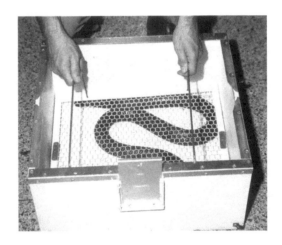

FIG. 30.62. Screen to fix the snake.

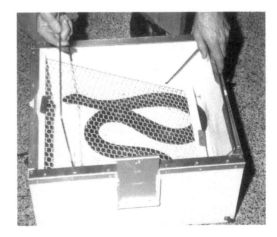

FIG. 30.63. The screen squeeze must be pressed straight down, otherwise the snake may escape.

sexing, and removal of caps from the eyes can be carried out with a great degree of safety on venomous snakes in a tube (Fig. 30.60).

It is sometimes difficult to induce flighty snakes such as cobras and other elapids to enter a tube, but with patience most of them can be successfully tubed. There are some exceptions. This technique is dangerous and unsuitable for handling large, extremely aggressive, and fast-moving snakes such as the boomslang or the king cobra. With all species of elapids, it is essential to hold the plastic tube with long forceps such as the Pilston tong.

The elapidae (cobra) family, in addition to being generally more aggressive and equipped with a more toxic venom, are flightier in temperament than vipers and consequently more dangerous to manipulate. The cobra's defensive posture is to raise the body to a vertical position with hood up. These snakes strike forward and downward from that position. Other venomous snakes have different striking patterns.

Squeeze boxes (Figs. 30.61, 30.62, 30.63) are more suitable than tubes for handling large, swift, and aggressive elapid snakes. Squeeze boxes may be incorporated directly into the permanent cage (Figs. 30.64, 30.65, 30.66). This is particularly important for a snake such as the king cobra or black mamba. Covering the squeeze cage with a solid top darkens it and creates a refuge for the snake, enticing it to crawl inside. Then a trap door is closed and the snake is contained. Removing the solid top permits pressing the snake with the screen squeeze, as illustrated in Figure 30.66. The screen permits the removal of eye caps and administration of intramuscular injections.

A versatile squeeze cage may be constructed with a removable top and slotted sides. The snake is hooked into the open box and a plastic or screen squeeze is inserted into a slot to press the animal (Figs. 30.67, 30.68). The squeeze is held

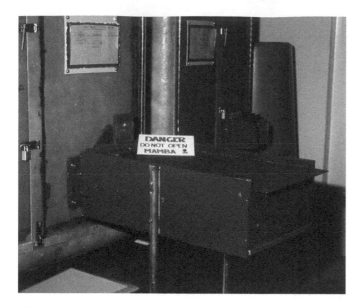

FIG. 30.64. A special snake squeeze box for handling mambas.

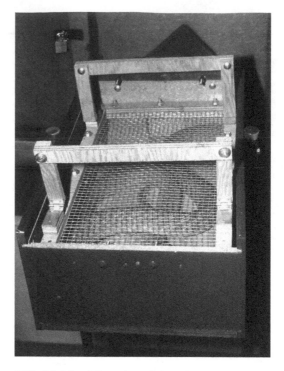

FIG. 30.66. When the solid top is removed, a screen squeeze may be pressed onto the snake.

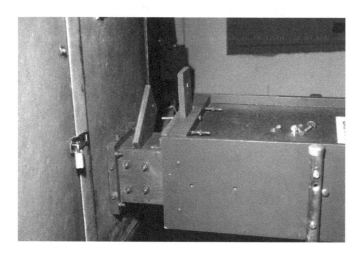

FIG. 30.65. Trap doors to restrict snake to the box.

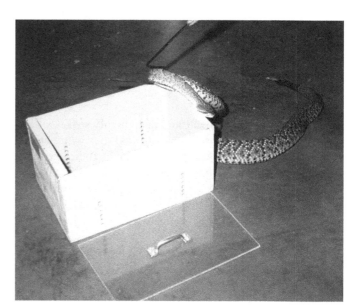

FIG. 30.67. Placing a rattlesnake in a homemade squeeze.

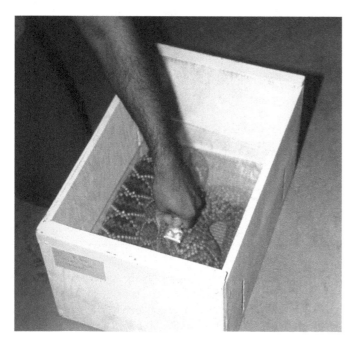

FIG. 30.68. Squeezing the snake in the box.

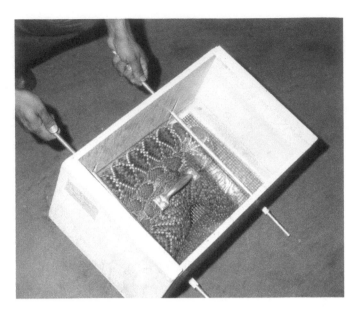

FIG. 30.69. Holding the squeeze with aluminum rods.

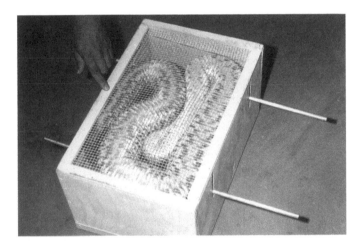

FIG. 30.70. Snake turned over to view ventral side.

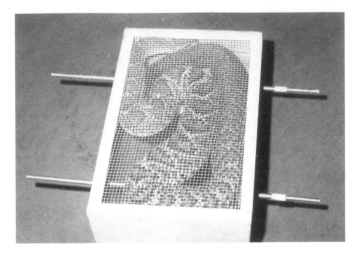

FIG. 30.71. Squeeze loosened to allow the snake to turn over for an intramuscular injection.

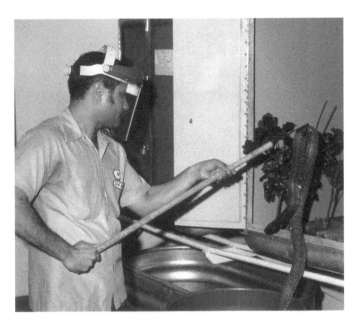

FIG. 30.72. Face shield for working with a spitting cobra.

in place with removable adjustable rods (Fig. 30.69). To examine anterior surfaces, tip the cage upside down, release the squeeze slightly to let the snake flip over, then retighten the squeeze (Figs. 30.70, 30.71).

A limited number of elapids are capable of forcibly ejecting venom from the fangs at the eyes of handlers, temporarily or permanently blinding the victim. Handlers of spitting cobras must use specialized equipment—usually a plastic shield or goggles—to protect the eyes (Fig. 30.72). Except for this equipment, spitting cobras are handled in the same manner as other cobra-type snakes. Come-along snares may be used on dangerous snakes such as the king cobra. Figure 30.73 illustrates using a come-along snare to restrain a king cobra. Figure 30.74 shows how to hold a king cobra.

Sea snakes present particularly difficult restraint problems. They have very short fangs, but the venom of these serpents is the most highly toxic known. Usually they are handled with small nets or squeeze cages as illustrated for other elapids. Figure 30.75 shows a commercial suction device for withdrawing serum and venom.

Special Procedures

Sexing snakes is a routine procedure. The male snake has paired hemipenes recessed into a diverticulum posterior or caudal to the vent. The sex of the animal can be determined by gently inserting a probe into the diverticulum (Figs. 32.76, 32.77, 32.78). In the male the probe can be inserted to a considerable depth (it should reach to the 7th to 15th subcaudal scales), depending on the size of the snake. In females the probe may be inserted only up to the 5th subcaudal scale.

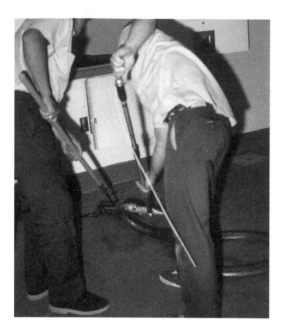

FIG. 30.73. Using a come-along snare to restrain a king cobra.

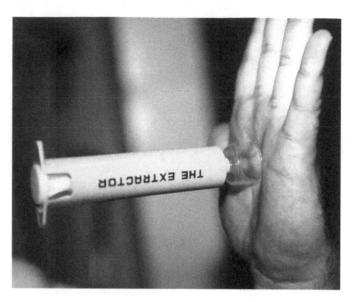

FIG. 30.75. Commercial suction device for withdrawing serum and venom.

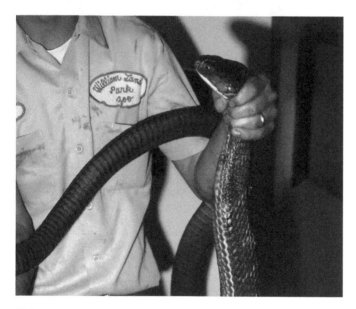

FIG. 30.74. Hand holding a king cobra.

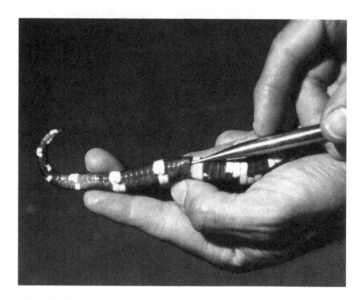

FIG. 30.76. Sexing a snake: Insert the probe into the lateral aspect of the vent and direct the probe caudally in the bursa.

Figure 30.79 is a diagram of the hemipenes of a male snake.

The length of the probe to be used is determined by the size of the snake. Probes are available commercially, or they can be improvised. It is important that the tip to be inserted into the diverticulum be a tiny ball and not a sharp point. In numerous instances straightened-out paper clips inserted to determine sex have penetrated the diverticulum, resulting in abscesses and frequently in the subsequent death of the snake.

Intramuscular injections may be given to a snake in the large muscles that parallel the vertebral column in the cranial

half of the body (Fig. 30.80). These muscles directly overlie the ribs, so care should be taken to avoid penetration of the abdominal or thoracic cavity and the subsequent injection of material into the lung or viscera. Hold the snake in the manner illustrated in Figure 30.80. Use the free hand to insert the needle beneath or between scales into the muscle in a diagonal direction.

Subcutaneous infusion in the snake can be carried out at the lateral side of the back muscles. There is a slight groove in this area, and the skin here is relatively free of underlying tissue, allowing more space for distribution of the fluid.

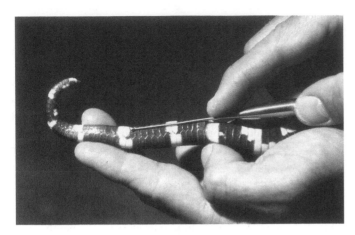

FIG. 30.77. Showing the depth of penetration of the probe: In a male it will penetrate to the 7th to 15th subcaudal scales; in a female it will penetrate to only the 5th subcaudal scale.

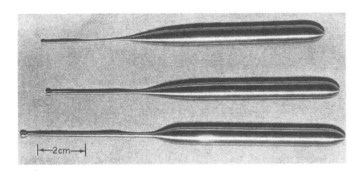

FIG. 30.78. Probes used for sexing snakes.

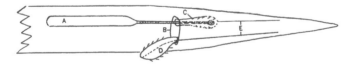

FIG. 30.79. Diagram of the hemipenes of a male snake: **A.** Probe. **B.** Vent. **C.** Bursa of the hemipenis. **D.** Erect hemipenis. **E.** Retractor muscles of the hemipenes.

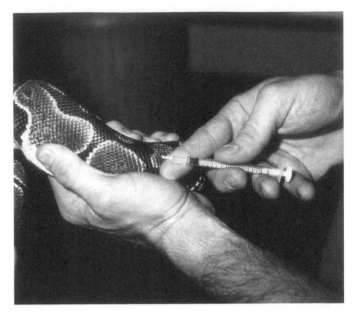

FIG. 30.80. Intramuscular injection may be given on either side of the vertebral column in the cranial half of the body.

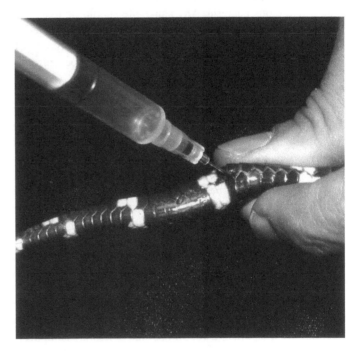

FIG. 30.81. Collecting blood from the tail vein of a snake.

Blood Collection[10]

Obtaining blood samples from a snake is not easy.

Venipuncture of the ventral coccygeal vein is performed as described for lizards (Fig. 30.81), but a direct cardiac puncture is more satisfactory for obtaining a blood specimen. Although the procedure may be carried out on an unanesthetized snake, it is safer to anesthetize the animal. After immobilization the snake is placed on its back. The heart can usually be seen pulsating at the junction of the anterior and middle portions of the snake's body. The heart is mobile and can be moved forward or backward, so it must be fixed between the thumb and the finger before proceeding. A 20-gauge, 3.8- to 7.6-cm (1.5- to 3.0-in.) needle is inserted between the scales over the heart. Insert the needle slowly until the heart is reached, a point defined by movement of the needle in the hand; then penetrate the ventricle with a quick jab. When the sample has been obtained and the needle withdrawn, apply slight pressure on the heart for a moment to assist in sealing the puncture.

Unextruded caps over the eyes are a common problem of snakes in captivity. The cap is an epithelial structure over the cornea of the eye, continuous with the skin, and should be shed with the skin. For various reasons the caps may fail to shed. As many as five or six may stack up if successive caps fail to shed. As the snake prepares to shed, the corneas of the eyes usually become opaque, making the snake relatively blind until the skin is shed. A snake is unlikely to feed during this period; if the caps are retained indefinitely, the snake may starve.

Reptile keepers usually try to loosen caps by soaking the animal, hoping the caps will come off without further treatment. If they do not come off, the caps must be removed manually. The snake should be restrained, either physically or with chemical immobilizers. Poisonous snakes must be partially anesthetized. The cap may then be gently removed with fine forceps.

Snakebite[6]

The bite from a nonpoisonous snake is rarely serious, except that the mouth of any snake is likely to harbor potentially dangerous bacteria. Any snakebite should be treated as a puncture wound. Initial bleeding should be encouraged to cleanse the tracts, and the area should be thoroughly washed with soap and water. Reptile handlers should be currently immunized against tetanus.

Small colubrid and boid snakes may bite and persist in their grasp. It is a mistake to attempt to tear away from them since this may lacerate the skin. Grasp the head and force the mouth open to disengage the snake, or keep a spray bottle of isopropyl alcohol to spray on the head of a reptile to encourage it to release its hold. Snakes that prey on birds frequently have long teeth to penetrate the feather layer and reach the bird's body. A bite from a green tree boa or an anaconda may result in a serious laceration. Prompt medical attention should be sought.

Those who handle poisonous snakes risk being bitten and must be prepared to apply first aid procedures to themselves or associates. The likelihood of being bitten is probably directly correlated with the number of snakes handled and the care exercised in working with the animals. The emotional response of a victim to a venomous snakebite may complicate first aid treatment. The bitten person may become hysterical, faint, hyperventilate, or suffer from neurogenic shock in addition to suffering from the effects of the venom.

The managers of most large reptile collections follow a planned protocol when dealing with snakebite emergencies.[5–10,12–14] Following is an example of such a protocol.

1. Return the snake to its own enclosure.
2. If returning the snake within 30 seconds seems improbable, kill the snake by a quick blow to the head with a hook or any other nearby object that will enable you to reach out without risking another bite.
3. Sound any alarm system in use or call for help.

4. If an identification slip is on the cage, remove this and keep it on your person.
5. Remove appropriate antivenin from refrigerated storage and place it nearby.
6. Lie down and rest until help arrives.
7. If others are present in the immediate area at the time of the bite, they should carry out steps 1–5 and the victim should lie down and rest.
8. Remove the victim to a health care facility for further medical attention.

It is difficult to recommend first-aid procedures when dealing with human envenomation if medical care is unavailable for hours. First-aid protocols change frequently with newer information on the pathophysiology of the effects of venoms. "Cut-and-Suction" techniques are no longer recommended. The use of constricting bands is discouraged unless the bite is from a highly toxic elapid snake such as the black mamba (*Dendroaspis polylepis*).

Commercially available suction devices may be helpful if applied immediately after a bite (Fig. 30.75). The device is placed on the site of a fang penetration and a vacuum applied to draw out serum and venom.

Immobilize the bite area, splinting limbs if possible. Keep the bite area below the heart level. Have the victim sit or lie down and avoid exertion. Fear and excitement may be alleviated by calm actions and reassurance on the part of the person giving the first aid.

Provide the physician with information about the species of snake involved and the time interval since the bite, report any unusual signs, and give details of any treatment given.

Antivenin is the only specific treatment for snake envenomation, but it should be administered only by trained persons with equipment and medication available to cope with anaphylaxis should the victim prove to be sensitive to horse serum. Additional information on venoms and snakebite may be found in the reference Veterinary Zootoxicology.[6]

Transport

Snakes are adept at escaping through tiny openings. Any shipping crate must be checked carefully for loose screens or doors. Glass or plastic cages may be used for short local trips, but wooden cages must be used for inter-zoo shipment. Cages for venomous species must be lockable.

Reptiles must be protected from extreme temperature variations. Styrofoam iceboxes make excellent temporary carrying cages for local trips, or foam rubber or styrofoam may be laminated onto the inside of wooden crates.

Snakes are commonly transported in sacks. A hoop sack (Fig. 30.82) is particularly desirable for transporting poisonous snakes, since a snake can be hooked into the sack while the handler remains at a safe distance. Once the snake is inside, the hoop is flipped over so the snake cannot crawl out (Fig. 30.83). Then a cord is tied around the sack. If the sack is constructed with a double bottom, it can be grasped to tip the snake out. The double bottom eliminates the danger of being bitten through the canvas sack.

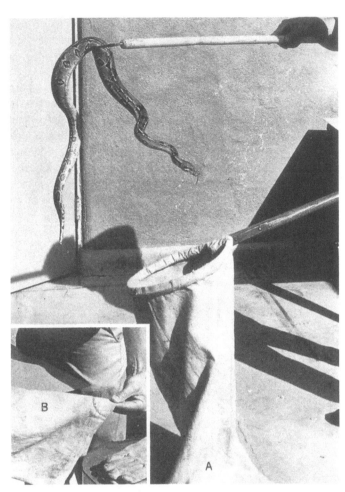

FIG. 30.82. **A.** Placing a snake on a hook into the snake sack. **B.** False bottom sewn into the sack allows grasping without danger of being bitten through the sack.

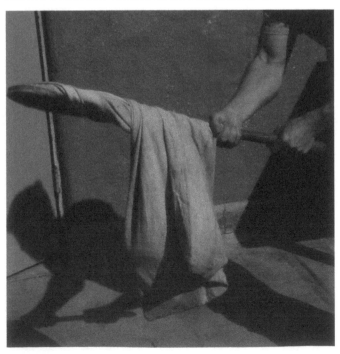

FIG. 30.83. Flip the hoop over to prevent the snake from climbing out.

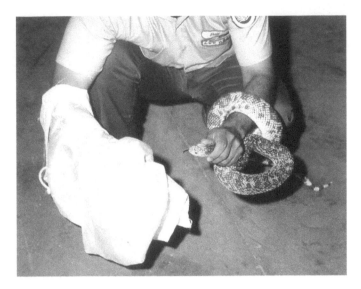

FIG. 30.84. Putting a docile nonpoisonous snake into sack. Sacking an aggressive nonpoisonous snake: Turn the sack inside out, keeping the hand in the inverted sack.

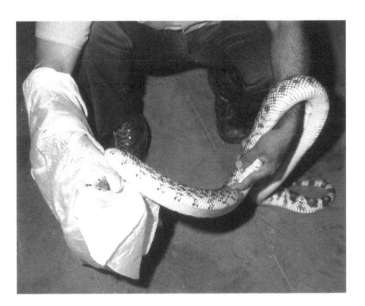

FIG. 30.85. Sacking an aggressive nonpoisonous snake. Re-grasp snake behind its head with the inverted sack. Sack is pulled over the body of the snake.

Tie a sack firmly at the top. Snakes easily force themselves through very small openings. Furthermore, it is important to check sacks to be certain there are no tiny holes that could be enlarged by a snake forcing its way through.

Docile nonvenomous snakes may be placed directly in the sack. With more aggressive non-venomous snakes, turn the sack inside out and grasp the head through it, everting the sack over the snake (Figs. 30.84, 30.85).

Be observant when placing a sacked snake in a strange place. Be sure that it will not get too hot or too cold. Additionally, do not place the sack on a chair or any other place where someone might unknowingly place a hand on it or sit on it.

In one instance, a rattlesnake in a sack was brought into my office in my absence and placed on a chair. When I returned, I did not notice the sack and, during the course of casual conversation, started to sit down. Fortunately those nearby alerted me before I sat on the snake.

Chemical Restraint[1,2,7–9,13,14,16]

Chemical restraint of venomous snakes is necessary to safely carry out many diagnostic and therapeutic procedures. Inhalation anesthesia using isoflurane in an anesthetic chamber (as shown in Fig. 30.86) is excellent but may require considerable time because of a snake's ability to hold its breath. Nonvenomous snakes may be intubated by holding the mouth open and waiting for the glottis to open. An endotracheal tube may be inserted (Figs. 30.87, 30.88) and connected to an anesthetic unit; the isoflurane/oxygen mixture is then forced into the lung by rebreathing-bag pressure or by use of a respirator. Figure 30.89 shows a puff adder intubated with the head restrained.

Injectable immobilization/anesthesia is also appropriate, as shown in Table 30.3. Currently tiletamine/zolazepam is recommended (4.0–8.0 mg/kg IM). Higher doses have been reported in the literature, but higher doses cause considerable delay in recovery. Ketamine is recommended (10.0–40.0 mg/kg). That dose is higher than the dose required for mammals of comparable weights. The drug produces mild sedation or profound anesthesia depending on the dose used. One of the first signs of a snake's impending immobilization after intramuscular injection of ketamine is a characteristic elevation of

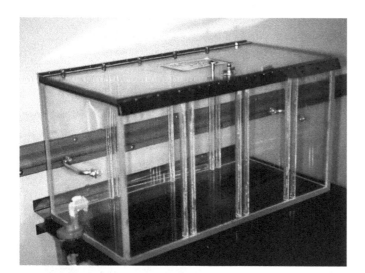

FIG. 30.86. An anesthetic or nebulizing chamber.

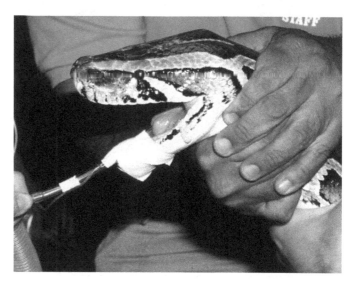

FIG. 30.88. Fixing the endotracheal tube in place with tape.

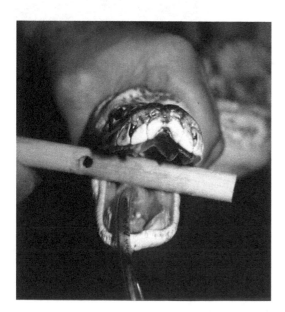

FIG. 30.87. Glottis of a snake with endotracheal tube in place.

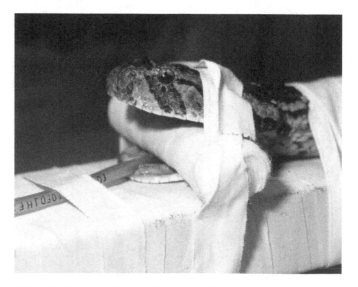

FIG. 30.89. A puff adder intubated with the head restrained.

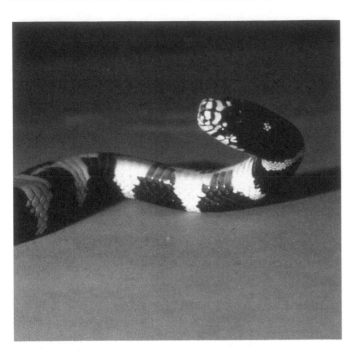

FIG. 30.90. Star gazing typical of ketamine immobilization.

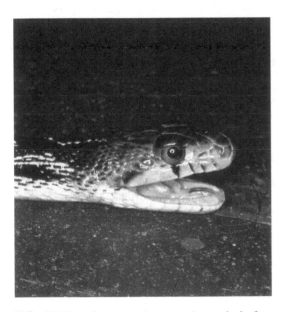

FIG. 30.91. Open-mouth stance also typical of ketamine hydrochloride anesthesia in a snake.

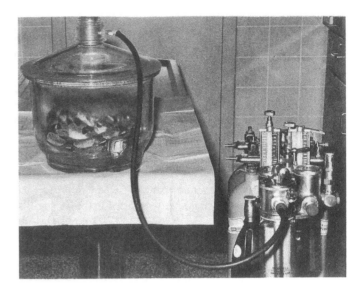

FIG. 30.92. Desiccating jar used as an anesthetic chamber to administer volatile anesthesia to a snake.

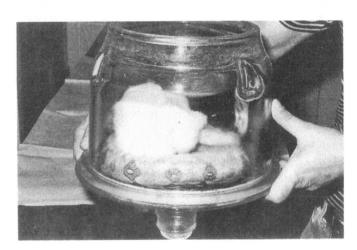

FIG. 30.93. Anesthesia is reached when the snake fails to right itself if inverted.

the head in a peculiar stargazing manner (Fig. 30.90), with the mouth held partially open (Fig. 30.91).

All snake immobilization procedures should be carried out with the snake on a heating pad or in a warm environment—not on a cold stainless steel table. Aftercare must include monitoring the environmental temperature to maintain sufficient body heat to allow the animal to metabolize the drug.

Snakes may be placed in an anesthetic chamber and a calibrated percentage of either isoflurane or halothane in oxygen flows into the chamber (Fig. 30.92).

The progression of anesthesia is determined by inverting the jar. If the snake is unable to right itself, it is probably anesthetized (Fig. 30.93).

Since a snake can hold its breath for 15–20 minutes, inhalant anesthesia induction may be prolonged. For this reason, apnea, a common concern of the mammalian restrainer, is not a serious problem of restrained reptiles. In fact it is sometimes difficult to ascertain whether a snake is actually alive during anesthetic procedures. However, it is easy to insert a tube past the glottis through the trachea, as described for administering anesthetic, and respire a distressed animal either manually, using mouth-tube respiration, or with inhalation equipment.

Once a snake is anesthetized, it is taped to a board (Fig. 30.94). Masking tape may be used on small snakes to minimize scale damage. Use only adhesive tape on large vipers.

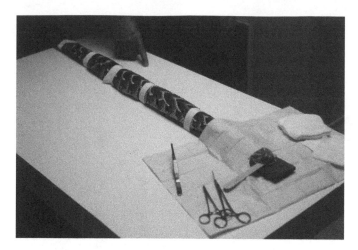

FIG. 30.94. Snake taped to a board for surgery.

Euthanasia of Reptiles

Numerous methods have been suggested for euthanasia of various taxa of reptiles. Many are unacceptable, especially if the owner of a pet wishes to be present at the time of euthanasia. One should follow the general principles of the AVMA Euthanasia Guidelines. The difficulty lies in determining when a reptile is dead. Breath holding is common in reptiles. The heart may continue to beat following death. Heart rate may slow from beats per minute to minutes per beat. Faced with the necessity of euthanizing, it would be well to consult a veterinarian with a specialty in reptile medicine. In lieu of such a contact, administer telazol 25.0 kg/kg, IM or ketamine 100.0 kg/kg, IM. Wait for 30 minutes and then administer a barbiturate euthanizing solution intracoelomicaly. If venous access is possible in larger species, saturated potassium chloride solution may be administered IV following the initial immobilization. See the Euthanasia section in Chapter 20.

REFERENCES

1. Bennett, R.A. 1996. Anesthesia. In: Mader, D.R., Ed. Reptile Medicine and Surgery. Philadelphia, W.B. Saunders, pp. 241–47.
2. Betelsen, M.F. 2007. Squamates (snakes and lizards). In: West, G., Heard, D., and Caulkett, N., Eds. Zoo Animal and Wildlife Chemical Immobilization and Anesthesia. Ames, Iowa, Blackwell Publishing, pp. 233–44.
3. Blake, D.K. 1993. The Nile Crocodile: Capture, care, accommodation, and transportation. In: McKenzie, A.A., Ed. The Capture and Care Manual, Pretoria: The South African Veterinary Foundation, pp. 653–76.
4. Esra, G.N., Benirschke, K., and Griner, L.A. 1975. Blood collecting technique in lizards. J Am Vet Med Assoc 167:555.
5. Fleming, G.J. 2007. Crocodilians. In: West, G., Heard, D., and Caulkett, N., Eds. Zoo Animal and Wildlife Chemical Immobilization and Anesthesia. Ames, Iowa, Blackwell Publishing, pp. 223–32.
6. Fowler, M.E. 1993. Veterinary Zootoxicology. Boca Raton, Fla., CRC Press.
7. Frye, F.L. 1991. Biomedical and Surgical Aspects of Captive Reptile Husbandry, 2nd ed., Malabar, Fla., Krieger Publishing, Vol. 1, p. 30, and Vol. 2, pp. 423–33.
8. Glenn, J.L., Straight, R., and Snyder, C.C. 1972. Clinical use of ketamine hydrochloride as an anesthetic agent for snakes. Am J Vet Res 33:1091–3.
9. Heard, D.J., and Stetter, M.D. 2007. Reptiles, amphibians and fish. In: Tranquilli, W.J., Thurman, J.C., and Grimm, K.A., Eds. Lumb and Jones' Veterinary Anesthesia and Analgesia, 4th Ed. Ames, Iowa, Wiley-Blackwell Publishing, pp. 869–90.
10. Jacobson, E.R. 1993. Blood collection techniques in reptiles laboratory investigations. In: Fowler, M.E., Ed. Zoo and Wild Animal Medicine, 3rd ed., Philadelphia: W.B. Saunders, pp. 144–52.
11. Lloyd, M.L. 2003. Crocodilia. In: Fowler, M.E., and Miller, R.E., Eds. Zoo and Wild Animal Medicine. 5th Ed. St. Louis, Saunders/Elsevier. pp. 59–70.
12. Lloyd, M.L. 1999. Crocodilian anesthesia. In: Fowler, M.E., and Miller, R.E., Eds. Zoo and Wild Animal Medicine. 4th Ed. Philadelphia, W.B. Saunders. pp. 215.
13. Page, C.D. 1993. Current reptilian anesthesia procedures. In: Fowler, M.E., Ed. Zoo and Wild Animal Medicine, 3rd ed., Philadelphia: W.B. Saunders, pp. 140–44.
14. Schumaker, J. 1996. Reptiles and amphibians. In: Thurmon, J.C., Tranquilli, W.J., and Benson, G.J., Eds. Lumb and Jones' Veterinary Anesthesia. 3rd Ed. Philadelphia, Lippincott Williams and Wilkens, pp. 670–80.
15. Schumacker, J. 2007. Chelonians. In: West, G., Heard, D., and Caulkett, N., Eds. Zoo Animal and Wildlife Chemical Immobilization and Anesthesia. Ames, Iowa, Blackwell Publishing, pp. 259–68.
16. Schumacker, J., and Yellen, T. 2006. Anesthesia and analgesia. In: Mader, D.R., Ed. Reptile Medicine and Surgery, 2nd Ed. St. Louis, Saunders/Elsevier, pp. 442–52.
17. Sleeman, J.M., and Gaynor, J. 2000. Sedative and cardiopulmonary effects of medetomidine and reversal with atipamezole in desert tortoises. J Zoo An Med 31(1):28–35.

CHAPTER 31
Amphibians and Fish

CLASSIFICATION

Class Amphibia (over 2,500 species)
    Order Anura (Salienta): frogs, toads
    Order Caudata (Urodela): salamanders, sirenids
    Order Gymnophonia (Caecilia): caecilians
Class Pisces (over 25,000 species ranging in length from a
    few millimeters to 18 m)

AMPHIBIANS
Danger Potential

All amphibians except pipid frogs and true toads have teeth of some description, but their size and location in the mouth vary. Large salamanders and a few of the large toads are capable of inflicting a painful bite with hardened cornified plates similar to those of turtles. A large amphibian's jaws are strong enough to give a sharp pinch.

No amphibian has a venomous bite. The secretion of the parotoid skin gland of certain toads, such as the Colorado River and marine toads, is toxic to dogs if ingested.[4] Parotoid does not refer to the parotid salivary gland but rather to being around or near (para, par) the ear (otoid) (Fig. 31.1). The

secretion irritates the human eye if it gets into the conjunctival sac. Hands must be thoroughly washed after handling a venomous toad lest a hand should inadvertently touch the mouth or rub an eye. In one unique instance a Colombian giant toad actually projected the secretion from the parotoid gland into the eye of a keeper who was holding the toad (Fig. 31.2). The keeper experienced an immediate burning sensation and quickly rinsed the secretion from his eyes, but the irritation persisted for an hour. No additional toxic manifestations were noted.

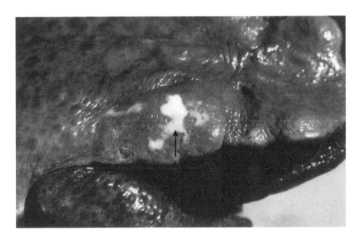

FIG. 31.2. Secretion from the parotoid gland of a Colombian giant toad (arrow).

The poison-arrow frogs Dendrobates and Phyllobates secrete highly toxic biotoxins from skin glands all over the body (Fig. 31.3). The skins of these frogs were used by indigenous peoples to make the substance used to coat arrowheads for hunting wild animals in specific locations in South America.[4] Restrainers must be careful to wash hands thoroughly following handling.

Anatomy and Physiology

Amphibians are obligate aquatic animals for at least the reproductive phase of the life cycle. A few species have evolved away from water and have developed the capacity to lay eggs that develop and metamorphose in minimal quantities of water, such as the amount that accumulates in the junctions of leaves and stems of plants in a rain forest.

The skin glands of amphibians produce a secretion that protects their skin from the deleterious effects of water.

These secretions prevent desiccation, inhibit the growth of microorganisms on the skin, and in specialized cases,

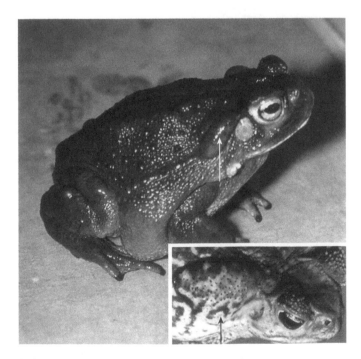

FIG. 31.1. Colorado River toad. Arrow points to the parotoid gland.

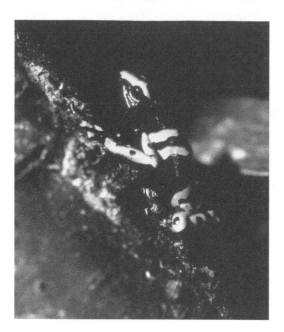

FIG. 31.3.   Poison arrow frog *Dendrobates leucomelas*.

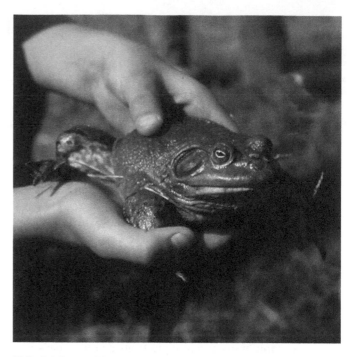

FIG. 31.4.   Bullfrog *Rana catesbeiana*.

discourage predators. The secretions may cause problems for the animal restrainer, because they make the animal slippery and difficult to grasp and hold. All species of toads secrete substances that are repulsive to animals that bite or mouth them. Puppies may bite toads once but usually resist the impulse a second time.

The skin of all amphibians functions as a supplementary respiratory organ, and in some species, it may be the primary organ of respiration.

Physical Restraint[3,7,10]

The hands should be moistened before handling any amphibian. Frogs can be captured from the water or while on a dry surface. Small species may be netted or grasped bare-handed (Figs. 31.4, 31.5, 31.6), but some of the larger may bite, so take precautions. Since the skin surface is slippery, the hand must surround the frog. If the animal is to be held for more than a few seconds, wrap the legs with gauze to assist in control (Figs. 31.7, 31.8, 31.9).

Small aquatic amphibians may be captured in a soft aquarium net. Small toads do not bite and can be handled like frogs (Fig. 31.10). The skin is usually not as slippery as that of frogs. Large frogs and toads may be picked up and held by the hind legs, with support of the body (Fig. 31.11).

Smaller species of salamanders may be grasped bare-handed (Fig. 31.12). One or both hands may be used. Moisten the hands first. Aquatic species are more slippery. Large salamanders like the hellbender or giant salamander should be handled more cautiously. The initial grasp should be

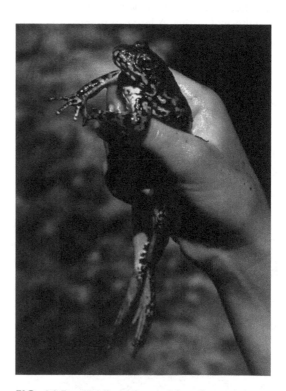

FIG. 31.5.   Holding a leopard frog *Rana pipiens*.

made quickly over the back, as one would grasp a crocodilian.

Caecilians are legless burrowing amphibians. They are seldom seen in the wild and are poor exhibit animals. Caecilians are docile and can be handled like a snake.

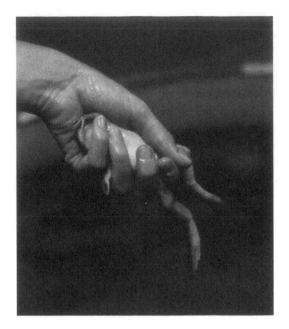

FIG. 31.6. **A.** Grasping clawed toad *Xenopus* sp. in a tank. One-hand method of holding a toad.

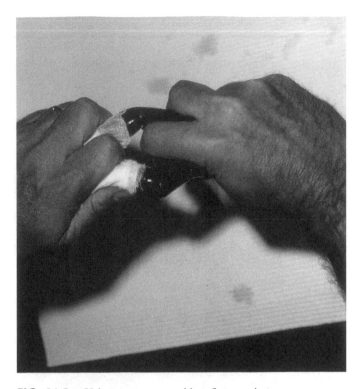

FIG. 31.8. Using gauze to provide a firmer grip.

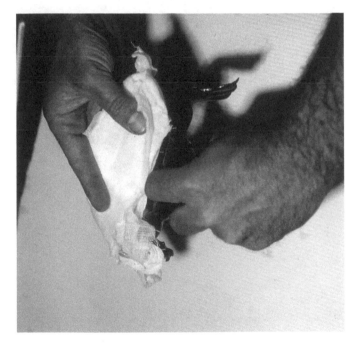

FIG. 31.7. Placing gauze on the legs to provide a firmer grip.

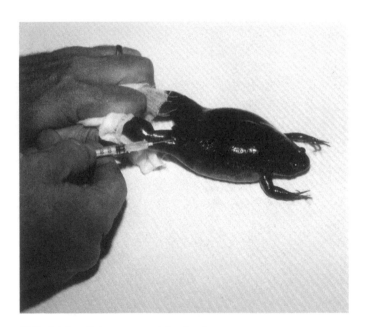

FIG. 31.9. Subcutaneous injection in an amphibian.

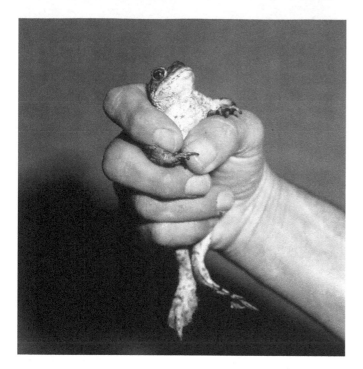

FIG. 31.10.   Method for holding a clawed frog.

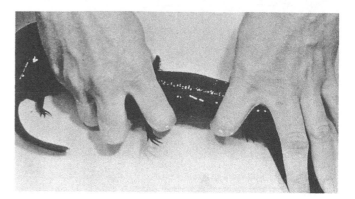

FIG. 31.12.   Grasping an axolotl salamander with moistened hands.

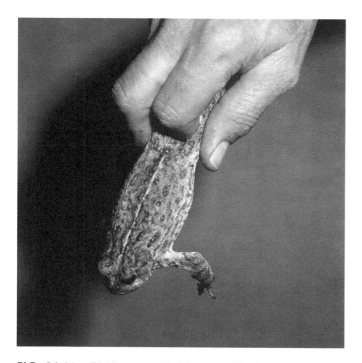

FIG. 31.11.   Picking up and holding a toad by its hind legs.

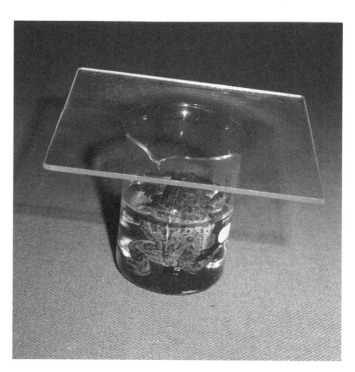

FIG. 31.13.   Emersing an amphibian in an anesthetic solution.

CHEMICAL RESTRAINT[3,7,8,10,13]

The chemical restraint agents and combinations mentioned in this chapter represent those used by the author or by experienced veterinarians with detailed knowledge of amphib-

ians or fish. Other protocols have been used, and no claim is made for including all possible drugs and combinations. For more detailed information, particularly for anesthesia, consult the references.[7,9,12,13]

The skin of amphibians is sufficiently permeable to allow absorption of anesthetic agents (Fig. 31.13). Table 31.1 lists selected immobilizing agents for use in amphibians. Tricaine

TABLE 31.1. Anesthetic agents for amphibians and fish

	Concentration (per liter H$_2$O)
Benzocaine	Stock solution, 100 g/L ethanol and add dropwise to water as required
Quinaldine	200 mg
Tricaine methanesulfonate Finquel (MS 222)*	0.25 to 0.5 g/L for amphibians with gills 1.0 to 2.0 g/L for frogs and salamanders 2.0 to 3.0 g/L for terrestrial toads 0.75 to 1.0 g/L for fishes
Isoflurane	5% isoflurane from a vaporizer bubbled through water bathing the amphibian 0.4 to 0.75 ml liquid isoflurane/L for induction of fishes 0.25 ml liquid isoflurane/L for maintenance of fishes

*Immobilizing drug of choice for amphibians.

methanesulfonate (Finquel, MS 222) is the agent of choice.

Water temperature has a profound bearing on induction, maintenance, and recovery times of anesthesia. Cool to cold water lengthens the times, while warmer water reduces the time. Amphibians should be kept moistened throughout anesthesia and recovery.

At a moderate to surgical plane of anesthesia, the respiratory rate is greatly depressed and may be imperceptible. If, however, the water temperature is low, cutaneous respiration will keep the animal oxygenated.

Intravascular injection may be administered into the dorsal lymph sac, which is a subcutaneous space in frogs and toads that connects with the cardiovascular system via either the cranial or caudal lymph hearts. The subcutaneous spaces cover large areas of both the dorsal and ventral surfaces of the body and may even extend onto the limbs.

Blood Collection

Blood samples are best obtained from the heart with the animal under sedation or anesthesia. Hold the animal in dorsal recumbency. Palpate the sternum and push it gently to one side. Insert a 22- to 26-gauge needle into the ventricle at a 30-degree angle. Large frogs and toads may have visible superficial veins that may be cannulated.

Transportation

Small aquatic species may be transported in sealed plastic bags containing one-third water and two-thirds oxygen. Terrestrial species should be placed in a moist, soft substrate such as peat moss or pieces of sponge. Avoid shaking, tipping, or dropping containers, and most importantly, avoid extreme temperatures. Either cold or heat may be directly or indirectly lethal. Styrofoam boxes are excellent receptacles for the primary container.

FISH

Fish culture for food and as a hobby has become a multimillion-dollar business. The industry is not new; food fish have been kept in home ponds or tanks for over 4,000 years.[11] The keeping of fish as pets dates back to the ancient Roman and Chinese empires.

Anatomy and Physiology

Streamlined fish with no demarcation between head and body are difficult to grasp or hold. The surface of the body is coated with a protective mucus, which further complicates handling.

Fish breathe via gills. They can live out of water for only a few minutes. Any handling procedure prolonged beyond this limit must provide oxygenated water to bathe the gills. Cold water contains more oxygen than warm water. If fish are held in small aquaria or transport tanks, the water must be aerated or the fish will die—especially if the water is warm.

Danger Potential[2,5]

Fish can bite, sting, and abrade the skin of handlers. The bite is not venomous, but carnivorous species are efficient predators with numerous teeth designed for grasping, shearing, and tearing flesh. Free-ranging sharks are notorious for their gruesome attacks on people. In captivity injuries are not as likely to occur, but these animals can and do bite if mishandled.

Smaller species may be equally aggressive. The diminutive piranha can inflict severe injury. A barracuda or a moray eel may inflict serious damage. The list of fish that may bite is long. It is important to keep hands clear of the mouths of fish.

Sharks have extremely rough skin that can abrade the skin of a handler.

Certain species of fish have developed the capacity to generate powerful electrical charges. Electric rays are found in three families distributed throughout the warm oceans of the world. Electrical discharges of over 200 volts and 2,000 watts have been measured from one of these rays.[4] This electricity is generated in one or more specialized organs. Electrical shock is used to procure food as well as to serve as an effective deterrent to predators.

Electric organs are also present in the electric catfish (Africa), the stargazer (USA), and the electric eel (South America).[4,5] The electric eel can develop a charge of 550 volts. Animals coming within the electrical field will be stunned. Touching the animal while it is discharging may be fatal to persons. Touching the eel simultaneously at two sites increases electrical conductivity and hence the hazard.

Many species of fish have venomous spines that inject secretions of varying degrees of toxicity. Very few venomous fish have been studied. Probably only a fraction of the actual number of venomous species are known.[2] Halstead[5] lists 4 sharks, 58 stingrays, 47 catfish, 4 weeverfish, 57 scorpion fish, 15 toadfish, 3 stargazers, 8 rabbitfish, and 8 surgeonfish species as venomous. The spines are usually associated with one or more of the fins, although in the case of the surgeonfish, the lancet-like spine is on the lateral surface of the base of the tail.

Tropical fish enthusiasts may be at risk of envenomation from small specimens of poisonous fish. One aquarist was injured while netting a small specimen of oriental catfish from a tank (Fig. 31.14). The fish flopped from the net, and he automatically reached out to grab it. A dorsal spine was driven into his hand. Pain was instantaneous and violent, and he was incapacitated within seconds. Sedation and general nursing care were required to effect recovery within 2 days. Another highly venomous aquarium fish is the zebra fish (Fig. 31.15).

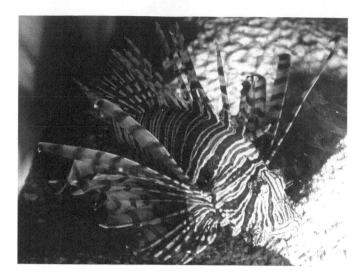

FIG. 31.15.   A zebra fish or turkey fish (*Pterois volitans*).

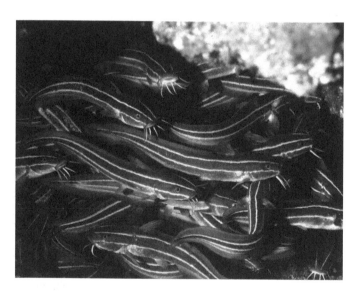

FIG. 31.14.   Oriental catfish (*Plotosus* sp).

The syndrome of envenomation by most stingray fish includes severe pain, inflammation of the wound, and temporary paralysis. There are no antivenins available.

Fish spines need not be venomous to inflict injury. The cartilaginous rays that keep the fins expanded may puncture a hand that grabs them. Those who must handle catfish repeatedly may wear light cotton gloves to minimize injuries from the spines. The value of the gloves as protection to the handler's hands must be balanced against the increased abrasion and trauma inflicted on the fish.

Being drenched is one unique hazard of working with certain fish. A small shark once swam up to the side of the tank and spit water all over my shirt. I was told this behavior is not unexpected for that species of shark.

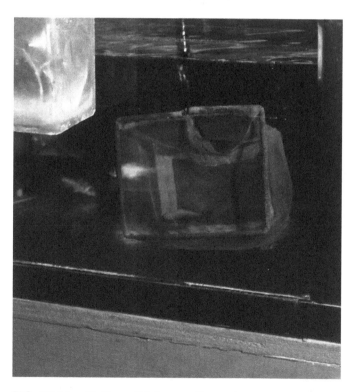

FIG. 31.16.   Netting a fish in a small aquarium.

Physical Restraint[11]

Nets are the primary tools for handling fish. The size of the net and the mesh vary from the lightweight, fine-meshed small nets used to transfer tropical fish (Fig. 31.16) to heavy, coarse commercial nets for harvesting tuna fish. All shapes and sizes in between are employed (Figs. 31.17 to 31.21). Plastic and wooden panels may be used to direct fish into a limited area to permit netting or into a smaller capture tank submerged in a large tank.

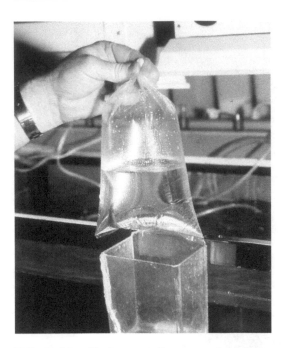

FIG. 31.17. Placing a small ornamental fish in a plastic bag for transport to a home.

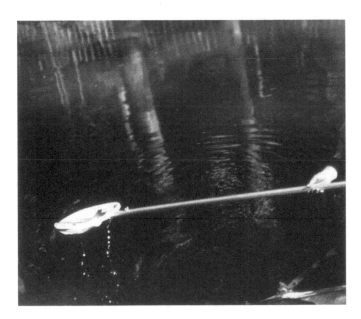

FIG. 31.18. Using a hoop net to capture a fish in a fish hatchery raceway.

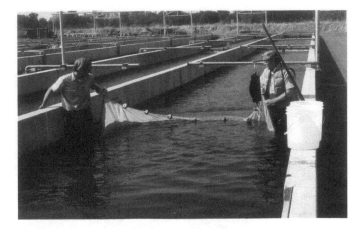

FIG. 31.19. Netting fish in a fish hatchery raceway.

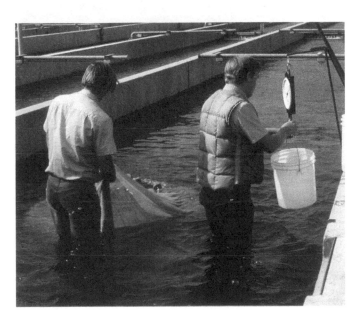

FIG. 31.20. Weighing fish in a fish hatchery.

Some fish have loosely adhered scales that can be easily scraped off by harsh handling. Mucous secretions on the surface of the skin plus the scales protect the epithelium from microbial infection. Avoid rubbing off the mucus or scales since this may allow penetration of pathogenic bacteria. Latex gloves on the hands minimize trauma. Harsh, prolonged, or repeated handling of fish may lead to heavy death loss as a result of stress and reduced resistance to bacterial infection.

Although nets are essential fish-handling tools, there are hazards associated with their use. Scales can be abraded and

fins entangled in the mesh. The lidless eyes of fish usually bulge from the surface of the body and are thus susceptible to abrasions if the net rubs tightly against the fish. Fish can also see the approaching net and may become traumatized as they dart about frantically to elude capture. Each net should be restricted to use in a single tank or be disinfected between tanks to avoid spreading infections or parasites from tank to tank.

Some tropical fish enthusiasts recommend the use of polyurethane plastic bags for fish capture instead of nets. The bag is transparent, thus the fish experience less fear and are not able to elude capture so readily. Another important benefit is that the disposable plastic bag is germ- and parasite-free, unlike nets used repeatedly between tanks. Small fish may also be transported in tightly sealed plastic bags containing one-third water and two-thirds oxygen.

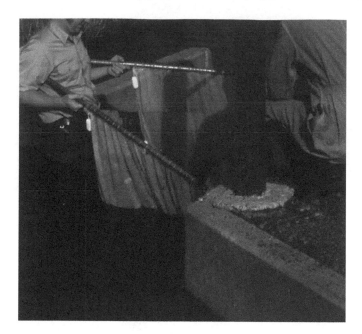

FIG. 31.21.   Lifting netted fish.

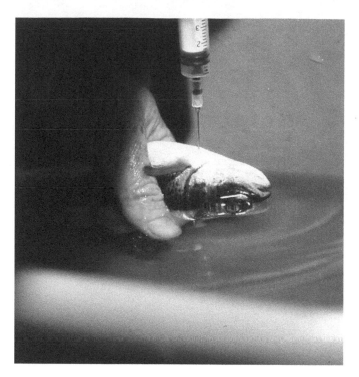

FIG. 31.23.   Collecting heart blood in an anesthetized trout.

Chemical Restraint[1,6,9,12]

Numerous chemical agents have been dissolved in water to anesthetize fish (Fig. 31.22). A few are listed in Table 31.1. Injectable anesthetic agents have also been used in fish including ketamine, ketamine/medetomidine, propofol, lidocaine, and xylazine.[9] A more detailed discussion of fish anesthesia is found in the references.[1,9,12] Figure 31.23 illustrates how to obtain an intracardial blood sample from an anesthetized trout.

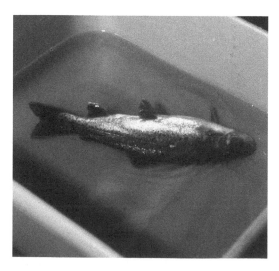

FIG. 31.22.   Trout in an anesthetic solution (MS 222).

REFERENCES

1. Brown, L.A. 1993. Anesthesia and restraint. In: Stoskopf, M.K., Ed. Fish Medicine, Philadelphia: W.B. Saunders, pp. 79–90.
2. Caras, R. 1974. Venomous Animals of the World, Englewood Cliffs, N.J., Prentice-Hall, p. 103.
3. Crawshaw, G.J. 1993. Amphibian medicine. In: Fowler, M.E., Ed. Zoo and Wild Animal Medicine, 3rd ed., Philadelphia: W.B. Saunders, pp. 131–40.
4. Fowler, M.E. 1993. Veterinary Zootoxicology. Boca Raton, CRC Press.
5. Halstead, B.W., and Cowville, D.A. 1965–1970. Poisonous and Venomous Marine Animals of the World, 3 vols. Washington, D.C.: U.S. Government Printing Office.
6. Healy, E.C. 1964. Anesthesia in fishes. In: Graham-Jones, O., Ed. Small Animal Anesthesia. Elmsford, N.Y., Pergamon Press.
7. Heard, D.J., and Stetter, M.D. 2007. Reptiles, amphibians and fish. In: Tranquilli, W.J., Thurman, J.C., and Grimm, K.A., Eds. Lumb and Jones' Veterinary Anesthesia and Analgesia, 4th Ed. Ames, Iowa, Wiley-Blackwell Publishing, pp. 869–90.
8. Letcher, J. 1992. Intracelomic use of tricaine methanesulfonate for anesthesia of bullfrogs and leopard frogs. Zoo Biol 11:243–52.
9. Neiffer, D.L. 2007. Bony fish (lungfish, sturgeon and teleosts). In: West, G., Heard, D., and Caulkett, N., Eds. Ames, Iowa, Blackwell Publishing, pp. 159–96.
10. Schumacher, J. 1996. Reptiles and amphibians. In: Thurmon, J.C., Tranquilli, W.J., and Benson, G.J., Eds. Lumb and Jones' Veterinary Anesthesia. 3rd Ed. Philadelphia, Lippincott Williams and Wilkens, pp. 670–80.

11. Spotte, S. 1970. Fish and Invertebrate Culture. New York, Wiley Interscience.

12. Stamper, M.A. 2007. Elasmobranchs (sharks, rays, and skates). In: West, G., Heard, D., and Caulkett, N., Eds. Ames, Iowa, Blackwell Publishing, pp. 197–204.

13. Stetter, M. 2007. Amphibians. In: West, G., Heard, D., and Caulkett, N., Eds. Ames, Iowa, Blackwell Publishing, pp. 205–10.

APPENDICES

APPENDIX A. DOMESTIC ANIMALS

Common Name	Scientific Name
Mammals	
Alpaca	*Llama pacos*
Ass (donkey)	*Equus asinus*
Banteng	*Bos javanicus*
Buffalo, water	*Bubalus bubalis*
Camel, bactrian	*Camelus bactrianus*
Camel, dromedary	*Camelus dromedarius*
Cat	*Felis catus*
Cattle, European	*Bos taurus*
Cattle, zebu	*Bos taurus var. indicus*
Dog	*Canis familiaris*
Ferret	*Mustela putorius*
Fox	*Vulpes vulpes*
Gayal	*Bos frontalis*
Goat	*Capra hircus*
Guinea pig	*Cavia porcellus*
Hamster, golden	*Mesocricetus auratus*
Horse	*Equus caballus*
Kouprey	*Bos sauveli*
Llama	*Llama glama*
Mink	*Mustela vison*
Mouse	*Mus musculus*
Mule	*Equus* sp.
Musk-ox	*Ovibos moschatus*
Rabbit	*Oryctolagus cuniculus*
Rat	*Rattus norvegicus*
Reindeer	*Rangifer tarandus*
Sheep	*Ovis aries*
Swine	*Sus scrofa*
Yak	*Bos grunniens*
Birds	
Budgerigar	*Melopsitticus undulatus*
Canary	*Serinus canarius*
Chicken	*Gallus gallus*
Duck, Muscovy	*Cairina moschata*
Duck, Pekin	*Anas platyrhyncos*
Goose	*Anser anser*
Goose, Canada	*Branta canadensis*
Guinea fowl	*Numida meleagris*
Peafowl	*Pavo cristatus*
Pheasant, ring-necked torquatus	*Phasianus colchicus*
Pigeon	*Columba livia*
Quail, coturnix	*Coturnix coturnix*
Swan, mute	*Cygnus olor*
Turkey	*Meleagris gallopavo*

APPENDIX B. WILD ANIMALS (SCIENTIFIC NAMES OF ANIMALS SPECIFICALLY MENTIONED IN THE TEXT)[1]

Common Name	Scientific Name
Monotremes and Marsupials	
Antechinus	*Antechinus stuarti*
Bandicoot	*Perameles* spp.
Echidna	*Tachyglossus aculeatus*
Glider, sugar	*Petaurus breviceps*
Kangaroo, gray	*Macropus giganteus*
Kangaroo, red	*Macropus rufus*
Koala	*Phascolarctos cinereus*
Kowaris	*Dasyuroides byrnei*
Opossum, Virginia	*Didelphis virginiana*
Phalanger, brush-tailed	*Trichosurus vulpecula*
Platypus	*Ornithorhynchus anatinus*
Quoll	*Dasyurus* spp.
Tasmanian devil	*Sarcophilus harrisii*
Wallaby, agile	*Macropus agilis*
Wallaby, red-necked	*Macropus rufogrisea*
Wallaroo	*Macropus robustus*
Wombat, common	*Wombatus ursinus*
Small Mammals	
Aardvark	*Orycteropus afer*
Agouti	*Dasyprocta* spp.
Anteater, giant	*Myrmecophaga tridactyla*
Armadillo, three-banded	*Tolypeutes tricinctus*
Armadillo, nine-banded	*Dasypus novemcinctus*
Armadillo, giant	*Priodontes giganteus*
Bat, fruit	Megachiroptera (suborder)
Bat, insectivorous	Microchiroptera (suborder)
Bat, vampire	*Desmodus rotundus*
Beaver	*Castor canadensis*
Capybara	*Hydrochaeris hydrochaeris*
Chinchilla	*Chinchilla laniger*
Flying lemur	*Cynocephalus* sp.
Golden mole	*Cryptochloris* spp
Hedgehog	*Erinaceus europaeus*
Hyrax, rock	*Procavia capensis*
Kangaroo rat	*Dipodomys* spp.
Mouse, deer	*Peromyscus* spp.
Muskrat	*Ondatra zibethius*
Pangolin	*Manis* spp.
Pika	*Ochotona* spp.
Porcupine, African crested	*Hystrix cristata*
Porcupine, Brazilian tree	*Coendou prehensilis*
Porcupine, North American	*Erethizon dorsatum*
Shrew, American short-tailed	*Blarina brevicauda*
Shrew, bicolored water	*Neomys fodiens*
Shrew, elephant	*Elephantulus* spp.
Shrew, European water	*Neomys fodiens*
Shrew, masked	*Sorex cinereus*
Sloth, three-toed	*Bradypus tridaclylus*
Solenodon, Haitian	*Solenodon paradoxus*
Springhaas	*Pedetes* sp.
Tamandua	*Tamandua tetradactyla*
Tenrec	*Tenrec ecaudatus*
Woodchuck	*Marmota* sp.

Common Name	Scientific Name
Carnivores	
Aardwolf	*Proteles cristatus*
Bear, American black	*Ursus americanus*
Bear, grizzly	*Ursus arctus horribilus*
Bear, polar	*Ursus maritimus*
Bear, sun	*Ursus malayanus*
Binturong	*Arctictis binturong*
Bobcat	*Felis rufus*
Cacomistle	*Bassariscus astutus*
Cat, leopard	*Felis bengalensis*
Cheetah	*Acinonyx jubatus*
Civet cat	*Viverra civetta*
Coatimundi	*Nasua nasua*
Coyote	*Canis latrans*
Fennec	*Fennecus zerda*
Fox, gray	*Urocyon cinereoargenteus*
Fox, red	*Vulpes vulpes*
Grison	*Galictis vittata*
Hyena, spotted	*Crocuta crocuta*
Kinkajou	*Potos flavus*
Leopard, clouded	*Neofelis nebulosa*
Lion	*Panthera leo*
Lion, mountain	*Felis concolor*
Mink	*Mustela vison*
Mongoose	Family Vivveridae (order Carnivora)
Ocelot	*Felis pardalis*
Otter, North American	*Lutra canadensis*
Otter, sea	*Enhydra lutris*
Otter, small clawed	*Amblonyx cinerea*
Panda, giant	*Ailuropoda melanoleuca*
Panda, lesser	*Ailurus fulgens*
Raccoon, North American	*Procyon lotor*
Skunk, striped	*Mephitis mephitis*
Tiger	*Panthera tigris*
Weasel	*Mustela* spp.
Wolf, gray	*Canis lupus*
Wolverine	*Gulo gulo*

Common Name	Scientific Name
Primates	
Baboon, yellow	*Papio cynocephalus*
Capuchin	*Cebus apella*
Chimpanzee	*Pan troglodytes*
Gibbon, white-handed	*Hylobates lar*
Gorilla	*Gorilla gorilla*
Langur	*Presbytis* spp.
Loris, slow	*Nycticebus coucang*
Macaque, Philippine	*Macaca philippinenon*
Macaque, rhesus	*Macaca mulatta*
Marmoset	*Callithrix jacchus*
Marmoset, pygmy	*Cebuella pygmaea*
Monkey, colobus	*Colobus* spp.
Monkey, green	*Cercopithecus aethiops*
Monkey, roloway	*Cercopithecus diana roloway*
Monkey, spider	*Ateles* spp.
Monkey, squirrel	*Saimiri sciureus*
Monkey, woolly	*Lagothrix* spp.
Orangutan	*Pongo pygmaeus*

Common Name	Scientific Name
Tamarin, cotton-topped	*Saguinus oedipus*
Tarsier	*Tarsius* spp.
Tree shrew	*Tupaia* sp.

Common Name	Scientific Name
Marine Mammals	
Dolphin, Atlantic bottle-nosed	*Tursiops truncatus*
Dugong	*Dugong dugon*
Manatee	*Trichechus manatus*
Seal, elephant	*Mirounga angustirostris*
Seal, harbor	*Phoca vitulina*
Seal, weddell	*Leptonychotes weddelli*
Sea lion, California	*Zalophus californianus*
Walrus	*Odobenus rosmarus*
Whale, blue	*Balaenoptera musculus*
Whale, killer	*Orcinus orca*

Common Name	Scientific Name
Elephants	
Elephant, African	*Loxodonta africana*
Elephant, Asian	*Elephas maximus*

Common Name	Scientific Name
Hoofed Stock	
Perissodactylids:	
Horse, Przewalski's	*Equus caballus przewalskii*
Rhinoceros, black	*Diceros bicornis*
Rhinoceros, Indian	*Rhinoceros unicornis*
Rhinoceros, white	*Ceratotherium simus*
Tapir, Brazilian	*Tapirus terrestris*
Tapir, Malayan	*Tapirus indicus*
Tapir, mountain	*Tapirus pinchaque*
Zebra, Grant's	*Equus burchelli*
Artiodactylids:	
Alpaca	*Lama pacos*
Aoudad	*Ammotragus lervia*
Antelope, roan	*Hippotragus equinus*
Antelope, sable	*Hippotragus niger*
Antelope, saiga	*Saiga tatarica*
Banteng	*Bibos javanicus*
Bison, American	*Bison bison*
Black buck	*Antilope cervicapra*
Bongo	*Tragelaphus euryceros*
Buffalo, Cape	*Syncerus caffer*
Buffalo, water	*Bubalus bubalis*
Bushbuck	*Tragelaphus scriptus*
Camel, bactrian	*Camelus bactrianus*
Camel, dromedary	*Camelus dromedarius*
Caribou	*Rangifer tarandus caribou*
Deer, fallow	*Dama dama*
Deer, mule	*Odocoileus hemionus*
Deer, muntjac	*Muntiacus muntjak*
Deer, sika	*Cervus nippon*
Deer, white-tail	*Odocoileus virginianus*
Eland	*Taurotragus oryx*
Elk (wapiti)	*Cervus elaphus canadensis*
Gazelle, Dorcas	*Gazella dorcas*
Gazelle, Thomson	*Gazella thomsoni*
Giraffe	*Giraffa camelopardalis*
Gnu, white-tail	*Connochaetus gnu*
Goat, Rocky Mountain	*Oreamnos americanus*
Guanaco	*Lama guanicoe*
Hippopotamus, Nile	*Hippopotamus amphibius*

Common Name	Scientific Name
Hippopotamus, pygmy	*Choeropsis liberiensis*
Ibex	*Capra ibex*
Impala	*Aepyceros melampus*
Klipspringer	*Oreotragus oreotragus*
Llama	*Lama glama*
Moose	*Alces alces*
Musk-ox	*Ovibos moschatus*
Nyala	*Tragelaphus angasi*
Okapi	*Okapia johnstoni*
Oryx, Arabian	*Oryx leucoryx*
Oryx, fringe-eared	*Oryx gazella callotis*
Peccary, collared	*Tayassu tajacu*
Peccary, white-lipped	*Tayassu albinostris*
Pronghorn	*Antilocapra americana*
Reindeer	*Rangifer tarandus*
Sheep, bighorn	*Ovis canadensis*
Sheep, Dall	*Ovis canadensis dalli*
Sheep, mouflon	*Ovis musimon*
Tahr	*Hemitragus jemlahicus*
Vicuna	*Vigugna vicugna*
Warthog	*Phacochoerus aethiopicus*
Yak	*Bos grunniens*

Birds

Aracari	*Pteroglossus* sp.
Bald eagle	*Haliaeetus leucocephalus*
Budgerigar (parakeet)	*Melopsittacus undulatus*
Canada goose	*Branta canadensis*
Canary	*Serinus canarius*
Cassowary, double-wattled	*Casuarius casuarius*
Cockatiel	*Nymphicus hollandicus*
Cockatoo	*Cacatua* sp.
Coly	*Colius* spp.
Crow	*Corvus* spp.
Crowned crane	*Balearica pavonina*
Crowned pigeon	*Goura cristata*
Duck, mallard	*Anas platyrhyncos*
Emu	*Dromaius novae-hollandiae*
Flamingo, American	*Phoenicopterus ruber*
Goose, spur-winged	*Plectropterus gambensis*
Golden eagle	*Aquila chrysaetos*
Great horned owl	*Bubo virginianus*
Hornbill	*Buceros* spp.
Kiwi	*Apteryx australis*
Macaw	*Ara* sp.
Macaw, hyacinth	*Anodorhynchus hyacinthinus*
Ostrich	*Struthio camelus*
Parrot, kea	*Nestor notabilis*
Peafowl	*Pavo cristatus*
Pelican, American white	*Pelecanus erythrorhynchos*
Penguin, Humboldt	*Spheniscus humboldti*
Pheasant	*Phaisanus coichicus*
Pigeon	*Columba livia*
Rhea, greater	*Rhea americana*
Saurus crane	*Grus antigone*
Screamer, horned	*Anhima cornuta*
Toucan	*Ramphastos* spp.
Trogan	*Trogon* spp.
Turaco	*Muso phagidae*

Common Name	Scientific Name

Reptiles

African puff adder	*Bitis arietans*
Anaconda	*Eunectes murinus*
Boa, California	*Lichanura roseofusca*
Boa, common	*Constrictor constrictor*
Boa, green tree	*Corallus caninus*
Boomslang	*Dispholidus typus*
Caiman	*Caiman* spp.
Cribo	*Spilotes pullatus*
Crocodile	*Crocodylus* spp.
Gila monster	*Heloderma suspectum*
Iguana, common green	*Iguana iguana*
King cobra	*Ophiophagus hannah*
Komodo dragon	*Varanus komodoensis*
Lizard, Mexican beaded	*Heloderma mexicana*
Lizard, sungazer	*Cordylus giganteus*
Rattlesnake	*Crotalus* spp.
Turtle, side-necked	Plerodira (suborder)
Turtle, snapping	*Chelydra serpentina*
Turtle, western pond	*Clemmys marmorata*
Viper, Russell's	*Vipera russellii*

Amphibians and Fish

Axolotl	*Ambystoma mexicanum*
Barracuda	*Sphyraena* sp.
Catfish, electric	*Malapterurus electricus*
Catfish, oriental	*Plotosus lineatus*
Eel, electric	*Electrophorous electricus*
Eel, moray	*Muraena helena*
Frog, poisoned-arrow	*Dendrobates* spp. and *Phylobates* spp.
Hellbender	*Cryptobranchus alleganiensis*
Rabbit fish	*Chimaera* sp.
Salamander, giant	*Andrias davidianus*
Scorpion fish	Scorpaenoidei (suborder)
Stargazer	*Astroscopus* spp.
Stingray	*Dasyatis* spp.
Surgeonfish	*Acanthurus triostegus*
Toad, Colombian giant	*Bufo blombergi*
Toad, Colorado River	*Bufo alvarius*
Toad, clawed	*Xenopus laevis*
Toad, marine	*Bufo marinus*
Toadfish	*Thalassophryne maculosa*
Tunafish	*Thunnus* spp.
Turkey fish	*Pterois volitans*
Weeverfish	*Trachinus* spp.
Zebra fish, lion fish	*Pterois volitans*

REFERENCES

1. Clements, J.F. 1974. Birds of the World: A Checklist. New York: Two Continents.
2. Grzimek, B., Ed. 1975. Grzimek's Animal Life Encyclopedia. New York: Van Nostrand Reinhold.
3. Norwalk, R.M. 1999. Walker's Mammals of the World, 6th Ed. Baltimore, Johns Hopkins University Press.
4. Wilson, D.E., and Reeder, D.A., Eds 2005. Mammal Species of the World, 3rd Ed. Baltimore, Johns Hopkins University Press.

APPENDIX C. GENERIC NAMES, COMMON OR TRADE NAMES, AND SOURCES OF DRUGS IN THE MENTIONED TEXT

GENERIC	COMMON OR TRADE	SOURCE*
Acepromazine maleate	Promace, ACE, aravet	9, 18
Alpha-chloralose		11, 19
Amobarbital, sodium	Amytal	8
Antivenin	Crotalid antivenin	10, 32
Atipamezole HCl	Antisedan	20, 30
Atricurium besylate	Tracrium	8
Atropine sulfate	Atropine	33
Azaperone	Stresnil	30
Butorphanol tartrate	Torbugesic	10, 30
Calcium borogluconate	Calcium borogluconate	33
Calcium gluconate	Calcium gluconate	33
Carfentanil citrate	Wildnil	30
Chloral hydrate	Chloral hydrate	9, 11
Chlorpromazine HCl	Thorazine	7
Desoxycorticosterone acetate	DOCA	19
Detomidine HCl	Domosedan	15
Dexamethasone	Azium	26
Diazepam	Vallium, Tranimal	24
Diprenorphine HCl	M50-50	30
Droperidol	Inapsine	22
Droperidol + fentanyl	Innovar-Vet	22
Doxopram HCl d-tubocurarine chloride	Dopram d-tubocurarine	22
Epinephrine	Adrenalin, epinephrine	33
Ether, diethyl	Ether	13
Etorphine HCl	M99, Immobilon	30, 34
Fentanyl citrate	Fentanyl, sublimaze	22
Flumazenil	Mazicon	24
Gallamine triethiodide	Flaxidil	2
Guaifenesin	Guailaxin, glycerol guaiacolate	12
Haloperidol	Haldol	24
Halothane	Fluthane	1
Hyaluronidase	Hyaluronidase	30, 34
Hydrocortisone sodium succinate	Solu-cortef	32
Isoflurane	Aerrane, isofluane	1, 3
Ketamine HCl	Vetalar, ketalar	5, 11, 21
Lactated Ringer's solution	Lactated Ringer's	33
Medetomidine	Domitor	20, 30, 34
Methoxyflurane	Metafane	21
Midazolam	Versed	24, 30, 34
Nalorphine HCl	Nalline	15
Naloxone HCl	Narcan	22, 30, 34
Naltrexone	Trexan	7, 12, 30
Pentobarbital sodium	Nembutal	1, 6
Perphenazine enanthate	Trilafon	26
Phenobarbital sodium	Phenobarbital	1
Phenylbutazone	Butazolidin	6
Prednisolone sodium succinate	Solu-Delta-Cortef	28
Quinaldine	Quinaldine	13
Secobarbital sodium	Seconal	1
Servoflurae	Utane, sevoflo	1
Sodium bicarbonate	Sodium bicarbonate	33
Sodium hypochlorite	Bleach (household)	33
Succinyicholine chloride	Anectine, Quelicin, Sucostrin	1, 11
Thiamyl sodium	Surital	21
Tiletamine/zolazepam	Telazol, Zolitil	10, 30, 34
Tolazoline	Tolazine	30, 34
Tribromoethanol	Avertin	31

GENERIC	COMMON OR TRADE	SOURCE
Tricaine methane sulfonate	Finquel, MS 222, Metacaine	4, 25
Tuberculin	Tuberculin	27
Xylazine HCl	Rompun, sedazine, tranquivet	12, 29, 30
Yohimbine	Antagonil, yobine	12, 30

APPENDIX D. FIRMS SUPPLYING DRUGS MENTIONED

1. Abbott Laboratories
Veterinary Division
P.O. Box 68
100 Abbott Park Rd.
North Chicago, Illinois 60064, USA
(312) 688-5109

2. American Cyanamid
One Cyanamid Plaza
Wayne, New Jersey 07470, USA
(800) 422-0222

3. Anaquest, Inc.
110 Allen Rd.
P.O. Box 804
Liberty Corner, New Jersey
07938-0804, USA

4. Argent Chemical Labs
8702 152nd Ave. N.E.
Redmond, Washington 98052 USA
(800) 426-6258
(800) 722-9292

5. Bristol Myers Squibb Co. (including
Mead Johnson)
P.O. Box 4500
Princeton, New Jersey 08543-4500,
USA
(609) 897-2000

6. Butler Animal Health Co. (Burns)
5600 Blazer Parkway
Dublin, Ohio 43017-7545, USA
(614) 761-9095

7. DuPont Pharmaceuticals
Willmington, Delaware, USA
(See Elanco)

8. Elanco Animal Health
Division of Eli Lily
2001 W. Main St.
N. Greenfield, Indiana 27408, USA

9. Fisher Scientific Co.
711 Forbes Ave.
Pittsburgh, Pennsylvania 15219,
USA
(412) 562-8300

10. Fort Dodge Laboratories
Division of American Home Products
P.O. Box 518
Fort Dodge, Iowa 50501, USA
(515) 955-4600

11. Glaxo Smith Kline
5 Moore Dr
Research Triangle Park, North
Carolina 27709, USA

12. Lloyd Laboratories
604 N. Thomas Ave
POB 86
Shenandoah, Iowa 51601, USA

13. Matheson Coleman & Bell
P.O. Box 7203
Los Angeles, California 90022,
USA
(213) 685-5280

14. McNeil Consumer Products Co.
Camp Hill Rd.
Fort Washington, Pennsylvania
19034, USA
(215) 233-7000

15. MSD Merck Sharp and Dohme
Merck Chemical Division
Whitehouse Station, New Jersey
07065, USA
(201) 574-4000

16. Miles Inc. Agricultural Division
Animal Health Products
12707 W. 63rd St. P.O. Box 390
Shawnee, Kansas 66201, USA
(800) 255-6517

17. Novartis
3200 Northline Ave. Suite 300
Greensboro, North Carolina 27408,
USA

18. Nutritional Biochemicals Corp.
26201 Miles Road
Cleveland, Ohio 44128, USA
(216) 831-3000

19. Organon, Inc.
375 Mt. Pleasant Ave.
West Orange, New Jersey 07052,
USA
(201) 325-4500

20. Orion Farmos Pharmaceuticals
Group, Ltd.
P.O. Box 65
FIN 20101 Espoo, Finland

21. Parke, Davis & Co. (with Pfizer)
201 Tabor Rd.
Morris Plains, New Jersey 07950,
USA
(201) 540-2000

22. Pitman-Moore Co.
P.O. Box 344
Washington Crossing, New Jersey
08560, USA
(609) 737-3700

23. A. H. Robins Co., Inc.
(with Wyeth)
1407 Cummings Drive
Richmond, Virginia 23220,
USA

24. Roche Laboratories
Division of Hoffman-LaRoche Inc.
Nutley, New Jersey 07110, USA
(201) 235-5000

25. Sandoz Pharmaceuticals
59 Rt. 10
East Hanover, New Jersey 07936,
USA
(201) 503-7500

26. Schering Plough Animal Health
10488 South 136th Street
Omaha, Nebraska 68138, USA
Merged with Glaxo

27. United States Department of
Agriculture APHIS-VSL
Ames, Iowa 50010, USA
(515) 239-8200

28. Upjohn Co.
7000 Portage Rd.
Kalamazoo, Michigan 49001, USA
(616) 323-4000

29. Vedco, Inc.
Rt. 6, Box 35A
5503 Corporate Dr.
St. Joseph, Missouri 64507, USA
(816) 238-8840

30. Wildlife Pharmaceuticals
1635 Blue Spruce Dr.
Fort Collins, Colorado 80524, USA
(303) 484-6267

31. Winthrop Laboratories
90 Park Ave.
New York, New York 10016, USA
(212) 907-2000

32. Wyeth-Ayerst
Division of Home Products Co.
555 Lancaster Ave.
St. Davids, Pennsylvania, 19087,
USA

33. Various pharmaceutical
and chemical supply companies

34. ZooPharm
Division of Wildlife Pharmaceuticals
1635 Blue Spruce Dr.
Fort Dodge, Colorado 80524,
USA

APPENDIX E. SOURCES OF RESTRAINT EQUIPMENT AND SUPPLIES

General Equipment

Nasco 901 Janesville Avenue
Fort Atkinson, WI 53538
(414) 563-2446
or
1524 Princeton Avenue
Modesto, CA 95352
(209) 529-6957

McMasters-Carr, wholesaler
P.O. Box 54960
Los Angeles, CA 90054
(213) 945-1311
or
P.O. Box 4355
Chicago, IL 60680
(312) 281-1010

Large hardware stores

Large mail order firms (ask for farm or tool catalogs) Montgomery Ward

Chemical Restraint Equipment

Syringes
Pneu-Dart, Inc.
15223 Route 87 Highway
Williamsport, Pennsylvania 17701, USA
(717) 323-2710

Pole syringes
Kay Research Products
1525 E. 53rd Street, Suite 503
Chicago, IL 60615, USA
(312) 643-9044

Weapons
Dan-Inject North America
P.O. Box 270837
Fort Collins, Colorado, 80527-0837, USA

Dist-inject
Peter Ott AG
Vet. Med. Gerate und Pharmazeutica
Postfach CH 4007
Basel, Switzerland
www.distinject.org

NASCO
1524 Princeton Ave.
Modesto, California 95352, USA
(209) 529-6957

Palmer Cap-Chur Equip. Inc
P.O.Box 867
Douglasville, Georgia, 39133-0867, USA

Telinject USA, Inc.
9316 Soledad Canyon Rd.

Saugus, California 91350, USA
(805) 268-0915

Zoolu Arms of Omaha
10315 Wright St.
Omaha, Nebraska 68124, USA
(402) 397-4983

Animal Care Equipment
613 Leebert Way
Crestline, California 92325, USA
(714)338-2799

Gloves

Routine animal-handling gloves
Ketch-all Co.
Department VMA
2537 University Avenue
San Diego, California 92104, USA
(714) 297-1953

Special order primate gloves
Lithgow Services
1205 S. Railroad Avenue
San Mateo, California 94402, USA
(415) 349-2310

Chain mail gloves
Butcher supply firms

Hooks

For elephants
John Beery Co.
2415 Webster Street
Alameda, California 94501, USA
(415) 769-8200

For reptiles
FurMont Reptile Hooks
Fuhrman Diversified
1212 W. Flamingo
Seabrook, Texas 77586, USA
(713) 272-4832

Horse Equipment

Colorado Saddlery
1411 Market Street
Denver, Colorado 80202, USA

H. Kaufman & Sons
Saddlery Co.
139–141 E. 24th Street
New York, New York 10010, USA

Nets

Hill & Hill Custom Veterinary Supplies
324 E. Shamrock
Rialto, California 92376, USA
(805) 268-1037

Beckman Net Co.
3729 Ross Street
Madison, Wisconsin 53707, USA
(608) 233-6991
Attn: Milo Beckman

Flexi-Nets
Fuhrman Diversified (FurMont Reptile Hooks also)
1212 W. Flamingo
Seabrook, Texas 77586, USA

West Coast Netting, Inc.
14929 Clark Avenue
City of Industry, California 91745, USA
(213) 330-3207

Ropes and Chains

ACCO
American Chain Division
454 E. Princess Street
York, Pennsylvania 17403, USA
(717) 741-0847

The Cordage Group
Division of Columbian Rope Co.
Auburn, New York 13021, USA
(315) 253-3221

Tubbs Cordage Co.
200 Bush Street
San Francisco, California 94104, USA
(415) 495-7155

Large hardware stores

Snares

Ketch-all Co.
Department VMA
2537 University Avenue
San Diego, California 92104, USA
(714) 297-1953

Squeeze Cages (for primates, carnivores, marine mammals)

Research Equipment Company, Inc.
P.O. Box 1151
Bryan, Texas 77801, USA
(713) 779-4459

Veterinary Equipment

Miles, Inc.
Haver-Lockhart Laboratories
Box 390
Shawnee Mission, Kansas 66201, USA
(913) 631-4800

APPENDIX F. ABBREVIATIONS USED IN THIS BOOK

U.S. Customary

av—avoirdupois
ft—foot, feet
gal—gallon(s)
in.—inch(es)
lb—pound(s)
mi—mile(s)
oz—ounce(s)
qt—quart(s)
sq—square
yd—yard(s)
ac—acre
apoth—apothecaries' weight
    (pharmaceutical)
sp.—species
spp.—species (plural)
b.w.—body weight
wt—weight

Metric

cc—cubic centimeter(s) = ml
cm—centimeter(s)
cu—cubic
g—gram(s)
ha—hectare(s)
kcal—kilocalorie(s)
kg—kilogram(s)
L—liter
m—meter(s)
mEq—milliequivalent
ml—milliliter = cc
mg—milligram
mm—millimeter(s)
t—metric ton(s)
μl—microliter
dl—deciliter = 100 ml

APPENDIX G. CONVERSION TABLES

Linear

1 millimeter = 0.039 inch	1 inch = 25.4 millimeters
1 meter = 3.281 feet	1 foot = 0.305 meters
1 meter = 1.094 yards	1 yard = 0.914 meter
1 kilometer = 0.621 mile	1 mile = 1.609 kilometers

Volume

1 liter = 33.815 fluid ounces	
1 liter = 1.057 quarts	
1 liter = 0.264 gallons US	

1 fluid ounce	= 29.573 milliliters
1 fluid ounce	= 0.03 liters
1 pint	= 0.473 liters
1 quart	= 0.946 liters
1 US gallon	= 0.83 Br. Imperial gal
	= 3.785 liters
1 British Imperial gal	= 4.545 liters
	= 1.2 US gallons

Area

1 hectare = 0.004 square miles	1 acre = (43,560 sq ft)
	= 0.405 hectare
1 hectare = 107,639.1 square feet	1 acre = 4046.86 sq meters
1 hectare = (10,000 sq miles) = 2.47 acres	

Mass

1 milligram	= 1/60 grain (apoth)	1 grain (apoth)	= 60 milligrams
1 gram	= 0.035 ounce	1 ounce (av)	= 28.35 grams
1 gram	= 15.432 grains (apoth)	1 pound	= 0.454 kilogram (454 grams)
1 kilogram	= 2.2 pounds	1 ton (2,000 lb)	= 0.907 metric ton (1,000 kg)
1 metric ton (1000 kg)	= 1.102 tons		
1 mg/kg	= 0.454 mg/lb	1 mg/lb	= 2.2 mg/kg

Temperature (degrees Celsius to degrees Fahrenheit)

C	F	C	F	C	F	C	F
25 — 77.0		33 — 91.4		38.5 — 101.3		43 — 109.4	
26 — 78.8		34 — 93.2		39 — 102.2		44 — 111.2	
27 — 80.6		35 — 95.0		39.5 — 103.1		45 — 113.0	
28 — 82.4		36 — 96.8		40 — 104.0		46 — 114.8	
29 — 84.2		36.5 — 97.7		40.5 — 104.9		47 — 116.8	
30 — 86.0		37 — 98.6		41 — 105.8		48 — 118.4	
31 — 87.8		37.5 — 99.5		41.5 — 106.7		49 — 120.2	
32 — 89.6		38 — 100.4		42.0 — 107.6		50 — 122.0	

I N D E X

CPSIA information can be obtained
at www.ICGtesting.com
Printed in the USA
BVHW060711081218
535068BV00005B/15